Foundations of Medical Physics

Covering topics in Radiobiology, Modern Physics, Medical Imaging and Radiation Therapy, *Foundations of Medical Physics* serves as an introduction to the field of Medical Physics, or Radiation Oncology Physics.

An overview of the history of cancer and cancer treatment along with a brief introduction to the fundamental principles of Radiobiology constitute Part I of this book, which serves as the motivation for the principles of Radiation Therapy, or cancer treatment with radiation. Part II contains the fundamental ideas from Modern Physics that form the foundation for an understanding of the approaches to treatment used in Radiation Therapy. Finally, Part III shows the applications of Parts I and II to Medical Imaging and Radiation Therapy.

This unusual introduction to Medical Physics is aimed at undergraduate physics majors along with other science majors who have taken at least one year of Physics and one year of calculus, although Medical Physics graduate students and radiation oncology residents may find this different approach to the subject illuminating. This text assumes that the instructor is a physicist who does not necessarily have a background in Medical Physics.

Victor J. Montemayor, PhD, teaches Physics and Advanced Mathematics at Germantown Academy (GA) in Fort Washington, PA. Dr. Montemayor has received numerous teaching awards, including the Ernest L. Boyer International Award for Excellence in Teaching, Learning, and Technology. Dr. Montemayor was chair of the Committee on Medical Physicists as Educators and a member of the Education Council of the American Association of Physicists in Medicine for 11 years.

George Starkschall, PhD, spent the majority of his medical physics career on the faculty at The University of Texas MD Anderson Cancer Center (MDACC), where he was instrumental in the development of one of the first three-dimensional radiation treatment planning systems in clinical use as well as a methodology for acquiring CT scans that captured respiratory motion. Since retiring from MDACC, he assumed the position of Executive Secretary on the Commission on Accreditation of Medical Physics Education Programs (CAMPEP). He is the recipient of the Edith H Quimby Lifetime Achievement Award of the AAPM and the Harold Johns Medal of the International Organization for Medical Physics (IOMP) for contributions to international medical physics education.

Foundations of Medical Physics

Victor J. Montemayor
George Starkschall

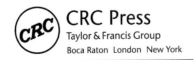

CRC Press
Taylor & Francis Group
Boca Raton London New York

CRC Press is an imprint of the
Taylor & Francis Group, an **informa** business

Designed cover image: Victor Montemayor, CC.

First edition published 2024
by CRC Press
2385 NW Executive Center Drive, Suite 320, Boca Raton FL 33431

and by CRC Press
4 Park Square, Milton Park, Abingdon, Oxon, OX14 4RN

CRC Press is an imprint of Taylor & Francis Group, LLC

ISBN: 978-1-498-74618-2 (hbk)
ISBN: 978-0-429-19476-4 (pbk)
ISBN: 978-1-003-47745-7 (ebk)

DOI: 10.1201/9781003477457

Typeset in Latin Modern font
by KnowledgeWorks Global Ltd.

*This book is dedicated to
all students of Medical Physics,
both present and future.*

Contents

Part III *Application:* **Imaging and Therapy**

Preface

"What kind of job can I get with a Physics degree, anyway?" One of us (VJM) was sitting with an undergraduate student who was considering switching their major to Physics. I gave my usual answer: "Physics graduates can get all kinds of jobs! They are excellent critical thinkers and problem solvers. They are good at math and computer programming. They are hardworking and driven. There are so many opportunities for Physics graduates!" The student was underwhelmed and, to be honest, so was I. I certainly appreciated the student's question; after all, when have you looked in the Jobs listings and seen, "Wanted: Physicist"? I had never seen one. Can a Physics graduate even get a job called "Physicist" without having a Ph.D. in Physics?

I got interested in the field of Medical Physics, or, more specifically, Radiation Oncology Physics—the physics behind the treatment of cancer with radiation—after I heard that the field needed Physics graduates and that someone with a Masters degree in Medical Physics could get a good-paying job in a clinic with the job title "Medical Physicist". I contacted the (then) head of the Medical Physics group at The Vanderbilt Clinic, Charlie Coffey, and asked if we could meet to discuss my thoughts of incorporating an introduction to the field of Medical Physics within an undergraduate Physics major curriculum.

At the time, I was a Professor of Physics at Middle Tennessee State University. I began the development of an upper-division course to introduce Physics and other interested science majors to the field of Medical Physics. I quickly learned that there was no introductory Medical Physics text geared toward undergraduate Physics majors, so I started putting together notes of my own. These notes, of course, were the genesis of this book.

I view Medical Physics as a fascinating and important application of Modern Physics, so I wanted to make sure the students understood those topics in Modern Physics that are of fundamental importance in Medical Physics. These topics, in my mind, form the foundation for an appreciation of the procedures in Medical Physics. As a result, Part II of the book (chapters 4 through 9), covering essential topics in Modern Physics, is titled "Foundation". These topics include a discussion of hydrogenic and multi-electron atoms, nuclear physics, and interactions of high-energy photons and charged particles with matter. Scattered throughout these chapters are examples and discussions showing how the physics can be applied in various areas of cancer treatment.

The whole point of treating cancer cells with radiation is to have the incident radiation cause strand breaks in the DNA within cancer cells. This topic is within the realm of Radiobiology. Whereas most introductory Medical Physics texts cover topics in Radiobiology at the end of the book, I wanted to put a discussion of Radiobiology at the front-and-center of the discussion of radiation therapy. Part I of the book (chapters 1 through 3), "Motivation", covers an introduction to cancer and to the field of Radiobiology. It provides the motivation for what we are doing in the rest of the book.

The third—and last—part of the book (chapters 10 through 25) introduces the field of clinical Medical Physics. It applies what has been covered in Parts I and II of the book to clinical cancer treatment and is therefore titled "Application". This application starts with a discussion of Medical Imaging, covering both projection and reconstruction imaging modalities. These imaging modalities can be considered one means of detecting cancer. The remainder of Part III covers Radiation Therapy—the treatment of cancer (as well as perhaps other diseases) with radiation. This includes discussions of ethics in Medical Physics, the equipment used to produce the radiation, topics in dosimetry, treatment planning, brachytherapy, radioisotope therapy, radiation protection, and quality assurance. The book ends with a view toward the future of Radiation Therapy, with discussions of informatics, radiomics, applications of machine learning, and FLASH radiotherapy.

While I (VJM) wrote Parts I and II of the book, along with the discussion of Medical Imaging at the beginning of Part III, the expertise of a well-rounded Medical Physicist was needed to work on the discussion of clinical Radiation Therapy. This person would also need to be an excellent teacher and communicator. I was therefore thrilled when George Starkschall agreed to join me on this project. George's vast expertise in Medical Physics, along with his reputation as an inspiring teacher at M.D. Anderson Cancer Center in Houston, has really served to raise the bar in the coverage of topics in Part III.

This book was started with the intent of introducing undergraduate, upper-division Physics majors to interesting topics in Modern Physics as they are used in clinical Medical Physics. Other science majors who have a year of introductory physics and calculus under their belts would also be an appropriate audience for this book. While most of the book does not use calculus, there are certainly some sections in various chapters that assume a familiarity with differential and integral calculus. Those not wanting to delve into the mathematics can simply skim the more mathematical sections and move on. Any homework problems involving calculus contain a note stating that calculus is needed in their solutions.

Although the intended audience for this book was originally undergraduates, the concise introduction to Radiobiology, the coverage of the fundamental physics, and the broad overview of topics in Medical Physics will also make this book of interest to Medical Physics graduate students and Radiation Oncology residents. For example, Ch. 22 on Brachytherapy and Ch. 23 on Radioisotope Therapy are very good, nearly self-contained overviews of those two topics for graduate students and residents, as is Ch. 25 on Evolving Topics in Medical Physics, which looks toward the future of Medical Physics.

The full content of this book is clearly too much to cover in a one-semester university course, but various chapters and sections can readily be pulled from its contents to cover desired topics. For example, an undergraduate course could cover chapters 4 through 7 on Atomic and Nuclear Physics rather quickly if the students have already studied Modern Physics, then a more thorough coverage of chapters 8 and 9 on interactions with matter could be included. The remaining time could then be spent on various topics in Radiation Therapy. Adding one or more visits to a local cancer clinic would then serve as an excellent introduction to Medical Physics for undergraduates. Or time could be spent more on Medical Imaging if that is of interest to the class or instructor.

On the other hand, an instructor may wish to cover the beginning chapters on cancer and Radiobiology and then hit various chapters of interest on cancer treatment in Part III, completely skipping the more mathematical treatment of Physics in Part II. (The coverage of topics in Parts I and II of the book are referenced in Part III in case the reader or instructor wishes to go back to cover or review that material.) A completely different approach would be to use Part II as an introduction to Modern Physics and then use selected portions of Part III, coupled with a visit to a local cancer clinic, as real-world, important applications of those topics in Modern Physics. Or the instructor could choose to simply cover the desired topics in Part III while referencing the earlier material as needed or desired. The topic coverage can be very flexible.

The invaluable help of numerous people in the creation of this book must be acknowledged. First, several experts have graciously and selflessly lent their time and expertise to this book. Joann Prisciandaro and Alex Moncion contributed the discussion of Brachytherapy in Ch. 22, and Jackie Zoberi and Jose Garcia contributed Ch. 23 on Radioisotope Therapy. In addition, Lisa Whitelock contributed the last section in Ch. 10 on Emerging Technologies in Medical Imaging, and Wendy Smith contributed the section on FLASH Radiotherapy at the end of Ch. 25. We are very grateful for the insightful contributions of these esteemed medical physicists.

Many thanks also go to those who gave useful comments or suggestions dealing with various portions of, or images in, this book: Rebecca Pizzino, Jay Burmeister, Michael Joiner, Wendy Smith, Lisa Whitelock, Manuel Morales, Brian Nett, Tyler Dolan, and David Ghalili. Their contributions and comments are very much appreciated.

This book has been a long-term project, and various people formerly or currently at Taylor & Francis have contributed greatly to it: Lou Chosen, Carolina Antunes, Lara Spieker, Betsy Byers, Emma Morley, Evie Evans, Shashi Kumar, and Haylie Allan.

Finally, the unwavering support from the administrations at both Middle Tennessee State University and Germantown Academy for work on this book is gratefully acknowledged.

This book was written assuming as little background in Medical Physics on the part of the instructor as possible, allowing Physics faculty with no background in Medical Physics to teach an introductory course in Medical Physics. It also assumes that the instructor and students do not have ready access to a Medical Physics department in a cancer-care clinic, so care has been taken to include as many images of equipment as possible. Nevertheless, it is recommended that the instructor of any course not associated with a Medical Physics department find a clinic somewhere in the area that can be visited by the students so they can see Medical Physics in action—Medical Physicists tend to be very busy, but they also tend to be very happy to give a tour of the clinic and to explain the equipment that can be found there to those interested in Medical Physics.

Regardless of whether this book is being used for a course taught by a faculty member with no Medical Physics background or by a Medical Physicist, or is being used by a student doing independent study, it is hoped that this book is found to be informative and readable. We hope that you enjoy working with it!

Victor J. Montemayor
George Starkschall
February, 2024

I

Motivation: Cancer and the Basics of Radiobiology

An Introduction to Cancer

CONTENTS

Significant resources are spent around the world each year on the diagnosis and treatment of cancer and on cancer research. A cancer report by Statista pointed out that, as of 2022, cancer was the second leading cause of death in the United States after heart disease. The report estimated that there were around 1.9 million new cases of cancer in the United States in 2022.[1] According to the U.S. Cancer Trends Progress Report,[2] it is estimated that $208.9 billion were spent on cancer care in the United States in the year 2020.

The mortality rate due to all types of cancer in both sexes has been in steady decline since the early 1990s. In 1991, the mortality rate due to cancer for both sexes in the United States was at an all-time high of 215.22 per 100,000; in 2019 the rate was at 146.14 per 100,000.[3] This reduction in cancer mortality rates was due to a decrease in smoking combined with earlier screenings for cancer and the subsequent earlier treatment. These changes have led to declines in the four major types of cancer: lung, colorectal, breast, and prostate.[4]

The purpose of this chapter is to provide some background on the topic of cancer along with some glimpses into how it is diagnosed and treated. The following two chapters will then delve into some of the details of the radiation biology that underlie the treatment of cancer with radiation.

1.1 AN HISTORICAL OVERVIEW OF CANCER AND CANCER TREATMENT

In around the year 400 BC, the Greek physician Hippocrates referred to the central mass and radiating veins of a breast tumor as a "crab", or καρκινος (*karkinos*) in Greek.[5] The Romans then later translated the Greek word into the Latin word for "crab": *cancer*. Cancer is a generic name given to many different diseases. In all cases, though, the disease is characterized by out-of-control cell growth.

Cancer in the Ancient World

Some people view cancer as a relatively modern disease caused by the plethora of processed foods in our diets, the inhalation of smoke, and the chemicals in our environment. While these factors from our modern lives certainly do contribute to the causes of cancer, the existence of cancer has been found by paleopathologists in prehistoric skeletal remains and the symptoms and even some treatments for cancer have been recorded for millennia.

The earliest documented incidence of cancer in human-lineage skeletal remains is an osteosarcoma (bone cancer) in the fifth metatarsal—the long bone running along the outside of the foot that connects to the small toe.[6] This cancerous bone segment was found in the area of South Africa called the Cradle of Humankind, which is about 30 miles northwest of Johannesburg. It is estimated to be about 1.6 million years old. Other findings of ancient cancer have also been found: the Kanam Man jaw bone found by Louis Leakey in 1932, cases from fifth-century Spain, a medieval cemetery in southern Germany,[7] and a startling find of an approximately 10-inch tumor on the left femur of a young adult Saxon male unearthed during an excavation at Standlake Down, England in 1954 (see Fig. 1.1.).[8] In addition, a generally agreed-upon example of a malignant tumor seen in a skeleton was found in Mauer, Austria, and dates from around 4000 BC.[9] Awareness of cancer and its effects have been documented in both ancient Greek and Egyptian writings. A papyrus, called the Edwin Smith Papyrus, suggests that surgery was performed to remove tumors from the breast dating back to about 3000 BC.[10]

Of course, many types of cancer form in the soft tissues, making detection of such disease very unlikely in skeletal remains unless the cancer spreads, or *metastasizes*, into the bone. The earliest example of secondary cancer in skeletal remains that resulted from the metastasis of cancer in soft tissue was found in 2013 in an archeological dig in Amara West, Sudan.[11] In this dig, the skeleton of a young man of age 25 to 35 years was found from carbon-14 dating to have been buried around 1200 BC. While only about 200 examples of cancer in skeletal remains around the world have been found to date,[12] it is nevertheless clear that cancer is certainly not a strictly modern disease.

For well over a thousand years, from the time of Hippocrates through the Middle Ages, the cause of cancer was believed to follow from an imbalance of the four types of body fluids, or *humors*. According to Hippocrates, the body contained blood, phlegm, yellow bile, and black bile—the four humors. A healthy body was one in which the four humors were balanced. If an imbalance occurred, an illness resulted. In particular, Hippocrates believed that an excess of black bile resulted in cancer.[13]

The Advent of Scientific Oncology

In the mid-1700s, the Italian physician and anatomist Giocanni Morgagni wrote about the link between anatomy, in particular as seen in autopsies, and the illness that led to the patient's death.[14] This link then led to the idea that the anatomical condition of a living patient could dictate a diagnosis of a patient's illness. A bit later in the

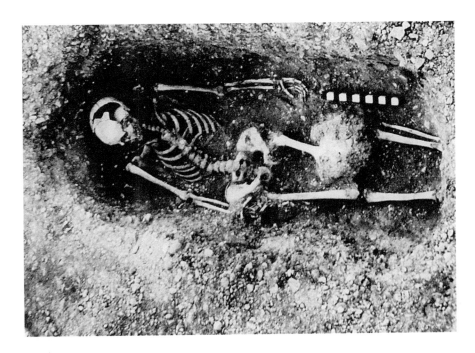

FIGURE 1.1: Skeleton of a young Saxon man from the seventh century, showing an approximately 10-inch tumor on the left femur. (Ashmolean Museum, Oxford, with permission.)

eighteenth century, the Scottish surgeon and lecturer John Hunter worked to base the treatment of patients and the practice of surgery on the results of experimental research and proposed that certain cancers might even be cured by means of surgery.[15] Despite this scientific approach, Hunter still held a belief of cancer formation resulting from fluids—specifically, a fluid known as *lymph*, which, along with blood, circulated throughout the body. Cancer was thought to result from the degeneration of lymph in the body.

The use of microscopes allowed Rudolf Virchow in the mid-1800s to study the cellular basis of disease, resulting in the creation of the field of cellular pathology.[16] He understood that cells come from other cells and, following Morgagni, correlated anatomical changes to disease, although Virchow's anatomical changes were studied at the microscopic level. Virchow was also the first person to recognize leukemia as a disease of the blood cells. The study of cancer at the cellular level allowed surgeons to study tissue removed from the patient, thereby allowing them to determine whether the disease had been completely removed during the surgery.

The relationship between estrogen and breast cancer was inferred in 1878 by the British physician Thomas Beatson, who found that breast-cancer patients could be helped by the removal of their ovaries (the hormone estrogen had not yet been discovered). This discovery laid the initial groundwork for what later became known as *hormone therapy*.[10]

The Discovery of Radiation
On 8 November 1895, the German physicist Wilhelm Röntgen discovered a new type of penetrating ray, which he called *x-rays*. Then, on 22 December 1895, Röntgen

took the now-famous x-ray image of his wife's hand,[17] showing the bones in her hand and her wedding ring. (See Fig. 11.3.) The x-rays were easily produced by the acceleration of electrons within evacuated glass tubes. Soon after the announcement of his discovery in December of 1895, Röntgen sent out copies of his announcement along with "x-ray pictures" to many of the leading physicists in Europe.[18] Word of these mysterious rays then quickly spread, and what resulted was an amazing progression of events that directly affected the field of medicine in general and the study of cancer in particular.

In January of 1896, two French physicians, Oudin and Barthélemy, presented x-ray photographs of the bones in a hand to the Académie Française.[8] In February of the same year, Thomas Edison in the United States published a paper on x-rays, and by May, he and his assistant, Clarence Dally, were showing Edison's newly developed fluoroscope at an exhibition in New York City where people could view their own bones with the new apparatus (see Fig. 1.2.).[19] The significant medical implications of the fluoroscope were apparent to anyone who saw Edison's exhibit.[20] Also in February of 1896, Henri Becquerel discovered radioactivity in a sample of uranium.[21]

By the year 1898, portable x-ray machines were being used to help diagnose traumatic injury by British military physicians in the Mahdist War in Sudan.[8] In that same year, Pierre and Marie Curie announced the discovery of two new radioactive elements: polonium (announced in July of 1898) and radium (announced in December of the same year).[22] Both of these elements emitted so-called "Becquerel rays", a generic term for radioactive emissions. (See Chapter 7 for a discussion of radioactive decay.)

Biological Damage due to Radiation

Despite their penetrating ability—or perhaps because of it—x-rays were initially widely thought of as harmless. People with access to a fluoroscope readily viewed their anatomy without any concerns. It soon became apparent, however, that x-rays were far from harmless.

In 1902 it was reported that irradiation of the skin by x-rays could cause skin cancer.[8] Numerous reports of skin damage, in particular by scientists who were working with x-radiation, soon followed. The seriousness of x-ray exposure was not fully appreciated and accepted, however, until Edison's assistant, Clarence Dally, displayed multiple signs of health issues associated with his exposure to x-rays.[23]

Dally had received regular doses of x-rays during his work for Edison, which took place with almost a complete lack of shielding from the radiation. By the year 1900, Dally had lost some of his hair, and his face and both of his hands displayed lesions. He was so dedicated to his research that he started using his right hand in his work instead of his left after developing significant swelling and pain in his left hand. By 1903 Dally's left arm had been amputated and four fingers were removed from his right hand. At this point, Edison not only stopped all experiments involving x-rays but vowed also to do no work involving the radiation emitted by the radioactive elements radium and polonium. Dally died of complications resulting from x-ray exposure in 1904.

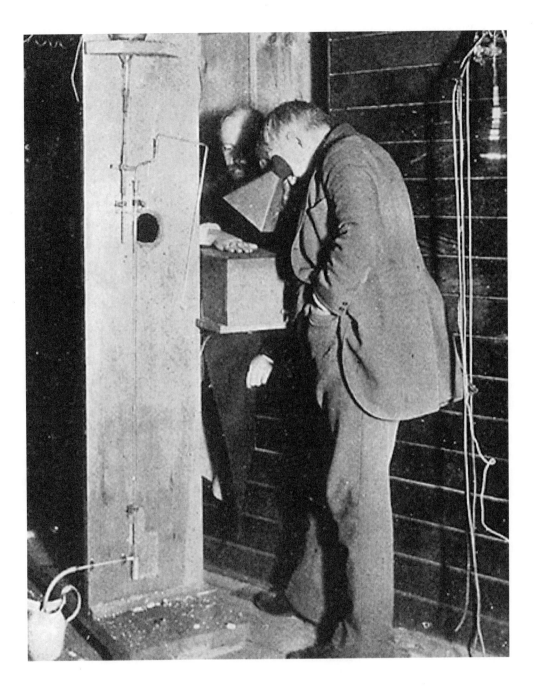

FIGURE 1.2: Thomas Edison examining the bones in the hand of his assistant, Clarence Dally, using Edison's newly invented x-ray imaging machine, the calcium tungstate flouroscope. This photograph was taken in 1896, the year following the discovery of x-rays by Wilhelm Röntgen. Dally later died of injuries resulting from the x-ray exposure that he received during his experiments carried out in Edison's labs. (Open Source: Wikimedia Commons.)

Not all biological damage caused by radiation is necessarily bad, however. The first application of x-rays to treat cancer was in 1896, when Émil Grubbé treated a woman with x-rays just several months after their discovery.[24,25] Then Alexander Graham Bell suggested in 1903 that a cancerous tumor could be treated by inserting a radioactive source directly into the tumor,[26,27] after which radium was used in a clinical setting that same year by Hermann Strebel,[22,28,29] who inserted radium into needles that had already been implanted into tissue. These treatment modalities for cancer performed by Grubbé and Strebel marked the beginnings of *external-beam radiation therapy* and *brachytherapy*, respectively.

1.2 MORE MODERN APPROACHES TO CANCER DETECTION AND TREATMENT

William Stewart Halsted, an American surgeon who was a pioneer in the field of anesthesiology, was interested in the treatment of breast cancer.[30] He did not believe that the cancer in the breast spread to other parts of the body through the blood vessels, so he concluded that breast cancer could be cured by the removal of the affected tissue. In 1889 he described a successful surgical cure for breast cancer: the *radical mastectomy*. His thinking guided the treatment of cancer with surgery for almost a century.[10]

On the other hand, the English surgeon Stephen Paget did believe that cancer cells could spread to other parts of the body and performed investigations into cancer that had metastasized, or spread. In 1889, he determined that not all tissues were equally susceptible to producing secondary cancer once a primary tumor had metastasized. He argued that, "When a plant goes to seed, its seeds are carried in all directions; but they can only live and grow if they fall on congenial soil".[31] Contrasted with the thinking of Halsted, these ideas not only pointed out the inherent limitations of surgery, but they also paved the way for systemic post-operative treatments for certain types of cancer. The aim of these treatments was to minimize the need for further operations associated with the spreading of the cancer by killing cancer cells that had metastasized.[10]

In the early 1900s, Paul Ehrlich proposed that drugs could be used to treat diseases, including cancer. He introduced the word *chemotherapy* for such a use of drugs.[32] Later, in 1939, Charles Huggins introduced the idea of *hormone therapy*. He used hormones to treat prostate cancer, with positive results. The idea of using drugs in an attempt to treat cancer was largely frowned upon, however, until successes with the treatment of childhood leukemia and advanced Hodgkin's disease were reported in the mid-1960s.[32]

Advances in Diagnostic Imaging

As the technical expertise of surgeons improved, it was found that less tissue removal was required for cancer treatment. Nevertheless, until better imaging techniques were developed for cancer diagnosis and tumor localization, surgery remained a primary component of not only the treatment but also the diagnosis of cancer. The role played by surgery in the diagnosis of cancer diminished as imaging techniques improved.

Advances in imaging were made in the 1950s when Russel Morgan, Edward Chamberlain, and John Coltman demonstrated a significant improvement in the quality of the image obtained in fluoroscopy[33] while at the same time reducing the corresponding dose to the patient. In 1958, Hal Anger invented the gamma camera,[34] which uses high-energy photons emitted in the radioactive decay of so-called *radiopharmaceuticals* to image the *physiology* of given regions inside the patient. This is to be contrasted with other imaging modalities that had been used up to that time that strictly produced images of the patient's *anatomy*.

In 1959, Ian Donald developed the technology that allowed ultrasound imaging to be used as a diagnostic tool. Then, in 1962, Sy Rankowitz and James Robertson invented the positron emission tomography (PET) transverse section scanner. As with the gamma camera, PET scans allow for the study of the physiology of certain tissues in the body. Further advances in imaging that led to alternate modes of cancer detection came in 1972. Godfrey Hounsfield and Allan Carmack invented the computerized axial tomography (CAT, or later, CT) scanner, which can produce cross-sectional or 3-D images of internal structure in the patient. In addition, in the same year, magnetic resonance imaging (MRI) was adapted to allow for its use as a medical imaging modality, allowing for an even more detailed image of soft tissue than that produced by a CAT scan.[33] (See chapters 10 through 12 for much more information about medical imaging modalities.)

Cancer Treatment with Radiation

The first use of x-rays to treat cancer was reportedly performed by Émil Grubbé,[24] who treated a woman for breast cancer in January of 1896 at the Hahnemann Medical College in Chicago.[35] (It should be noted that there is not complete agreement as to who performed the first cancer treatment with x-rays. Victor Despeignes,[36] among others,[37] also claim to have performed the first such treatment.) Radiation therapy continued to be performed in the early 1900s with the use of the radioactive emissions of the element radium and with low-voltage x-ray machines that worked by slamming high-energy electrons into a dense target material. X-rays are then produced as the electrons collide with the target atoms in a process known as *bremsstrahlung*. (See Chapter 9 for more information.) The technology to produce and precisely deliver energy to the desired location within the body using radiation has continually improved since that time.

In 1946, Robert R. Wilson proposed that a beam of high-energy protons could produce a distribution of dose within the patient that would have advantages over that produced by x-rays.[38] In particular, whereas x-rays deliver a significant dose to the patient throughout a whole range of depths, a beam of protons would produce a dose that was more locally distributed around a particular depth. This means that protons would tend to deliver less dose to healthy tissue surrounding the tumor than x-rays. He also suggested that high-energy carbon atoms might also one day be therapeutically useful. Cancer treatment using high-energy proton beams and carbon beams are both part of today's cancer-treatment modalities using radiation. (See Chapter 9 for a discussion of the physics of charged particle interactions with matter and Chapter 19 for information about cancer treatment with charged particles.)

Prior to 1951, most x-ray treatment machines used voltages in the kilo-volt range to accelerate electrons that were then used to produce bremmstrahlung x-rays.[39] Such x-rays have very limited penetration ability into the body and were therefore often used to treat skin cancers. Then, in 1951, the first cobalt-60 units were used for cancer treatment in Canada. These machines used a radioactive cobalt-60 source to produce high-energy (1.17 and 1.33 MeV) gamma rays.

Linear accelerators, or *linacs*, were then developed to deliver even higher-energy x-ray photons to the cancer patient. This was important, as higher-energy x-rays are able to penetrate deeper into the patient and therefore deliver dose to a tumor at depth. In 1953, a linac using an accelerating voltage of 8 MV became operational in London.[39] Today, linacs produce x-rays using voltages up to about 25 MV for cancer treatment. (A detailed discussion of the machines used to produce radiation can be found in Chapter 15.)

When we speak of cancer treatment with radiation, we do not always mean irradiating the patient with high-energy photons or charged particles from a source of that radiation that is *outside* the patient's body. *Brachytherapy* is that mode of radiation therapy in which a radioactive source is actually inserted into the body in order to irradiate a tumor *from within*. Whether the radiation treatment for a given tumor should involve radiation from an external or internal source of radiation, or even a combination of the two, is dictated by the location of the tumor and by the oncologist in charge of the treatment. (See Chapter 22 for more information on brachytherapy.)

Some Other Cancer Treatment Modalities

There are three primary ways of approaching the treatment of cancer: surgery, chemotherapy, and radiation therapy. It is not uncommon for an oncologist to use a combination of treatment modes in the treatment plan for a particular patient.

But these three modes are not the only approaches that have been taken in the treatment of cancer. We have already mentioned *hormone therapy* in the treatment of cancers whose growth is influenced by hormones. In this approach, the effects of hormones are blocked with certain medicines given to the patient. These medicines act to either stop the associated hormones from being produced, or stop the influence of the hormones on the growth of the tumor. Hormone therapy is sometimes used in the treatment of breast, prostate, ovarian, uterine, and kidney cancers.[40]

Another type of cancer treatment is generically called *biological therapy*, and includes such approaches as *immunotherapy* and *targeted therapy*.[40] In immunotherapy, biologic agents, whether naturally occurring in the body or produced in the lab, are used to either mimic or to influence the body's immune system response in controlling cell growth. As opposed to chemotherapy drugs that kill any rapidly growing cells in the body, targeted therapy drugs specifically target the growth of cancer cells. These drugs typically achieve this goal in one of three ways: they act to block the signals that tell cancer cells to grow, they stop the production of new blood vessels that carry the blood needed by tumor cells to grow, or they can simply signal the cancer cells to die.[10]

In the treatment of certain types of leukemia, lymphoma, or myeloma, it may be necessary to administer very high doses of chemotherapy or radiation in order to kill the cancer cells. But in such treatments, the stem cells within the bone marrow or the bone marrow cells themselves may be killed. In this case, a *transplant* of stem cells or bone marrow cells will then be necessary in order for the patient to survive after the chemotherapy or radiation treatment.[40]

Finally, we simply mention in passing some other modes of cancer treatment. In *heat therapy*, the patient's body is exposed to high temperatures in an attempt to mimic the effects of a fever in fighting disease in the body.[41] In a somewhat related treatment, *radiofrequency ablation* (RFA), radiofrequency waves are administered by means of a probe that is inserted into the tumor. These waves result in energy being deposited into the tumor cells, which results in the cells being heated up to an extent that kills them. This same type of effect is attempted in *high intensity focused ultrasound* (HIFU), in which high frequency sound waves are focused on the tumor. At the opposite end of the temperature spectrum, *cryotherapy* attempts to kill cancer cells by freezing them. As with all modes of cancer treatment, the use of these modes of treatment are being carefully studied.[40]

The alternate modes of cancer treatment discussed in this section will in general not be discussed any further in this book.

1.3 SOME CELL AND DNA FUNDAMENTALS

Cells form the basic unit of all living matter (see Fig. 1.3).[42] All cells can be broadly divided into two categories: *prokaryotes* and *eukaryotes*. Bacteria are prokaryotes, while plants and animals are made up of eukaryotic cells. For our purposes, the primary difference between prokaryotic and eukaryotic cells is that most of the DNA in a eukaryotic cell are contained within a *nucleus*, while the DNA in a prokaryotic cell are not.

The nucleus of a human eukaryotic cell contains almost all of the DNA for the entire organism. (There are also some DNA molecules located inside mitochondria, which are found in the cytoplasm of the cell outside of the nucleus.) A DNA molecule consists of a series of *nucleotides* arranged in the form of a double helix (see Fig. 1.4).[43] Each nucleotide consists of a base, a sugar (deoxyribose), and a phosphate group. There are four types of nucleotides in DNA, named according to the base that they contain. Two of the bases, *adenine* (A) and *guanine* (G), consist of double-ringed structures of atoms and are referred to as *purines*. The remaining two bases, *thymine* (T) and *cytosine* (C), consist of single rings of atoms called *pyrimidines*.[44] Within the structure of the DNA, a nucleotide containing a *single-ringed* base on one strand of the DNA helix is always bonded *via* hydrogen bonds to a nucleotide containing a *double-ringed* base on the other strand. Such a grouping of two bases is called a *base pair*. See Figs. 1.4 and 1.5.

A section of nucleotides along a DNA molecule that often corresponds to an inheritable trait is called a *gene*[a] (see Fig. 1.6).[45] By a *human genome*, we mean the

---

[a]More officially, a *gene* is a sequence of nucleotides that codes for a specific *product*. A gene product could be a protein, but it could also be any type of RNA molecule (tRNA, mRNA, or rRNA).

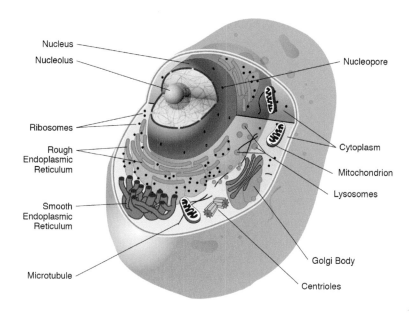

FIGURE 1.3: A typical animal cell. (Courtesy of the National Human Genome Research Institute.)

complete set of all DNA contained within a human. While all humans have genomes that are largely very similar if not almost identical, there are also some small portions of the genome that vary wildly from one person to the next.[46]

The human genome consists of about three billion base pairs (one purine paired with one pyrimidine) within the human DNA molecules. These DNA are almost exclusively found within the nuclei of typical human cells, although they are also found in a small chromosome in the cell's mitochondria.[47] However, not all base pairs are associated with genes. All sections of a DNA molecule that comprise a gene provide the codes for producing certain proteins. According to the results of the Human Genome Project, the human genome consists of about 30,000 genes.[48] But, amazingly enough, these genes only comprise about 2% of the total human genome— the rest of the genome in the DNA consists effectively of spacers, or non-coding DNA sequences, between the protein-building information of the genes.[49]

As mentioned above, a nucleotide containing a *single-ringed* base (T or C) on one strand of the DNA helix is always bonded to a nucleotide containing a *double-ringed* base (A or G) on the other strand *via* hydrogen bonds. (This bonding of bases is called *complementary base pairing*.) More specifically, two hydrogen bonds always join an A on one strand to a T on the other strand, while a G is always joined to a C on the opposite strand with three hydrogen bonds. This formation of the base pairs $A–T$ and $G–C$ from opposite strands of the DNA helix means that, if we know the sequence of nucleotides on one strand of the helix, then we can immediately specify the corresponding sequence required on the other strand. This idea of nucleotide

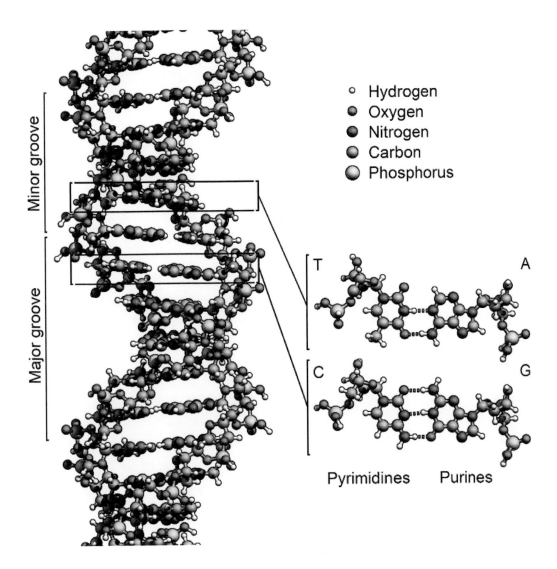

FIGURE 1.4: The 3-D structure of DNA showing with detail the structure of the four bases, adenine (A), cytosine (C), guanine (G) and thymine (T). (Creative Commons: Created by Richard Wheeler.)

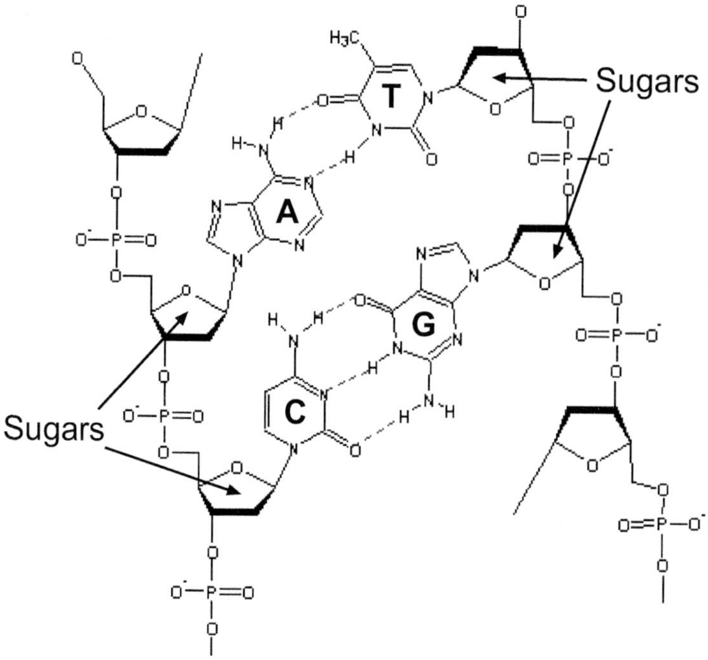

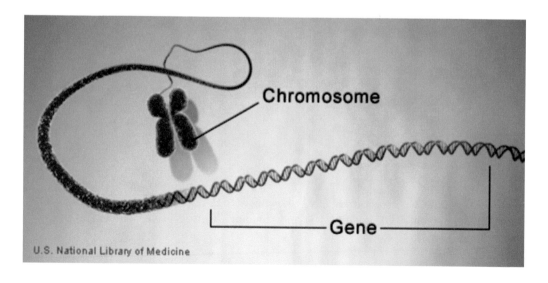

FIGURE 1.5: A 2-D view of a segment of a DNA molecule, showing the phosphate groups, the sugars, the bases (A, T, C, and G), and the associated hydrogen bonds. The sugar-phosphate bonds and the hydrogen bonds between the bases are often sites of cell-killing DNA damage—so-called *strand breaks*. (See Chapter 2.)

FIGURE 1.6: A gene is a segment of a DNA molecule that is often associated with an inheritable trait. The DNA coils up into a rod-shaped chromosome in preparation for cell reproduction. (Courtesy of MedlinePlus from the U.S. National Library of Medicine.)

matching, coupled with the inherently weak nature of the hydrogen bonds, comprise the fundamental concepts associated with the replication of the DNA within the cell during cell reproduction.

If the DNA in the human genome were stretched out into a straight line, it would reach a length of about two meters. But somehow this length of DNA must fit within the nucleus of almost every cell in the human body, which is at most about $10\,\mu m$ in diameter.[50] This means that somehow the DNA molecules have to be compacted to fit into such a small space and they have to be organized in such a way that will make DNA replication and subsequent separation of the two copies possible.

Some Chromosome-Related Terminology

A DNA molecule within the nucleus of a cell ordinarily appears as long, thread-like mass, as long as the cell is not preparing for cell division. (See the discussion of the cell cycle in §1.4 below.) In this state, the contents of the nucleus—the DNA, proteins, and RNA—is collectively referred to as a *chromatin*. The DNA molecules within the chromatin are wrapped around proteins called *histones*. A section of about two loops of DNA wrapped around a group of histones forms a nodule along the length of the DNA called a *nucleosome*. Nucleosomes are formed along the entire length of the DNA (see Fig. 1.7).[51] In some sense, the idea of the DNA molecule wrapping around successive histone groups is like a string wrapping around successive pearls to form a pearl necklace if the pearls were tightly packed. Despite the organized nature of the DNA, they still appear as long threads within the nucleus when it is not undergoing cell division.

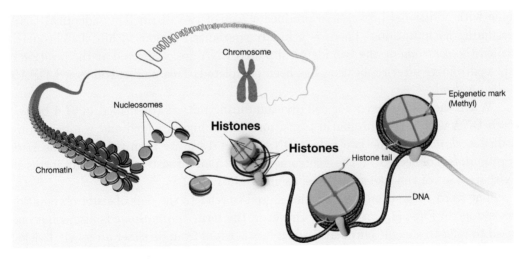

FIGURE 1.7: The DNA molecule wraps around histone proteins in order to make the DNA more compact, thereby allowing the DNA to fit inside the cell nucleus. (Courtesy of the National Human Genome Research Institute.)

Prior to cell division, the DNA must first be replicated. DNA replication takes place when the DNA are in the form of the semi-condensed, long thread-like structures described above.[50] This loosely organized structure allows for the orderly replication

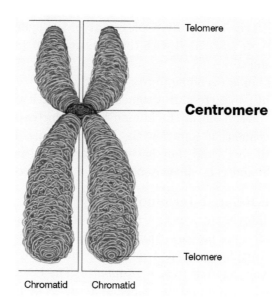

FIGURE 1.8: The highly compact form of a DNA molecule is called a *chromatid*. When the two paired DNA, joined at the centromere, transition to compact chromatids, as shown above, they are called *sister chromatids*. (Courtesy of the National Human Genome Research Institute.)

of the DNA molecule. As the DNA within the chromatin are replicated, they combine with additional histones to produce a pair of two distinct but identical DNA, assuming no mutations. There is a highly specialized region within the chromatin called the *centromere*; the two identical paired DNA are connected at the position of the centromere after replication has been completed. This pair of connected DNA is called a *dyad*.

When the cell prepares for cell division during mitosis (described in §1.4 below), each DNA within the chromatin transitions into a highly folded and compact state, called a *chromatid*. The two paired DNA in the dyad are then referred to as *sister chromatids*, connected at the centromere. This pair of sister chromatids forms an X-shaped set of rod-like structures, as shown in Fig. (1.8).[52]

The word *chromosome* is sometimes used to refer to the pair of sister chromatids, as is done in Figs. (1.6) and (1.7). However, the term *chromosome* is also sometimes used to refer to a single chromatid when it is isolated from its sister after cell division, as in Fig. (1.9). In an attempt to avoid confusion, we shall refer to a paired set of DNA connected at a centromere as a *dyad*, whether they are in the thread-like state in a chromatin or in the form of sister chromatids. By a *chromosome* we shall mean a single DNA molecule—either in the form of an isolated single chromatid, or in the corresponding isolated, partially unraveled form of DNA wrapped around histones in the chromatin. This means that there is a one-to-one correspondence between a chromosome and its corresponding DNA molecule. Thus, the nucleus of a typical human cell contains 46 chromosomes, as shown in Fig. (1.9).[53]

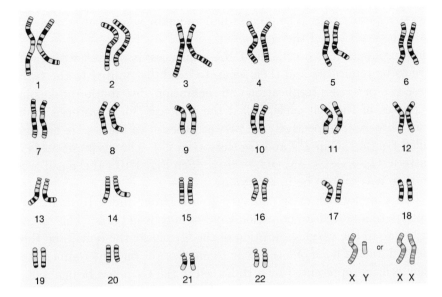

FIGURE 1.9: The 46 chromosomes found in a normal human cell: 22 pairs of autosomes, plus the X and possibly Y sex chromosomes. One chromosome (or DNA) in each pair is from the mother and one is from the father. (Courtesy of the National Human Genome Research Institute.)

In order to guarantee that each daughter cell contains a complete set of chromosomes, the two sister chromatids in a dyad are pulled apart and distributed to opposite ends of the cell before the cell splits into two daughter cells. (See the next section for more details about the cell cycle.) The centromere provides the assembly position for the *kinetochores*, which are the plate-like sites where spindle fibers attach to pull the duplicate chromatids apart during mitosis.[54] As mentioned above, each of the separated sister chromatids constitutes a *chromosome*.

A normal cell from a human contains 23 pairs of chromosomes, one chromosome in each pair from the mother, and one from the father. One of these 23 pairs consists of two sex chromosomes. There are two types of sex chromosomes, referred to as X and Y. The cell of a typical male will have one X sex chromosome and one Y sex chromosome, while a typical female cell will have two X sex chromosomes. The remaining twenty-two pairs of chromosomes are called *autosomes*, and are each referred to by an assigned number, between *1* and *22*. (See Fig. 1.9.) Thus, each normal human cell contains a total of 46 chromosomes. It then follows that, when the cell is not busy with cell division, the chromatin in each typical human cell contains 46 loosely organized, thread-like DNA molecules, also called chromosomes, in addition to various proteins and RNA.

1.4 CELLULAR REPRODUCTION AND THE CELL CYCLE

In order for one cell to reproduce and form two effectively identical cells, the cell must first double in size and duplicate its DNA; it must then partition the DNA and split into two separate cells. The process undergone by a cell that starts with one cell and ends with two is called the *cell cycle*.

In the reproduction of a cell, the DNA sequences associated with each chromosome have to be replicated and then separated and distributed to the two daughter cells. These two processes (replication and separation/distribution) take place in two separate phases of the cell cycle, called the S phase (for "Synthesis") and the M phase (for "Mitosis"), respectively. In between these two phases are two gaps in the cycle, called G_1 (for "Gap 1") and G_2 (for "Gap 2"). The cycle proceeds according to the pattern: $G_1 \rightarrow S \rightarrow G_2 \rightarrow M \rightarrow G_1 \rightarrow S \rightarrow$ .... (See Fig. 1.10.) If the cell is not in the M phase, then it is said to be in *interphase*.

The total time for one cycle can vary greatly, from about 10 hours for hamster cells in culture to hundreds of hours for some stem cells in tissue. This large variation is primarily due to the varying duration of the G_1 phase; the remaining three phases vary little in duration from one cell type to another, or one environment to another. In a human cell, as represented by a HeLa cell,[55] the G_1 phase lasts about 11 hours, the S phase lasts 8 hours, the G_2 phase 4 hours, and the M phase lasts 1 hour, for a total time-per-cycle of about 24 hours.[37]

The progression of the cell through the cell cycle is governed by many proteins, but it is primarily regulated by so-called *cyclin-dependent kinases* (Cdks), which are proteins found in the cell's cytoplasm.[56] There are Cdks associated with the G_1, S, and G_2/M phases. These Cdks promote the progress into and/or through the corresponding phase, but only when bound to a corresponding *cyclin*. One way the cell guarantees that the various phases of the cell cycle are followed in the correct order is to vary the abundance of the cyclins corresponding to each phase as the cycle progresses.[57] Figure (1.10) maps out the regions of influence of the primary cyclin-Cdk complexes that guide the cell through the cell cycle. The 2001 Nobel Prize in Physiology or Medicine went to Leland Hartwell, Timothy Hunt, and Sir Paul Nurse for their discoveries associated with this regulation of the cell cycle by cyclins and Cdks.[58]

In what follows, we will overview the main characteristics of the four phases of the cell cycle.

G_1: The First Growth Phase

This phase is characterized by active cell growth, as manifested by the duplication of various cell constituents such as proteins, ribosomes (for making proteins), mitochondria (for producing useable energy), and endoplasmic reticulum (for intracellular protein transport), among others. Progress through the G_1 phase is mediated by the binding of a protein called cyclin D to the corresponding Cdks (Cdk4 and Cdk6). The protein cyclin E is also synthesized during this period.[59] These cyclin-Cdk bindings signal that the cell should prepare for chromosome replication.[60]

Before the cell ends the G_1 phase, it undergoes a check for the integrity of the DNA—a so-called *DNA damage checkpoint*. If no DNA damage is detected, then an S-phase cyclin (cyclin E) binds with the S-phase Cdk (Cdk2—the cell-cycle checkpoint kinase[59]) to form an S-phase promoting factor (SPF). The SPF enters the nucleus of the cell and signals for the preparation of DNA and centrosome duplication, which

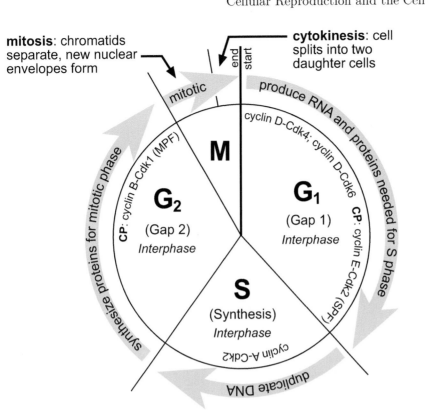

FIGURE 1.10: The main stages of the cell cycle. Also shown are the primary cyclin-Cdk complexes that guide the cell through the cell cycle. **CP** stands for a checkpoint for DNA integrity within the cycle.

ushers the cell into the S-phase. (The *centrosome* contains two *centrioles*, which are the origin of the mitotic spindle; the mitotic spindle is responsible for separating the sister chromatids during cell division. See the discussion of the mitotic phase below.)

On the other hand, if DNA damage is detected, then the production of SPF is inhibited. Since the production of SPF is necessary in order for the cell to move into the S phase, it follows that the progress of the cell cycle is halted if DNA damage is found. The cell cycle does not resume until the damage is repaired and the cyclin E-Cdk2 binding resumes. If the damage is too extensive for repair, then the cell kills itself by *apoptosis*[60]—a process that is exploited in the use of radiation therapy to treat cancer. (See Chapters 18 through 21 in Part III of this book for a discussion of radiation therapy.)

Apoptosis can be thought of as a pre-programmed cellular suicide. It is used in developing human embryos to get rid of, for example, the cells forming the webbing between the fingers and toes. In healthy people, apoptosis is used to get rid of cells that are older and not functioning properly, thereby making way for new cells. Humans lose tens of billions of cells each day to apoptosis (see Fig. 1.11).[61]

If, on the other hand, the biochemical processes of apoptosis do not function properly, the worn-out cells will not die off. These cells will then continue to replicate,

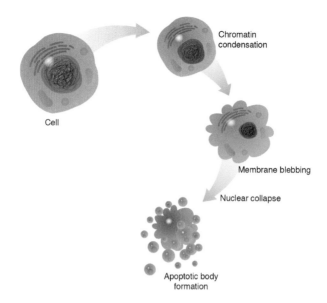

Cell

Chromatin
condensation

Membrane blebbing

Nuclear collapse

Apoptotic body
formation

FIGURE 1.11: The process of *apoptosis*, in which a cell kills itself. During apoptosis, the nuclear contents fragment, the chromatin condenses and the cell shrinks. *Blebbing*, or a blistering of the cell's plasma membrane, makes the cellular structure flexible enough to allow it to bulge and separate into pieces called *apoptotic bodies* that are subsequently absorbed into the surrounding tissue. (Courtesy of the National Human Genome Research Institute.)

forming an over-abundance of cells called a *tumor*, and the resulting disease is called *cancer*. (See Fig. 1.13.) Cancer is the result of certain DNA mutations, themselves resulting from errors made during the process of replication or from environmental factors such as smoke or radiation from the sun or other sources. Unfortunately, some mutations in germ cells that can lead to cancer can also be inherited.

S: The Synthesis Phase
During the S phase, the centrosome in the cell is replicated, as is the DNA in each chromosome.

The replication of the DNA starts with the partial unwinding and separation of a portion of the two strands in the double helix. These processes are accomplished by a group of enzymes, including DNA *helicases* and DNA *polymerases*. These enzymes use energy from ATP molecules in the cell to break the weak hydrogen bonds that connect the bases between the two DNA strands.[62] The cytoplasm in the cell contains nucleotides that are used to match up the corresponding bases to form the required base pairs on each of the two separated DNA-strand segments. The DNA helicase then unwinds and separates the parent DNA further, and the process continues.[44]

Once the duplication process is complete, the cell contains two of each of the 46 original DNA in the chromatin, each pair comprising a dyad with the two DNA connected at their centromeres. Each DNA molecule has one strand from the original DNA molecule, and one strand that has been generated from cytoplasmic nucleotides—a result that is referred to as *semi-conservative replication*.

The protein cyclin A is produced early in the S phase. The cyclin A-Cdk2 complex then regulates the progression through the S phase[63] and allows for the transcription of the genes[59]. During the replication of the DNA, a cyclin called *cyclin E*, which is an S-phase initiating cyclin, is degraded. This degradation means that the activity of the corresponding S-phase Cdk (Cdk2) will be progressively reduced so that, by the time the DNA replication is completed, additional replication of DNA will not be initiated.[59]

G_2: The Second Growth Phase

Immediately following the S-phase, this second phase of growth is characterized by the production of numerous proteins, including cyclin B. This cyclin combines with Cdk1 to produce the *Maturation Promoting Factor* (MPF), which prepares the cell for entry into the M phase.[59] However, as in the G_1 phase, there is a DNA damage checkpoint in the G_2 phase. If no DNA damage is detected, then the cell cycle proceeds as normal. But if the integrity of the DNA is found to be compromised, then the action of Cdk1 is inhibited, which means that the production of the MPF is stopped, and the cell will be prevented from entering the next phase until the repairs have been completed.[60]

M: The Mitotic Phase

Mitosis is actually only one of two parts, or *sub-phases*, that comprise the M-phase.

Mitosis is the first sub-phase of the mitotic phase. It can be sub-divided into the following five distinct parts: (i) **prophase**: the two centrosomes move to opposite ends of the cell to form the two poles, the mitotic spindle is generated from the two centrioles within each centrosome, and the paired DNA making up each dyad become more tightly folded and compact, forming sister chromatids; (ii) **prometaphase**: the nuclear envelope disintegrates, a kinetochore forms on each chromatid at the location of the centromere of each dyad, the mitotic spindle fibers attach to the kinetochores and to the arms on each of the chromatids in a dyad such that one chromatid gets attached to one pole and the other chromatid gets attached to the other pole; (iii) **metaphase**: the highly compact dyads are pulled to a plane midway between the two poles, called the *metaphase plate*; (iv) **anaphase**: the two kinetochores in each dyad separate, and the spindle fibers pull the identical chromatids (or chromosomes) apart and toward opposite poles; and (v) **telophase**: two new nuclear envelopes appear around the separated sets of chromosomes, which then de-compact into the necklace-like form of DNA within the chromatin (see Fig. 1.12).[64,65]

Cytokinesis is the second sub-phase during which a belt of filaments made of a protein called *actin* forms around the edge of the metaphase plate. The interaction of the filaments with the motor protein myosin II causes a constriction of the filaments,[66] which results in the formation of a furrow on the surface of the dividing cell. Further interactions result in a deepening of the furrow, until the two sides of the cell are pinched apart, resulting in two distinct daughter cells.[67]

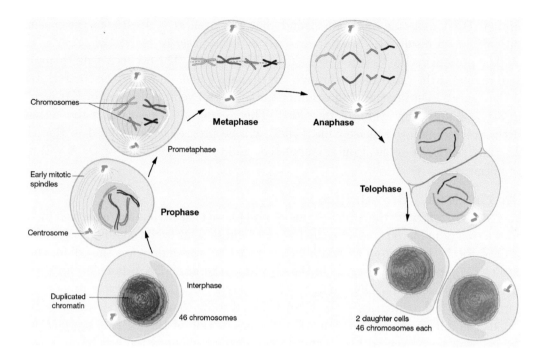

FIGURE 1.12: The process of *mitosis*, during which the paired DNA (or chromosomes) in each dyad condense into sister chromatids, still connected at the centromere (prophase); the nuclear envelope disintegrates and the spindle fibers connect each chromatid in a dyad to one of the two opposite poles, which are defined by the centrosomes (prometaphase); the dyads are pulled to and lined up along the metaphase plate (metaphase); the sister chromatids in each dyad are separated by the spindle fibers, thus forming two separated chromosomes (or DNA), which are then pulled to their respective poles (anaphase); and, finally, two new nuclear envelopes are formed, one around each of the two sets of chromosomes, which then unwind into the loose form of DNA that is characteristic of the chromatin (telophase). *NOTE:* Despite the fact that each human cell undergoing mitosis contains 46 dyads, for clarity and simplicity, this figure shows only 4 dyads, with 4 corresponding chromosomes in each of the daughter cells. (Courtesy of the National Human Genome Research Institute.)

During mitosis, the cyclin B-Cdk1 (MPF) complex interacts with various proteins. These interactions serve to *phosphorylate* (that is, add a phosphate group to) those proteins, which subsequently serve various functions within the cell cycle. For example, the phosphorylation of the *condensin* proteins results in compacting the loosely-formed DNA within the chromatin into chromatids. In like manner, the cyclin B-Cdk1 enzymes affect the stability of the nuclear membrane, as well as the construction of the spindle fibers used to separate the sister chromatids.[56]

During anaphase, the B cyclins are destroyed or rendered ineffective, which means that the M phase cannot be re-initiated. In addition, the synthesis of cyclin D begins, which prepares the cell for the G_1 phase of the next cycle.[60]

The G_0 Phase

Not all cells are in one of the phases of the cell cycle discussed above. Some cells, after completing mitosis and cytokinesis, enter a so-called quiescent stage in which they do not undergo cell division. Such cells are said to be in a third gap phase, called the G_0 **phase**. Certain cells undergo what is called *terminal differentiation*, in which their function is dictated and they simply live out the rest of their lives performing that function without further cell division.[68] For example, mature cardiac muscle cells and nerve cells never exit the G_0 phase, and simply continue to perform their function until undergoing apoptosis (cell death).[69]

Other cells are only temporarily in the G_0 phase, however, and can re-enter the cell cycle in the G_1 phase when signaled to do so. For example, white blood cells—B cells and T cells—typically remain in the G_0 phase. However, they can be activated by particular antigens—along with a second signal from an *antigen-presenting cell* (APC)—at which point they enter the cell cycle in the G_1 phase and undergo repeated duplications,[70] thereby producing an immune-system response to the presence of the antigen within the body.

1.5 REGULATION OF THE CELL CYCLE AND CANCER

When you cut your finger, the damaged cells around the edges of the cut release proteins called *growth factors* that can stimulate the growth and division of cells. These cells then grow rapidly from the edge of the wound inward until they meet with the cells growing from the other side of the cut, at which point the cell growth and division stop.

This type of behavior in cell growth and division is also observed when mammalian cells are placed on a microscope slide, for example. Stimulated by appropriate growth factors, the cells will grow and divide until they come into contact with other cells. Once the entire slide is covered with a single layer of cells, cell duplication ceases. If a section of cells is subsequently wiped from a region of the slide, the cells on the edges of the cleared region start to grow and divide until the slide is once again covered by a monolayer of cells.

We thus see that, in addition to stimulated growth, cells also exhibit *contact inhibition*, in which cell growth and division stop when cells contact other cells.[67] Clearly there have to be some sort of chemical factors released by the cells that regulate the cell cycle—factors to promote the cycle when cells are damaged and other factors to stop the repetition of the cycle when a sufficient number of cells have been produced.

Cancer

Normal cells divide more rapidly in a young person than in an old person. Once a person becomes an adult, cell division takes place only to replace old cells or to repair injuries. Normal cells seem to be able to grow and divide a finite number of times—typically between about 20 and 50 times—before they die from apoptosis.[67]

Some cells, on the other hand, outlive normal cells and are found to continue to grow and multiply indefinitely. Put another way, some cells never enter the G_0 phase. Such cells are called *cancer* cells. A result of the non-stop duplication of cancer cells is that they do not stop reproducing once contact with other cells takes place. This means that there will be a pile-up of cancer cells on top of other cancer cells. The resulting excess tissue that develops is called a *tumor*, as shown in Fig. (1.13).[71] Not all tumors are cancerous, however. Some cells display uncontrolled growth for a period of time, and then stop or reduce their rate of duplication.

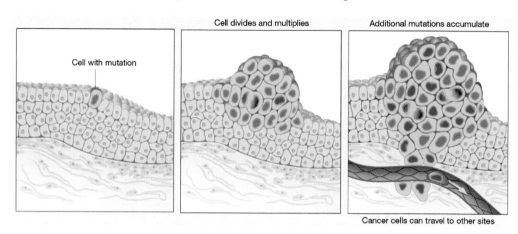

FIGURE 1.13: Cancer is the result of DNA mutations that allow for the uncontrolled growth of certain cells, leading to the possible formation of a tumor. The spreading of cancer cells to other parts of the body is called *metastasis*. (Courtesy of the National Human Genome Research Institute.)

A Quick Note on Terminology

The prefix *onc-* comes from the Greek word $o\nu\kappa o\sigma$ *(onkos)*, meaning *mass*. The field of *oncology* is therefore the study of tumors, or undesirable masses of cells that may result from uncontrolled cell reproduction. An *oncogene* is a gene having the potential to cause a normal cell to become cancerous. *Oncogenesis* is the induction or formation of cancer cells, or a tumor. Likewise, *oncogenicity* is the capacity to form or induce tumors, and an *oncologist* is a medical doctor who specializes in treating cancer.

Underlying Causes of Cancer

We have seen in our discussion of the cell cycle that there are some cyclin-Cdk complexes that promote the cell's progress through the cell cycle and others that serve to stop the cycle if certain DNA checkpoints are not passed. It is clear that the conditions for cancer can be achieved by having too much promotion for cell growth, or too little inhibition of the cell cycle, or both. It thus should be no surprise to find out that abnormalities in the behaviors of cyclins or Cdks that are associated with the cell cycle could lead to cancer. But we pointed out earlier that cyclins, which are produced during the cell cycle, enable the activities of the Cdks; variations in the abundance of the different cyclins throughout the cell cycle promote or stop the progress of the cell through the cycle. Therefore, an alteration of the cyclins can lead to uncontrolled cell proliferation.[59]

Any normal genes that are associated in any way with the promotion of the cell cycle—or, more specifically, with the promotion of mitosis—are referred to as *proto-oncogenes*. The reason they are called proto-oncogenes is that, if they are copied incorrectly during DNA duplication in the cell cycle—that is, if they are *mutated*—the resulting gene can contribute to cancer. The mutated version of the normal gene is referred to as an *oncogene*.[72] These mutations can be caused by anything that can penetrate the nucleus of a cell and interact with the DNA—specifically, high-energy radiation and certain chemicals. In general, any alteration in a DNA sequence that occurs during DNA replication is a type of *mutation*. Mutations occur randomly during the DNA-duplication process in the cell cycle.[73]

It is worth noting at this point that not all mutations are bad: they are responsible for evolution as well as for the death of cancer cells during cancer treatment. Mutations can be neutral (no effect), beneficial, or detrimental. All humans have cells with mutated genes in them. Indeed, certain types of mutations, called *passenger mutations*, seem to have no effect on cells becoming cancer cells and are just as likely to be found in healthy cells as they are in cancer cells. However, other mutations, called *driver mutations*, are frequently found in cancer cells and are therefore associated with a normal cell becoming cancerous. Mutations of genes associated with the regulation of the cell cycle are driver mutations. It takes more than one driver mutation in a cell to make it a cancer cell, however—cancer cells often have two to eight driver mutations in them.[74]

Tumor Suppressor Genes

All genes that are proto-oncogenes can contribute to the formation of cancer if they are mutated. However, not all genes whose mutations can contribute to the formation of cancer are proto-oncogenes. It is important to remember that proto-oncogenes are genes associated with *promoting mitosis*. But certainly mutations in other genes associated with the cell cycle can lead to uncontrolled cell proliferation.

We mentioned in our discussion of the cell cycle that certain cyclins are associated with the *inhibition* of the cell cycle. In particular, cyclins associated with the DNA checkpoints within the cell cycle can stop the progression of the cycle—and therefore stop cell growth—when combined with the appropriate Cdk.

We can therefore break genes down into three categories as far as the cell cycle is concerned. The first is genes that result in the production of proteins that *promote mitosis*. As already mentioned, such genes are referred to as *proto-oncogenes*. The second is genes whose proteins *inhibit mitosis*. These genes are called *tumor suppressor genes*. The third category is genes that are not associated with the promotion or inhibition of the cell cycle. Mutations of these genes will not lead to cancer.

When proto-oncogenes are mutated and become oncogenes, they can produce proteins that will result in the cell constantly being pushed into cell duplication. When tumor suppressor genes are mutated, their proteins will not act to stop the progression of the cell cycle. Some types of cancer require both of these types of mutations in order to become established.[73]

It should be pointed out that many other genes can be associated with cancer if they are mutated. For example, if the genes associated with apoptosis are mutated, they can help induce cancer since the cells will then effectively become immortal. For example, some genes, such as *Bcl-2*, produce proteins that act to inhibit apoptosis. If the action of this gene is over-expressed, then it could lead to B-cell cancer.[72]

(B cells are a type of white blood cell, as mentioned previously in the discussion of the G_0 phase of the cell cycle.) It should also be pointed out that the action of tumor suppressor genes can be altered by means other than mutations, with the same result of allowing the cell cycle to continue when damage has been detected.[75]

p53

One of the most important tumor suppressor genes in our body is the gene associated with the production of the protein called *p53*.[b] The p53 gene is a very important gene in the body's fight against cancer. It is found that over half of the tumors associated with lung, ovarian, and colorectal cancers have no normally active p53 proteins as a result of mutations of the associated gene.[75] Indeed, it appears to be nearly impossible for a cell in the human body to become cancerous without the inactivation of the p53 protein.[76]

It has been found that the action of the p53 protein is induced whenever general cell damage or, more specifically, DNA damage is detected. The p53 protein interacts with another protein called p21 to inhibit the actions of the cyclin E-Cdk2 complex, which is the S-phase promoting factor (SPF).[68]

More generally, if cell damage is detected and the damage can be repaired, then p53 will prevent the completion of the cell cycle until the repair is completed. On the other hand, if irreparable cell damage is detected, then p53 acts to force the cell into apoptosis.[75] As a result, p53 is often called the "guardian of the genome".

1.6   TWO BASIC TYPES OF TUMORS

The word *tumor* simply refers to a *mass*. The actual condition or contents of the mass do not matter—we could still call it a tumor. The word "tumor" is typically used to mean a *neoplasm*, which can be defined as a mass of tissue resulting from an abnormal growth of cells. The cells in a neoplasm tend to be rapidly growing cells that will continue to undergo mitosis unless treated.[77] When we speak of a "tumor" in this book, we will mean a neoplasm.

There are generally two types of tumors: *benign tumors* and *malignant tumors*. *Benign tumors* tend to be slow growing masses that serve no purpose, but typically do not directly affect the health of the host.[78] Benign tumors tend to be localized, and do not spread to other parts of the body.[77] That is not to say that benign tumors cannot pose a health risk, however. If allowed to grow, such tumors may reach a size that causes them to press against and interfere with the functions of other tissues, which can then result in health complications. For example, if a benign tumor pushes against a blood vessel or a nerve, it is possible for serious complications to result unless the tumor is treated.[79] Benign tumors tend to respond well to treatment and tend not to reoccur when successfully removed.[78]

On the other hand, *malignant tumors* can lead to the death of the host if left untreated. Cells in malignant tumors tend to be more rapidly duplicating than those in benign tumors. The cells in a malignant tumor can invade and destroy nearby

---

[b]The term *p53* comes from the fact that the associated protein has a mass of 53 thousand atomic mass units.

tissues and they can metastasize and cause secondary cancers in other parts of the body distant from the primary tumor.[78] It is these secondary cancers that result from the metastasization of the primary tumor that actually tend to lead to the death of the host.[74]

In summary: benign tumors are non-cancerous and non-malignant; malignant tumors are cancerous—they can spread to other parts of the body (metastasize) and they can result in the death of the host.

1.7 PUTTING THINGS IN PERSPECTIVE

There are about 3 billion DNA base pairs in the human genome,[49] which means that every time a cell divides, the S phase of the cell cycle must correctly match 6 billion base pairs when reproducing the DNA in the cell. During an average human lifetime, it is estimated that there are about 10^{16} cell divisions.[74] It is further estimated that there is an error in matching the base pairs in DNA replication on average once every ten thousand to one million bases.[23] This means that roughly 6×10^{20} errors are made in matching base pairs in DNA synthesis throughout our lifetime. Given all of this, it's amazing how well our cells work in catching errors and reducing the onset of cancer!

1.8 QUESTIONS, EXERCISES, & PROBLEMS

1-1. Compare and contrast the approaches to cancer treatment of Halsted and Paget. Base your discussion not only on reading in this chapter but also on information from online professional websites. As always, be sure to cite your references. (And, as always, *Wikipedia* is not an acceptable professional reference.)

1-2. Do an online search for information on HeLa cells, which were mentioned in the text in the discussion on the cell cycle. (a) What are these cells, and where did they come from? (b) What is controversial about them? (c) What are your thoughts on the controversy? As always, be sure to cite your references. (And, as always, *Wikipedia* is not an acceptable professional reference.)

1-3. Figure (1.10) shows a diagram of the cell cycle. Is the diagram reasonably to scale for a HeLa cell? If yes, explain why. If no, make a sketch that is reasonably to scale for a HeLa cell. (*Hint:* angles.)

1-4. Research the roles played by cyclins D, E, A, and B in the cell cycle. Then discuss the variations in the abundances of these cyclins throughout the cell cycle, and explain how these variations guide the cell through the cell cycle. As always, be sure to cite your references. (And, as always, *Wikipedia* is not an acceptable professional reference.)

1-5. Figure (1.10) shows that there is a DNA checkpoint at the end of the G_1 phase of the cell cycle. Why is there a checkpoint for the integrity of the DNA *before* the DNA are even synthesized during the cycle?

1-6. Research and explain the formation of and role played by the *kinetochore* during the mitotic phase of the cell cycle. As always, be sure to cite your references. (And, as always, *Wikipedia* is not an acceptable professional reference.)

1-7. Explain the differences between the chromatin, the chromosomes, and the chromatids within a cell. Your explanations should include appropriate sketches.

1-8. Compare and contrast proto-oncogenes and oncogenes. How are they related to cyclins?

1-9. Discuss the role of mutations in the formation of cancer.

1-10. Compare and contrast proto-oncogenes and tumor-suppressor genes.

1-11. Explain the significance of apoptosis in the cell cycle.

1-12. Research the process of apoptosis. (a) What happens during this process? (b) What is a *caspase*? Explain. (c) Which caspases are involved in apoptosis? What roles do they play in this process? As always, be sure to cite your references. (And, as always, *Wikipedia* is not an acceptable professional reference.)

1-13. The following statement can be found in the discussion of DNA replication in this chapter: "Each DNA molecule has one strand from the original DNA molecule, and one strand that has been generated from cytoplasmic nucleotides—a result that is referred to as *semi-conservative replication*". In your own words, clearly explain this statement.

1-14. Using data given in this chapter, compute a rough estimate of the number of base-pair matches made per second during the S phase of the cell cycle for a typical human cell. Be sure to state your assumptions.

1-15. "All genes that are proto-oncogenes can contribute to the formation of cancer if they are mutated. However, not all genes whose mutations can contribute to the formation of cancer are proto-oncogenes". Explain.

1-16. Discuss the significance of the protein p53 in the cell cycle. Do some research to extend your discussion beyond the discussion found in this chapter. Why is p53 called the "guardian of the genome"? As always, be sure to cite your references. (And, as always, *Wikipedia* is not an acceptable professional reference.)

1-17. It is stated in the last section of this chapter, *Putting Things in Perspective*, that there are roughly 6×10^{20} errors in copying the base pairs during DNA duplication throughout an average human lifetime. Use the other data in that paragraph to show where this rough approximation comes from. Your answer should also address the following: Why are there *6* billion base-pair matches made per cycle when there are only *3* billion base pairs in the human DNA? After all, if there are 3 billion base pairs in the human DNA, then shouldn't it take just 3 billion base-pair matches to make duplicate copies of the DNA?

1-18. Using information given at the end of this chapter, estimate the average amount of time it takes for an error to be made in copying the base pairs during DNA duplication. Express your answer in *seconds*.

1.9 REFERENCES

1. National Cancer Institute. Cancer in the U.S. - Statistics & Facts (2022). https://www.statista.com/topics/1192/cancer-in-the-us/#topicHeader___wrapper. Accessed June 14, 2022.
2. National Cancer Institute. Cancer Trends Progress Report: Financial Burden of Cancer Care (2022). https://progressreport.cancer.gov/after/economic_burden. Accessed June 14, 2022.
3. National Cancer Institute (2022). Cancer Trends Progress Report: Mortality. https://progressreport.cancer.gov/end/mortality and (graph details). https://progressreport.cancer.gov/sites/default/files/graphs/lbox_emo1.jpg. Accessed June 14, 2022.

4. American Cancer Society (2019). Cancer Mortality Milestone: 25 years of Continuous Decline. https://pressroom.cancer.org/Statistics2019. Accessed June 14, 2022.

5. Carpenter A. Anatomy Words: Cancer. http://anatomyalmanac.blogspot.com/2007/08/cancer-latin-word-for-crab.html. Accessed February 11, 2015.

6. Odes EJ, Randolph-Quinney PS, Steyn M, Throckmorton Z, et al. Earliest hominin cancer: 1.7-million-year-old osteosarcoma from Swartkrans Cave, South Africa. *S Afr J Sci*. 2016;112(7/8):5. https://doi.org/10.17159/sajs.2016/20150471. Accessed June 14, 2022.

7. Johnson, G. Cancer Has Afflicted People Since Prehistoric Times. *Discover magazine online*. July/August issue, 2013. https://www.discovermagazine.com/health/cancer-has-afflicted-people-since-prehistoric-times. Accessed March 18, 2017.

8. Dickinson TM. Excavations at Standlake Down in 1954: The Anglo-Saxon Graves. *Oxoniensia*. 1973;XXXVIII:239-259. http://oxoniensia.org/volumes/1973/dickinson.pdf. Accessed March 18, 2017.

9. Strouhal E. Myeloma Multiplex versus Osteolytic Metastatic Carcinoma: Differential Diagnosis in Dry Bones. *International Journal of Osteoarchaeology*. 1991;1:219-224. doi: 10.1002/oa.1390010314

10. American Cancer Society. Cancer Basics. https://www.cancer.org/cancer/understanding-cancer/history-of-cancer/cancer-treatment-hormone-therapy.html. Accessed February 9, 2015.

11. Binder M, Roberts C, Spencer N, Antoine D, Cartwright C. On the Antiquity of Cancer: Evidence for Metastatic Carcinoma in a Young Man from Ancient Nubia (c. 1200BC). *PLoS ONE*. 2014;9(3):e90924. doi:10.1371/journal.pone.0090924

12. Johnson J. Unearthing Prehistoric Tumors, and Debate. *The New York Times*. December 28, 2010. p.D1.

13. Sudhakar A. History of Cancer, Ancient and Modern Treatment Methods. *J Cancer Sci Ther*. 2009 Dec 1;1(2):1-4. doi: 10.4172/1948-5956.100000e2. PMID: 20740081.

14. Encyclopædia Britannica. Giovanni Battista Morgagni. http://www.britannica.com/EBchecked/topic/392171/Giovanni-Battista-Morgagni. Accessed Februrary 11, 2015.

15. The Royal College of Surgeons of England. John Hunter. https://www.rcseng.ac.uk/museums/hunterian/history. Accessed February 11, 2015.

16. Schultz MG. Photo Quiz. Emerging Infectious Diseases. 2008;14(9):1479-1481. doi:10.3201/eid1409.086672.

17. Deutsches Röntgen Museum. 100 Years of Diagnostic Radiology. http://www.roentgenmuseum.de/fileadmin/bilder/PDF/ChronikDiagnostik.pdf. Accessed July 3, 2016.

18. Alpen E. *Radiation Biophysics*. 2nd ed. San Diego: Academic Press; 1998.

19. anonymous (https://commons.wikimedia.org/wiki/File:Edison_using_a_calcium_tungstate_flouro-scope._Wellcome_M0015487.jpg), https://creativecommons.org/licenses/by/4.0/legalcode.

20. King G. Clarence Dally—The Man Who Gave Thomas Edison X-Ray Vision. http://www.smithsonianmag.com/history/clarence-dally-the-man-who-gave-thomas-edison-x-ray-vision-123713565/. Accessed February 12, 2015.

21. CERN. 26 February 1896: Becquerel discovers radioactivity https://timeline.web.cern.ch/becquerel-discovers-radioactivity. Accessed August 15, 2023.

22. Mazeron J-J and Gerbaulet A. The centenary of discovery of radium. *Radiation and Oncology*. 1998;49(3):205-216

23. Forsheir S. *Essentials of Radiation Biology and Protection*. 2nd ed. Clifton Park: Delmar/Cengage Learning; 2009.

24. News of Science. Pioneer in X-Ray Therapy. *Science*. 1957;125(3236):18-19. https://www.science.org/doi/10.1126/science.125.3236.18. Accessed August 21, 2022.

25. Grubbe EH. X-rays in the treatment of cancer and other malignant diseases. *Medical Record*. 1902;62:692-695.

26. Bell AG. The uses of radium. *Am. Med*. 1903;6:261.

27. Brenner DJ. Radiation biology in brachytherapy. *Journal of Surgical Oncology*. 1997;65(1):66-70. doi: 10.1002/(sici)1096-9098(199705)65:1<66::aid-jso13>3.0.co;2-q. PMID: 9179271.

28. Strebel H. Vorrschläge zur Radium Therapie. *Dtsch Med Z*. 1903;24:1145-6

29. Mould RF. Priority for radium therapy of benign conditions and cancer. *Curr Oncol*. 2007;14(3):118-122. doi: 10.3747/co.2007.120. PMID: 17593984; PMCID: PMC1899356.

30. The Johns Hopkins Health System. A Brief Sketch of the Medical Career of Dr. William Stewart Halsted. https://www.hopkinsmedicine.org/about/history/history-of-jhh/founding-physicians. Accessed February 18, 2015.

31. Paget S. The distribution of secondary growths in cancer of the breast. *The Lancet*. 1889;133(3421):571-573.

32. DeVita VT Jr, Chu E. A history of cancer chemotherapy. *Cancer Res*. 2008;68(21):8643-8653. doi: 10.1158/0008-5472.

33. National Academy of Engineering. Greatest Engineering Achievements of the 20th Century. http://www.greatachievements.org/?id=3753. Accessed February 18, 2015.

34. Tuller D. Hal Anger Dies at 85; Invented Diagnostic Cameras. *New York Times*. Nov. 21, 2005. http://www.nytimes.com/2005/11/21/science/21anger.html?_r=0. Accessed February 18, 2015.

35. Grubbé É. *X-ray Treatment—Its Origin, Birth and Early History.* Saint Paul:Bruce Publishing Co.; 1949.

36. Sgantzos MN, Tsoucalas G, Konstantinos L, Androutsos G. The physician who first applied radiotherapy, Victor Despeignes, on 1896. *Hellenic Journal of Nuclear Medicine.* 2014;17(1):45-46.

37. Hall E, Giaccia A. *Radiobiology for the Radiologist.* 6th ed. Philadelphia: Lippincott Williams & Wilkins; 2006.

38. Wilson R. Radiological Use of Fast Protons. *Radiology.* 1946;47:487-491.

39. Perez C, Brady L, Halperin E, and Schmidt-Ullrich R. *Principles and Practice of Radiation Oncology.* Philadelphia: Lippincott Williams & Wilkins; 2004.

40. Cancer Research UK. Cancer Treatments. https://www.cancerresearchuk.org/about-cancer/treatment/hormone-therapy/for-cancer. Accessed February 22, 2015.

41. American Cancer Society. Heat Therapy. https://www.cancer.org/cancer/managing-cancer/treatment-types/hyperthermia.html. Accessed February 22, 2015.

42. National Human Genome Research Institute. https://www.genome.gov/genetics-glossary/Cell. Accessed March 18, 2023.

43. Richard Wheeler. https://en.wikipedia.org/wiki/File:DNA_Structure%2BKey%2BLabelled.pn_NoBB.png. Accessed March 27, 2023.

44. Tortora G, Berdell F, and Case C. *Microbiology: An Introduction.* 4th ed. Redwood City: The Benjamin/Cummings Publishing Company, Inc.; 1992.

45. MedlinePlus. https://medlineplus.gov/genetics/understanding/basics/gene/. Accessed February 17, 2022.

46. Hesman Saey T. We finally have a fully complete human genome. Science News, 31 March 2022. https://www.sciencenews.org/article/human-genome-complete-dna-genetics. Accessed June 14, 2022.

47. National Human Genome Research Institute. Genome. https://www.genome.gov/genetics-glossary. Accessed March 18, 2023.

48. National Human Genome Research Institute, NIH. Human Genome Project FAQ. https://www.genome.gov/human-genome-project/Completion-FAQ. Accessed June 14, 2022.

49. U.S. Department of Energy Human Genome Project. The Science Behind the Human Genome Project: Understanding the Basics. http://web.ornl.gov/sci/techresources/Human_Genome/project/info.shtml. Accessed February 28, 2015.

50. Cooper G. *The Cell: A Molecular Approach.* 2nd ed. Sunderland, MA: Sinauer Associates; 2000.

51. National Human Genome Research Institute. (Figure cropped.) https://www.genome.gov/genetics-glossary/histone. Accessed March 18, 2023.

52. National Human Genome Research Institute. https://www.genome.gov/genetics-glossary/Centromere. Accessed March 18, 2023.

53. National Human Genome Research Institute. https://www.genome.gov/genetics-glossary/Karyotype?id=114. Accessed March 18, 2023.

54. O'Connor C. Chromosome segregation in mitosis: The role of centromeres. *Nature Education.* 2008;1(1):28. www.nature.com/scitable/topicpage/chromosome-segregation-in-mitosis-the-role-of-242. Accessed March 1, 2015.

55. Skloot R. *The Immortal Life of Henrietta Lacks.* New York:Crown Publishing Group; 2010.

56. Nature Education. CDK. http://www.nature.com/scitable/topicpage/cdk-14046166. Accessed March 6, 2015.

57. The JigCell Project, Virginia Tech. Generic Model of Eukaryotic Cell Cycle Control: Biological Details. http://jigcell.cs.vt.edu/generic_model/GenericBio.html. Accessed February 26, 2015.

58. Nobel Media. The Nobel Prize in Physiology or Medicine 2001. http://www.nobelprize.org/nobel_prizes/medicine/laureates/2001/. Accessed March 4, 2015.

59. SABiosciences. Cyclins and Cell Cycle Regulation. http://www.sabiosciences.com/pathway.php?sn=Cyclins_Cell_Cycle_Regulation. Accessed February 27, 2015.

60. Kimball J. Kimball's Biology Pages: The Cell Cycle. http://www.biology-pages.info/C/CellCycle.html. Accessed February 25, 2015.

61. National Human Genome Research Institute. https://www.genome.gov/genetics-glossary/apoptosis. Accessed March 18, 2023.

62. Nature Education. Helicase. http://www.nature.com/scitable/definition/helicase-307. Accessed February 26, 2015.

63. Strausfeld U, Howell M, Descombes P, et al. Both cyclin A and cyclin E have S-phase promoting (SPF) activity in Xenopus egg extracts. *J. Cell Sci.* 1996;109:1555-1563.

64. Kimball J. Kimball's Biology Pages: Mitosis. http://www.biology-pages.info/M/Mitosis.html. Accessed February 25, 2015.

65. National Human Genome Research Institute. https://www.genome.gov/genetics-glossary/Mitosis. Accessed March 18, 2023.

66. Lodish H, Berk A, Zipursky S, Matsudaira, P., Baltimore, D., Darnell, J., *Molecular Cell Biology*. 4th ed. New York: W. H. Freeman; 2000. Section 18.3, Myosin: The Actin Motor Protein. Accessed March 1, 2015 at http://www.ncbi.nlm.nih.gov/books/NBK21724/

67. Postlethwait, J. and Hopson, J. The Nature of Life, McGraw-Hill, New York (1989).

68. King, M. (2015) The Medical Biochemistry Page: Eukaryotic Cell Cycles. Accessed March 2, 2015 at http://themedicalbiochemistrypage.org/cell-cycle.php

69. Boundless. "The Mitotic Phase and the G0 Phase." Boundless Biology. Boundless, 02 Jan. 2015. Retrieved 28 Feb. 2015 from https://bio.libretexts.org/Bookshelves/Introductory_and_General_Biology/Book%3A_General_Biology_(Boundless)/10%3A_Cell_Reproduction/10.02%3A_The_Cell_Cycle/10.2B%3A_The_Mitotic_Phase_and_the_G0_Phase

70. Kimball J. Kimball's Biology Pages: B Cells and T Cells. http://www.biology-pages.info/B/B_and_Tcells.html. Accessed March 2, 2015.

71. National Human Genome Research Institute. Cancer. https://www.genome.gov/genetics-glossary/Cancer. Accessed March 18, 2023.

72. Kimball J. Kimball's Biology Pages: Oncogenes. http://www.biology-pages.info/O/Oncogenes.html. Accessed March 6, 2015.

73. Washington C, Leaver D. *Principles and Practice of Radiation Therapy*. 3rd ed. St. Louis:Mosby; 2010.

74. Kimball J. Kimball's Biology Pages: Cancer. http://www.biology-pages.info/C/Cancer.html. Accessed March 6, 2015.

75. Kimball J. Kimball's Biology Pages: Tumor Suppressor Genes. http://www.biology-pages.info/T/TumorSuppressorGenes.html. Accessed March 6, 2015.

76. Nature Education. p53: The Most Frequently Altered Gene in Human Cancers. http://www.nature.com/scitable/topicpage/p53-the-most-frequently-altered-gene-in-14192717. Accessed March 6, 2015.

77. Johns Hopkins University/The Sol Goldman Pancreatic Cancer Research Center. What Are Tumors. https://pathology.jhu.edu/pancreas/types-of-tumors. Accessed March 4, 2015.

78. New Health Guide. Two General Types of Tumors. http://www.newhealthguide.org/Two-General-Types-Of-Tumors.html. Accessed March 4, 2015.

79. WebMD. Benign Tumors. http://www.webmd.com/a-to-z-guides/benign-tumors-causes-treatments. Accessed March 4, 2015.

CHAPTER 2

Ionizing Radiation and Cell Survival

CONTENTS

Radiation therapy is the treatment of cancer using radiation. The very basic idea in radiation therapy is that, if a cancerous tumor is irradiated with sufficient ionizing radiation, then it will at least result in bringing the spread of the cancer cells under control and contain the effects of the cancer. If we can manage to do this without killing neighboring healthy tissue, then we may be able to prolong the life of the patient. In radiation therapy, the radiation is effectively used as a surgical knife to cut out the cancer cells. It would then seem to follow that, if we get better at using radiation—that is, if we can get better at putting the radiation where we want it while keeping it away from where we don't want it—then we should see an increase in patient survival after treatment.

2.1 WHERE WE'RE HEADED

Part I of this book is titled *Motivation* since it explains the motivation for attempting to treat cancer with radiation. This motivation comes in the form of *radiobiology*, which shows how, under the right circumstances, ionizing radiation can be used to kill cancer cells. In this chapter and the next we shall cover some of the fundamentals of radiobiology. These fundamentals will then help us understand the underlying

DOI: 10.1201/9781003477457-2

design of some approaches to treating cancer with radiation discussed later in the book.

With this groundwork in radiobiology under our belts, we will then move on to *Part II*, titled *Foundation*. This part covers the basics of modern physics that are needed to understand how radiation interacts with matter and, more specifically, how energy is deposited in tissue by different types of radiation. *Part III*, titled *Application*, then applies these fundamentals by delving into the heart of the matter: a study of imaging modalities that aid in the diagnosis of cancer and the basic ideas behind the treatment of cancer with radiation.

2.2 THE BEGINNINGS OF RADIOBIOLOGY

Radiobiology can be defined as the study of the effects of ionizing radiation on living cells, tissues, and organisms. The beginning of radiobiology is usually cited as the accidental exposure of Henri Becquerel to radiation from radium.[1,2] Evidently, Becquerel carried around a vial of radium in his waistcoat pocket for demonstration purposes. Marie Curie reported in her biography of Pierre Curie[3,4] that Becquerel had told her and Pierre that he had carried around a glass tube of radium salt and had warned them of the dangers associated with its radiation.

But Becquerel himself, in his paper with Pierre Curie,[5] gives credit for the first observations of the biological effects of radiation on living tissue to F. Walkhoff and F.O. Giesel. They reported in 1900 on the effects of radiation due to radium on the skin.[6,7] Giesel had attached a sample of radium bromide to his arm for two hours, and reported on the radiation burn that appeared on his skin that lasted for weeks. Hearing about Giesel's findings, Pierre Curie then performed his own radiobiological experiment by placing a sample containing radium on his arm for 10 hours, resulting in the production of reddening, scabs, and eventually an open wound. Curie reported that, after fifty-two days, a one centimeter-square gray-colored patch of skin remained where the skin had been irradiated.[4,5]

Curie's experimentation on his arm was quickly followed by further experimentation by Becquerel and even by Marie Curie, who irradiated herself for 30 minutes with a few centigrams of radium bromide that had been placed in a small tube that was then placed inside a thin metallic box.[4,5] She reported the formation of a red spot fifteen days after irradiation, which eventually formed a blister; the irradiated area was healed after another fifteen days.

News of these biological effects produced by irradiation of the skin by radium convinced H. Danlos and P. Block to try treating skin lesions with radiation from radium sources.[8,9] The field of radiobiology was thereby born.

At the beginning of this section, radiobiology was defined as the study of the biological effects of *ionizing radiation*. This naturally leads to the questions, what is ionizing radiation and how does it produce these biological effects? These are the topics of the upcoming sections in this chapter.

2.3   TYPES OF INTERACTIONS

By *radiation* we mean photons, charged particles (such as electrons, protons, or nuclei), or neutrons. When high-energy radiation is incident on atoms, it can in general deliver some of its energy to the atoms. How this energy delivery takes place may be the result of one or more of the following processes:

electron excitation, in which an electron is promoted to a higher-energy state within the atom;

electron ionization, in which an electron in a target atom is given sufficient energy to be promoted to a free state, which means that it is no longer bound to the atom;

nuclear fission, in which the nucleus of a target atom absorbs (typically) a neutron and subsequently becomes unstable; and

nuclear fusion, in which an incident high-energy nucleus joins with a target nucleus to produce a larger nucleus.

Of these, only electron excitation and ionization are important in interactions with atoms in biological tissue, and only ionization is really important in delivering relatively large amounts of energy to surrounding tissue.[2] We therefore typically divide incoming radiation into two classes: ionizing radiation and non-ionizing radiation.

Ionizing radiation itself can be subdivided into two types: directly ionizing and indirectly ionizing. *Directly ionizing radiation* consists of incident *charged* particles (electrons, protons, nuclei). Due to their charge, these radiation particles interact with and can continuously deliver energy to the target atoms as they pass through the material. As a result, we can speak of an average energy delivered to the target medium per unit length of that medium traversed. (For example, we can speak of the joules delivered to the target medium per centimeter of tissue traversed by the particles.) This quantity is called the *linear energy transfer*, or *LET*.

The other type of ionizing radiation is called *indirectly ionizing radiation*, which consists of *uncharged* incident particles (photons and neutrons). As opposed to charged particles that continuously interact with the target atoms as they traverse the target, photons, for example, tend to give up their energy in discrete amounts via occasional interactions with sporadic target atoms—indeed, sometimes a photon travels some distance through the target medium before giving up all of its energy in a single interaction. In such an interaction, a high-energy electron can be released from the atom, which can then go on to continuously interact with the target atoms, delivering energy to the target medium along its trajectory. This results in a certain amount of energy being absorbed by the medium.

In radiation therapy, the medium we are interested in is typically tissue. When we speak of energy being absorbed in tissue, we are really speaking of the *absorbed dose*, or simply the *dose*, in the tissue, denoted D. *Dose* is defined to be the energy absorbed into the tissue from the incident ionizing radiation, E_{abs}, divided by the mass m of the tissue into which the energy is absorbed:[10]

$$D = \frac{E_{abs}}{m}.$$ (2.1)

The SI units of dose are J/kg. This combination of units associated with dose is called the *gray* (Gy): $1\,J/kg = 1\,Gy$. It is this dose that can disrupt the proliferation of cancer cells and cause cell death in tumors. Dose is delivered by charged particles moving through the tissue.

2.4 THE AVERAGE ENERGY ABSORBED PER ION PAIR

A fundamental quantity in radiobiology associated with radiation therapy is the average amount of energy absorbed (or *expended*) in the tissue per ionization; this quantity is denoted $\overline{W}$. (The symbol W is often used to represent the amount of energy, or *work*, required to remove an electron from an atom. On the other hand, we are using the symbol $\overline{W}$ to represent the average total amount of energy absorbed by the medium associated with a single ionization event. These are two associated, but different, quantities. We will discuss this point in more detail at the end of this section.) When an atom is ionized, what results is an ion and a free electron. This pair of particles, one of charge $+e$ and the other of charge $-e$, is often referred to as an *ionization pair* (ip). We can thus say that $\overline{W}$ is equal to the average energy absorbed by the medium per ionization pair produced:

$$\overline{W} = \frac{\overline{E}_{abs}}{ip}.$$ (2.2)

When discussing $\overline{W}$, many books on medical physics give the average energy absorbed in dry air per ionization pair, $\overline{W}_{air}$:[11,12]

$$\overline{W}_{air} = \frac{33.97\,eV}{ip},$$ (2.3)

where $1\,eV = 1.6 \times 10^{-19}\,J$ is called an *electron-volt*. This value of $\overline{W}_{air}$ is a very well known and fundamental quantity. But what we are interested in at this point is determining an approximate value for the average energy absorbed per ionization pair *in tissue*, $\overline{W}_{tissue}$.

We have some work ahead of us to get a rough value for this quantity, but in case you'd like to jump to the punch line and move on to the next section without going through all of the work, the result is given below in Eq. (2.4). This is an approximate result, but it will nevertheless give us a rough idea of the amount of energy imparted to the medium when an ionization event occurs. Since dose is delivered to the medium by charged particles—typically electrons—the number given here is for electrons moving through the medium. It will be shown below that, for electrons traveling through tissue,

$$\overline{W}_{tissue} \approx \frac{37\,eV}{ip}.$$ (2.4)

This average value is obtained for electron energies in the range from 0.01 to 10 MeV. Again, the work leading up to this value for tissue is far from rigorous, but it will

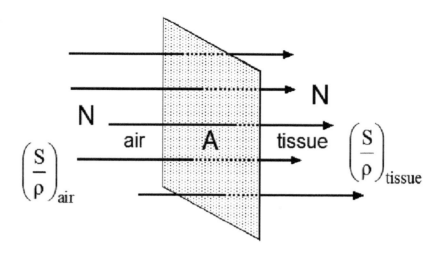

FIGURE 2.1: Fluence is the number of particles, N, passing per unit area, A. The mass stopping power, S/ρ, is the energy lost per unit distance traveled into the medium divided by the density of that medium. The figure shows electrons moving through a border between air and tissue.

nevertheless lead us through some important concepts and definitions. The approximate result shown above is one that is good enough to serve our purposes.

The Calculation Details for $\overline{W}_{tissue}$

In this section we will find out how the result shown in Eq. (2.4) is obtained.

When discussing radiation traveling through a medium, it is convenient to discuss the fluence of the particles making up the radiation. The radiation *fluence* is just the number of radiation particles passing through a medium per unit area (for example, the number of particles per cm^2).

Consider Fig. (2.1) that shows some number N of electrons incident on a border of area A between air and tissue. We will be making a number of approximations in this discussion—here is the first one: we will assume that the number of electrons N passing through the region of air is equal to the number passing through the area A and continuing on into the tissue. The *fluence* of the electrons, Φ, is then equal to

$$\Phi = \frac{N}{A} \tag{2.5}$$

in both the air and the tissue near the border.

We are fundamentally interested in the amount of energy absorbed by the medium (either air or tissue) when an incident electron interacts with and ionizes an atom. This energy absorbed by the medium is associated with the *stopping power* of the electrons in the medium, S. If an electron (or any charged particle) loses an amount of energy E_{lost} as it travels a distance ℓ through the medium, then the stopping power of that electron is defined to be

$$S = \frac{E_{lost}}{\ell}. \tag{2.6}$$

Much of the energy lost can be absorbed into the medium, but some of it may not be—in particular for electrons, energy may be given off in the form of radiation when the incident electrons interact with the nuclei of the medium through which they are traveling. (This type of radiation is called *Bremsstrahlung*, which will be discussed in more detail in Chapter 9.) We will assume that this radiated energy is negligible, so that the energy lost by the electrons as they traverse the medium is equal to the energy absorbed by the medium at that location. In this case, the stopping power becomes equal to the linear energy transfer that was mentioned in the previous section.

The problem with the stopping power is that the amount of energy lost by the incident electrons per unit distance through the medium depends critically on how many atoms the incident electrons encounter within that distance. In other words, the value of S depends critically on the density of the medium, ρ. In an attempt to remove the density dependence from the energy-loss considerations (although it does so only partially[10]), the *mass stopping power* S/ρ is often used instead of the stopping power. This enables us to more meaningfully compare energy losses of charged particles in different media (especially in different media with such vastly different densities as air and tissue). The *mass stopping power* for each charged particle (electron) is therefore given by

$$\frac{S}{\rho} = \frac{E_{lost}}{\rho \ell}. \tag{2.7}$$

We will delve much more deeply into the topic of mass stopping powers for electrons as well as for heavy charged particles in Chapter 9.

In the homework you will be asked to show that several relationships are true using the definitions stated so far in this section and the last, along with the approximations that have been discussed. As a result, those relationships will simply be stated here. First, using the definition of *dose* in Eq. (2.1) along with the definitions of *fluence* and *mass stopping power* from this section, it can be shown that

$$D = \Phi \left(\frac{S}{\rho} \right). \tag{2.8}$$

Also, using the definition of $\overline{W}$ along with the quantity J_m, which is the number of ionization pairs produced by the incident electrons per unit mass of the medium,

$$J_m = \frac{\# ip}{m}, \tag{2.9}$$

it can also be shown that the dose can be written as

$$D = \overline{W} J_m. \tag{2.10}$$

You will also be asked to argue in the homework problems that, if the number of ionization pairs produced per unit volume in a given medium is proportional to the density of the medium, then, for air and some other medium,

$$J_{m, medium} = J_{m, air}. \tag{2.11}$$

Equations (2.8) and (2.10) give us two equations for dose, so we can set these two expressions for dose equal to one another. Doing so, then writing down the resulting equation twice, once for a general medium and once for air, and then dividing the two resulting equations will result in the following equation (after some simplifications):

$$\overline{W}_{medium} = \left[\frac{(S/\rho)_{medium}}{(S/\rho)_{air}} \right] \overline{W}_{air}. \tag{2.12}$$

It should be pointed out once more that this result is only an approximation—there has been no attempt to be rigorous in this derivation. But keep in mind that all we want is to obtain a rough idea of the amount of energy absorbed by the tissue per ionization event in that tissue. The result in Eq. (2.12) will allow us to do that.

All that remains is for us to get some values for the mass stopping powers and use them in Eq. (2.12) to find an approximate value for $\overline{W}_{tissue}$. This task is also delegated to the homework problems, where mass stopping power values for dry air, water, muscle, and fat are given as a function of incident electron energy. The result of the calculations, averaged over electron energies, is given in Eq. (2.4).

Energy Absorbed is Less Than Energy Transferred

It should be kept in mind that, as stated at the beginning of this section, the value of $\overline{W}$ is not equal to the energy required to ionize an atom and free an electron. In general, when an incident charged particle undergoes a collision with an atom via the Coulomb interaction and ionizes an electron, some average amount of energy $\overline{\delta E}$ is transferred to the atom. Some of this energy obviously goes into releasing the electron; the rest of the energy is carried off as kinetic energy of the electron. If the kinetic energy of the emitted electron is high enough, that electron may carry some of its energy far from the region where it was ionized. This means that not all of its energy will be absorbed locally into the medium. Some of the energy of the released electron may go into ionizing electrons in other atoms. Or some of its energy may cause electronic excitation in other atoms, or simply end up as extra energy of motion (translational, vibrational, or rotational) in other atoms, which represents thermal energy. In general, the energy of the originally ionized electron may go into any combination of these possible results which may take place either locally or far from the location of the original ionization event, depending on the energy of the ionized electron.

In addition, as mentioned previously, some energy may be lost from the released electron in the form of bremsstrahlung (photons emitted as the electron accelerates), which may travel some (relatively large) distance from the site of the original ionization. The energy associated with this radiation is not included in the energy absorbed by the medium; the same is true of the energy from high-energy electrons that carry their energy away from the ionization site. In general, the value of $\overline{W}$ includes only that portion of the energy transferred to the ionized atomic electron that ends up being absorbed by the medium in the vicinity of the ionization event.

2.5   LINEAR ENERGY TRANSFER

We are now familiar with the idea that incident charged particles deliver energy to the target material as they pass through that material. How much energy is delivered depends on the type and energy of the particles. What is of particular interest as far as damage to cells is concerned is the amount of energy absorbed by the target material per unit length of the incident particle's trajectory. We mentioned this quantity in the previous section, but we now give it a more formal introduction.

Consider an incident charged particle moving through some medium. If the incident particle loses an amount of energy E_{lost} as it travels a distance ℓ through the medium, then the *unrestricted linear energy transfer*, denoted LET or simply L, is given by

$$L = \frac{E_{lost}}{\ell} . \tag{2.13}$$

This may seem a bit strange to you if you remember Eq. (2.6), which was the definition of the stopping power S—these two definitions are exactly the same! Why do we define two different quantities to be the same thing?

The reason is that we are not typically interested in the unrestricted linear energy transfer. Rather, we tend to be interested in a closely related quantity called the *(restricted) linear energy transfer*, denoted L_Δ:[10]

$$L_\Delta = \frac{E_{lost,\Delta}}{\ell} . \tag{2.14}$$

The "Δ" in the subscripts of L and E_{lost} refers to the fact that there is an *energy cut-off* in the energy lost that we will count toward the linear energy transfer. What does this energy cut-off really mean and why do we worry about it?

In the last section we discussed the ways in which energy can be delivered to a medium: it can cause ionizations, excitations, thermal energy, and (photon) radiation. We also discussed that, if the kinetic energy of an ionized electron is too large, then that electron might carry its energy far from the ionization site, meaning that its energy will not be deposited in the region of the original ionization event. Since we are interested in determining the dose to a region of tissue, we want to ensure that the energy contributing to the dose calculation is only the energy absorbed within that region.

The purpose of the "Δ" cut-off value is to say that only energy going to those ionized electrons with kinetic energies *less than* "Δ" will be included in the value of L_Δ. This effectively limits the energy lost by the incident charged particle to include only those interactions that will deposit the energy in the region close to where the interaction took place. It is this energy that will contribute to the dose delivered to a given region of the target medium, as given in Eq. (2.1), and, perhaps more significantly for our purposes, result in the localized energy deposition that can lead to the killing of cancer cells.[1]

Unless specified otherwise, when we speak of linear energy transfer (LET), we will mean the value L_Δ, with Δ equal to $100\,keV$—the standard value for Δ. Likewise, the value of $E_{lost,\Delta}$ in Eq. (2.14) will be understood to include only the energy lost per interaction that does not deliver more than $100\,keV$ to ionized electrons. The resulting restricted energy loss can then be associated with the region close to the point of interaction.

If, however, we want to consider the LET for *all* energy loses of the incoming electrons (with no cut-off), then would set $\Delta = \infty$. Since the stopping power S includes all lost energy, no matter how much kinetic energy might go to an ionized electron, it follows that the stopping power and the linear energy transfer are related by the simple equation $S = L_\infty = L$, the unrestricted linear energy transfer in Eq. (2.14).

2.6 RADIATION EFFECTS IN CELLS

The purpose of using radiation in radiation therapy is to keep tumor cells from reproducing. Recall that cancer cells are cells that undergo duplication indefinitely. It is this uninhibited reproduction that leads to the formation of a tumor. How can we stop tumor-cell reproduction? Very basically, this is accomplished by causing sufficient damage to the DNA molecules within the cell such that repair, and therefore the reproduction of the cell, is rendered very difficult if not impossible.

Recall from Chapter 1 that the DNA molecule is in the form of a double helix. The backbone of each strand in the helix is comprised of alternating sugar (deoxyribose) and phosphate groups. The "rungs" of the helical DNA ladder consist of the base pairs A–T or C–G. The combination of a phosphate group, a sugar, and a base constitute a nucleotide. The bases A and T are connected by two hydrogen bonds, while C and G are connected by three hydrogen bonds. These hydrogen bonds are the only things holding the two strands of the DNA molecule together, which is what makes the strands so easy to separate during DNA replication.

DNA damage caused by incident radiation tends to be described in terms of "strand breaks". These strand breaks tend to result from damage to the sugar-phosphate backbone to the DNA or to the hydrogen bonds connecting the bases.[13] See Fig. (1.5).

Direct Action
Incident radiation can damage DNA in two ways. One way is for the radiation to interact directly with the DNA molecules within the cells. In particular, if the incident radiation causes damage to a sugar in a DNA molecule, it may result in a strand break. Recall from §2.4 that the average energy absorbed by tissue in a single ionization event, $\overline{W}_{tissue}$, is in the range $30-40\,eV$. Since the average chemical bond in biological tissue is about $4-5\,eV$,[13] one ionization event can result in multiple chemical-bond breaks within in a DNA molecule.

The mode of incident radiation damaging DNA just discussed is referred to as *direct action* and tends to be the dominant mode for high linear energy transfer (LET) radiation such as neutrons or alpha particles.[2] (An alpha particle is a helium nucleus: 2 protons and two neutrons.) However, these types of radiation are not typically used in radiation therapy for cancer patients. Instead, radiation therapy typically uses high-energy photons (x-rays or γ-rays) or electrons, and sometimes protons. In these lower-LET particles, direct action accounts for only 30–40% of cell killing (within the laboratory and in aerobic conditions). The remaining 60–70% is attributed to a mode called *indirect action*.[13]

Indirect Action

About 80% of a cell is composed of water, so when we are speaking of processes inside a cell, we are basically talking about those processes taking place in water. A water molecule contains two hydrogen atoms—each containing one electron—and an oxygen atom, which contains eight electrons. The water molecule therefore contains a total of ten electrons. Electrons can have their spin angular momenta *up* or *down*. (See Chapters 4 and 5 for discussions of the spin angular momentum of electrons.) When two electrons are in the same atom or molecule, it is energetically favorable for them to have their spins opposite to one another, one spin *up* and the other spin *down*; such electrons are said to be *paired*. Since there is an even number of electrons in the water molecule, all of the electrons in water can be paired.

If incident ionizing radiation removes one of the electrons from a water molecule, it forms a water ion, H_2O^+. This ion is then a *free radical*, meaning that it has an unpaired orbital electron. Paired electrons in atomic or molecular orbitals have a high degree of chemical stability relative to atoms or molecules that have an unpaired electron. Free radicals are highly reactive, with lifetimes on the order of $10^{-5}\,s$. Free radicals that are also ions are extremely reactive, with lifetimes around $10^{-10}\,s$.[14] As a result, the water ion H_2O^+ almost immediately combines with a neutral water molecule to produce a hydronium ion (H_3O^+) and a hydroxyl radical $(\cdot OH)$:

$$H_2O^+ + H_2O \rightarrow H_3O^+ + \cdot OH\,. \tag{2.15}$$

It is the hydroxyl radical that can interact with the sugars in the DNA molecule and cause strand breaks. Indeed, it is thought that about two thirds of DNA damage resulting from irradiation of human tissue cells by x-rays is caused by the hydroxyl radical.[2]

The DNA helix has a width of about $2\,nm$ and a hydroxyl radical can diffuse a distance of about 1 nm during its average time before undergoing an interaction. This means that the hydroxyl radical will have a chance of interacting with a sugar in a DNA molecule and potentially cause a strand break as long as it is formed within a circle of radius 2 nm centered on the DNA molecule,[2] as shown in Fig. (2.2).[15]

DNA Repair and Types of Strand Breaks

An issue that must be addressed at this point is that, despite the formation of strand breaks in DNA by hydroxyl radicals or by direct damage caused by the incoming radiation, cells tend to be very good at repairing DNA damage. As a result, about 50% of single strand breaks in a DNA molecule tend to be repaired on average within a few minutes, depending on the amount of incident radiation; the repairs then continue, albeit at a slower rate, after that point.[16,13] This should not be too surprising keeping in mind how well cells can match up missing bases after a DNA has been ripped apart during duplication!

So, if DNA can be repaired, how can radiation result in cell death? There are basically three types of strand breaks: single strand breaks, double strand breaks at a distance, and paired double strand breaks. We've already mentioned that single strand breaks can be readily repaired. Double strand breaks at a distance consist of two strand breaks that are so far removed from one another that they basically act like two independent single strand breaks and are readily repaired. The type of strand break that can result in cell death is most often the paired double strand break, in which two strand breaks occur directly or almost directly (within a few base pairs) across from one another within the DNA helix.

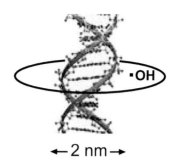

FIGURE 2.2: As long as a hydroxyl radical is formed within a circle centered on the DNA molecule of radius about equal to the 2 nm width of the DNA molecule, it can diffuse to and interact with a sugar in the DNA and possibly cause a strand break. DNA image created by Richard Wheeler. (Creative Commons.)

In this case, the DNA molecule may actually snap in two. While it appears to still be possible for the cell to repair double strand breaks, it is the paired double strand break that appears to lead to cell death most often. We will therefore assume that a lethal double strand break must result from the formation of two or more hydroxyl radicals, each within about 1 nm of opposite sides of the two DNA strands. This is perhaps not so unlikely as it might at first seem.

When energy is deposited into cells from radiation, the energy deposition tends to be very nonhomogeneous. In particular, the energy tends to be deposited in high concentrations in very localized regions. One such region, called a *spur*, can contain a high concentration of free radicals. Since the $\cdot OH$ radicals can migrate distances up to $1\,nm$, it follows that spur formation in the proximity of the double DNA helix, resulting in a high concentration of $\cdot OH$ radicals within that region, most likely explains how double DNA strand breaks are formed. In addition, delayed strand breaks may appear in so-called *potential strand breaks*, which may evolve in time as a result of a slow hydrolysis of DNA sugar molecules that have received $\cdot OH$ damage, but not severe enough damage to result in an immediate strand break.[13]

2.7 RELATIVE BIOLOGICAL EFFECTIVENESS (RBE)

We saw in §2.4, where we discussed $\overline{W}$ (the average absorbed energy per ionization pair), that a given type of radiation can have different effects in different media. But do different types of radiation have different effects within the same medium? More specifically, do incoming particles having different charges, masses, or energies but supplying the same amount of dose affect biological tissue differently?

Radiation Quality

By the *quality* of radiation what we will mean is the type of particles in the radiation beam and their energy. We might *a priori* think that the quality of the incoming radiation beam should not matter as long as the amount of energy deposited into the medium is the same—after all, depositing the same amount of energy should mean (on average) producing the same number of ionizations, the same number of hydroxyl radicals, and the same amount of DNA damage within the cells. So why should the details of the radiation delivering the energy matter? The answer is that the beam quality *does* matter—very much—and LET is a part of the reason why.

RBE

Since different qualities of radiation can affect tissue very differently, it is important to have some kind of measure of the biological effect that characterizes a particular quality of radiation. While an increase in LET tends to correspond to an increase in biological effectiveness for lower values of LET, this does not hold true for higher values of LET. A different kind of measure is needed. That measure is called the *relative biological effectiveness*, or *RBE*.

The "relative" part of RBE refers to the fact that we need to compare the biological effectiveness of a particular quality of radiation to a reference quality—some sort of standard quality of radiation. The reference radiation is typically taken to be 250 kVp x-rays, although it is sometimes taken to be the γ-rays from Co-60 radiation or some other low-LET radiation. ("250 kVp" stands for "250 kilo-volt peak", meaning that a 250 kVp x-ray beam consists of a continuous distribution of photon energies up to a maximum (peak) energy of 250 keV.) Letting "Q" stand for the quality (type and energy) of the radiation whose RBE value is being determined and letting "*ref*" stand for the reference radiation (we will assume that it is 250 kVp x-rays unless noted otherwise), the RBE is defined to be[17]

$$RBE = \frac{D_{ref}}{D_Q} , \qquad (2.16)$$

where D_{ref} and D_Q are the doses of the reference radiation and the quality radiation being studied that both result in the same (average) endpoint of biological damage in the same kind of target. For example, the target being used may be seedlings of a given age from a certain type of plant and the biological endpoint may be the death of half of the seedlings. (Such a dose resulting in the death of half of the population being studied is called the *lethal dose-50*, denoted LD_{50}.) The radiation being studied might be 10 MeV protons. Then the RBE for the protons is the dose of 250 kVp x-rays that results in the death of just 50% of the plant seedlings divided by the dose of the 10 MeV protons that results in the same fraction of seedling death. In this way, the RBE of various qualities of radiation can be determined.

Variation of RBE with LET

Consider the graphs in Fig. (2.3)[18] showing RBE as a function of LET. This graph is worth some careful consideration as there is a good bit of important information contained within it.

We first note that a given LET value corresponds to a given quality of radiation—that is, a given particle with a given energy has a fixed corresponding value of LET, so we can think of the various points on the LET axis as corresponding to different qualities of radiation. We also note the general trend that, over a rather large range,

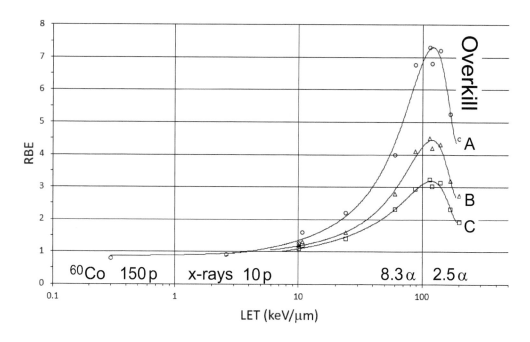

FIGURE 2.3: Relative biological effectiveness (RBE) as a function of linear energy transfer (LET) for three different cell survival fractions: A = 0.8, B = 0.1, and C = 0.01. Several qualities of radiation are listed just above the LET axis. From the left: Co-60 (1.17 and 1.33 MeV γ-rays), 150 MeV protons, $250\,kVp$ x-rays, 10 MeV protons, 8.3 MeV α-particles, and 2.5 MeV α-particles.

increasing LET from low LET values means increasing RBE. But then we hit the most prominent feature of the graph: the peaks at an LET value of approximately $100\,keV/\mu m$, after which the RBE drops rather quickly.

There are three plots shown in the graph corresponding to three different surviving fractions of the cell population being studied (human tissue cells in this case). Plot A corresponds to a surviving fraction (SF) of cells equal to 0.8, so that 80% of the initial population of cells survived. Plot B corresponds to $SF = 0.1$ and plot C corresponds to $SF = 0.01$. Since a higher surviving fraction corresponds to a lower dose of radiation, we see that lower doses of the same quality of radiation and therefore the same LET value have higher RBE values.

Table (2.1) lists several qualities of radiation and their corresponding LET values. Each of these beam qualities is shown just above the LET axis in Fig. (2.3). We note that, for a given particle type (photon, proton, or alpha particle), increasing the particle energy decreases the LET and, therefore, generally decreases the RBE.

Let's dig a bit more deeply into the characteristics in Fig. (2.3) mentioned above. First: as LET increases, so does RBE. This should make sense, since, as the LET increases, the density of ionization-event locations should increase, thereby increasing the likelihood of DNA paired strand breaks and associated cell death.

Second: the pronounced peaks in the *RBE vs. LET* plots. As just mentioned, an increasing LET increases the density of ionization sites, which in turn increases

TABLE 2.1: LET values for various radiation beam qualities

Quality	LET ($keV/\mu m$)	Reference
Photons		
250 kVp x-rays	2.0	Hall & Giaccia[2]
Co-60 (1.17 and 1.33 MeV)	0.2	
Protons		
10 MeV	4.7	Hall & Giaccia[2]
150 MeV	0.5	
α-particles (helium nuclei)		
2.5 MeV	165	Joiner & van der Kogel[19]
8.3 MeV	61	

the density of damage-causing hydroxyl radicals within the cell. This results in an increased likelihood of cell death. For a given type of cell, there will be an optimal ionization-site density in the cell that will result in maximal cell death. For human cells, this occurs at an LET value of $100\,keV/\mu m$, which results in ionization events separated by a distance of about $2\,nm$—the width of the DNA helix. (See Fig. 2.2.) This will then maximize the probability of having a double-strand break with DNA breaks on opposite sides of the helix—a paired double-strand break.[2] If more energy is deposited into a cell than is needed to kill the cell, the cell will still be dead but the RBE will decrease since more energy will have been expended in order to achieve the same end result. This is termed *overkill*. The result of all of this is a peak in the plots of *RBE vs. LET*.[19]

Third: As the energy of the radiation increases, the LET, and therefore the RBE, tends to decrease. For charged-particle radiation this makes sense since the higher energy means a faster speed, which, in turn, means less time that the incident particles spend in the region around the target atoms. For the uncharged particle radiation this is a result of the decreased probability of interaction as the energy of the radiation increases.

Fourth and final point: for a given value of LET, as the surviving fraction (SF) values decrease and the corresponding dose to the tissue increases the RBE values decrease. This is an interesting characteristic that results from the behavior displayed in a plot of *SF vs. D* (dose). The curves displayed in such plots are called *cell survival curves* and are the topic of the next section. We will return to this fourth point after discussing the behavior of cell survival curves.

2.8   CELL SURVIVAL CURVES

Consider a population of a certain type of cell. As this population of cells is irradiated with a given quality of radiation (charge, mass, energy), some of the cells will die due to damage to their DNA. Recall from Eq. (2.1) that the dose to the cell population increases with the increased energy absorbed by the cells from the incident radiation. Therefore, as the cell population acquires more dose D, the surviving fraction (*SF*) of the original cell population will decrease. A plot of surviving fraction *versus* dose is called a *cell survival curve*.

Two examples of cell survival curves are shown in Fig. (2.4). (The data in these plots were taken from Tubiana *et al.*[14], p. 276.) The data displayed in the plots are for intestinal cells from mice irradiated with high LET neutrons and with low LET cobalt-60 γ-ray (gamma-ray) photons. The top graph in the figure shows the data plotted using linear (*regular*) axes. Note the rapid decrease in cell survival with dose for the high-LET neutrons as contrasted with the low-LET γ-rays. The lower graph shows the same data, but plotted with the vertical *Surviving Fraction* axis set up using a logarithmic scale as opposed to a linear scale. (Look closely at the axes on the two graphs. See if you can tell that the *Surviving Fraction* values for each data point are the same on the two graphs. The *Dose* axes have not been changed.) Such a plot is called a *semi-log plot*. The bottom graph in Fig. (2.4) is the standard way of presenting a cell survival curve.

Why RBE Decreases as Dose Increases for a Given LET

Recall that we postponed from the end of the last section the discussion of why the RBE (*Relative Biological Effectiveness*) decreases as the dose increases for a given incident quality of radiation (that is, for a fixed value of LET). We are now in a position to see why this is the case.

As given in Eq. (2.16), the RBE of a given quality of radiation is equal to the ratio of the dose of a reference radiation beam to the corresponding dose of the given quality radiation beam, where the reference radiation corresponds to a low-LET radiation and both doses end up with the same biological endpoint. We can now apply this definition in order to determine the RBE of the neutrons in Fig. (2.4).

Taking the reference radiation in this discussion to be the Co-60 γ-rays, and taking the biological endpoint to be the surviving fraction of the initial cell population, we can see from Fig. (2.4) that, for example, for $SF = 0.5$, $D_{neutrons} = 1.3\,Gy$, and $D_{Co-60} = 3.3\,Gy$. (Make sure that you see how to read these values off of the bottom cell survival curve shown in Fig. 2.4.) It then follows that, for a biological endpoint of SF $= 0.5$, $RBE_{neutrons} = D_{Co-60}/D_{neutrons} = 3.3/1.3 = 2.5$. (Note that, by definition in this discussion, $RBE_{Co-60} = 1.0$.) Likewise, for $SF = 0.3$, we get that $RBE_{neutrons} = D_{Co-60}/D_{neutrons} = 4.8/2.1 = 2.3$. This then demonstrates that, as the SF value decreases and the dose increases, the RBE value also decreases. The homework will ask you to further verify this numerically.

2.9   THE LINEAR-QUADRATIC MODEL FOR CELL SURVIVAL

We now wish to develop a mathematical model that can be used to quantitatively describe the effects of dose on cell survival. In order to do this, we will have to work through some fundamental ideas of probability theory associated with the Poisson probability distribution.

The Probability of Cell Killing

Consider a criterion that either *is* or *is not* true, and consider a large number of systems each of which either *may* or *may not* satisfy the criterion. Let μ denote the

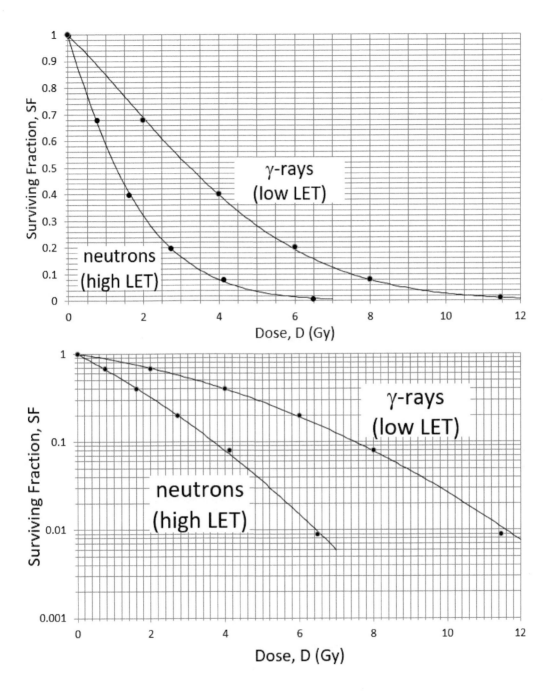

FIGURE 2.4: Cell survival curves for high (neutrons) and low (cobalt-60 gamma rays) LET radiations. (Top) Surviving fraction of cells as a function of absorbed dose, D, on standard linear axes. (Bottom) The same data plotted with a logarithmic *Surviving Fraction* axis.

average number of systems that satisfy the stated criterion. The probability that some number n of the systems will satisfy the criterion, given the value of μ, is then given by

$$P(n; \mu) = \frac{\mu^n}{n!} \, e^{-\mu}, \tag{2.17}$$

where e is the base of the natural logarithm. (Remember that the *factorial of n*, denoted $n!$, is defined to be $n! = n \cdot (n-1) \cdot (n-2) \cdots 2 \cdot 1$. Thus, for example, $4! = 4 \cdot 3 \cdot 2 \cdot 1 = 24$.) This probability distribution is called the *Poisson distribution* and applies as long as one system satisfying the criterion does not influence the probability of another system satisfying the criterion.

We are interested in the probability of incident radiation killing cancer cells. For us, this will mean that paired double strand breaks have been formed. The particles in the radiation beam are incident on the numerous cells in a tumor. We wish to come up with a criterion for the cells, and then use the Poisson distribution above to tell us the probability that the cells will *survive*. This will then give us a model for the cell survival curves discussed in the previous section. The model that we will now introduce is a very simplistic model, but it typically gives reasonable agreement with experiment, and it has a very physical interpretation that is easy to grasp.

The Linear Term

Again, we are interested in cell-killing double strand breaks within cells. We will take as a system a cell that has a particle of radiation passing through it. A cancerous tumor is therefore composed of many systems. We then consider the following criterion: a single radiation particle passes close to a DNA molecule within the nucleus of a cell and causes a paired double strand break in the DNA. (Remember that a paired double strand break means that two strand breaks have taken place more-or-less right across from one another on the DNA helix, so that the DNA is effectively broken into two pieces.)

We will make the reasonable assumption that the average number of cells satisfying the criterion, μ, is proportional to the dose, so that, if the dose is doubled, then the average number of cells acquiring paired double strand breaks from the incoming radiation will also be doubled. We can then write that $\mu = \alpha D$, where α is a proportionality constant, and D is the dose. Since the average number of cells being killed is proportional to D^1 (D raised to the power 1), this model is said to be *linear* in the dose, D.

We can now apply the Poisson distribution, Eq. (2.17). The probability that some number n of cells will satisfy the criterion—that is, they will receive paired double strand breaks and subsequently die—is given by

$$P(n; \mu) = P(n; \alpha D) = \frac{(\alpha D)^n}{n!} \, e^{-\alpha D}. \tag{2.18}$$

The Quadratic Term

We must now acknowledge that having a single radiation particle traverse the cell's DNA is not the only way to get a paired double strand break. Another—perhaps more likely—way to get a paired double strand break is to have two different particles traverse the same DNA molecule within the same cell and cause the paired strand breaks. This, then, is a different criterion, but one leading to the same result—the death of the cell.

In this new model there will have to be two different incident beam particles interacting with the same DNA molecule—that it, there will have to be two separate events. Since the occurrence of one of the two events does not affect the occurrence of the other event, it follows that these two events are *independent* of one another. Probabilities for independent events are *multiplicative*, meaning that, if $P(A)$ is the probability of event A occurring and $P(B)$ is the probability of event B occurring, then the probability of events A and B occurring is given by $P(A\,and\,B) = P(A)P(B)$.

Remembering that the probability for one particle to interact with the DNA is proportional to D, it follows that the probability for *two* particles to interact must be proportional to D^2, since these two events are independent of one another. Then, since the average number of events occurring can be written as the total number of possible events times the probability of occurrence of a single event, the average number of cells satisfying this new criterion must also be proportional to D^2.

We can thus write that, for this two-interaction model, $\mu = \beta D^2$, where β is again a proportionality constant. Since this value of μ is proportional to D^2, this model is said to be *quadratic* in D. The probability that n cells will be killed by two different particles causing a paired double-strand break in the cell's DNA is therefore given by

$$P(n; \mu) = P(n; \beta D^2) = \frac{(\beta D^2)^n}{n!}\, e^{-\beta D^2} . \tag{2.19}$$

The Probability of Cell Survival

The behavior that we are trying to model is that shown in the cell *survival* curves, not the cell *death* curves! This means that we need an equation to show us the behavior of *SF*—the surviving fraction of the original population of cells—as the dose D is increased. If $P(n)$ represents the probability that n cells will be killed, then $P(0)$ must tell us the probability that *no cells* will be killed—that is, the cells *survive*. It therefore follows that the probability that the cells survive a single-particle double strand break is

$$P(n = 0; \mu) = P(0; \alpha D) = \frac{(\alpha D)^0}{0!}\, e^{-\alpha D} = e^{-\alpha D} , \tag{2.20}$$

and the probability that the cells survive a two-particle double strand break is given by

$$P(n = 0; \mu) = P(0; \beta D^2) = \frac{(\beta D^2)^0}{0!}\, e^{-\beta D^2} = e^{-\beta D^2}. \tag{2.21}$$

(Remember that, by definition, $1! = 1$ and $0! = 1$.)

A cell can be killed by a paired double strand break, whether that paired double break is caused by one or two of the incoming radiation particles. Therefore, in order for the cells to *survive* irradiation, they must survive both a single-particle double strand break *and* a two-particle double stand break. Since a cell surviving a single-particle double strand break has nothing to do with whether it will survive a two-particle double strand break, the total probability that the cells will survive a paired double strand break, $P(0)$, must be given by (again, remember that independent probabilities are multiplicative)

$$P(0) = P(0; \alpha D)P(0; \beta D^2) = e^{-\alpha D}\,e^{-\beta D^2}\,. \tag{2.22}$$

The Linear-Quadratic Model

If there were N cells in the original population, then $NP(0)$ must represent the average number of original cells that were *not* killed by the radiation beam after a dose D was deposited. To get the *fraction* of cells surviving, *SF*, we must then divide this number by the original population, N. This means that the probability $P(0)$ is the same thing as the surviving fraction. Since $P(0)$ is a function of the dose, D, it follows that the surviving fraction of original cells is also a function of D, *SF(D)*, which is exactly what we wanted:

$$SF(D) = e^{-\alpha D - \beta D^2}\,. \tag{2.23}$$

Since this function depends both linearly and quadratically on the dose, D, this result is called the *Linear-Quadratic model for cell survival*. The solid lines in the cell survival curves shown in Fig. (2.4) are the linear-quadratic fits to the data. (The values of the parameters α and β used to generate the displayed curves are: $\alpha_{neutrons} = 0.50\,Gy^{-1}$, $\beta_{neutrons} = 0.033\,Gy^{-2}$, $\alpha_{\gamma-rays} = 0.14\,Gy^{-1}$, and $\beta_{\gamma-rays} = 0.022\,Gy^{-2}$.)

Let's look a bit more closely at the linear and quadratic terms in Eq. (2.23). Fig. (2.5) shows the Co-60 γ-ray cell survival data from Fig. (2.4). Again, the solid line is the linear-quadratic model fit to the data. The graph also shows two other curves—one corresponding to the linear term, Eq. (2.20), and the other to the quadratic term, Eq. (2.21).

Note that the exponential linear term actually appears linear since the curve has been drawn on a semi-log plot and the linear term is a pure exponential function involving D in its exponent. Likewise, the exponential quadratic term looks quadratic since it has a D^2 in its exponent. (One way to see why this is the case is to consider the function $f(D) = e^{KD^n}$ for some constant K. In a semi-log plot we are effectively looking at the behavior of the *logarithm* of the function. Since $ln[f(D)] = KD^n$, we can see that the behavior shown on a semi-log plot for the linear term ($n = 1$) will be $-\alpha D$, a linear plot, and that for the quadratic term ($n = 2$) will be $-\beta D^2$, a quadratic plot.)

The Crossover Dose, $D_{\alpha\beta}$

Note that the linear and quadratic curves in Fig. (2.5) intersect. This means that there must be s special value of dose, denoted $D_{\alpha\beta}$, where the linear and quadratic terms contribute the same amount to cell death. But the linear and quadratic terms will only be equal when $\alpha D = \beta D^2$, from which it follows that $D_{\alpha\beta} = \alpha/\beta$. For the values of α

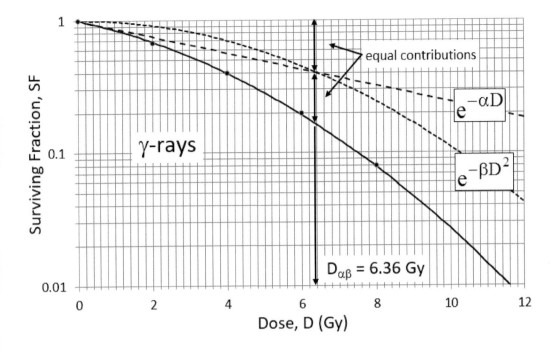

FIGURE 2.5: This graph shows the same cell survival curve associated with the beam of Co-60 γ-rays shown in Fig. (2.4). The solid line is the linear-quadratic model fit to the data. (See the text for the parameters for the fit.) Also shown are the linear- and quadratic-term contributions to the full linear-quadratic result, and the crossover dose $D_{\alpha\beta}$ at which these two contributions are equal.

and β given above for the Co-60 γ-rays, we get that $D_{\alpha\beta} = 0.14\,Gy^{-1}/0.022\,Gy^{-2} = 6.36\,Gy$. This special dose is shown in Fig. (2.5).

At this value of dose the linear and quadratic terms contribute exactly the same amount to the full value from the linear-quadratic model. We will refer to the dose $D_{\alpha\beta}$ as the *crossover dose* since, as the dose to the cell population increases past $D_{\alpha\beta}$, the dominant contributor to cell death switches from the linear single-particle term (for smaller values of D) to the quadratic two-particle term (for larger values of D) within the linear-quadratic model. This behavior is clearly shown in Fig. (2.5). (Keep in mind that more cell death means a lower value of SF.)

2.10   RISKS IN IMAGING AND RADIATION THERAPY

We have been discussing in this chapter the radiobiology associated with the killing of cancer cells in tumors. We have seen that incident radiation particles can kill such cells either by direct or indirect means. But what we have not mentioned so far is that, in order to get radiation to the cells in a tumor, we almost always have to pass that radiation through *healthy* cells. This means that the radiation can kill not only tumor cells but also healthy cells in the vicinity of the tumor.

We have focused on cell death caused by radiation. But, for each cell killed by an incoming radiation beam, many more cells are typically damaged. This damage is often quickly repaired within the cell, but not always. Cell damage that is not repaired can lead to cell mutations. In Chapter 1, we discussed the cell cycle and the roles played by cyclin-Cdk complexes that serve to promote or stop the cell's progression through the cell cycle. If any part of these complexes are mutated, or if any genes associated in any way with cell mitosis are mutated, it can lead to uncontrolled cell growth—in other words, cancer. This means that, in an attempt to kill cancerous cells, the radiation used in radiation therapy can at the same time cause new cancer. This is a risk associated with any form of ionizing radiation.

But ionizing radiation is not only used in radiation therapy—that is, in the treatment of cancer with radiation. Before the cancer is treated, it must first be detected. This is often done with imaging modalities such as CT or PET scans, for example, that also involve ionizing radiation. (Imaging modalities will be discussed at the beginning of *Part III* of this book.) In order to obtain the images in which the presence of cancer can be detected in CT or PET scans, ionizing radiation must be passed through the body. The energy associated with the imaging radiation—and therefore the dose delivered to the body from that radiation—tends to be much less than that associated with radiation therapy, but that doesn't change the fact that the radiation used in imaging can still cause cell damage, cell mutations, and cell death. (This is true, for example, whenever you get an x-ray at the dentist's or the doctor's office.)

Much effort is put into protecting the body from unnecessary radiation, but this unfortunately does not completely eliminate the risk of the imaging or treatment radiation causing cancer. Fortunately, the risk of developing cancer from the radiation associated with radiological imaging or radiation therapy tends to be far outweighed by the cancer detection and treatment benefits associated with these procedures.

2.11   QUESTIONS, EXERCISES, & PROBLEMS

2-1. What is the difference between *linear energy transfer* and *stopping power*?

2-2. Consider some number N of charged particles passing through an area A and into a mass m of tissue. Assuming that the energy absorbed in the mass m is equal to the total energy lost by all of the charges within that mass, derive Eq. (2.8). That is, assuming that $E_{abs} = N\,E_{lost}$, where E_{lost} is the average energy lost in the tissue per charged particle, show that $D = \Phi \cdot S/\rho$.

2-3. Show that $D = \overline{W} \cdot J_m$.

2-4. Show that, if the number of ionization pairs produced in a given volume of a medium is proportional to the density of that target medium ρ, then $J_{m,\,air} = J_{m,\,tissue}$.

2-5. Following the discussion in the text, show that Eq. (2.12) must be true given the approximations stated.

2-6. The purpose of this problem is to verify the value of $\overline{W}_{tissue}$ given in Eq. (2.4). Table (2.2) below lists values of the total mass stopping power, S/ρ, for electrons in air, water, muscle, and fat (in units of MeV·cm^2/g) as a function of incident electron energy (in MeV). (These data are taken from Appendix E in Attix.[11]) We wish to use these data, along with Eq. (2.12) and other information given in the chapter, to compute the value for $\overline{W}_{tissue}$ given in Eq. (2.4). We will do this as follows: *(i)*

Compute the ratio of the mass stopping powers for water, muscle, and fat relative to dry air for each of the energy values given in Table (2.2). *(ii)* Then compute $\overline{W}_{medium}$ for each of the values computed in *(i)* using the value of $\overline{W}_{air}$ given in Eq. (2.3). *(iii)* Average the $\overline{W}$ values for water over the various energy values to compute $\overline{W}_{water}$. Do the same for all of the muscle and fat values *combined* to compute $\overline{W}_{muscle \& fat}$. Your calculations should give you the following values:

$$\overline{W}_{water} \approx \frac{37.2\,eV}{ip} \quad \text{and} \quad \overline{W}_{muscle \& fat} \approx \frac{37.4\,eV}{ip}. \tag{2.24}$$

(It is interesting to note that the values for water and for muscle-and-fat combined are very close to one another. It is for this reason that a tank of water is often substituted for the human body in clinical tests and quality assurance procedures.) *(iv)* Finally, to find the approximate value for $\overline{W}_{tissue}$ given in Eq. (2.4), we simply average the two values given in Eq. (2.24). (Note that the value given in Eq. (2.4) was only kept to two significant figures due to the approximations involved.)

TABLE 2.2: Total Mass Stopping Power Values (in units of MeV·cm^2/g) as a function of incident electron energy (in units of MeV)

E (MeV)	Dry Air	Water	Muscle	Fat
0.01	19.76	22.57	22.31	23.47
0.1	3.637	4.12	4.075	4.241
1	1.674	1.862	1.839	1.891
10	2.159	2.149	2.125	2.151

2-7. The following statement appears at the end of §2.5: "...it follows that the stopping power and the linear energy transfer are related by the simple equation $S = L_\infty = L$, the unrestricted linear energy transfer in Eq. (2.14)". Explain this statement and how it follows from the discussion in that section.

2-8. Explain in your own words why the value of the average energy absorbed by the medium per ionization pair, $\overline{W}$, is not equal to the average energy required to ionize an atom or molecule in that medium.

2-9. Explain the difference between *directly ionizing* and *indirectly ionizing* radiation. Give two examples of each.

2-10. The text mentions the formation of "spurs" associated with the nonhomogeneous deposition of energy into cells, resulting in localized regions of high concentrations of ·OH radicals. Assume that the energy associated with the formation of a spur is $60\,eV$.[20] For each of the qualities of radiation given in Table (2.1), compute the average distance between spurs, assuming that all of the energy given up by the radiation particles is in the form of spurs.

2-11. It was shown in Fig. (2.3) that the peak in the *RBE vs. LET* curves tends to be around $LET = 100\,keV/\mu m$. Following the procedure in the previous problem, find the average distance between spurs at the LET value of the *RBE* peak.

2-12. We have discussed cell killing due to particles of radiation interacting directly or indirectly with DNA molecules. Either way, the cell is traversed by a radiation particle that causes the damage to the cell. Research and explain in your own words the phenomenon called *the bystander effect*, which involves biological effects in cells that were not traversed by a beam particle. As always, be sure to cite your references. (And, as always, remember that *Wikipedia* is not an acceptable professional reference.)

2-13. Compute *RBE* values for the neutron radiation beam whose cell survival curve is shown in Fig. (2.4) for the biological endpoints given by *SF* = 0.2, 0.4, 0.6, and 0.8, using the Co-60 γ-rays as the reference radiation. Then explain the order of the three *RBE vs. LET* curves shown in Fig. (2.3) (*A above B above C*).

2-14. The fact that some probabilities are multiplicative and not additive was used multiple times in the discussion of the Linear-Quadratic Model. (a) Explain what "multiplicative and not additive" means within the context of probabilities. When are probabilities multiplicative? ... additive? (b) Give a simple, everyday example in which the calculation of a probability is multiplicative. (c) Give a simple, everyday example in which the calculation of a probability is additive.

2-15. (a) Explain in your own words the concept of *overkill* within the context of *RBE* and *LET*. That is, what is meant by the term "Overkill" shown in Fig. (2.3)? (b) Explain the existence of a peak in the plot of *RBE vs. LET*.

2-16. Figure (2.5) shows the linear and quadratic contributions to the full linear-quadratic curve (the solid line). Consider the following statement: *The sum of the linear and quadratic curves is equal to the full linear-quadratic curve.* How can this statement be true? After all, it is the *product* of the two terms $e^{-\alpha D}$ and $e^{-\beta D^2}$ that gives the full linear-quadratic curve as specified by the function *SF(D)* in Eq. (2.23). Secondly, the *sum* of the two dashed curves shown in the figure will give a curve *above* the two curves, not *below* them! However, we note the following: if we take the $SF = 1$ line at the top of the plot to represent the starting point for measuring distance and if we measure distance from the starting point at the top downward in the graph, then the statement above is true. For example, if we consider $D = 8\,Gy$, using a ruler to measure the distance from the $SF = 1$ line down to the linear plot and then add that to the distance from the starting point down to the quadratic curve, you will find that this sum is equal to the distance from the starting point down to the full cell-survival curve. (All distances, in case, are measured along the line $D = 8\,Gy$.) This can be done for one value of D after another, showing that the statement above is indeed true. Carefully explain why this is so. (*Hint:* Remember that the cell survival graph is a semi-logarithmic plot.)

2.12   REFERENCES

1. Alpen EL. *Radiation Biophysics.* 2nd ed. San Diego: Academic Press; 1998.
2. Hall EJ, Giaccia AJ. *Radiobiology for the Radiologist.* Philadelphia: Lippincott Williams & Wilkins; 2006.
3. Curie M, Curie P. Kellogg VL, Kellogg C, trans. New York: The Macmillan Company; 1923.
4. Mould RF. Pierre Curie, 1859-1906. *Curr Oncol.* 2007;14(2):74-82. https://www.ncbi.nlm.nih.gov/pmc/articles/PMC1891197/. Accessed June 16, 2022.
5. Becquerel H, Curie P. L'action physiologique des rayons du radium. *Comptes Rendus Hebdomadaires des Séances de L'Academie des Sciences.* 1901;132(22):1289-1291.
6. Walkoff F. Unsichtbare, photographisch wirksame Strahlen. *Photographische Rundsch Z Freunde Photographie.* 1900;14:189-191
7. Giesel FO. Über radioactive Stoffe. *Ber Dtsche Chem Ges.* 1900;33:3569-3571.

8. Danlos H, Bloch P. Note sur le traitement du lupus érythèmateux par desapplications de radium. *Ann Dermatol Syphil.* 1901;2:986-988.

9. Diamantis A, Magiorkinis E, Papadimitriou A, and Androutsos G. The contribution of Maria Sklodowska-Curie and Pierre Curie to Nuclear and Medical Physics, A hundred and ten years after the discovery of radium. *Hellenic journal of nuclear medicine.* 2008;11(1):33-38.

10. International Commission on Radiation Units and Measurements. Fundamental Quantities and Units for Ionizing Radiation (Revised). *Journal of the ICRU.* 2011;11(1):Report 85.

11. Attix FH. *Introduction to Radiological Physics and Radiation Dosimetry.* New York: John Wiley & Sons; 1986.

12. Khan FM. *The Physics of Radiation Therapy.* 4th ed. Philadelphia: Wolters Kluwer/Lippincott Williams & Wilkins; 2010.

13. Ward JF. Some Biochemical Consequences of the Spatial Distribution of Ionizing Radiation-Produced Free Radicals. *Radiation Research.* 1981;86(2):185-195.

14. Tubiana M, Dutriex J, Wambersie A. *Introduction to Radiobiology.* London:Taylor & Francis; 1990.

15. Created by Richard Wheeler. Available through the Creative Commons Attribution-Share Alike 3.0 Unported license. Image cropped and labels added. https://en.wikipedia.org/wiki/File:DNA_Structure%2BKey%2BLabelled.pn_NoBB.png. Accessed March 27, 2023.

16. Frankenberg-Schwager, M. Review of repair kinetics for DNA damage induced in eukaryotic cells in vitro by ionizing radiation. *Radiother. Oncol.* 1989;14:307-320.

17. National Council on Radiation Protection and Measurements. The Relative Biological Effectiveness of Radiations of Different Quality. 1990: NCRP Report No. 104.

18. Data for this figure were taken from Barendsen GW. Responses of cultured cells, tumors, and normal tissues to radiation of different linear energy transfer. *Curr Top Radiat Res Q.* 1968;4:293-356.

19. Joiner MC, van der Kogel AJ, eds. *Basic Clinical Radiobiology.* 5th ed. Boca Raton, FL: CRC Press, Taylor & Francis Group; 2019.

20. Committee on the Biological Effects of Ionizing Radiation. Health Effects of Exposure to Low Levels of Ionizing Radiation: BEIR V. National Academy of Sciences; 1990.

Cellular Repair and Fractionation

CONTENTS

In the last chapter, we discussed the effects of ionizing radiation on living cells. We saw how the linear energy transfer (LET) affects the biological endpoint and thus the relative biological effectiveness (RBE). And we deduced how, for a given quality of radiation and therefore for a given LET, as the dose increases, the RBE decreases—contrary to what we might at first expect. All of these behaviors are manifest in the cell survival curves.

In this chapter, we will continue our discussion of the effects of radiation on living cells, as well as our examination of the behavior exhibited in the cell survival curves and our analysis of those behaviors with the linear-quadratic model of cell survival. This analysis will then lead us to some important conclusions that are used every day in treatment planning for cancer patients.

3.1   THE EFFECT OF OXYGEN ON CELL SURVIVAL

We saw in the last chapter that a cell survival curve, in general, slopes downward as the dose to the cells increases. The higher the LET of the radiation, the more rapid the downward slope. Fig. (3.1) below is copied from Chapter 2 for reference.

For a given type of cell, the rate of decrease in the cell survival curve is influenced by a variety of factors: total dose, time duration for the delivery of the dose, type of radiation particles, and energy of those particles, to name just a few.

Another important factor that can affect the surviving fraction of cells after irradiation is the presence of oxygen. Indeed, while other chemical and pharmacological substances have been found to affect the sensitivity of tissue to radiation, none is as dramatic, ubiquitous, and clinically valuable as oxygen.[1,2]

DOI: 10.1201/9781003477457-3

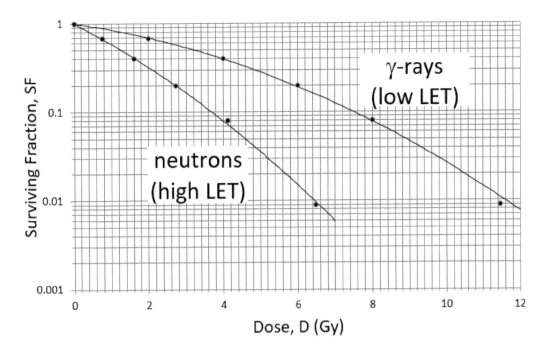

FIGURE 3.1: Cell survival curves for high (neutrons) and low (cobalt-60 gamma rays) LET radiations. (From Chapter 2.)

The Oxygen Enhancement Ratio (OER)

Cells are generally found to be more susceptible to radiation damage in the presence of oxygen (*oxic*) than in an environment that has a deficiency of oxygen (*hypoxic*). This effect is quantified with the *oxygen enhancement ratio (OER)*, which is defined to be the ratio of the dose required for a given biological endpoint in the absence of oxygen divided by the dose required for the same biological endpoint with oxygen.

Typical tissue values for OER range from about 2.5 to 3.0 for high doses of low-LET radiation such as x-rays and gamma-rays. The higher the LET of the incoming radiation, the lower the OER value; $OER = 1.0$ for high-LET α-particles. The OER values for cells vary with the phase of the cell cycle, with lower values of OER for cells in the G_1 phase, and relatively higher values of OER in the S phase.[3]

The increased sensitivity to ionizing radiation in the presence of oxygen results from the oxygen molecules reacting with free radicals to produce unrepairable peroxy radicals.[4] In particular, as discussed in Chapter 2, electrons released by the incident particles of ionizing radiation travel through the tissue, producing ionization pairs along their paths. The production of these ion pairs can result in free radicals that can cause damage to the DNA molecules. If this damage is a single strand break, then it can be readily repaired. However, if molecular oxygen is present, then an organic peroxide associated with the DNA damage can be formed, resulting in DNA damage that cannot be easily repaired. The presence of oxygen can thereby render DNA damage effectively permanent.[3]

It should be noted that healthy tissue tends to have sufficient blood flow to keep it well oxygenated, while tumors tend to lack a good blood flow, leaving them in a relatively hypoxic state. This greater supply of oxygen to healthy tissue renders it more susceptible to radiation damage than cancerous tissue. This unfortunate situation must be addressed in the development of any treatment plan involving radiation for a cancer patient.

3.2 RADIOSENSITIVITY AND CELL-CYCLE PHASE

The cells in any tissue or tumor can be thought of as an *asynchronous* population of cells in that the cells represent all stages of the cell cycle. That is, cells in the tissue can be found in each of the phases of the cell cycle. Not all phases of the cell cycle are equally susceptible to damage from incident ionizing radiation, however.

Consider the histogram shown in Fig. (3.2). The plot shows the relative susceptibility of the various phases of the cell cycle to cell killing by incident ionizing radiation. The data for this histogram come from a plot by Withers and Peters[5] showing the surviving fraction of

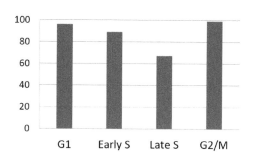

FIGURE 3.2: The relative radiosensitivity of cells in the various phases of the cell cycle. The numbers are only intended to give a rough idea of the relative susceptibility of a sample cell population to cell death caused by incident ionizing radiation.

a population of Chinese hamster cells that had been synchronized in the various stages of the cell cycle prior to irradiation by varying doses of radiation. The data in this histogram correspond to a dose of about $570\,cGy$. Since the values for susceptibility can vary greatly with dose (although the susceptibility ranking for each phase does not change), the numbers shown in the plot are only intended to give a very rough idea of the relative susceptibilities of the various phases of the cell cycle to radiation damage. Nevertheless, it is clear from the figure that the G_2/M phase is significantly more susceptible to radiation damage than is the late S phase. This non-uniformity in radiosensitivity among the cell-cycle phases has an interesting consequence in radiation therapy.

As tumor cells are irradiated, those cells in the most sensitive phases will be more likely to be damaged and, potentially, killed. Therefore, as the irradiation proceeds, the fraction of the remaining cells in more radioresistant phases increases. The subsequent radiation will then be less effective than the initial incident radiation. This results in what is called a *partial synchronization* of the surviving cells after irradiation, since the surviving cells will tend to be in the less radiosensitive phases.

Since different cells progress through the cell cycle at a variety of rates, it follows that the cell population will eventually return to its original state of asynchronicity, thereby becoming overall more susceptible to the killing effects of ionizing radiation than it was immediately after irradiation. We will return to this important point shortly.

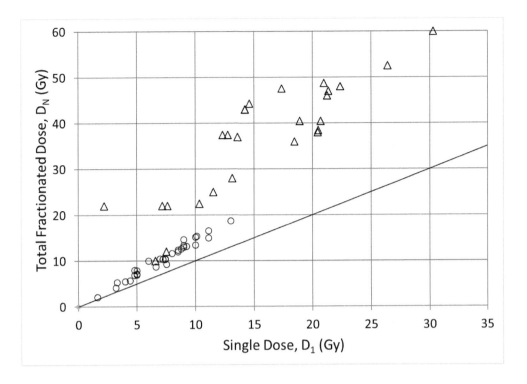

FIGURE 3.3: A plot showing the total dose, D_N, delivered in N fractions as a function of the single-fraction dose, D_1, such that the two doses have the same biological endpoint. $\circ : N = 2$; $\triangle : N = 10$. The solid line corresponds to $D_N = D_1$.

3.3 STRAND BREAKS AND CELLULAR REPAIR

It is found that, after a cell receives a dose of about $1\,Gy$ from high-energy photon irradiation, approximately 1000 strand breaks have been formed in DNA. However, if the same DNA are examined a few hours later, fewer than 20 strand breaks are found to remain.[6] Clearly, a DNA repair mechanism has been hard at work since the incident radiation ceased. This finding introduces two new concepts to our discussion of cell survival: *time* and *repair*. The upcoming sections will address the issue of time. In this section, we will focus on DNA repair.

Radiation damage is thought to fall into one of three categories: *lethal*, in which the damage results in cell death, *potentially lethal*, in which the damage may be repaired depending on the cellular environment, and *sublethal*, which may be repaired given sufficient time for the repair mechanisms to take place and given the lack of any further radiation damage.[3] We will simplify our discussion by including the potentially lethal damage in with the sublethal damage and referring to this combined category as simply *sublethal damage*.

The Fractionation of Dose
To see the effects of DNA repair on tissue that has been irradiated with ionizing radiation, consider the plot of D_N *vs.* D_1 shown in Fig. (3.3). (The data in this plot

were calculated from data given in Tables I and II in Withers.[7]) In this plot, the quantity D_1 is the total dose delivered to cells in a single treatment session. On the other hand, the dose D_N is also the total dose delivered to the cells, but this dose is divided up into N equal parts, or *fractions*, each fraction delivered in a separate treatment session. The *dose-per-fraction*, or dose delivered during each treatment session, is then simply D_N/N.

The plot shows two sets of data corresponding to two different values for N: $N = 2$ (circles) and $N = 10$ (triangles). For each data point, the dose D_2 or D_{10} is that total dose that yields the same biological end effect as the single dose D_1. (For example, the end effect could be LD_{50}—a lethal dose delivered to 50% of the cell population.) The various data in Fig. (3.3) correspond to many different end effects as well as dose durations (that is, different *dose rates*) and different times between fractions, varying from 3 to 24 hours. Despite all of the variation in the data, we see one characteristic that they all share: they all lie above the solid line, which represents the line $D_N = D_1$. Let's think about this a little more.

If $D_N = D_1$, then it does not matter if the dose is divided up into fractions or not—the same total dose is required for a given end effect. But the data show us that this is not the case. Since *all* of the data fall above the $D_N = D_1$ line, this means that, whenever the dose is divided up into pieces—that is, whenever the dose is *fractionated*—it will always take more total dose to acquire the same biological end effect. Why would this be the case? Clearly, this is because of DNA repair—if the dose is fractionated, then time is allowed for sublethal damage to be repaired.

If some of the two-hit double strand breaks are repaired during the time between fractions, then the surviving fraction of the cell population will *increase*. This means that we are backtracking, and will have to "re-damage" some of the cells to get back to the lower surviving fraction value that we had achieved by the end of the previous fraction. It should therefore make complete sense that it must take more total dose to achieve a given biological end effect if the dose is fractionated as a result of DNA repair.

There is one more thing that should be pointed out about the data plotted in Fig. (3.3)—namely, all of the data correspond to *in vivo* hypoxic experimental conditions in animals in which the blood supply to the tissue was stopped before and during irradiation. This results in eliminating reoxygenation effects in the data.

As we've already discussed, it has been found that the repair of sublethal damage is oxygen dependent—the more oxygen in the cell environment, the less readily repairs will take place and the more cell damage will become permanent. Since tumors are typically less oxygenated than healthy tissue, tumor cells may be able to more readily repair sublethal damage compared to healthy cells.[8] Since the data in Fig. (3.3) were obtained under relatively hypoxic conditions, repair of sublethal damage should readily be able to take place.

Repair and the Linear-Quadratic Model

Many models have been produced in an attempt to understand and explain the observed cell survival curve behavior. No one model is considered the superior model, but the linear-quadratic model is often referred to, so we will continue our discussion with that model.

We saw in Chapter 2 that the surviving fraction, SF, of a cell population as a function of the dose, D, of ionizing radiation can be modeled by the equation

$$SF(D) = e^{-\alpha D - \beta D^2} = \left[e^{-\alpha D} \right] \left[e^{-\beta D^2} \right] . \tag{3.1}$$

In this equation, the first term in brackets represents cell death that results from a single incident particle of radiation causing a deadly double-strand break. This effect is clearly illustrated by high-LET α-particles, for example, in which each incident particle produces a high density of ionization events near the DNA. This high density of ionizations from the passage of a single α-particle results in numerous paired double-strand breaks in DNA and subsequent cell death. The cell-survival curves for such single-particle cell-killing interactions are found to be quite linear.[9] As a result, the first bracketed term in Eq. (3.1) is taken to represent irreparable cell damage as a result of a single-particle interaction.

The second bracketed term, on the other hand, represents the case in which two independent incident particles produce strand breaks at different positions on the same DNA molecule that can, nevertheless, result in cell death. When taking DNA repair into consideration in this model, we acknowledge that it is possible in this two-particle case for the strand breaks to eventually be repaired. As a result, the second bracketed term in Eq. (3.1) is considered to be the term associated with *sublethal* damage to the DNA. This sublethal damage may lead to cell death if left unrepaired.

A Linear Cell Survival Curve means No DNA Repair

Let's consider a tumor being irradiated, and let's pretend for a moment that only lethal, single-particle double strand breaks occur. If this is the case, then the only term that would contribute in Eq. (3.1) would be the first bracketed term. We noted in our discussion of Fig. (2.5) in Chapter 2 that the first term in Eq. (3.1) actually appears to be linear on a semi-log plot such as the cell survival curve plot. We can therefore conclude that a linear behavior displayed on a cell survival curve means that no DNA repairs are taking place—all damage to DNA results in cell death.

But two-particle events *are* taking place in the tumor that result in double strand breaks that may be considered sublethal damage if they are relatively close within the DNA molecule. In this case, either enzymes present in the cell will have time to repair the breaks before the cell advances in the cell cycle, or else the breaks may remain unrepaired, in which case the cell will die. This situation is represented by the second bracketed term in Eq. (3.1) and is responsible for the curved shoulder that is seen in the typical cell survival curve.[3] See, for example, the curves shown in Fig. (3.1).

Of course, what is found in typical cell survival curves is that the curve starts off fairly linearly for low doses well below the crossover dose $D_{\alpha\beta}$ since the linear term is dominant for cell killing in that region. As $D_{\alpha\beta}$ is approached and crossed in the SF *vs.* D plot, the dominant cell-killing term switches and the quadratic term becomes more important, resulting in the shoulder region of the curve. (See the discussion in Chapter 2 associated with Fig. (2.5) if this discussion does not sound familiar to you.) Then, for very high doses beyond typical treatment doses, the curve is often

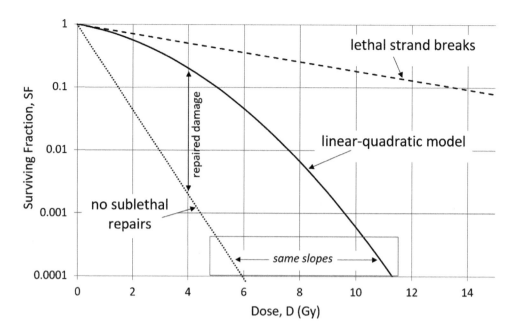

FIGURE 3.4: By drawing a linear behavior starting at the beginning point of a cell-survival curve and having the same slope as the high-dose portion of the full cell-survival curve, the amount of DNA repair can be approximated. The amount of repair is shown in this figure for the dose $D = 4.0\,Gy$.

seen to become linear again. But we have already concluded that a linear behavior on the semi-log *SF vs. D* plot represents a region in which no cellular repair is taking place—*all* strand breaks result in cell death.

Let's dig into this a bit more.

The Extent of Sublethal Repair

The solid line in Fig. (3.4) represents the standard cell survival curve resulting from the linear-quadratic model. The long-dashed line shows the linear-term contribution to the linear-quadratic result—the single-particle lethal strand breaks. (This is the same as the longer-dashed line in Fig. 2.5.)

It was stated above that, experimentally, the *SFvs.D* curve is found to become linear for very large doses. This linear behavior represents, of course, no repair of radiation damage, just as the linear behavior of the low-dose limit represents no repairs—only imminent cell death. These two linear behaviors represent two very different things, however. While the low-dose linear behavior represents no repair of cell damage resulting from single-particle interactions that produce lethal paired double-strand breaks, the high-dose linear behavior is in the region in which double strand breaks resulting from interactions with two incident beam particles dominate. This means that the high-dose linear behavior must represent no DNA repair for damage that results from two independent particle interactions—the type of damage that would be sublethal at lower doses.

The solid line in Fig. (3.4) representing the linear-quadratic model never becomes linear once the dose is larger than the crossover dose $D_{\alpha\beta}$—this is one of the disadvantages of this model. Nevertheless, we can still use the slope of the high-dose portion of the curve to give an indication of the slope of a large-dose linear behavior. This high-dose slope gives us the rate of decrease of the *Surviving Fraction* with *Dose* that we would get if there were no repairs of sublethal damage at any dose. If we draw in a linear behavior in the *SF vs. D* plot starting at the point *(D,SF) = (0,1)* having the same slope as the high-dose linear-quadratic slope, then we can see the cell-survival behavior that we would have if there were *no sublethal repairs* of the irradiated cells. (This linear behavior is shown as the dotted line in the figure.) It then follows that the difference between the full cell survival curve (solid line) and the no-repairs line (dotted line) for a given value of dose, D, must represent the amount of sublethal damage that was repaired during the delivery of that dose.

But how can we explain what is going on if the cell survival curve becomes linear for high D values, implying that all strand breaks result in cell death? Why would DNA repair cease for high doses?

There are different thoughts about how to interpret the high-dose linear behavior observed in typical (experimental) cell survival curves. One is that, for high doses, the mechanism for DNA repair simply becomes saturated and can't perform any more repairs.[7] Another way of looking at this is that the repair enzymes themselves may become unresponsive or damaged for high doses.[6] Whatever the reason, DNA repair seems to become negligible for high values of dose.

So—it appears that we have found the answer that so many researchers have been seeking: to completely kill a tumor, all we have to do is deliver a very large dose to the cancerous cells. All DNA strand breaks will then result in cell death, and the cancerous cells will all be dead. Our concerns about cancer are at an end!

Of course, things cannot be that simple. The problem is that we have no way of ensuring that all of the incident radiation hits only the cancerous cells—some of it will also hit healthy cells. This is one of the biggest issues in the treatment of cancer with radiation: you will always be causing damage to healthy tissue when you try to irradiate cancerous tissue. If you deliver a sufficiently high dose of radiation to ensure the death of *all* of the cancer cells, as discussed above, then you have not only killed the tumor, but you have also most likely killed the patient. This is, of course, not the desired result!

The Fundamental Principle of Radiation Therapy

The fundamental principle in radiation therapy can be simply stated as follows: "Kill the tumor, but spare the healthy tissue". In reality, this can never be completely achieved, but it is always the goal. As with so many things in life in general, and in medicine in particular, it all boils down to compromise.

So how can we compromise the treatment of cancer with radiation in an attempt to most closely fulfill the fundamental principle stated above? That is the subject of the upcoming sections.

3.4   THE IDEA OF CELL SURVIVAL

We have been discussing cell survival curves showing the fraction of the original cell population that survives irradiation as a function of dose. We've been implicitly taking *cell survival* to mean that, after irradiation, the cell is either alive or dead. Unfortunately, it's not quite that simple. At this point, it is important for us to understand exactly what is meant by cell *survival*. That is the purpose of this brief section.

Consider two identical cells that have been placed in two culture dishes within a nurturing environment and maintained at a temperature that is conducive to cell proliferation. The two dishes are represented by the top and bottom boxes in Fig. (3.5). After one cell cycle there are two cells present in each dish; after two cycles, there are four cells. The length of the solid vertical lines in the figure represent the duration of the cell cycle; the dotted horizontal lines connect the two daughter cells resulting from the mitosis of the parent cell. As the third cycle is being completed, producing eight cells in each dish, the second dish shown in the lower box is irradiated with $2\,Gy$ of radiation, as represented by the thick horizontal line with arrows in the bottom box; nothing is done to the cells in the top box.

The cells in the top box that were not irradiated reproduce as normal. After the five cell cycles shown, there are $2^5 = 32$ cells in the dish, as expected. All of these cells are viable—that is, they continue to reproduce as normal. Viable cells are represented by black-filled circles in the diagram.

This is to be contrasted with the cells in the lower dish in Fig. (3.5). Immediately after irradiation, we can see that, of the eight cells that were irradiated, two have died, as represented by the empty circles. But this means that six of the eight irradiated cells continue to grow and divide in the cell cycle. But, by following their progress through successive cell cycles, we can see that not all of the six remaining cells continue to reproduce as normal. Three of the six show signs of being nonviable as progeny one or more cells cycles later die.

When we speak of *cell survival* after irradiation, we man that the cell line continues to proliferate as normal for five or six cell cycles after irradiation. Cells that had sublethal damage after irradiation that was partially repaired, allowing them to progress through the cell cycle one or more times until the cell was no longer able to reproduce are counted as nonviable after irradiation and are therefore said not to have survived, even though they were able to reproduce to a limited extent after they were irradiated.

For the irradiated cells in Fig. (3.5), we can say that the surviving fraction is, at best, $SF = 3/8 = 0.38$. We say "*at best*" since only two cell cycles are shown after irradiation—we would really have to see what happens after about five cell cycles in order to make a good determination of the SF value.

3.5   THE RATIONALE FOR FRACTIONATION

We have already mentioned the idea of *fractionation*: breaking up a treatment dose into pieces, or fractions. In particular, we saw the effect of fractionation in Fig. (3.3)

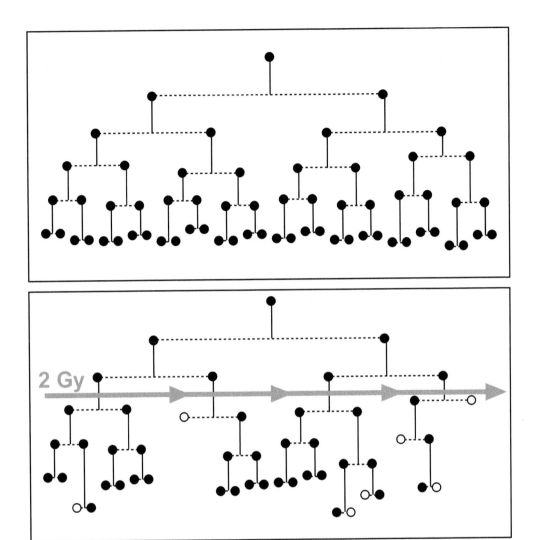

FIGURE 3.5: Two cells are placed in two culture dishes (at the top of the top and bottom boxes) and allowed to proliferate. Time progresses as we move lower in each of the two boxes. The cells in the bottom dish are irradiated with $2\,Gy$ of radiation at the end of three cell cycles. While the cells in the top dish are allowed to reproduce unaffected, it can be seen that some of the cells in the bottom dish die, as represented by the empty circles. It can be seen that all eight of the cell lines after the initial three cell cycles in the top dish continue to proliferate as normal, but only three of the eight irradiated cells in the lower dish continue to proliferate as normal. For this example, we thus have that, at best, $SF = 3/8 = 0.38$.

when we were discussing DNA repair. In that figure, we noted that it always takes more total dose to achieve the same biological end effect if we break the dose up into fractions than if we deliver all of the dose in a single fraction. As a result, fractionation may seem to be quite an inefficient means of achieving the same result: since allowing time to pass between successive fractions of the total dose also allows for DNA repair and for repopulation as cells continue to progress through the cell cycle between fractions. This means that, by the time the next fraction of dose is being administered, the viable cell population is greater than it was at the end of the previous fraction. It may therefore come as a surprise to find out that fractionation tends to be a very common practice in clinical treatment plans for radiation therapy. The purpose of this section is to convince you that this is a very reasonable thing to do.

Early and Late Responding Tissues

Of course, not all tissues respond in the same way to the same dose of radiation. We have already discussed different factors that can change the dose response: the quality of the ionizing radiation (the type of ionizing particle and its energy), the amount of oxygen in the tissue, and fractionation are just a few. Different tissues can also respond differently in terms of the amount of time between the irradiation and when the effects of the radiation are observed.

Some tissues show the effects of radiation within several days to several weeks after the start of irradiation.[1,10] Such tissues are referred to as *early responding*, or *acute responding* tissues. On the other hand, some radiation effects can appear several months to years after irradiation; these effects are referred to as *late effects*, and the tissues in which these effects appear are called *late responding* tissues. Of course, late effects are the result of early effects that were not repaired and which were progressive.[8] Examples of early reacting organs are the skin, colon, testes, and the small and large intestines, while examples of late-responding organs are the spinal cord, kidneys, lungs, and the urinary bladder.[3,11]

It has been pointed out[1] that the early/late terminology can be misleading, since tissues and organs can contain a great variety of cell types. As a result, a single tissue type can be both early and late responding, depending on the type of radiation effect being considered. Nevertheless, we will follow common usage and refer to radiation effects and the associated tissues in which those effects are observed as *early* or *late responding*.

The Crossover Dose and Cell Survival Curves for Early and Late Responding Tissues

There has been much clinical evidence that one way in which early and late responding tissues and organs differ is in their values of the crossover dose, $D_{\alpha\beta} = \alpha/\beta$: it is typically found that $D_{\alpha\beta\,(late)} < D_{\alpha\beta\,(early)}$. More specifically, crossover dose values for late responding tissues tend to vary from 1.5 Gy up to about 7 Gy, but more often tend to be in the range 3–5 Gy, while early responding tissues tend to have $D_{\alpha\beta}$ values around 10 Gy.[2] As far as the linear-quadratic model parameters are concerned, the α values do not vary much for early and late tissues, with

$0.06\,Gy^{-1} \leq \alpha_{(late)} \leq 0.23\,Gy^{-1}$, and $0.03\,Gy^{-1} \leq \alpha_{(early)} \leq 0.13\,Gy^{-1}$. These values are basically saying that the lethal single-particle double strand breaks affect early and late tissues more-or-less equally. The β values differ more radically, however: $0.02\,Gy^{-2} \leq \beta_{(late)} \leq 0.064\,Gy^{-2}$, while $0.001\,Gy^{-2} \leq \beta_{(early)} \leq 0.008\,Gy^{-2}$.[6] Standard cell survival curves for late and early responding tissues are shown in Fig. (3.6).

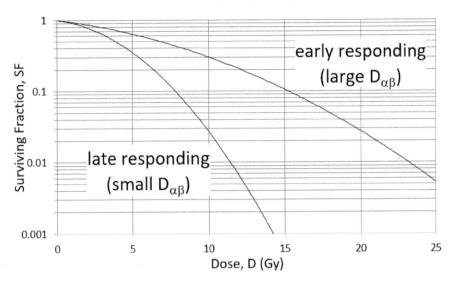

FIGURE 3.6: Typical examples of cell survival curves for early- and late-responding tissues. The linear-quadratic parameter values that were used for the plots are the following: $\alpha_{(late)} = 0.06\,Gy^{-1}$, $\beta_{(late)} = 0.03\,Gy^{-2}$, $D_{\alpha\beta\,(late)} = 2\,Gy$; $\alpha_{(early)} = 0.06\,Gy^{-1}$, $\beta_{(early)} = 0.006\,Gy^{-2}$, and $D_{\alpha\beta\,(early)} = 10\,Gy$. Note that the two α values are the same in this example, meaning that the single-particle damage is the same, so the two initial slopes are the same. This means that the only difference between the two curves shown is the contribution from the β term, which represents the repairable sublethal damage caused by two-particle double strand breaks.

Recall from our discussion of Fig. (3.4) that the initial linear portion of the cell survival curve represents a region of dominance for the lethal single-particle paired double strand breaks to the DNA. On the other hand, the curved shoulder of the cell survival curve represents sublethal damage in the form of two-particle paired double strand breaks—the more steeply sloped the curved portion, the more sublethal damage takes place at a lower dose. In light of this discussion, we can see from Fig. (3.6) that the small $D_{\alpha\beta}$, late-responding tissue has much sublethal damage waiting for repair, while the large $D_{\alpha\beta}$, early-responding tissue does not deviate much from the linear single-particle damage behavior, and therefore does not have much unrepaired sublethal damage.

Why Does Early-Responding Tissue Have a Large Value of $D_{\alpha\beta}$?

It's important to keep in mind that the quantities α and β in the linear quadratic model are simply parameters—their values are chosen so that the observed behavior of *SF vs. D* for the tissue under consideration is fit by Eq. (3.1) as closely as possible. Late-response tissue—tissue in which the radiation response cannot be seen for months or possibly years later—has an *SF vs. D* curve that rapidly bends downward with increasing dose, as shown in Fig. (3.6). This behavior is modeled most closely with the β term in Eq. (3.1) being dominant. As mentioned previously, the β term is associated with two-particle hits causing two independent strand breaks resulting in sublethal damage.

On the other hand, early-responding tissue—tissue that displays the effects of radiation exposure within days or weeks—drops down only slowly with increasing dose relative to the early-responding tissue curve. This behavior is modeled best with the α term being dominant, meaning that single particle damage resulting in paired-double strand breaks dominates the cell killing for early-responding tissues.

But what makes a tissue early or late responding? Why does it take so long for late-responding tissue to show radiation effects while early-responding tissue effects show up so quickly? The reason, of course, is the duration of the cell cycle for the tissue at hand. If the cell cycle is short—as it is for early-responding tissue—then numerous cell cycles can rapidly take place during which sublethal damage can be repaired. As a result, the primary cause of cell death is, by default, the single-particle double-strand break hits. For long cell-cycle duration, late-responding tissues, however, significant sublethal damage can remain unrepaired over time, resulting in cell death dominated by two-hit, two particle double strand breaks.

The cross over dose, $D_{\alpha\beta} = \alpha/\beta$, gives an indication of the dose at which the dominant mode of cell killing switches from single-particle double strand breaks (α) to double strand breaks caused by two incident particles (β). (See the dashed line showing the α-behavior corresponding to lethal strand breaks in Fig. 3.4.) Since sublethal damage in early-responding tissue can be readily repaired, the single-hit double-strand break α-behavior is what remains for the dominant cell killing modality. This means that the cell-survival curve for early responding tissue will tend to follow the linear α-behavior until higher doses, at which point the large amount of sublethal damage becomes too great to be repaired and the β term starts becoming dominant.

It should therefore make sense that the value of $D_{\alpha\beta}$ for early-responding tissue is large compared to that for late-responding tissue.

Bringing Tumors into the Discussion

We have already stated that the time delay between the irradiation and observing the effects of the radiation on tissue is a reflection of the time interval required for the cell population to be replaced by apoptosis (cell death) and cell regeneration. More rapidly regenerating cells will have a quicker turn-over rate, and therefore will show damage from radiation more quickly; these are cells associated with early-responding tissues. On the other hand, late-responding tissues have cells that have very low regeneration rates, and take a long time for the cell population to be replaced.

Examples of tissues or organs that have a slow turn-over rate tend to be well-differentiated, such as the spinal cord, the brain, kidneys, the bowel and the lungs. Tissues and organs with a fast turn-over rate—that is, tissues consisting of rapidly preproducing cells—tend to be more undifferentiated. For example, the skin, mucous membranes, and the bone marrow.[12]

But we have talked previously about structures with a rapidly reproducing cell population—these structures were called *tumors*, and the rapid, uncontrolled reproduction of cells is what characterized cancerous cells. This means that tumor cells are expected to have relatively large $D_{\alpha\beta}$ values like early responding tissues. Indeed, growing tumors have a range of $D_{\alpha\beta}$ values varying from about 5 Gy up to about 30 Gy, although they more typically vary from 10 to 20 Gy.[2] Everything said about early responding tissues in our previous discussion can therefore also generally be applied to typical tumors. (This is, of course, not strictly true, however. For example, prostate cancer has a $D_{\alpha\beta}$ value of about 1.1 Gy.[13])

Healthy organs must be spared when a nearby tumor is being irradiated. We thus refer to the tissue in these well-differentiated organs as *dose-limiting tissue*. Since healthy, dose-limiting tissue tends to be late-responding tissue with a small $D_{\alpha\beta}$ value, while most tumors tend to be tissues with relatively large $D_{\alpha\beta}$ values, it is reasonable for us to now shift our discussion from one involving *late* and *early* responding tissue, to one involving *healthy, dose-limiting tissue* and *tumors*.

The Effects of Fractionation

As discussed previously, *fractionation* means breaking up the dose to tissue into pieces, or fractions. It was pointed out in the discussion associated with Fig. (3.3) that, when the dose is fractionated, the total dose required to achieve the same biological end effect must increase; it was argued that this was due to the repair of sublethal damage during the interval between successive fractions.

We are now led to an important conclusion—namely, that fractionation will help more healthy (late-responding) tissue survive than cancerous (early-responding) tissue. Fractionation spares all types of tissue—that is, it reduces the killing of cells in all types of tissue. But it tends to spare healthy tissue more than tissue in tumors. This is, of course, because there is more sublethal damage that can be repaired during the time between fractions in late-responding tissue than there is in early-responding tissue.

We are now at the crux of the matter. Figure (3.7) shows a very important distinction between the effects of fractionation on healthy tissue and on typical malignant (growing) tumors. The two curves are called *isoeffect curves*. Each isoeffect curve shows how the total dose to the tissue must change in order to achieve the same biological end effect as the number of fractions is increased in a fractionated treatment plan. The end effects for the two curves need not be the same. For example, the end effect for the healthy tissue may be maintaining a dose to the tissue that is a fixed number of grays below the limiting-dose value for sparing the tissue, while the end effect for the tumor may be a tight control on the growth of the tumor.[12]

The behavior suggested by Fig. (3.7) explains why fractionation is often a critical means of approaching treatment planning for cancer—namely, that for a suitably large number of fractions, the healthy tissue can be spared while still getting enough dose to the tumor to achieve the desired end effect. This is a result of the fact that the slopes of the isoeffect curves for healthy (late) tissues tend to be steeper than the isoeffect curve slopes for the cancerous (early) tissue. This means that, using the end effects stated above, as the number of fractions increases, the dose needed to control the tumor dose not increase by much, but the limiting dose for sparing the healthy

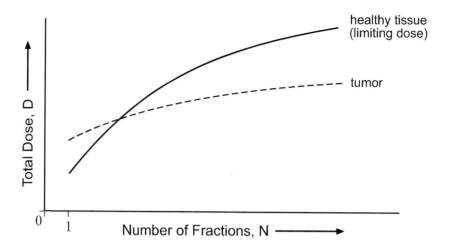

FIGURE 3.7: General behavior of isoeffect curves as the number of fractions is increased for tumors (early responding, high $D_{\alpha\beta}$) and healthy, dose-limiting tissues (late responding, low $D_{\alpha\beta}$).

tissue gets much higher, meaning that we can more readily control the tumor growth while not getting close to the limiting dose to the healthy tissue. In other words, achieving the goals becomes easier. Let's examine these ideas a little more closely.

Breast Cancer: An Example in Fractionation

Let's consider as an example the case of breast cancer. The radiation oncologist has prescribed a treatment regime in which a total of $N = 25$ fractions of equal dose are to be administered to the whole breast—healthy tissue and cancerous tissue alike. The cell survival curves for both the healthy breast tissue (solid lines) and the cancerous tissue (dashed lines) are shown in Fig. (3.8). (Values for the crossover dose $D_{\alpha\beta}$ are from Joiner and van der Kogel.[14] The value of the linear-quadratic parameter α follows Hall.[3])

As always in radiation therapy, we wish to spare the healthy tissue while treating the tumor. For the sake of this discussion only, let's imagine the *very hypothetical* situation in which the healthy breast tissue can withstand a reduction in surviving fraction (SF) down to a value of 0.001 and still be able to recover fully. Thus, we assume that the healthy breast tissue can withstand a biological end effect of $SF = 0.001$ and still be spared. (*We make this assumption purely for instructional purposes—these are not clinical numbers.*) Let's see what this says about the dose to the tumor in the case of a single treatment dose ($N = 1$) and the fractionated treatment plan prescribed by the oncologist ($N = 25$).

Let's first consider the case of unfractionated treatment ($N = 1$). Examination of Fig. (3.8) shows that, for $SF = 0.001$, the healthy breast tissue can withstand a dose of up to $5.9\,Gy$. At this dose value, the cancerous tissue in the breast will have an SF value of 0.018.

Now let's look at the curves for the prescribed fractionation ($N = 25$). For the minimum SF value of 0.001 for sparing the healthy tissue, a dose of $17\,Gy$ can be

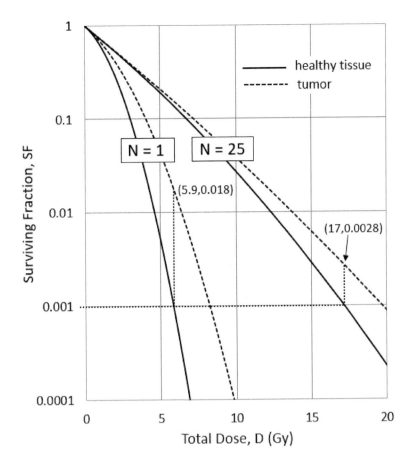

FIGURE 3.8: Cell survival curves for healthy breast tissue (solid lines) and for cancerous breast tissue (dashed lines) for unfractionated ($N = 1$) and fractionated ($N = 25$) treatments. Linear-quadratic parameter values used: $\alpha_{healthy} = 0.3\,Gy^{-1}$, $D_{\alpha\beta\,(healthy)} = 2\,Gy$; $\alpha_{tumor} = 0.3\,Gy^{-1}$, $D_{\alpha\beta\,(tumor)} = 4.6\,Gy$.

administered to the breast. For this dose value, the resulting surviving fraction of cancerous tissue cells is 0.0028.

You should now be able to appreciate the value of fractionation: for the same biological end effect—sparing the healthy breast tissue—the surviving fraction of cancer cells has decreased from 0.018 for a single fraction, to 0.0028 for 25 fractions. This is a decrease by a factor of about 6.4 in the surviving fraction of cancerous cells because of the fractionated administration of radiation. Clearly, a fractionated treatment plan is a good option as long as the crossover dose for the cancerous tissue is significantly greater than that for the healthy tissue being spared.

A few comments are now in order.

First: The values of $D_{\alpha\beta}$ for the healthy and cancerous breast tissues used in Fig. (3.8) are $2\,Gy$ and $4.6\,Gy$, respectively.[14] These values are not significantly different, and yet there was still a clear advantage for using a fractionated treatment plan. Remember that the value of the crossover dose for cancerous tumors is typically around $10\,Gy$—if cancerous breast tissue had this more typical value of $D_{\alpha\beta}$ the effect of fractionation would have been even more dramatic.

Second comment: In treatment plans involving fractionation, the tumor and the healthy tissue do not receive the same dose. Rather, the beam of incident radiation is shaped so that it mimics the shape of the tumor. A treatment plan involving *intensity-modulated radiation therapy (IMRT)* will accomplish this. (IMRT will be discussed in Part III of this book.) If this is the case, then the radiation to the healthy tissue to be spared will be just a fraction of the dose delivered to the tumor. This will result in an even greater benefit from the use of fractionation.

Third comment: The formalism that we have used here—based on the linear quadratic model—is an extremely simplistic one. Clinical treatment plans use very complicated treatment-planning software packages to help plan precisely how the treatment of each patient should proceed. The purpose of our simplistic approach has simply been to help motivate the use of fractionation.

Lastly, if the breast cancer being treated were a localized tumor in the breast, then the treatment plan would not just be the whole-breast exposure to dose as was discussed in this example. Typically, extra dose would be administered to the localized region around the tumor itself—a so-called *boost* in dose to the tumor.

3.6   THE FIVE RS OF RADIOTHERAPY

In 1975, Withers published an article titled *The Four R's of Radiotherapy*.[7] The "Four R's" listed were *repair, reoxygenation, redistribution,* and *regeneration*. Then in 1989, Steel *et al.* published an article titled "The 5Rs of Radiobiology", in which they criticized Withers' use of an "ungrammatical apostrophe", and argued that *radiosensitivity* should be added to the list.[15] In what follows, we will discuss the five *Rs (no apostrophe)* of radiotherapy.

Repair We have already extensively discussed the importance of sublethal dose repair, especially for late-responding tissue. This repair is associated with the quadratic (β) term in the linear quadratic model and plays a major role in the advantage of fractionation for many cancer treatment plans.

Reoxygenation The fact that an oxic environment increases the likelihood of unrepairable DNA damage during radiation treatment was also discussed earlier in this chapter. This does not serve as an advantage to healthy, vital organs, which tend to have a good blood flow and therefore remain well oxygenated. Tumors, on the other hand, tend not to be as well oxygenated. Therefore, when they are irradiated, it tends to be the cells near a source blood flow within the tumor that are killed, leaving behind the more radioresistant hypoxic cells.[1] The idea of reoxygenation is that, given appropriate time between fractions in a fractionated treatment plan, oxygen can diffuse to otherwise hypoxic regions in the tumor, thereby rendering the cells more radiosensitive and easier to kill.[3]

Redistribution The various phases of the cell cycle are not equally radiosensitive. We have already discussed the fact that the growth phases are most susceptible to radiation damage, while the late S phase is least susceptible to damage. (See Fig. 3.2.) *Redistribution* refers to that fact that, after irradiation, those cells in the G phases were more selectively killed, leaving behind a semi-synchronized cell population in which a larger-than-normal fraction of the cell population is in the S phase. A delay between fractions then allows the tumor cells to progress through the cell cycle. They will then redistribute themselves among the various phases, thereby repopulating the more radiosensitive G phases.[7]

Regeneration Of course, cells in the tissues being irradiated can still progress through the cell cycle as the radiation treatment and the breaks between fractions proceed. This means that the change in the cell population during irradiation can have a positive contribution due to cell regeneration as well as a negative contribution as the cells are killed by the incident radiation. The repopulation of tumor cells can be significant if the fractionated treatment plan extends for weeks.[4] There is also evidence that the repopulation of tumor cells can actually accelerate if the treatment extends beyond about 5 weeks after the initial irradiation.[16,17] Thus, for extended treatment plans, regeneration may be a significant effect.

Radiosensitivity The term *radiosensitivity* can be interpreted in different ways.[15] We shall use the term to mean the initial slope of the cell survival curve which, as discussed previously, represents the rate of cell death due to lethal single-particle double strand breaks caused by the incident radiation. Radiosensitivity can vary not only from one tissue type to another but also, for a given tissue type, from one individual to another.[4] Everything that we have discussed associated with fractionated treatment hinges on the radiosensitivity of the tissues involved. The greater the radiosensitivity, the greater the effects of the treatment. The variations in radiosensitivity can be a result of the integrity of the DNA repair mechanisms within the cells, or even the effectiveness of the cyclins that regulate the progression of the cells through the cell cycle[4] (see Chapter 1).

3.7   THE LINEAR-QUADRATIC MODEL AND FRACTIONATION

We will now delve a bit further into the effects of fractionation on the cell survival curves, and, in the process, deepen our understanding of the behavior of the curves as the number of fractions is increased for late- (healthy) and early-responding (cancerous) tissues. We will exploit the linear-quadratic model formalism that we developed in Chapter 2 to help us understand the effects of fractionation.

Recall that the surviving fraction, SF, of a given cell population is given as a function of dose, D, according to

$$SF = e^{-\alpha D - \beta D^2} . \tag{3.2}$$

Now, let's consider the case of fractionation, in which a total dose D is divided up into N equal fractions, $d = D/N$. If sufficient time is allowed between successive fractions for reoxygenation of the tumor and a redistribution of the tumor cells among the phases of the cell cycle to take place, then the effects of the successive fractions should be basically the same. This means that we can treat each of the dose fractions as being described by the same function, in analogy with Eq. (3.2):

$$sf = e^{-\alpha d - \beta d^2} ,\tag{3.3}$$

where we have used sf to represent the surviving fraction contribution of a single fraction of dose d. It then follows that the surviving fraction of the cell population after all N fractions have been administered is given by

$$SF = (sf)^N = \left[e^{-\alpha d - \beta d^2} \right]^N .\tag{3.4}$$

Using the definition of d then allows us to rewrite Eq. (3.4) in the form

$$SF = e^{-\alpha D - \beta \frac{D^2}{N}} .\tag{3.5}$$

It is this equation that was used to plot the curves in Fig. (3.8). We note that only the β term is affected by the number of fractions, N. This explains why late-responding tissue, whose behavior tends to be dominated by two-particle, two-hit sublethal strand breaks as characterized by β, is most affected by increasing values of N in fractionation, as indicated in Figure (3.7).

Let's take a look at some more curves plotted using Eq. (3.5).

An Example: Treating a Lung Tumor While Sparing the Spinal Cord

Figure (3.9) shows cell survival curves for healthy tissue and for cancerous tissue for three values of the number of fractions, N: $N = 1$, 2, and 10. The parameter values α and $D_{\alpha\beta}$ (and, hence, β) were chosen under a scenario in which a cancerous lung tumor is to be irradiated, but close attention has to be paid to the nearby spinal cord, which has to be spared. The α and $D_{\alpha\beta}$ values used for the healthy tissue therefore correspond to the spinal cord, and those for the tumor correspond to lung tumor values. The value of $D_{\alpha\beta}$ for the spinal cord was obtained from Schultheiss[18] and that for the cancerous lung tissue was obtained from Karagounis et al.[19] The value $\alpha = 0.3\,Gy^{-1}$ is a common average value suggested by Hall[3] in lieu of a documented better value.

We first note that, as expected, the small value of $D_{\alpha\beta}$ for the spinal cord and the corresponding large value of β cause the cell survival curves for the spinal cord to slope down steeply, and to be capable of quite a bit of repair of sublethal DNA damage as a result of fractionation. Note the large change in the spinal cord curves as N changes from 2 to 10. On the other hand, the large value of the crossover dose for the cancerous lung tissue and its relatively small value of β ensure that not much DNA repair will be taking place since the damage is dominated by the single-particle damage represented by the linear (α) term in Eq. (3.5).

Further inspection of Fig. (3.9) shows that it also contains a dotted line not corresponding to a cell survival curve. This is what the plot of a cell survival curve would look like if we were to set $\beta = 0$ in Eq. (3.5). In other words, this is what a cell survival curve would look like if there were only lethal single-particle double strand

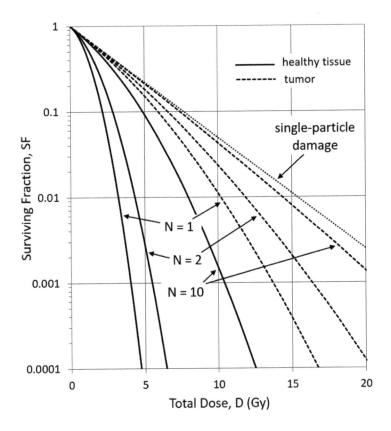

FIGURE 3.9: Cell survival curves for various total number of fractions, N. The linear-quadratic parameter values used correspond to the values for the spinal cord (*healthy tissue*) and cancerous lung tissue (tumor): $\alpha_{spinal\,cord} = 0.3\,Gy^{-1}$, $\beta_{spinal\,cord} = 0.35\,Gy^{-2}$, $D_{\alpha\beta\,(spinal\,cord)} = 0.87\,Gy$; $\alpha_{lung} = 0.3\,Gy^{-1}$, $\beta_{lung} = 0.015\,Gy^{-2}$, $D_{\alpha\beta\,(lung)} = 20\,Gy$. The dotted line shows the behavior of a cell survival curve with only lethal single-particle double strand break damage.

breaks produced by the radiation. This means that there is no sublethal damage repair at all. Note that the high-$D_{\alpha\beta}$ lung cancer curves in Fig. (3.9) approach the single-particle damage dotted line as N increases. This makes sense since the tumor tissue does not sustain much sublethal damage. As a result, after each fraction, there is less and less sublethal damage to repair, meaning that the lethal single-particle damage becomes more and more dominant. This can also be seen mathematically in Eq. (3.5): as N increases, its presence in the denominator of the β term makes that term smaller, resulting in a behavior that is more dominated by the single-particle lethal-damage term containing α.

3.8 RADIATION THERAPY

The use of radiation to treat cancer can be broadly divided into two categories: external beam radiotherapy and brachytherapy. Both of these forms of radiation therapy will be discussed in depth in Part III of this text. The topics discussed in this chapter have been associated with radiotherapy, typically with x-rays and gamma-rays. In particular, much discussion in this chapter revolved around the idea of fractionation—breaking the treatment dose up into fractions with some amount of delay time between fractions.

As far as sparing the healthy tissue is concerned, the point of fractionation is to allow for repair of sublethal dose, especially in late-reaction tissues which tend to be the healthy tissue in the vicinity of the tumor being treated. In terms of killing the tumor cells, fractionation allows for the reoxygenation of the otherwise hypoxic tumor cells after irradiation, as well as for the redistribution of cells among the phases of the cell cycle. Both of these consequences of fractionation improve the ability for the radiation to kill tumor cells.

We have seen that increasing the number of fractions, N, tends to increase the sparing effect of the healthy tissue. So, are real treatment plans being developed in the cancer-treatment clinics that involve larger and larger numbers of fractions with sufficient time between each fraction for reoxygenation and redistribution of the tumor cells?

The answer is *no*. There are really two parts to the reason for this. The first part is that, while increasing the total time for the treatment plan has little impact on late effects, it has a detrimental effect on the treatment of early responding tumors due to regeneration, as discussed previously.[3] The second part is that there is a minimum dose per fraction, called the *flexure dose*, d_f, below which there is no change in the biological endpoint.[20,2] In other words, any reduction in the dose-per-fraction d below d_f provides no additional benefit from fractionation. The combination of these two reasons tells us that there is no point in going crazy with the number of fractions beyond certain limits.

As far as the cell survival curves are concerned, the flexure dose can be thought of as that (low) dose where the cell survival curve leaves the linear behavior representing the single-particle lethal component of the dose. For example, inspection of the cell survival curve shown in Fig. (2.5) shows that $d_f \cong 0.8\,Gy = 0.13\,D_{\alpha\beta}$. The value of the flexure dose varies from tissue to tissue, but its value tends to lie approximately in the range $0.05\,D_{\alpha\beta} \leq d_f \leq 0.15\,D_{\alpha\beta}$.[21]

The typical treatment of cancer by fractionated radiotherapy usually means daily doses per fraction of $1.8 \leq d \leq 2.0\,Gy$ delivered 5 days per week.[12] This approach does not work for all tumors, however, and there are alternate approaches that may be overtaking the standard treatment mentioned above. For example, in *hyperfractionation*, smaller values of d are used with more frequent administrations, while in *hypofractionation*, fewer fractions but larger doses per fraction are used,[1] which can be advantageous for tumors having small values of $D_{\alpha\beta}$ such as prostate cancer[14].

Moving Forward

This concludes our discussion of radiobiology. The purpose of this discussion was to show how energy deposited into tissue by incident radiation particles can result in damage to the DNA in the tissue cells and how the characteristics of this damage can be exploited to produce treatment plans to effectively treat cancerous tumors. We will now move on to Part II of this book, which delves into the physics behind how energy gets deposited into the tissue by the incident radiation particles. An understanding of how radiation particles deposit energy will then prepare us for Part III, which discusses imaging modalities and finally some of the fundamental procedures in the practice of radiation therapy for cancer.

3.9 QUESTIONS, EXERCISES, & PROBLEMS

3-1. It is stated in this chapter that it is unfortunate that healthy tissue is kept well oxygenated by a good blood flow, while the typically poor flow of blood through tumors tends to keep them in a hypoxic state. Explain what is so unfortunate about this situation.

3-2. At the end of the section on the sensitivity of the various phases of the cell cycle to ionizing radiation, it is stated that, " ...it follows that the cell population will eventually return to its original state of asynchronicity, thereby becoming overall more susceptible to the killing effects of ionizing radiation than it was immediately after irradiation". Explain why returning to its original asynchronous state will make the cell population more susceptible to radiation damage than it was immediately after irradiation ceased.

3-3. It was stated in the text that a linear portion of the cell survival curve corresponds to a region in which DNA repair is negligible. There are two such linear—or nearly linear—regions: one is at the beginning of the curve for very low doses, and the other is at the other end of the curve for very high doses. If both of these portions of the curve represent regions of very little, if any, DNA repair, why are the corresponding rates of change in surviving fraction with dose—that is, the slopes of the tangent lines at the two ends of the curve—so different?

3-4. The chapter contains the following statement toward the end of the discussion about the treatment of breast cancer and Fig. (3.8): "Clearly, a fractionated treatment plan is a good option as long as the crossover dose for the cancerous tissue is significantly greater than that for the healthy tissue being spared". Explain in your own words why this condition on the values of $D_{\alpha\beta}$ must be true in order for fractionation to be a good option for a treatment plan.

3-5. In the second comment after the discussion of the breast cancer example, it is stated that the use of an IMRT treatment plan will result in an even greater benefit from fractionation. Clearly explain why.

3-6. Explain how the *changes* in the curves for the healthy tissue and the cancerous tumor as N increases from 1 to 10 in Fig. (3.9) are related to the healthy tissue and tumor curves in Fig. (3.7).

3-7. List the "five Rs" of radiotherapy and, in your own words, state their significance as far as fractionated radiotherapy is concerned.

3-8. Fill in the steps to show how Eq. (3.5) follows from Eq. (3.4).

3-9. Research the term *hyperfractionation*. What does it mean? What are its advantages and disadvantages as far as radiation treatment of cancer is concerned? Cite a particular case from your research in which a hyperfractionated treatment plan resulted in positive results for the patient. As always, be sure to cite your references.

(And, as always, remember that *Wikipedia* is not an acceptable professional reference.)

3-10. Consider the following two quotes:

Quote 1: (from the Journal of the American Medical Association–Oncology, October 2015)[22]

> "Hypofractionation not only improves convenience but also may reduce acute pain, fatigue, and the extent to which patients are bothered by dermatitis in patients with breast cancer undergoing whole-breast radiotherapy."

Quote 2: (from a press release by the American Society of Radiation Oncology (ASTRO) for its 2016 annual meeting summarizing work done by A. Widmark *et al.* involving 1200 men with prostate cancer)[23]

> "Extremely hypofractionated radiation therapy shows promising toxicity results for intermediate risk prostate cancer patients."

(a) Research the term *hypofractionation*. What does it mean? What are its advantages and disadvantages as far as radiation treatment of cancer is concerned?

(b) The value of $D_{\alpha\beta}$ for prostate cancer is $1.1\,Gy$.[14] Use the discussions in this chapter to explain why it would be expected to get a more positive result for a hypofractionated treatment of prostate cancer over the standard fractionated treatment schedule.

As always, be sure to cite your references. (And, as always, remember that *Wikipedia* is not an acceptable professional reference.)

3.10   REFERENCES

1. Perez C, Brady L, Halperin E, Schmidt-Ullrich R. *Principloes and Practice of Radiation Oncology.* Philadelphia: Lippincott Williams & Wilkins; 2004.
2. Alpen E. *Radiation Biophysics.* 2nd ed. San Diego:Academic Press; 1998.
3. Hall EJ, Giaccia AJ. *Radiobiology for the Radiologist.* Philadelphia: Lippincott Williams & Wilkins; 2006.
4. Bomford CK, Kunkler IH. *Walter and Miller's Textbook of Radiotherapy: Radiation Physics, Therapy and Oncology.* 6th ed. Edinburgh: Churchill Livingstone; 2003.
5. Withers HR, Peters LJ. Biological aspects of radiation therapy. In: Fletcher GH, ed. *Textbook of Radiotherapy.* 3rd ed. Philadelphia: Lea & Febiger; 1980.
6. Tubiana M, Dutriex J, Wambersie A. *Introduction to Radiobiology.* London: Taylor & Francis; 1990.
7. Withers HR. The Four R's of Radiotherapy. *Advances in Radiation Biology.* 1975;5:241-271.
8. Washington C, Leaver D. *Principles and Practice of Radiation Therapy.* 3rd ed. St. Louis:Mosby; 2010.
9. Barendsen GW. Responses of cultured cells, tumours and normal tissues to radiations of different linear energy transfer. *Curr Topics Radiat Res Q.* 1968;4:293-356.
10. Thames HD, Withers HR, Peters LJ, and Fletcher GH. Changes in Early and Late Radiation Responses with Altered Dose Fractionation: Implications for Dose-Survival Relationships. *Int. J. Radiation Oncology Biol. Phys.* 1982;8:219-226.
11. Hobbie RK. *Intermediate Physics for Medicine and Biology.* 3rd ed. New York: Spring-Verlag; 2001.
12. Shrieve DC, Loeffler JS. *Human Radiation Injury.* Philadelphia: Lippincott Williams & Wilkins; 2011.
13. Bentzen SM, Ritter MA. The alpha/beta ratio for prostate cancer: what is it, really? *Radiother Oncol.* 2005;76:1-3.
14. Joiner MC, van der Kogel AJ, eds. *Basic Clinical Radiobiology.* 5th ed. Boca Raton, FL: CRC Press, Taylor & Francis Group; 2019.
15. Steel GG, McMillan TJ, Peacock JH. The 5Rs of Radiobiology. *International Journal of Radiation Biology.* 1989;56(6):1045-1048.

16. Withers HR, Taylor JM, Maciejewski B. The hazard of accelerated tumor clonogen repopulation during radiotherapy. *Acta Oncol.* 1988;27(2):131-146.
17. Maciejewski B, Majewski S. Dose fractionation and tumour repopulation in radiotherapy for bladder cancer. *Radiother. Oncol.* 1991;21(3):163-170.
18. Schultheiss TE. The Radiation Dose-Response of the Human Spinal Cord. *International Journal of Radiation Oncology Biology/Physics.* 2008;71(5):1455-1459.
19. Karagounis IV, Skourti EK, Liousia MV, Koukourakis MI. Assessment of Radiobiological α/β Ratio in Lung Cancer and Fibroblast Cell Lines Using Viability Assays. *Vivo.* Mar-Apr 2017;31(2):175-179.
20. Withers HR. Response of Tissues to Multiple Small Dose Fractions. *Radiat. Res.* 1977;71:24-33.
21. Tucker SL, Thames HD Jr. Flexure dose: the low-dose limit of effective fractionation. *Int J Radiat Oncol Biol Phys.* 1983;9(9):1373-1383.
22. Jagsi R, Griffith KA, Boike TP, et al. Differences in the Acute Toxic Effects of Breast Radiotherapy by Fractionation Schedule: Comparative Analysis of Physician-Assessed and Patient-Reported Outcomes in a Large Multicenter Cohort. *JAMA Oncol.* 2015;1(7):918-930. doi:10.1001/jamaoncol.2015.2590
23. American Society for Radiation Oncology. https://www.astro.org/News-and-Publications/News-and-Media-Center /News-Releases/2016/Extremely-hypofractionated-radiation-therapy- shows-promising-toxicity-results-for-intermediate-risk-prostate- cancer-patients/. Accessed March 21, 2017.

II

Foundation: Modern Physics Fundamentals

Atomic Physics I: Hydrogenic Atoms

CONTENTS

Atoms are the basic building blocks of matter. In radiation oncology, we are interested in the interactions between incident radiation and matter found in the body—namely tissue. By *radiation* we mean uncharged particles such as photons (bundles of light energy) or neutrons, and charged particles such as electrons, protons, or heavier nuclei. (In radiation therapy, "heavier nuclei" typically means carbon nuclei.) We can therefore conclude that, in radiation oncology, we are interested in the interactions between particles and atoms. In order to understand these interactions, and therefore understand how to exploit the characteristics of these interactions in coming up with imaging and treatment modalities for cancer patients, we must first understand the structure and properties of atoms.

In this chapter we will study the structure of atoms containing only a nucleus and a single electron—so-called *hydrogenic atoms*. Once we understand the structure of these simplest of atoms, we will then be able to move on into the next chapter where we will be introduced to the more complicated—but more relevant for imaging and treatment—discussion of multielectron atoms.

4.1 ATOMS—THE BASICS

An *atom* consists of a *nucleus* surrounded by an *electron cloud*. Atoms have diameters on the order of 10^{-10} m (called one *angstrom*, 1 Å), while nuclei have diameters on the order of 10^{-15} m (called one fermi, 1 F). The nucleus is composed of *protons* and *neutrons*, which are collectively referred to as *nucleons*. Since protons are positively charged and electrons are negatively charged, we see that the negatively charged

DOI: 10.1201/9781003477457-4

electrons in the electron cloud are held in the region around the positively charged nucleus by the attractive electrical force—the *Coulomb force*. The charge magnitudes (that is, the absolute value of the charges) of the electron and proton are equal and are each denoted e:

$$e = 1.602\,176\,487 \times 10^{-19}\,\text{C}. \qquad (\text{C} = \text{Coulombs}) \qquad (4.1)$$

A proton has the charge $+e$, and an electron has the charge $-e$. A neutron contains both positive and negative charge, but has zero net charge.

When we refer to an *atom*, we will typically mean a neutral (zero net charge) system consisting of a single nucleus and a bound cloud of electrons. That is, in what we will call an atom, the number of protons in the nucleus will typically equal the number of electron charges in the electron cloud surrounding the nucleus. A system consisting of a single nucleus and a bound cloud of electrons that has a non-zero net charge will be called an *ion*. An ion may be positively or negatively charged, meaning that the corresponding atom has lost or gained one or more electrons, respectively. (An exception to this nomenclature is the term "hydrogenic atom", which will be explained in the next section.) An atom with all of its electrons removed will be called a *bare nucleus*, or simply a *nucleus*.

The Atomic Number Defines the Element

An *element* is a substance that contains only one kind of atom. An atom, and therefore an element, can be characterized by the number of protons in its nucleus. This characteristic number is called the *atomic number* and is denoted Z. The value of the atomic number for various elements can typically be found in the top or upper-left corner of the box corresponding to the element shown in the periodic table of the elements. For example, for hydrogen (H), $Z_H = 1$; for helium (He), $Z_{He} = 2$; while for carbon (C), $Z_C = 6$.

In Chapter 6 we will be discussing nuclear physics. Within that discussion, we will refer to the atomic number of an *electron*. In this case, we will treat the atomic number Z as meaning the number of *proton charges* instead of the number of protons. Since the electron charge is negative the proton charge, we will use $Z = -1$ for an electron.

The *neutron number*, N, is the number of neutrons in the nucleus, and the *mass number*, A, is the number of neutrons plus the number of protons in the nucleus. Therefore,

$$A = Z + N. \qquad (4.2)$$

Note that the mass number can also be thought of as the number of nucleons in the nucleus.

Isotopes

Atoms of the same element need not all be identical. As mentioned previously, an atom is associated with a particular element by virtue of the number of protons in its nucleus—that is, by its atomic number, Z. It then follows that atoms of the same element may have different numbers of neutrons in their nuclei, despite the fact that they must have the same number of protons. Atoms of a particular element that have different numbers of neutrons are called *isotopes* of that element.

Because of the existence of different isotopes of the same element, it is important to have a notation that can unambiguously denote a particular isotope. Such a notation is called *isotopic notation* and is given by ^{A}X, where A is the mass number of the isotope and X is a generic letter representing the chemical symbol for that element, as given in the periodic table: H for hydrogen, He for helium, *etc.* Note that the chemical symbol specifies the element, which in turn specifies the value of the atomic number, Z. Therefore, given the isotopic notation for an isotope, we can determine the corresponding values of A, Z, and N. It is also possible to express the isotopic notation in the form X–A, so that ^{4}He, representing that isotope of helium that contains four nucleons, means the same thing as He–4, for example. If we wish to be completely explicit about the mass number as well as the atomic number, then we can use *full isotopic notation* to specify the isotope: $^{A}_{Z}X$. For example, the carbon isotope C–12 can more explicitly be specified as $^{12}_{6}$C.

4.2 SOME NOTES ABOUT HYDROGEN

The adult human body is on average about 50% water by mass (somewhat more for males, and slightly less for females). Hydrogen comprises about 67% of a water molecule by the number of atoms, but only about 11% by mass. The remaining 89% of the mass of water is, of course, in oxygen. It should therefore come as no surprise that, out of all of the elements, oxygen accounts for most of the mass of the average human body, while hydrogen accounts for the greatest fraction of the number of atoms in the body.

Hydrogen is the Simplest Element

Hydrogen is the most abundant element in the universe. It is also the simplest atom in the universe since it consists of a very small and dense positive charge—the nucleus—surrounded by the electron cloud associated with a single electron. (We will discuss the quantum mechanical probability distribution of the electron in an atom, or the *electron cloud*, later in this chapter.) Therefore, studying the basic structure of hydrogen amounts to studying what is called the *two-body problem* in physics: a system consisting of two mutually interacting particles. In the case of the hydrogen atom, the interaction between the two particles (the nucleus and the electron) is the attractive Coulomb interaction—the electrical force between the two charged particles. We can readily solve the equations describing such a two-particle system, which means that we understand the properties of the hydrogen atom very well.

The Three-body Problem is Unsolvable

It is interesting to note that, if we were to add just one more particle to a two-particle system to produce a system of three mutually interacting particles, then the equations cannot in general be solved.[1] This means that taking one step across the periodic table and going from hydrogen to helium results in going from a two-particle system whose equations can be solved exactly (hydrogen) to a three-particle system whose equations can only be solved given certain special conditions or approximations (helium). Matters only get worse as we work our way down the periodic table to lithium, beryllium, *etc*. This shows us the fundamental and theoretical importance of the hydrogen atom: it is the only atom whose structure is completely understood analytically (that is, using equations). Every other atom in the periodic table is understood in terms of our understanding of the hydrogen atom.

Hydrogenic Atoms

Of course, in the world of atomic physics, hydrogen is not the only two-particle system around. If we take a helium atom, for example, and remove one of its two electrons, then we are left with a nucleus of charge $+2e$ (since there are two protons in the nucleus of a helium atom, each having a charge of $+e$) and one electron orbiting the nucleus. This is a positively charged ion that is also a two-particle system, just like hydrogen. Because of this, we could refer to this ion as *hydrogen-like helium*, or we could say that it is a *hydrogenic ion* or a *hydrogenic atom*.

We will define a *hydrogenic atom* to be a two-particle system consisting of a positively charged nucleus having atomic number Z and one electron. For any value of $Z > 1$ we can see that, according to our earlier definition of *atom*, this is not really an atom, but rather a positive ion. But we will relax our definition of an *atom* in this case to allow us to speak of *hydrogenic atoms*, which include the (neutral) hydrogen atom as well as (positively charged) ions that have only one electron remaining. Regardless, hydrogenic atoms are two-particle systems whose equations of motion can be solved.

Isotopes of Hydrogen

Since there is only one proton in the nucleus of a hydrogen atom, we must have that the atomic number for hydrogen is equal to 1: $Z_H = 1$. There are three important isotopes of hydrogen: ^{1}H, ^{2}H, and ^{3}H. Since hydrogen is an element of such fundamental importance, these three isotopes are given special names. The first, ^{1}H, is simply referred to as *hydrogen*, although officially, all three isotopes are of course isotopes of hydrogen. The second, ^{2}H, is called *deuterium*. Hydrogen and deuterium occur naturally on Earth. The third isotope, ^{3}H, called *tritium*, is a radioactive isotope that undergoes radioactive decay into an isotope of helium, ^{3}He, and so is not found naturally occurring on Earth. (We'll learn about radioactive decay in our study of nuclear physics in Chapter 7 of this book.) These three isotopes of hydrogen are sometimes written in the special forms ^{1}H, ^{2}D, and ^{3}T. Since the neutron number, N, is equal to $A - Z$, it follows that hydrogen has $1 - 1 = 0$ neutrons in its nucleus, deuterium has $2 - 1 = 1$ neutron, and tritium has $3 - 1 = 2$ neutrons in its nucleus.

4.3 ATOMIC MASSES

The mass of an atom is cleverly called the *atomic mass*. More specifically, unless specified otherwise, the atomic mass is taken to be the mass of a neutral atom in its ground state. If the atom is not in its ground state, then it must have absorbed enough energy ΔE to be in an excited state. It then follows from Einstein's energy-mass relationship, $E = mc^2$, that the mass of the atom must have increased by an amount Δm, where $\Delta m = \Delta E/c^2$. Thus, the mass of an atom in an excited state must be slightly larger than the mass of the same atom in its ground state.

Since the atomic mass depends on the number of nucleons in the nucleus, it follows that the atomic mass of one isotope of an element will be different from the atomic mass of another isotope of the same element. When we speak of an atomic mass, therefore, we are referring to a specific isotope. We shall let m denote atomic mass, or, if we wish to be very specific, we'll write $m(^A X)$ or $m(^A_Z X)$, showing explicitly the isotope whose mass is being specified. For example, the atomic mass of tritium is $m(^3 H) = 5.008\,267\,01 \times 10^{-27}\,kg$.

The Atomic Mass Unit

Since atomic masses are so tiny, the kilogram is not a particularly convenient unit of mass to use in specifying them. The *unified atomic mass unit*, denoted u, is defined to be exactly 1/12 of the atomic mass of the isotope ^{12}C (remember that this is the mass of a neutral C–12 atom in its ground state). The current value of the unified atomic mass unit given in the *National Institute of Standards and Technology (NIST)* data tables[2] is

$$1\,u \equiv \frac{1}{12}\,m(^{12}C) = 1.660\,538\,86 \times 10^{-27}\,kg, \tag{4.3}$$

where we take the symbol " $\equiv$ " to mean "is defined to be". Thus, for example, the mass of a (neutral) tritium atom in unified atomic mass units is

$$m(^3 H) = 5.008\,267\,01 \times 10^{-27}\,kg \left(\frac{1\,u}{1.660\,538\,86 \times 10^{-27}\,kg} \right)$$

$$= 3.016\,049\,27\,u. \tag{4.4}$$

Relative Atomic Mass

Using the terminology currently recommended by *NIST*, the ratio of the mass of an isotope (the neutral atom in its ground state) to 1/12-th the mass of the ^{12}C atom (the atomic mass unit, u) is called the *relative atomic mass* of an isotope (since it gives the mass *relative to* that of the ^{12}C atom) and is denoted $A_r(^A X)$ (this was formerly called the *atomic weight*):

$$A_r(^A X) \equiv \frac{m(^A X)}{\frac{1}{12}\,m(^{12}C)} = \frac{m(^A X)}{1\,u}. \tag{4.5}$$

Note that the relative atomic mass must be a unitless quantity since it is defined to be the ratio of two masses. Thus, for example, we can immediately see from Eq. (4.4) that the relative atomic mass of tritium is $A_r(^3 H) = 3.016\,049\,27$.

We can see that the value of the relative atomic mass is very close to the mass number, A. (For tritium, $A = 3$.) This is because the masses of the neutron and proton are very close to $1\,u$:[10]

$$\text{Proton:} \quad m_p = 1.007\,276\,466\,88\,u\,; \tag{4.6}$$

$$\text{Neutron:} \quad m_n = 1.008\,664\,915\,60\,u\,. \tag{4.7}$$

We also note that the mass of the electron is[10]

$$\text{Electron:} \quad m_e = 0.000\,548\,579\,909\,45\,\text{u}, \tag{4.8}$$

so the mass of the electron cloud surrounding the nucleus in an atom contributes very little to the mass of the atom.

Example 4.1: Ionization Energy and Relative Atomic Mass

Ionization plays a very important role in both imaging and radiation therapy. Indeed, the majority of the dose delivered to a patient comes from the energy delivered by ionized electrons. The *ionization energy* of an atom, E_I, is defined to be the least amount of energy required to release an electron from the atom—that is, to *ionize* an electron. The ionization energy of a C–12 atom (in its ground state) is $E_I = 11.260\,3\,\text{eV}$, where *eV* stands for *electron-volt*, a small unit of energy commonly used in atomic and nuclear physics. Using this information, compute the relative atomic mass of a singly-ionized C–12 atom. Note that $1\,\text{eV} = 1.602\,189 \times 10^{-19}\,\text{J}$ and that the speed of light in a vacuum is $c = 299\,792\,458\,\text{m/s}$. Comment on the result.

Solution:
To find the relative atomic mass of any particle, we simply need to find the mass of the particle in atomic mass units, and then divide by $1\,\text{u}$. We will start by putting the given ionization energy in *SI* units:

$$E_I = 11.260\,3\,\text{eV} \left(\frac{1.602\,189 \times 10^{-19}\,\text{J}}{1.0\,\text{eV}} \right)$$
$$= 1.804\,112 \times 10^{-18}\,\text{J}. \tag{4.9}$$

This is the minimum amount of energy that must be added to the (neutral) C–12 atom in order to release an electron. This amount of energy has an associated ionization-energy mass, m_I, given by Einstein's energy-mass relationship:

$$m_I = \frac{E_I}{c^2} = \frac{1.804\,112 \times 10^{-18}\,\text{J}}{(299\,792\,458\,\text{m/s})^2} = 2.007\,346 \times 10^{-35}\,\text{kg}, \tag{4.10}$$

or, in atomic mass units using Eq. (4.3),

$$m_I = 2.007\,346 \times 10^{-35}\,\text{kg} \left(\frac{1\,\text{u}}{1.660\,538\,86 \times 10^{-27}\,\text{kg}} \right)$$
$$= 1.208\,8522 \times 10^{-8}\,\text{u}. \tag{4.11}$$

From the definition of relative atomic mass in Eq. (4.5), it then follows that the relative atomic mass associated with the ionization mass, which we can denote $A_r(m_I)$, is given by

$$A_r(m_I) = \frac{m_I}{1\,\text{u}} = 1.208\,8522 \times 10^{-8}. \tag{4.12}$$

Likewise, we can define the relative atomic mass of an electron, $A_r(e)$, to be

$$A_r(e) = \frac{m_e}{1\,\mathrm{u}} = 0.000\,548\,579\,909\,45, \tag{4.13}$$

where we have made use of Eq. (4.8). In addition, we can see from Eq. (4.3) that the relative atomic mass of (neutral) C–12 is $A_r(^{12}\mathrm{C}) = 12$.

We are finally ready to get our answer. Noting that the $^{12}\mathrm{C}^+$ ion is obtained by starting with a (neutral) $^{12}\mathrm{C}$ atom, adding the ionization energy, and then removing an electron, we can see that the relative atomic mass corresponding to the $^{12}\mathrm{C}^+$ ion is found by taking the relative atomic mass of the $^{12}\mathrm{C}$ atom, adding to it the relative atomic mass corresponding to the ionization energy, and then subtracting the relative atomic mass of the electron:

$$A_r\left(^{12}\mathrm{C}^+\right) = A_r\left(^{12}\mathrm{C}\right) + A_r(\mathrm{m_I}) - A_r(e)$$

$$= 12.000 + 1.208\,852 \times 10^{-8} - 0.000\,548\,579\,909\,45 \tag{4.14}$$

or,

$$\boxed{A_r\left(^{12}\mathrm{C}^+\right) = 11.999\,45.} \tag{4.15}$$

Comment:

Take a look at the numerical values of the three terms that contribute to the value of $A_r\left(^{12}\mathrm{C}^+\right)$ in Eq. (4.14). The first term is the relative atomic mass of the neutral C–12 atom—this establishes the rough value of $A_r\left(^{12}\mathrm{C}^+\right)$. The next term is the very small correction to this value due to the energy added to the atom to ionize an electron. Finally, there is the reduction in $A_r\left(^{12}\mathrm{C}^+\right)$ due to the removal of the mass of the electron.

The first term has a value on the order of 10^1, the second term is on the order of 10^{-8}, and the last term is on the order of 10^{-3} (rounding up). If you take the first value and subtract the third value, you will get the answer given in Eq. (4.15) to seven significant figures. The correction term due to the addition of the ionization energy is totally negligible compared to the other terms in the equation, and won't make a difference in our answer unless we keep the answer to eight decimal places (or ten significant figures)!

Our conclusion from this example is the following: unless we are doing *very* precise calculations, it is totally reasonable for us to neglect any contributions to mass from binding energy corrections.

$$\boxed{End\ of\ solution\ to\ Example\ 4.1.}$$

Standard Atomic Weight

The *relative atomic mass of an element*, also called the *standard atomic weight* and denoted $A_r(X)$, is defined to be the average relative atomic mass of all of the naturally occurring isotopes of an element weighted by their relative abundance in nature.

This relative abundance is listed in the NIST tables of *Atomic Weights and Isotopic Compositions* under the heading *Isotopic Composition*.[10]

| Example 4.2: Using the *NIST* Tables |

From the NIST tables[10] we can find the data shown in the table below for the isotopes of hydrogen. The numbers given in parentheses in the various columns gives the uncertainties associated with the values listed; these digits would follow the digits shown before the parentheses.

Isotope		Rel. Atomic Mass	Isotopic Comp.	Stand. Atomic Wt.
H	1	1.007 825 032 07(10)	0.999 885(70)	1.007 94(7)
D	2	2.014 101 7778(4)	0.000 115(70)	
T	3	3.016 049 2777(25)		

(a) What is the significance of the column of numbers that have no heading after the *Isotope* column? (b) Why is there no value for *Isotopic Composition* listed for tritium (T) in the table of data? (c) Why are there no values for *Standard Atomic Weight* given for deuterium (D) and tritium (T)? (d) Use the data to compute the relative atomic mass (or standard atomic weight) of naturally occurring hydrogen, $A_r(\text{H})$, thus verifying the value of the standard atomic weight listed in the table.

Solution:

(a) Keep in mind that hydrogen (H), deuterium (D), and tritium (T) are all isotopes of the hydrogen atom. This means that they all have one proton in the nucleus ($Z = 1$), but differing numbers of neutrons. Hydrogen has no neutrons ($N_H = 0$), so that the mass number for hydrogen is $A_H = Z_H + N_H = 1 + 0 = \boxed{1}$. Likewise, deuterium has one neutron ($N_D = 1$), so that $A_D = Z_D + N_D = 1 + 1 = \boxed{2}$. Finally, tritium has two neutrons, so that $A_T = Z_T + N_T = 1 + 2 = \boxed{3}$. These are the three values in the unlabeled column, so this column must be the values of the mass number, A.

(b) Note that the sum of the two numbers in the column of Isotopic Composition gives 1, to seven significant figures. Since the isotopic composition gives the fractional contribution of the various isotopes found in nature, this means that the isotopic composition of tritium must be zero, since it is not naturally occurring on Earth.

(c) Remember that the standard atomic weight of an element is the weighted average of the relative atomic masses of all of the naturally occurring isotopes of that element on Earth. Therefore, the value shown is not the value corresponding to the ^1H isotope of hydrogen, but rather it is the value of $A_r(H)$ for all of the isotopes of hydrogen naturally occurring on Earth. (If you look further down in the NIST tables online you will see that there is always only one value of A_r listed for each element.)

(d) Examining the isotopic composition values listed in the table above, we can see that 99.988 5% of naturally occurring hydrogen found on Earth is ^1H, 0.011 5%

is ^{2}D, and 0% is ^{3}T. The relative atomic mass of hydrogen, $A_r(\text{H})$, is equal to the abundance-weighted average of the relative atomic mass values for the various naturally occurring isotopes of hydrogen. This may sound complicated, but it's really not. All you have to do is multiply the A_r value for each listed isotope by its isotopic composition value (its fractional contribution to naturally occurring hydrogen—or its abundance), and add up the values that you get. The result will give the value of $A_r(\text{H})$ listed in the last column in the table above. Let's try it and see what we get:

$$(1.007\,825\,032\,07)(0.999\,885) + (2.014\,101\,777\,8)(0.000\,115)$$
$$+(3.016\,049\,2777)(0) = 1.007\,940\,754 \qquad (4.16)$$

which rounds to $\boxed{1.007\,94 = A_r(\text{H})}$, the value listed in the table (to six significant figures).

$$\boxed{\textit{End of solution to Example 4.2.}}$$

Gram Atomic Mass

The *gram-atomic mass of an element*, which we shall denote $A_g(X)$ (NIST does not recommend a symbol for this quantity, so we'll make up our own), is defined to be the mass in grams of one mole of atoms of the given element. The numerical value of the gram-atomic mass is equal to the numerical value of the relative atomic mass of that element, $A_r(X)$, although the former has units of grams (g) while the latter has no units. It therefore follows that

$$A_g(X) = A_r(X) \cdot (1\,\text{g}) . \qquad (4.17)$$

Thus, from Ex. 8.2, we see that one mole of hydrogen atoms has a mass of $1.007\,94$ g. Note that it makes sense to use the relative atomic mass of an *element*—which is a weighted average of naturally occurring isotopes—when specifying the gram-atomic mass of that element. This is because the gram-atomic mass involves a very large number of atoms—on the order of *moles* (Avogadro's number, $N_A = 6.022\,141\,5 \times 10^{23}\,\text{mol}^{-1}$)—within which the naturally occurring isotopes will most likely be present with the listed fractions.

We have already argued that, in order to understand how radiation interacts with matter so that we can understand the ideas behind imaging and cancer treatment with radiation, we must first understand atoms. But the physics that explains the behavior and structure of atoms is *quantum mechanics*. For this reason, we will spend the next few sections becoming acquainted with some of the concepts of and results from the quantum mechanics of atoms.

4.4 QUANTUM MECHANICS—AN INTRODUCTION

Quantum Mechanics is that branch of physics that deals with very small systems or collections of very small systems, where, by *very small*, we typically mean atomic size or smaller. Since we will be very interested not only in the properties of atoms but also in how atoms can interact with incident radiation, it will be important for us to get some basic understanding of quantum mechanics. But before we can come to an understanding of some fundamentals of quantum mechanics, we will first need to take a little detour into the physics of special relativity.

We start by considering a particle of mass m traveling through deep space with velocity $\vec{v}$. That the particle is moving through *deep space* means that we may assume that there are no external forces acting on the particle, and therefore no energies associated with those forces. (Remember that conservative forces such as gravity and the electrical force can result in a potential energy function associated with the particle experiencing the force and the system exerting the force.)

Classical Momentum and Energy

In 1687, Newton published his seminal work referred to as *The Principia* in which he outlined his theory of what became known as *classical mechanics*. (We will put the subscript *"cl"* on a symbol when we wish to stress that it corresponds to Newton's theory of *classical* mechanics.) Within the framework of Newton's mechanics, the *linear momentum* of the particle is given by

$$\vec{p}_{cl} = m\vec{v}. \tag{4.18}$$

Newton then goes on to tell us that the momentum of the particle will change if there is a net force exerted on the particle by its surroundings. In particular, the *rate of change* of the particle's momentum at any time is dictated by the net force acting on the particle at that time, according to

$$\vec{F}_{net} = \frac{d\vec{p}_{cl}}{dt}. \tag{4.19}$$

This equation for the net force $\vec{F}_{net}$ is sometimes called the *equation of motion* for the particle, since it describes how the momentum (or *motion*) of the particle changes according to the net force acting on it. Note that, if the mass of the particle is constant, then the equation of motion can be written in the form $\vec{F}_{net} = d\vec{p}_{cl}/dt = m\,d\vec{v}/dt = m\vec{a}$, which we recognize as Newton's second law.

The energy of the particle is given in classical mechanics by

$$E_{cl} = \frac{1}{2}mv^2 = \frac{p_{cl}^2}{2m}, \tag{4.20}$$

which is, of course, the energy associated with the particle's *motion*—the *kinetic energy*, $E_{K,cl}$. From this equation we see that the energy of the particle when it is stationary—the so-called *rest energy*—is given in classical mechanics by

$$E_{cl,0} = 0, \tag{4.21}$$

since in this case $v = 0$ (which accounts for the "0" subscript on the rest energy).

Relativistic Momentum and Energy

In the year 1905, Albert Einstein published an article[3] in which he outlined the *special theory of relativity*, which is the theory describing particles that are moving close to the speed of light in a vacuum, $c = 299\,792\,458\,\text{m/s} \cong 3.00 \times 10^8\,\text{m/s}$. By "*close*", we typically mean that the speed of the particle is at least $0.1\,c$. If you are doing very precise calculations, then you may need to worry about relativistic equations at lower speeds. For very low speeds the classical and relativistic results will be effectively the same.

There are two quantities typically defined in relativistic physics, denoted β and γ, that tend to make the equations associated with the motion of a relativistic particle look a little simpler. These quantities are defined as follows:

$$\beta \equiv \frac{v}{c} \qquad and \qquad \gamma \equiv \frac{1}{\sqrt{1 - \beta^2}}\,. \tag{4.22}$$

In terms of these quantities, the relativistic linear momentum and its rate of change are given by

$$\vec{p}_{rel} = \gamma m \vec{v} \tag{4.23}$$

and

$$\vec{F}_{net} = \frac{d\vec{p}_{rel}}{dt}\,, \tag{4.24}$$

where we have used the subscript "*rel*" to denote the relativistic expressions and, again, $\vec{F}_{net}$ is the net force acting on the particle. As in the classical case, Eq. (4.24) is referred to as the *equation of motion* for the relativistic particle.

We note the close similarities between the classical and the relativistic expressions for the linear momentum and its rate of change. These similarities seem perhaps misleading, however, when we examine the relativistic expression for the total energy of the particle,

$$E_{rel} = \sqrt{p_{rel}^2 c^2 + m^2 c^4}\,, \tag{4.25}$$

which looks completely different from the equation for the classical energy, E_{cl}, in Eq. (4.20).

As in the classical case, we examine the expression for the rest energy of the particle. To this end, we start by examining the relativistic factors given in equations (4.22) when $v = 0$:

$$\beta \equiv \frac{v}{c} = 0 \qquad and \qquad \gamma \equiv \frac{1}{\sqrt{1 - \beta^2}} = \frac{1}{\sqrt{1 - 0^2}} = 1\,. \tag{4.26}$$

It then follows that $p_{rel,0} = \gamma m v = 0$, so that, from Eq. (4.25), it follows that the relativistic rest energy is given by

$$E_{rel,0} = \sqrt{p_{rel,0}^2\, c^2 + m^2 c^4} = mc^2\,. \tag{4.27}$$

We note that, in complete contradiction to the classical result in which the rest energy is equal to zero, the relativistic rest energy is *not* equal to zero. Indeed, the relativistic equation for the rest energy is the famous Einstein equation $E = mc^2$. (The mass m in this equation is often called the *rest mass*, which simply means the value of mass you would measure if you were at rest relative to the mass. Since this is the way we typically measure mass, this is really nothing new.) Evidently, in relativistic physics, a particle has energy simply by virtue of its mass.

Example 4.3: Relativistic Results for Classical Motion

A rock of mass $m = 1.20\,\text{kg}$ is dropped from the top of a building of height $H = 32.0\,\text{m}$. By the time it reaches ground level the rock is moving with a speed $v = 25.0\,\text{m/s}$. (a) What are the classical and relativistic values of the rock's rest energy? (b) What are the classical and relativistic values of the rock's momentum magnitude just before it hits the ground? (c) What are the classical and relativistic values of the rock's energy just before it hits the ground?

Solution:

(a) The two rest energy values of the rock are $E_{cl,0} = \boxed{0\,\text{J}}$, and $E_{rel,0} = mc^2 = (1.20\,\text{kg})(3.00 \times 10^8\,\text{m/s})^2 = \boxed{1.08 \times 10^{17}\,\text{J}}$.

(b) The classical value of the rock's momentum magnitude is simply $p_{cl} = mv = \boxed{30.0\,\text{kg} \cdot \text{m/s}}$, while the relativistic value comes from the equation $p_{rel} = \gamma mv$. Thus, in order to compute the relativistic momentum value, we must first compute β and γ: $\beta = v/c = 8.33 \times 10^{-8}$ and $\gamma = (1 - \beta^2)^{-1/2} = 1.000$. The relativistic momentum is therefore equal to $p_{rel} = \gamma mv = \boxed{30.0\,\text{kg} \cdot \text{m/s}}$, the same as the classical value. This is because the speed of the rock is so small compared to c, so that γ is just basically equal to 1.

(c) The classical value of the rock's energy is equal to $E_{cl} = mv^2/2 = p_{cl}^2/(2m) = \boxed{375\,\text{J}}$, while the relativistic value is $E_{rel} = \sqrt{p_{rel}^2 c^2 + m^2 c^4} = \sqrt{p_{rel}^2 c^2 + E_{rel,0}^2} = \boxed{1.08 \times 10^{17}\,\text{J}}$. The stark difference in the two energy values is, of course, due to the fact that the relativistic energy includes the rock's rest energy, which we can see from part *(a)* is huge! To "compare apples with apples", we should look only at the rock's *kinetic* energy, since the classical value is really just the kinetic energy value. The relativistic kinetic energy is simply the total relativistic energy minus the rest energy: $E_{K,rel} = E_{rel} - E_{rel,0}$. If we keep *lots* of significant figures in our calculations, we will find that $E_{K,rel} = 375\,\text{J}$, the same as the classical result. This is again due to the very small speed of the rock relative to the speed of light.

End of solution to Example 4.3.

Example 4.4: Relativistic High-Energy Electron Calculations

An oncologist prescribes a dose of 10 MVp x-rays for a cancer patient. The "MVp" stands for *mega-volt peak*, and refers to the fact that the electrons are accelerated through a potential difference (or *voltage difference*) of 10 MV (*mega-volts*). These high-energy electrons are then incident on a tungsten block inside the head of the clinic's linac (*linear accelerator*). The accelerated electrons have a kinetic energy of 10 MeV as they hit the tungsten target. This then results in a beam of x-ray photons emerging from the head of the linac. These x-rays have energies ranging from very low energies up to a peak value of 10 MeV—hence the "mega-volt peak" terminology and notation. (All of this will be discussed in much more detail in Part III of this book.) The mass of an electron is $m_e = 9.109\,38 \times 10^{-31}$ kg, and its charge magnitude is 1.602×10^{-19} C. Also, recall that $1\,\text{eV} = 1.602 \times 10^{-19}$ J. (a) What are the classical and relativistic values of the rest energy of an electron? (b) What is the speed of the electrons just before they collide with the tungsten target inside the head of the linac? (c) What are the classical and relativistic values of the electrons' momentum magnitude just before they collide with the tungsten?

Solution:

[Note that the value $c = 299\,792\,458\,m/s$ is used in the following calculations. Use of $3.00 \times 10^8\,m/s$ can result in surprisingly different results, especially in part (c).]

(a) The rest energies are $E_{cl,0} = \boxed{0\,\text{J}}$, and $E_{rel,0} = m_e c^2 = (9.109\,38 \times 10^{-31}\,\text{kg})(3.00 \times 10^8\,\text{m/s})^2 = \boxed{8.187 \times 10^{-14}\,\text{J}}$. Note that the relativistic energy is small compared to rock's rest energy in the previous example due to the tiny mass of the electron. Nevertheless, this is still a large energy at the atomic level.

(b) We are told that the kinetic energy of the electrons just before they collide with the tungsten is 10 MeV. We need to use this energy to find the corresponding speed of the electrons. This means that we first must convert the units from *MeV* to the *SI* units of *joules*:

$$E_K = 10\,\text{MeV}\left(\frac{10^6\,\text{eV}}{1\,\text{MeV}}\right)\left(\frac{1.602 \times 10^{-19}\,\text{J}}{1\,\text{eV}}\right) = 1.602 \times 10^{-12}\,\text{J}. \qquad (4.28)$$

To find the speed, we must solve the energy equation for v—but which energy equation should we use—the classical or the relativistic equation? Since we're not sure, let's try the (*easier!*) classical equation $E_{cl} = E_K = m_e v^2/2$. Solving for v is easy: we get that $v = \sqrt{2E_{cl}/m_e} = 1.875 \times 10^9\,\text{m/s}$. Remember the relativistic "rule-of-thumb": if v is less than $0.1\,c \cong 3 \times 10^7\,\text{m/s}$, then classical equations can generally be used. But there is another absolute rule that we have not yet mentioned but that we all know: no material object can move as fast as, let alone faster than, the speed of light in a vacuum. (You will show this in the homework at the end of this chapter.) In terms of the relativistic factor β, this means that $\beta \equiv v/c < 1$—*always* for *any* object with mass. But for the linac electrons, we see that $v > c$, or, more specifically, that $\beta = v/c \cong 6.3$. *There is clearly something wrong!* What's wrong, of course, is that the motion of the electrons is *very* relativistic, which means that relativistic equations must be used to find the speed v.

We are given that the kinetic energy is $E_K = 10\,\text{MeV} = 1.602 \times 10^{-12}\,\text{J}$. This means that the total relativistic energy is given by $E_{rel} = E_K + E_{rel,0} = 1.684 \times 10^{-12}\,\text{J}$. From Eq. (4.25) for the relativistic energy, we get that

$$p_{rel} = \frac{\sqrt{E_{rel}^2 - E_{rel,0}^2}}{c} = 5.611 \times 10^{-21}\,\text{kg} \cdot \frac{\text{m}}{\text{s}}. \qquad (4.29)$$

We wish to solve for the speed v, which is buried inside the momentum equation $p_{rel} = \gamma m_e v$. (Remember that γ has a v inside of it since it contains $\beta = v/c$.)

You will be asked to show in the end-of-chapter problems that the speed is given by

$$v = \frac{p_{rel}c}{\sqrt{p_{rel}^2 + m_e^2 c^2}} = \boxed{2.994 \times 10^8 \, \frac{\text{m}}{\text{s}}}. \tag{4.30}$$

We see that this value is less than $c = 2.998 \times 10^8$ m/s (rounded to four significant figures), as required.

(c) The magnitude of the classical momentum is equal to $p_{cl} = m_e v = (9.109\,38 \times 10^{-31}$ kg$)(2.994 \times 10^8$ m/s$) = \boxed{2.727 \times 10^{-22} \, \text{kg} \cdot \text{m/s}}$, while the relativistic momentum magnitude is equal to $p_{rel} = \gamma m_e v = \gamma p_{cl} = p_{cl}/\sqrt{1 - (v/c)^2} = \boxed{5.331 \times 10^{-21} \, \text{kg} \cdot \text{m/s}}$. These two results are very different, again resulting from the fact that the motion of the electrons within the linac is very relativistic. The correct answer is therefore the relativistic one. Note that, in general, the relativistic result is always the correct result. It agrees with the (approximate) classical result only when the particle speed is small compared to the speed of light, which is the regime within which the classical results are valid.

$$\boxed{\textit{End of solution to Example 4.4.}}$$

The Energy and Momentum of a Photon

As we've seen, Eq. (4.27) shows us that we can write the energy of a relativistic particle as given in Eq. (4.25) in terms of the relativistic rest energy $E_{rel,0} = mc^2$ as follows:

$$E_{rel} = \sqrt{p_{rel}^2 c^2 + m^2 c^4} = \sqrt{p_{rel}^2 c^2 + E_{rel,0}^2} \,. \tag{4.31}$$

A *photon* is a packet of light-energy with a rest energy equal to zero: $E_{photon,0} = 0$. This of course means that it must also have a rest mass equal to zero: $m_{photon} = 0$. Since this is the case, shouldn't the linear momentum of the photon also equal zero? To answer this question, we will use the equation for the relativistic energy, Eq. (4.31), since the photon is certainly a relativistic particle (its speed is not only *close to* the speed of light in a vacuum, it's *equal to* that speed since a photon *is* light!). Using $m_{photon} = 0$, we get that the relativistic energy for a photon, which we shall denote E_{photon}, is given by

$$E_{photon} = \sqrt{p_{photon}^2 c^2 + E_{photon,0}^2} = \sqrt{p_{photon}^2 c^2 + 0^2} = p_{photon} c, \tag{4.32}$$

where p_{photon} is the relativistic linear momentum of the photon. It thus follows that the photon does indeed have a non-zero linear momentum in special relativity—a momentum given by

$$p_{photon} = \frac{E_{photon}}{c}. \tag{4.33}$$

In 1905, Einstein proposed what is now called the *Einstein-Planck relation*, which gives the energy of a photon in terms of its linear frequency ν (the Greek letter "nu"; this is the same as the frequency f in your first-year physics course):

$$E_{photon} = h\nu, \tag{4.34}$$

where h is a universal constant called *Planck's constant*,

$$h = 6.626 \times 10^{-34} \, \text{J} \cdot \text{s} \,. \tag{4.35}$$

The frequency ν satisfies the typical equation for traveling waves,

$$\text{speed} = (\text{wavelength})\,(\text{frequency}) \quad \text{or} \quad c = \lambda_{photon}\nu \,, \tag{4.36}$$

where λ_{photon} is the wavelength of the photon (in a vacuum) and c is the speed of the photon (the speed of light—also in a vacuum).

Combining equations (4.36) and (4.34) gives the photon energy in terms of the photon's wavelength,

$$E_{photon} = h\nu = \frac{hc}{\lambda_{photon}} \,, \tag{4.37}$$

which, when combined with Eq. (4.33) for the relativistic photon linear momentum, yields

$$p_{photon} = \frac{E_{photon}}{c} = \frac{1}{c} \frac{hc}{\lambda_{photon}} = \frac{h}{\lambda_{photon}} \,. \tag{4.38}$$

Thus, the linear momentum is inversely proportional to the wavelength of the photon.

The deBroglie Wavelength

Louis deBroglie was a doctoral student in physics in 1924 when he proposed that not only photons, but indeed *all* particles should obey an equation of the form of Eq. (4.38):

$$p_{rel} = \frac{h}{\lambda} \,. \tag{4.39}$$

In this equation, p_{rel} is the relativistic momentum of the particle, h is Planck's constant as given in Eq. (4.35), and λ is some sort of wavelength associated with the particle. Equation (4.39) is called the *deBroglie relation*.

Don't worry if you are bothered by the idea of a wavelength associated with a particle—you are in very good company, as many physicists in deBroglie's time were also very bothered by this idea. The important thing to keep in mind about the deBroglie wavelength for a particle is that the wavelength does *not* mean that the particle will move up and down as it travels (like a water wave), but rather that the wavelength associated with the particle will result in *interference and diffraction effects*, which are characteristic of all waves and are governed by the wavelength of the waves. These interference and diffraction effects for particle waves have been experimentally observed and numerically verified many times since deBroglie made his proposal in 1924.

Example 4.5: Calculating the deBroglie Wavelength

Consider the rock in example (4.3) and the electrons in example (4.4). What are the deBroglie wavelengths associated with these objects?

Solution:

In order to find the deBroglie wavelength of a particle, we first need to find its relativistic momentum. In Ex.(4.3) we found that, for the rock, $p_{rock} = 30.0 \, \text{kg} \cdot \text{m/s}$, while in Ex.(4.4) we found for the electrons that $p_{electron} = 5.331 \times 10^{-21}$ kg · m/s. (Remember that we must use the correct relativistic value for the momentum in order to get the correct value of the deBroglie wavelength.) It then follows from Eq. (4.39) that the deBroglie wavelengths are equal to:

$$\lambda_{rock} = \frac{h}{p_{rock}} = \frac{6.626 \times 10^{-34} \, \text{J} \cdot \text{s}}{30.0 \, \text{kg} \cdot \text{m/s}} = \boxed{2.21 \times 10^{-35} \, \text{m}}, \tag{4.40}$$

and

$$\lambda_{electron} = \frac{h}{p_{electron}} = \frac{6.626 \times 10^{-34} \, \text{J} \cdot \text{s}}{5.331 \times 10^{-21} \, \text{kg} \cdot \text{m/s}} = \boxed{1.24 \times 10^{-13} \, \text{m}}. \tag{4.41}$$

$$\boxed{\textit{End of solution to Example 4.5.}}$$

Reality of the deBroglie Wavelength

The results in the previous example are interesting for the following reasons.

As may have been discussed in your introductory physics course, waves exhibit certain phenomena that are exhibited by nothing else—namely, *interference* and *diffraction* effects. When a wave passes through an aperture that is roughly the same size or smaller than the wavelength of the wave, then the wave displays a pattern of maxima and minima as it passes through the aperture. This is called *diffraction*, and the maxima and minima result from the constructive and destructive *interference* of the various portions of the wave as they emerge from the aperture. A similar phenomenon is observed if the wave passes through a series of many very narrow apertures (or *slits*) in which the spacing between the apertures is likewise roughly the same size or smaller than the wavelength of the wave. Such a series of apertures is known as a *diffraction grating*.

Noting that a nucleus has a size of about 10^{-15} m while an atom has a size of about 10^{-10} m = 1 Å, we see that the wavelength of the rock is a tiny fraction of the size of a nucleus. This means that there is no way for us to find something that can act like a diffraction grading to show the wave-like properties of a rock—the deBroglie wavelength is simply much too small.

But for the electrons the story is different. The wavelength of the accelerated electrons in Ex.(4.5) is smaller than but not too far from the size of an atom. If instead of using clinical treatment energies of about 10 MeV we used much smaller electron energies—say around 100 eV—then the deBroglie wavelength would be around 1.2 Å, which is about the size of an atom. Perhaps more significantly from an experimental point of view, this is also close to the separation between the planes of atoms that form a crystal, which means that the ordered arrays of atoms in a crystal could be used as a naturally occurring diffraction grating to observe interference effects for a beam of relatively low-energy electrons if deBrogie's hypothesis is correct.

This is exactly what was done by Davisson and Germer in 1927. Their results showed that electrons do indeed have wave-like properties in that they display diffraction effects when incident on a crystal, and the wavelength determined from the electron diffraction pattern agreed with the value of the deBroglie wavelength, thereby experimentally verifying the deBroglie relation.

Davisson and Germer showed that deBroglie's relation was correct—at least for electrons. (It has since been shown to be true for other particles.) But where does this relation come from? Is it good enough in physics to simply propose a relation and, if it turns out to be true, then to claim that you've come up with a new law and move on to something else? The answer, of course, is *no*. Physics is a fundamental and mathematical science in that it strives to boil down relations like deBroglie's to a more fundamental level—one that enables us to answer other questions like, "Where does the deBroglie relation and the associated wavelength come from?", or "What is the physical significance of the wavelength?" This more fundamental level of understanding came a couple of years after deBroglie's proposal and is the subject of the next section.

4.5 THE SCHRÖDINGER EQUATION

One problem with deBroglie's proposal was that, at the time, there was no underlying formalism that implied that a wave-like character should be associated with a moving particle. However, such a formalism was presented in 1926 by Erwin Schrödinger with his introduction of the quantum mechanical equation of motion for a particle.

Recall that, in the classical equation of motion, Newton asks us to specify all of the forces acting on a particle in order to determine the net force. His equation of motion then tells us how the momentum of the particle changes with time, thereby tracing out step-by-step the future motion of the particle. In Schrödinger's formalism of quantum mechanics, the equation of motion is not specified in terms of forces, but rather in terms of *energies*. Noting that conservative forces such as the electrical force or the gravitational force can be used to compute corresponding potential energy functions, we can see that specifying a potential energy function E_P experienced by a particle within the formalism of quantum mechanics is analogous to specifying the forces acting on a particle in classical mechanics.

For the special case of a particle of mass m moving in one dimension along the x-axis under the influence of a potential energy function $E_P(x)$, the quantum mechanical equation of motion, more commonly called the *Schrödinger equation*, is given by

$$\frac{-\hbar^2}{2m} \frac{\partial^2 \Psi(x,t)}{\partial x^2} + E_P(x)\Psi(x,t) = i\hbar \frac{\partial \Psi(x,t)}{\partial t} . \tag{4.42}$$

Again, as in classical mechanics, we are required to specify the forces acting on a particle or system of particles in quantum mechanics, but we must do so within the realm of *energies*. Indeed, the Schrödinger equation is really just a quantum mechanical means of specifying the *total energy* of a particle or system of particles.[a]

---

[a]Remember that the total energy of a particle is just the sum of its kinetic and potential energies. It's easy enough to find the potential energy term in the Schrödinger equation—it's just the term with $E_P(x)$ in it. However, since quantum mechanics expresses the total energy in terms of quantum mechanical *operators*, we would be hard-pressed at this point to find the *kinetic energy* term. It's actually the first term in Eq. (4.42).

The Meanings of the Symbols in the Schrödinger Equation

Let's examine the various symbols within the Schrödinger equation, Eq. (4.42). Starting from the beginning of the equation, we have the constant $\hbar$, which is pronounced "h-bar" and is called the *reduced Planck constant*. This constant has the value $\hbar \equiv h/2\pi = 1.055 \times 10^{-34} \, \text{J} \cdot \text{s}$. We've already stated that m is the particle's mass, and $\partial^2/\partial x^2$ is the second partial derivative with respect to the position x. What we are taking a derivative of is the function $\Psi(x,t)$, which is called the *wavefunction* of the particle. We see that, for this 1-D case, the wavefunction is a function of *position* and of *time*. (If we are working in 3-D, as we will be when discussion the hydrogen atom, then the wavefunction will be a function of 3-D position and time: $\Psi(\vec{r},t) = \Psi(x,y,z,t)$.) It is the wavefunction, $\Psi(x,t)$, that we wish to solve for in the Schrödinger equation, since the wavefunction contains all dynamical information about the allowed states of the particle within the formalism of quantum mechanics.

Continuing on through the symbols in Eq. (4.42), we next get to the potential energy function $E_P(x)$, the pure imaginary number denoted i, where $i \equiv \sqrt{-1}$, and finally the partial derivative of the wavefunction with respect to time, $\partial\Psi(x,t)/\partial t$.

Partial Derivatives

A word is perhaps in order about *partial derivatives*. When we write something like $\partial\Psi(x,t)/\partial x$ or $\partial\Psi(x,t)/\partial t$, all we are saying is that we wish to take the derivative of the function $\Psi(x,t)$ with respect to x or with respect to t, just like you did in your first-semester calculus class. So why the fancy notation with the curly "d"s? The reason is to acknowledge that, unlike in your first-semester calculus class, the function that we are taking a derivative of is a function of *more than* one variable—in this case, it is a function of two variables: the position x and the time t. So when we take the partial derivative of $\Psi(x,t)$ with respect to x for example, $\partial\Psi(x,t)/\partial x$, all the notation is doing is first of all reminding us that there are more variables around than just x (t in this case), and that, when taking the derivative with respect to x, we should treat any other variables as *constants*. Of course, $\partial^2\Psi(x,t)/\partial x^2$ just tells us to take two consecutive partial derivatives of the wavefunction $\Psi(x,t)$ with respect to x while treating t as a constant. For example, if $f(x,t) = 2x^2 t + 5t$, then $\partial f(x,t)/\partial x = 4xt$, and $\partial^2 f(x,t)/\partial x^2 = 4t$. Likewise, $\partial f(x,t)/\partial t = 2x^2 + 5$, and $\partial^2 f(x,t)/\partial t^2 = 0$.

The Wavefunction

The Schrödinger equation in the form of Eq. (4.42) is said to be a *differential equation* since it involves *derivatives* of the unknown function $\Psi(x,t)$. More specifically, it is said to be a *partial differential equation* since it involves *partial* derivatives of the desired function $\Psi(x,t)$.

As mentioned previously, the wavefunction $\Psi(x,t)$ contains all *dynamical information* about the state of the particle under study—that is, the wavefunction contains information about the particle's probable position, linear momentum, energy, *etc.* In order to extract this information about the particle, we first must solve the Schrödinger equation for the unknown function $\Psi(x,t)$ given the appropriate potential energy function $E_P(x)$, as dictated by the forces acting on the particle. We must also take into account any *boundary conditions* that must be satisfied by the wavefunction.

The Schrödinger equation is a differential equation involving derivatives of the wavefunction $\Psi(x,t)$. In order to solve this equation for the wavefunction we must effectively integrate the Schrödinger equation using the methods of solving differential equations. (We will not be needing these special methods in this book.) The *boundary conditions* for the wavefunction $\Psi(x,t)$ are essentially like the limits on an integral, and in general contain information about the *confinement* of the particle in question. That is, the forces acting on the particle often tend to hold the particle within a certain region of space. As we'll see, there is something very important that emerges from the mathematics involved with the solution to the Schrödinger equation when boundary conditions that correspond to a confinement of the particle are imposed.

Even though you may not have any experience in actually solving differential equations, you nevertheless have some experience with physical solutions to differential wave equations with boundary conditions. What's more, you have already seen how such physical solutions are characterized by something very important that emerges from the solution of the Schrödinger equation with boundary conditions— namely, *quantum numbers*.

4.6   A MATHEMATICAL ANALOGY: QUANTUM NUMBERS

Quantum numbers play a fundamental role in quantum mechanics in general, and in the structure of atoms in particular. But where do these quantum numbers come from, and what kind of role do they play? In this section we will try to get a feel for the answers to these questions within the context of a simple and familiar system: standing waves on a string.

Consider a string of length L stretched horizontally between two support posts. If the string is at rest, it is simply stretched horizontally between the two posts, as shown in Fig. (4.1a). This is the so-called *equilibrium position* of the string. If we were to pluck the string, we would find that a number of different standing wave patterns could be produced on the string—see Figs. 4.1*b*, *c*, and *d*. Labeled on the figures are the positions of *antinodes*, A (positions of maximum displacement from the equilibrium position of the string) and *nodes*, N (positions of zero displacement from equilibrium).

Quantum Numbers Come From Boundary Conditions

Waves traveling on a string are described by functions that are called *wavefunctions*. These wavefunctions are solutions to equations called the (classical) *wave equation*. The problem in physics is to solve the wave equation given certain constraints that are specified with so-called *boundary conditions*. These boundary conditions tell the mathematics what must be going on with our system (the waves on the string in this case) at the edges, or *boundaries*, of the region of space available to it.

For example, in the case of the plucked string, the boundary conditions say that the ends of the string cannot move since they are attached to the two posts—in other words, the two ends of the string must be *nodes*. These boundary conditions for the string effectively confine the waves on the string to a 1-D region of length L (the string).

As a result, it is found that a variable called a *quantum number* naturally arises out of the mathematics associated with solving the wave equation for the string. For vibrating strings, the quantum number n is called the *harmonic number*, and specifies the frequency of the standing wave. In the quantum mechanical description of the hydrogen atom, on the other hand, the quantum number n is called the *principal quantum number*, and dictates the energy of the atom.

Quantum numbers can only take on certain specific values with no allowed values in between. The quantum number for standing waves on a string tells us that only certain frequencies (or wavelengths) of oscillation of the waves on the string can be sustained—namely, those that satisfy the boundary conditions at the ends of the string. Note that the standing wave patterns shown in Fig. (4.1) all satisfy the boundary conditions that the two ends of the string are *nodes*.

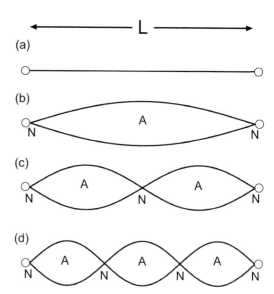

FIGURE 4.1: Standing waves on a string of length L stretched between two posts. (a) No wave. (b) The first harmonic (n = 1). (c) The second harmonic (n = 2). (d) The third harmonic (n = 3). (A = antinode; N = node).

The Quantum Number Quantizes the Frequency and the Energy

If the frequency of the *first harmonic* wave shown in Fig. (4.1b) is denoted ν_1, then it is found that the frequency of the second allowed wave, or *second harmonic*, is given by $\nu_2 = 2\nu_1$, so that its frequency is twice that of the first harmonic and its wavelength is half as big, as shown in Fig. (4.1c). Likewise, the frequency of the third wave satisfying the imposed boundary conditions is called the *third harmonic*, given by $\nu_3 = 3\nu_1$. Its frequency is equal to three times the fundamental frequency, and its wavelength is one-third that of the fundamental, as shown in Fig. (4.1d).

It is now easy to see that, in general, the frequency of the nth harmonic wave is given by

$$\nu_n = n\,\nu_1 \qquad for \qquad n = 1, 2, 3, \ldots, \infty. \tag{4.43}$$

The various frequencies given in Eq. (4.43) are characteristic of the different allowed *vibrational states* of the vibrating string. The quantum number n specifies which state the system is in, and dictates with which frequency the string vibrates when it is in that state. We could then say that the allowed frequencies on the vibrating string as specified in Eq. (4.43) are *quantized*—that is, they can only have certain discrete values ($\nu_1, 2\nu_1, 3\nu_1$, *etc*). But the greater the value of the frequency, the greater the corresponding energy of that vibrational state of the string. Thus, the existence of the quantum number n results not only in the quantization of the frequency but also in the energy of the standing wave. This is an extremely important consequence of the appearance of a quantum number in the formalism of standing waves.

The reason for this discussion of standing waves on a string is that it is completely analogous to the situation in quantum mechanics. In quantum mechanics, the wave equation to be solved is given a special name: the Schrödinger equation. The solution to the 1-D Schrödinger equation given the applicable boundary conditions is called the wavefunction and is denoted $\Psi(x, t)$. This wavefunction contains all of the information about the state of the system, which is specified by one quantum number. If we were to denote that quantum number by n, then we could express the wavefunction by $\Psi_n(x, t)$, explicitly showing that the state is dictated by the value of the quantum number n.

Returning to the consideration of standing waves on a string, we note that the value of n for the harmonic waves corresponds to the number of *antinodes* (or positions of maximum displacement) in the corresponding wavefunction (the standing wave patterns shown in Fig. 4.1). This is actually not a coincidence—it often shows up for 1-D systems of a confined particle—and we shall see it surface again in our discussion of the hydrogen atom, a 3-D system.

The Dimensionality Gives the Number of Quantum Numbers

We see that there is only *one* quantum number for the standing wave on the vibrating string. This is because the wave is confined to only *one* dimension—the x-direction along the string's length. Likewise, in quantum mechanics, the solution to the Schrödinger equation for a particle confined to a 1-D region of space involves just *one* quantum number—for example, an electron confined to a length of a thin conducting wire so that it can only move back-and-forth along the length of the wire. Furthermore, the solution of the Schrödinger equation for a particle confined to a 2-D region of space—such as an electron confined to a thin rectangular metal plate—involves *two* quantum numbers, and a 3-D quantum system, such as an electron confined to the inside of a rectangular metal block, has a solution that is characterized by *three* quantum numbers. We conclude that the dimensionality of the confined quantum system tells us how many quantum numbers to expect in the wavefunction describing the available states of that system.

For the vibrating string, the quantum number (or harmonic number) n specifies the vibrational state of the system: the greater the value of n, the higher the frequency. But higher frequencies are associated with higher energies. Therefore, the quantum number n specifies not only the state and the associated wavefunction for the system, but it also specifies the *energy* of the system. This is of fundamental importance in quantum mechanics in which these same ideas hold true: the three quantum numbers that come from the solution of the 3-D Schrödinger equation determine the state, the corresponding wavefunction, and the associated energy of the atom in that state. (Actually, only *one* of the three quantum numbers—the principal quantum number, n—is needed to determine the energy of the state for an isolated hydrogen atom. We will see how this works in the next section.)

This concludes our introduction to the general ideas of quantum mechanics and the Schrödinger equation. It's now time to return to the purpose of this introduction—namely, the quantum mechanical description of atoms. Since hydrogen is the simplest of the atoms, we will finish up this chapter with a discussion of hydrogen and atoms similar to it. The next chapter will then focus on more complex atoms.

4.7 ENERGY LEVELS IN HYDROGENIC ATOMS

Hydrogen is an atom consisting of a nucleus containing one proton ($Z = 1$) surrounded by an electron cloud that contains one electron charge. A *hydrogenic atom* is an atom whose nucleus contains Z protons (where $Z \geq 1$) but still has a surrounding electron cloud consisting of only *one* electron charge. Thus, in hydrogenic atoms, the only interaction is between one nucleus and one electron—in particular, there are no other electrons around to cause other interactions. Multielectron atoms, on the other hand, are much more complicated since each electron in the atom interacts not only with the nucleus but also with each of the other $Z - 1$ electrons in the atom. We will discuss the case of multielectron atoms and the complications associated with them in the next chapter.

Three Classical Atomic Quantum Numbers

Let's consider a hydrogenic atom with Z protons in its nucleus and one electron charge in the surrounding electron cloud. Since the electron moves in 3-D space around the nucleus, the Schrödinger equation describing the energy of this atomic system is an equation involving three spatial variables (x, y, z) and one temporal variable t. The electrical Coulomb force effectively constrains the motion of the electron to the 3-D region of space around the nucleus. As a result, as was mentioned in the previous section, there arise three quantum numbers (one for each dimension of space) to characterize the allowed states of the electron in the atom. These quantum numbers are: i) the *principal quantum number, n*; ii) the *orbital angular momentum quantum number, ℓ*; and iii) the *z-component of orbital angular momentum quantum number* (also called the *magnetic quantum number*), denoted m_ℓ. The mathematics used in obtaining the solution to the Schrödinger equation for a hydrogenic atom leads naturally to the allowed values for the quantum numbers shown in Table (4.1).

TABLE 4.1: The hydrogenic Schrödinger quantum numbers

Symbol	Possible Values
n	$1, 2, 3, \ldots, \infty$
ℓ	$0, 1, 2, 3, \ldots, n - 1$
m_ℓ	$-\ell, -\ell + 1, \ldots, 0, \ldots, \ell - 1, \ell$

Four Relativistic Atomic Quantum Numbers

As a result of the work of Paul Dirac in 1929 incorporating special relativity into the formalism of quantum mechanics, there emerged a fourth quantum number. This fourth quantum number can be more readily appreciated once it is realized that, in special relativity, the fourth dimension—*time*—is treated equally with the three spatial dimensions. The fourth quantum number is, therefore, simply a result of the incorporation of an additional dimension into the formalism of quantum mechanics. This fourth quantum number is called the *z-component of spin angular momentum quantum number* (or simply the *spin quantum number*) and is denoted m_s. The mathematics of the relativistic version of the Schrödinger equation, called the *Dirac equation*, leads to only two possible values for the spin quantum number: $m_s = +1/2$ and $-1/2$. These values are given in the revised list of quantum numbers shown in Table (4.2).

TABLE 4.2: The complete set of hydrogenic quantum numbers resulting from relativistic quantum mechanics

Symbol	Possible Values
n	$1, 2, 3, \ldots, \infty$
ℓ	$0, 1, 2, 3, \ldots, n-1$
m_ℓ	$-\ell, -\ell+1, \ldots, 0, \ldots, \ell-1, \ell$
m_s	$-\frac{1}{2}, +\frac{1}{2}$

To demonstrate the application of the range of quantum-number values listed in Table (4.2), let's consider the case of $n = 3$. Since, from the table, ℓ can have any value from 0 up to $n-1$, it follows that, for $n = 3$, ℓ can have any one of the possible values $\ell = \{0, 1, 2\}$. Each value of ℓ can have different possible values for m_ℓ varying from the smallest value $m_\ell = -\ell$, up to the largest possible value of $m_\ell = +\ell$, in increments of 1. Thus, for $\ell = 0$ we can only have $m_\ell = 0$, while for $\ell = 1$ we can have $m_\ell = \{-1, 0, 1\}$, and for $\ell = 2$ we can have $m_\ell = \{-2, -1, 0, 1, 2\}$. For any of these n, ℓ, and m_ℓ values, we can have $m_s = +\frac{1}{2}$ or $m_s = -\frac{1}{2}$. Since the quantum state of a hydrogenic atom is specified by the values of the four quantum numbers n, ℓ, m_ℓ and m_s, it follows that, for the case of $n = 3$, we can have any of the following quantum states for the hydrogenic atom (excluding the value of the spin quantum number for just a moment):

$$(n, \ell, m_\ell) = \begin{array}{l} (3,0,0) \\ (3,1,-1), (3,1,0), (3,1,1) \\ (3,2,-2), (3,2,-1), (3,2,0), (3,2,1), (3,2,2) \end{array} \qquad (4.44)$$

For each of these listed states, m_s can have a value of either $+\frac{1}{2}$ or $-\frac{1}{2}$. We can therefore see that, for the $n = 3$ shell, there is a total of 18 possible quantum states for the atom.

Specifying Quantum States

Specifying a value for each of the four quantum numbers for the hydrogenic atom specifies a unique quantum state for that atom. This state is described by the wavefunction for the atom evaluated at the given values of the four quantum numbers: $\Psi_{n,\ell,m_\ell,m_s}(x, y, z, t)$. Note that this wavefunction is a function of the position of the electron in space (relative to the position of the nucleus), (x, y, z), and of the time, t. We use the list of quantum numbers as subscripts for the wavefunction in order to label the quantum state characterized by that wavefunction.

In the relatively simple case of an isolated hydrogenic atom, the energy of each state is determined solely by the value of the principal quantum number n, so we will focus our attention on this quantum number in the remainder of this section. (We'll say more about the other quantum numbers in the next chapter on multi-electron atoms.)

The principal quantum number n basically plays the same role in atomic physics as the harmonic number played for standing waves on a string mentioned in the previous section: it can take on the values 1, 2, 3, $\ldots, \infty$, and higher values of n are associated with higher energies. For the electron in a hydrogenic atom, these higher energy states are associated with a more spread-out electron cloud around the nucleus, resulting in a larger atom.

Radial Probability Densities

The wavefunction $\Psi_{n,\ell,m_\ell,m_s}(x,y,z,t) = \Psi_{n,\ell,m_\ell,m_s}(\vec{r},t)$ can be a complicated function of the position and time variables and of the values of the quantum numbers. When we say that the state of the atom is specified by the set of four quantum numbers n, ℓ, m_ℓ, and m_s, all we mean is that the values of these quantum numbers specify precisely which function describes the atom when it is in that state. This function contains all of the information concerning the state of the atom.

In particular, the wavefunction contains information about the energy of the atom in the state specified by the set of quantum numbers (n, ℓ, m_ℓ, m_s), as well as information about the probability of finding the electron at various positions around the nucleus. It is this idea of *probabilities* of finding the electron around the nucleus that leads to the picture of an electron *cloud* around the nucleus in a quantum mechanical illustration of the atom—the greater the probability, the more dense or opaque the cloud.

We can therefore get some idea of the *size* of a hydrogenic atom by examining the probability of finding the electron at various distances from the nucleus. This type of probability function comes directly from the wavefunction and is called the *radial probability density function* for the electron in the hydrogenic atom, denoted $P_{n\ell}(r)$. The subscript "$n\ell$" reminds us that the radial probability density function depends only on the values of two of the four quantum numbers to specify a state of the atom, n and ℓ. The "r" in parentheses denotes the fact that the value of the function $P_{n\ell}(r)$ depends on the (radial) distance $r = \sqrt{x^2 + y^2 + z^2}$ from the nucleus.

In general, the actual function $P_{n\ell}(r)$ for hydrogenic atoms can be a rather complicated function of r, but it takes on a relatively simple form if ℓ has its largest possible value for a given value of the principal quantum number n—that is, $P_{n\ell}(r)$ takes on a particularly simple form if $\ell = n - 1$. In this case, a plot of $P_{n\ell}(r)$ vs. r shows a smooth curve having a single maximum. The value of r at which the maximum occurs represents the distance from the nucleus at which the probability for locating the electron is a maximum—we are *most likely* to find the electron at that distance from the nucleus. Figure (4.2) shows three plots of radial probability densities for hydrogen for the cases $n = 1, 2$, and 3, and for $\ell = n - 1$.

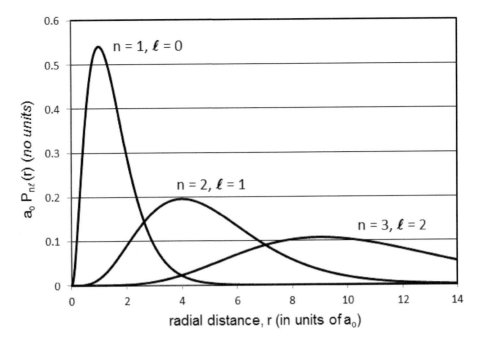

FIGURE 4.2: Hydrogen radial probability densities $P_{n,\ell}(r)$ for $(n = 1, \ell = 0)$, $(n = 2, \ell = 1)$, and $(n = 3, \ell = 2)$. The radial variable r is given in units of the Bohr radius, a_o. (See Eq. (4.47).)

The Size of Hydrogenic Atoms

We can see from the plots in Fig. (4.2) that the distance r at which $P_{n\ell}(r)$ has its peak—that is, the distance from the nucleus at which we are most likely to find the electron—increases as the principal quantum number n increases. Indeed, it can be shown that the maximum value of $P_{n\ell}(r)$ occurs at the distance r_n from the nucleus (the subscript signifies that the result depends on the value of the principal quantum number, n), where

$$r_n = \left(\frac{4\pi\varepsilon_o\hbar^2}{m_e e^2}\right)\frac{n^2}{Z}. \tag{4.45}$$

In this equation, $\varepsilon_o = 8.854\,187 \times 10^{-12}\,\mathrm{C^2/(N \cdot m^2)}$ is the *electric permittivity of free space*, $\hbar = h/(2\pi) = 1.054\,571\,596 \times 10^{-34}\,\mathrm{J \cdot s}$ is the reduced Planck constant, $m_e = 9.109\,381\,88 \times 10^{-31}\,\mathrm{kg}$ is the electron mass, $e = 1.602\,176 \times 10^{-19}\,\mathrm{C}$ is the fundamental charge (the charge magnitude of the electron or proton), Z is the number of proton charges in the nucleus (the atomic number), and n is the principal quantum number. It is important to keep in mind that Eq. (4.45) is only valid for states in which $\ell = \ell_{max} = n - 1$, corresponding to states in which the radial probability density has a single maximum, as shown in Fig. (4.2).

The Bohr Radius
We note from Eq. (4.45) above that, for $n = 1$ and $Z = 1$ (the ground state of hydrogen),

$$r_1^{(H)} = \frac{4\pi\varepsilon_o\hbar^2}{m_e e^2} = 5.291\,77 \times 10^{-11}\,\text{m}. \qquad (4.46)$$

This special value of r for hydrogen is called the *Bohr radius* and is typically denoted by the symbol a_o:

$$a_o \equiv r_1^{(H)} = \frac{4\pi\varepsilon_o\hbar^2}{m_e e^2} = 5.291\,77 \times 10^{-11}\,\text{m} = 0.529\,177\,\text{Å}. \qquad (4.47)$$

(Note, as pointed out earlier, that an atom has a diameter of about $10^{-10}\,\text{m}$.) We can then rewrite Eq. (4.45) in terms of a_o as simply

$$r_n = a_o\,\frac{n^2}{Z}. \qquad (4.48)$$

This equation gives us a rough idea of the size of a hydrogenic atom having an atomic number Z and with its single electron in a quantum state with principal quantum number n.

Hydrogenic Energies
As mentioned previously, we can also determine the energy of the electron in a given quantum state from the wavefunction $\Psi_{n,\ell,m_\ell,m_s}(\vec{r},t)$. The result is, again for hydrogenic atoms,

$$E_n = -\left(\frac{m_e e^4}{32\pi^2\varepsilon_o^2\hbar^2}\right)\frac{Z^2}{n^2}. \qquad (4.49)$$

Note that, since the largest value of n is ∞, the largest value that E_n can have is 0 (the other values of E_n are all negative). An electron in the $n = \infty$ state is said to be *ionized*.

For the ground state of *hydrogen* ($n = 1$, $Z = 1$) we get the ground-state energy

$$E_1^{(H)} = -\frac{m_e e^4}{32\pi^2\varepsilon_o^2\hbar^2} = -2.178\,70 \times 10^{-18}\,\text{J} \qquad (4.50)$$

or, in units of *electron volts*,

$$E_1^{(H)} = -2.178\,70 \times 10^{-18}\,\text{J}\left(\frac{1\,\text{eV}}{1.602\,176 \times 10^{-19}\,\text{J}}\right)$$
$$= -13.598\,4\,\text{eV} \cong -13.6\,\text{eV}. \qquad (4.51)$$

We can thus write Eq. (4.49) in the simpler form for hydrogenic atoms:

$$E_n = E_1^{(H)}\,\frac{Z^2}{n^2}. \qquad (4.52)$$

Bound Systems and Energy-Level Diagrams
It's important to note that $E_n < 0$ in Eq. (4.52) due to the fact that, from Eq. (4.50) or (4.51), $E_1^{(H)} < 0$. Whenever the total energy of a system is *negative* (as is the case

for an atom or a solar system), it means that the system has internal forces (electrical or gravitational, respectively) that hold the components of the system together. The fact that $E_n < 0$ in Eq. (4.52) is a result of the fact that the electron is bound to the nucleus by the electrical Coulomb force of attraction.

In quantum mechanics, whenever particles are held together in a system by internal forces, the allowed energies of the system are always negative and they are always *quantized*—that is, the energy can only have certain *discrete* values. This means that the hydrogenic atom would have to "*jump*" from one state to another if it were to make a transition from some state with an initial energy to a final state having a different energy. (This discrete nature of energy levels in atoms is a natural consequence of the solution of the Schrödinger equation for the atom.)

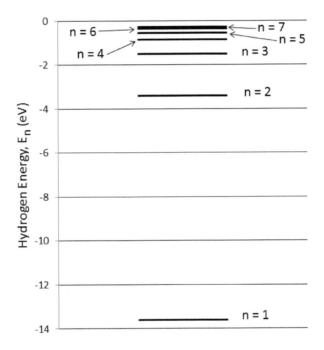

FIGURE 4.3: Hydrogen energy level diagram for the states $n = 1$ through $n = 7$, drawn to scale. Note that the maximum possible energy is $E = 0$, corresponding to $n = \infty$ (*not shown*). An atom in this state is said to be *ionized*.

Given that quantum states with different principal quantum numbers n have different energies E_n, it follows that we can construct an *energy-level diagram* showing the energies for various quantum states. Such a diagram is shown in Fig. (4.3) for hydrogen. Note that the highest energy shown for the hydrogen atom in Fig. (4.3) is $E = 0$, which is at the very top of the diagram since all of the other energies $(E_1, E_2, \ldots, E_7)$ are negative. We can see from Eq. (4.52) that $E_n \to 0$ as $n \to \infty$. If we give the atom enough energy (from an incident photon, or from a collision with an incident charged particle), then it can make a transition to the $n = \infty$ quantum state—a state in which $E = 0$. Since the energy would then no longer be negative, the electron would no longer be bound to the nucleus—it would be *ionized*, and could wander off to do as it pleased.

The Ionization Energy, E_I

The minimum energy required for an electron to undergo a transition to the $E = 0$ ($n = \infty$) state and therefore ionize that electron is called the *ionization energy* (or *binding energy*) of that electron, E_I. (This was discussed in Ex.(4.1) on p.88). If the atom were given enough energy so that E actually became *positive*, then that positive amount of energy would appear in the form of extra kinetic energy that would move the electron away from the nucleus faster than would be needed to simply ionize it. This idea was used in Chapter 2 in our discussion of the linear energy transfer (LET) being the restricted linear electronic stopping power, L_Δ. In that discussion, we were concerned about ionized electrons possibly carrying energy far from the site of the ionization, and therefore not contributing to the dose to the tissue at that location. We can now see that these are electrons that were given significantly more energy than what was needed to simply ionize them—electrons whose final energy was a relatively large positive number.

Example 4.6: Approximate Ionization Energy Calculations

The dominant process involved in medical imaging with x-rays is called the *photo-electric effect*. In this process, a lower-energy x-ray photon—a photon with energy in the range from about $100\,\text{eV}$ to about $100\,\text{keV}$—is incident on an atom. If the photon has barely enough energy to ionize an electron that is close to the nucleus in the atom, then that photon will have a relatively high probability of being absorbed and its energy used to ionize the electron from the atom. (The ejected electron is called a *photo-electron*). The photon has thus been removed from the beam of incident x-ray photons moving through the tissue. The greater the number of photons removed, the darker that part of the x-ray image will appear.

The whole reason for using lower-energy x-rays in imaging is that, as opposed to other regions of the electromagnetic spectrum, these x-rays interact to a different extent with atoms having different Z values. Therefore, lower-energy x-rays interact differently with soft tissue (average Z of around 7.4) than they do with bone (average Z-value of around 12). (See Chapter 8 for more information on the photo-electric effect.) As a result, the region of an x-ray image representing soft tissue will look different from a region representing bone. It is the resulting contrast between regions corresponding to different average Z-values that makes x-ray imaging useful for medical imaging. (We'll discuss this topic in much more detail in Chapter 11.) For this example, let's use nitrogen (N) with $Z_N = 7$ to represent soft tissue, and magnesium (Mg) with $Z_{Mg} = 12$ to represent bone. Compute an *approximate* value for the ionization energy associated with the photoelectric effect in these two atoms, and comment on your answers.

Solution:

We first note that nitrogen and magnesium are far from hydrogenic with 7 and 12 electrons surrounding their nuclei, respectively. However, note in the discussion of the photoelectric effect above that this process has the greatest chance of occurring if the electron is close to the nucleus. Looking at the plots in Fig. (4.2), we are reminded of the fact that, in general, the electrons having the lowest values of the principal quantum number n will be closest to the nucleus. As we'll see in the next chapter, these electrons will be the ones that behave energetically the most like electrons in a hydrogenic atom, so we're going to come up with an *approximate* answer by assuming that there is only one electron in its ground state ($n = 1$) surrounding the nucleus in each atom—that is, we're going to assume that we can ignore the presence of the other electrons in the atom.

From Eq. (4.52), we have that

$$E_1^{(N)} = E_1^{(H)} \frac{Z_N^2}{1^2} = (-13.6\,\text{eV})\frac{7^2}{1^2} = \boxed{-666.4\,\text{eV}}, \tag{4.53}$$

and

$$E_1^{(Mg)} = E_1^{(H)} \frac{Z_{Mg}^2}{1^2} = (-13.6\,\text{eV})\frac{12^2}{1^2} = \boxed{-1.958\,\text{keV}}. \tag{4.54}$$

Remember that the ionization energy is the minimum energy required to ionize an electron from the atom in question. Recall also that a hydrogenic atom that is barely ionized has an energy $E_\infty = 0\,\text{eV}$. If we wish the nitrogen atom, for example, to make a transition from its ground-state energy of $-666.4\,\text{eV}$ to its ionization state energy of $0\,\text{eV}$, we will need to give it $666.4\,\text{eV}$ of energy from an incident x-ray photon. Therefore, according to our approximate model for these atoms, we would expect that x-ray photons of energies slightly above $670\,\text{eV}$ and $2.0\,\text{keV}$ to have the best chances of undergoing the photoelectric process and contributing to an x-ray image containing soft tissue and bone.

$$\boxed{\textit{End of solution to Example 4.6.}}$$

We have now concluded our discussion of hydrogenic atoms. The ideas of quantum numbers specifying the possible states of the atom, and the idea that those states are described by wavefunctions that give us information about probabilities and allowed energies of the atom, are all important for us to keep in mind as we move on to a discussion of multielectron atoms in the next chapter. It is these atoms that are responsible for many of the behaviors that are exploited in imaging modalities and in cancer treatment planning that we'll be discussing later in this book.

4.8 QUESTIONS, EXERCISES, & PROBLEMS

You will need to be able to access data for various elements in order to complete some of the problems below. You have already been referred to the NIST tables for Atomic Weights and Isotopic Compositions within this chapter.[10] A wealth of information on the various elements can be found in other NIST tables. If you do an online search for *NIST Elemental Data Index and Periodic Table*, one of the first entries should take you to a page on the NIST website with a periodic table on the left. If you click on any element in the table, the box on the right will show you the atomic weight, the ionization energy, and the electron configuration of the atom in its ground state (we'll cover this in the next chapter). Under *Nuclear Physics Data* and then *Isotopic* you will find the same data for that element that you will find in the Atomic Weights table referred to above. Clicking on other links in the box will lead you to lots of other data on the element. Finally, doing an online search for *Fundamental Physical Constants from NIST* will lead you to the latest values for all types of physical constants (Planck's constant, electron mass, proton mass, *etc.*). You will be most interested in *Universal* and *Frequently Used Constants*.

4-1. Use the NIST tables to show that the relative atomic mass (standard atomic weight) of uranium is $A_r(U) = 238.0289$.

4-2. Show that the relative atomic mass (standard atomic weight) of iron is $A_r(Fe) = 55.845$.

4-3. Use Einstein's mass-energy equation, along with the conversion from electron-volts (eV) to joules (J), to show that the mass equivalent of $931.494\,\text{MeV}$ is approximately equal to $1\,\text{u}$.

4-4. Oxygen has an ionization energy of $13.6181\,\text{eV}$. By what percent are we off (that is, find the percent difference) in a calculation of the relative atomic mass of the singly ionized oxygen isotope $^{16}_{8}O^{+}$ if we neglect the mass-energy corresponding to the ionization energy of the ejected electron in the calculation? [*Answer:* approximately $1 \times 10^{-7}\%$—this is *totally* negligible!]

4-5. You find a 65-gram chunk of "pure" copper while out visiting the "ole west". Use data from the NIST Atomic Weights tables to compute the average values of the following: (a) the mass of a single copper atom; (b) the number of atoms per gram of copper; (c) the total number of electrons per gram of copper; and (d) the approximate total number of copper atoms in your 65-g sample. Also, (e) write out in full isotopic notation (including the atomic-number subscript) the naturally occurring isotopes of copper, and, for each isotope, list the number of protons, the number of nucleons, the number of neutrons, and the number of electrons. (These would most conveniently be shown in a table.) [*Answers:* (a) $1.0552 \times 10^{-25}\,\text{kg}$ (b) $9.4770 \times 10^{21}\,\text{atoms/g}$ (c) $2.7483 \times 10^{23}\,\text{electrons/g}$ (d) $6.1601 \times 10^{23}\,\text{atoms}$]

4-6. For an electron traveling at $500\,\text{m/s}$, find its (a) classical value of linear momentum magnitude, (b) classical value of total energy, (c) relativistic value of momentum magnitude, and (d) relativistic value of total energy. [*Answers:* (a) $4.554691 \times 10^{-28}\,\text{kg} \cdot \text{m/s}$ (b) $1.138673 \times 10^{-25}\,\text{J}$ (c) $4.554691 \times 10^{-28}\,\text{kg} \cdot \text{m/s}$ (d) $8.18752 \times 10^{-14}\,\text{J}$]

4-7. For an electron traveling at half the speed of light, find its (a) classical value of linear momentum magnitude, (b) classical value of total energy, (c) relativistic value of momentum magnitude, and (d) relativistic value of total energy. [*Answers:* (a) $1.365496 \times 10^{-22}\,\text{kg} \cdot \text{m/s}$ (b) $1.023439 \times 10^{-14}\,\text{J}$ (c) $1.576739 \times 10^{-22}\,\text{kg} \cdot \text{m/s}$ (d) $9.454132 \times 10^{-14}\,\text{J}$]

4-8. A linac used for radiation therapy accelerates electrons for treatment in a cancer treatment center. (a) Find the speed v of the electrons at which their relativistic momentum is twice their classical momentum. (b) What would the energy setting of the linac have to be (in *MeV*) in order for the electrons to have the speed in part (a)? [*Answers:* (a) $0.866\,c = 2.596 \times 10^{8}\,\text{m/s}$ (b) $0.511\,\text{MeV}$]

4-9. A very important mode of cancer treatment has been treatment using the radiation given off by radioactive cobalt-60 nuclei. The cobalt-60 nucleus ($^{60}_{27}\text{Co}$) is an unstable isotope that decays into an isotope of nickel along with the emission of two electrons and two high-energy photons. The electrons tend to be absorbed by the equipment housing the radioactive cobalt sample and result in a very small dose to the patient. The useful treatment beam is the beam of photons emitted in the decay. These photons have energies of 1.17 MeV and 1.33 MeV. The emitted electrons have a maximum kinetic energy of 0.32 MeV.[4] (a) What are the wavelengths of the emitted photons (in air)? (b) What are the momenta of the emitted photons? (c) What is the maximum momentum of the emitted electrons? (d) What is the minimum deBroglie wavelength of the emitted electrons? [*Answers:* (a) 1.06×10^{-12} m and 9.33×10^{-13} m (b) 6.24×10^{-22} kg · m/s and 7.10×10^{-22} kg · m/s (c) 3.50×10^{-22} kg · m/s (d) 1.89×10^{-12} m]

4-10. The radioactive iodine isotope $^{125}_{53}$I is often used in the treatment of ocular melanoma (eye cancer),[5,6] and is also commonly used in the treatment of prostate cancer[7]. This isotope decays with the emission of a 35.5 keV photon.[4] (a) What is the wavelength of the emitted photon? (b) What would the relativistic kinetic energy of an electron have to be in order for the electron to have the same wavelength as the photon emitted in the decay of I–125? (c) What is the speed of such an electron? [*Answers:* (a) 3.50×10^{-11} m (b) 1.967×10^{-16} J = 1.228 keV (c) $0.0698\,c = 2.09 \times 10^7$ m/s]

4-11. *Mycosis fungoides* is a form of skin disease in which lesions can cover large areas of the body, if not the total body surface. Relatively low energy electron beams only penetrate the body to a depth of about 1 cm and are therefore useful in treating skin lesions. In the case of large-area lesions such as mycosis fungoides, the pre-scribed treatment may involve a total skin irradiation by electron beams. Consider a treatment beam consisting of electrons having a kinetic energy of 3.0 MeV. (a) What is the speed of the electrons in this beam? (b) What is the momentum of the electrons? (c) What is the deBroglie wavelength of the electrons? [*Answers:* (a) $0.989\,c = 2.97 \times 10^8$ m/s (b) 1.86×10^{-21} kg · m/s (c) 3.57×10^{-13} m]

4-12. In the solution to Ex.(4.4b) starting on p.94, the relativistic momentum of electrons in a linac was found from the relativistic energies. The speed of the electrons was then solved for in terms of the relativistic momentum. Derive the analytical result that was given in that solution. That is, starting with the equation for the relativistic momentum $p_{rel} = \gamma m_e v$, show that $v = p_{rel}c/\sqrt{p_{rel}^2 + m_e^2 c^2}$.

4-13. It was stated in this chapter that, in general, relativistic equations should be used when determining momentum and energy values of a particle if the speed of the particle satisfies $v \gtrsim 0.1\,c$. Show that this is equivalent to the following relation for the relativistic kinetic energy of the particle in terms of its rest energy: $E_{K,rel} \gtrsim 0.02\,E_{rel,0}$.

4-14. Recall that an atom has a size of about 10^{-10} m = 1 Å. It was stated in the solution to Ex.(4.5) that electrons having a kinetic energy of about 100 eV have a corresponding deBroglie wavelength that is about the same size as an atom. Perform calculations to prove that this is true. (Davisson and Germer used electrons of en-ergy 54 eV to demonstrate diffraction effects using nickel, which has a crystal lattice spacing of about 0.091 nm.) *Hint:* Do you need to use relativistic equations to solve this problem? (See the previous problem statement.)

4-15. *Fact 1:* There is a fundamental theorem in introductory physics called the *Work-Energy Theorem*. This theorem simply states that the net work done on an object is equal to the change in kinetic energy of the object. This theorem is valid whether the motion of the object is classical or relativistic. Also remember that "*work done on*" an object is the same thing as "*energy transferred to*" that object. ***Fact 2:*** We don't know how much mass/energy there is in the universe, but we do know one thing about it: *it is finite*. Use these two facts to determine the amount of work it would take to accelerate a particle of mass m from rest up to the speed of light, c. Then reason that it must be concluded from your result that no material object can be accelerated up to, let alone beyond, the speed of light in a vacuum.

4-16. Figure (4.3) on p.109 shows a scaled energy-level diagram for an isolated hydrogen atom for the states having principal quantum numbers $n = 1, 2, \ldots, 7$. Verify the energy levels shown in the figure by computing the energies for each of the listed states. Also compute the energy difference between adjacent energy states. Note how quickly the energy differences decrease with increasing principal quantum number, as can be seen in the figure.

4-17. (**This problem involves calculus.**) The wavefunctions for hydrogenic atoms can be broken up into three parts: a radial wavefunction, $R_{n\ell}(r)$, that depends only on the radial distance r between the nucleus and the electron, an angular wavefunction, which we can symbolically denote $\Omega_{\ell m}(angles)$ and depends only on the angular position of the electron relative to the nucleus, and a temporal part, $T(t)$, which depends only on the time t. We can thus write that $\Psi_{n\ell m}(\vec{r}, t) = R_{n\ell}(r)\Omega_{\ell m}(angles)T(t)$. (We are not concerned with the spin part of the wavefunction here.) For the ground state $(n = 1, \ell = 0)$, the radial wavefunction is given by[8]

$$R_{10}(r) = 2\left(\frac{Z}{a_o}\right)^{3/2} e^{-Zr/a_o}, \tag{4.55}$$

where Z is the atomic number of the atom and a_o is the Bohr radius. (a) Construct a computer plot of the ground-state radial wavefunction $R_{10}(r)$ for hydrogen. To keep the numbers on the axes nicer, plot $a_o^{3/2} R_{10}(r)$ on the vertical axis, and plot r/a_o on the horizontal axis (this gives r values in units of a_o). Your horizontal axis should extend from $r/a_o = 0$ up to $r/a_o = 6$. (Be careful of your axis labels.) (b) It was stated in this chapter that the radial probability density, $P_{n\ell}(r)$, can be obtained from the wavefunction for the state of interest. It turns out that the radial probability density comes from the radial part of the full wavefunction according to the equation $P_{n\ell}(r) = r^2 R_{n\ell}^2(r)$. Using this information, construct a computer plot of the ground-state radial probability density, $P_{10}(r)$, for hydrogen. Again, to make the axis numbers nicer, on your vertical axis you should plot $a_o P_{10}(r)$, and on the horizontal axis you should once more plot r/a_o. The horizontal axis should again extend from 0 up to 6. (Be careful of your axis labels.) Does the resulting plot agree with what is shown in Fig. (4.2) on p.107? (c) Use the equation for $P_{10}(r)$ from part *(b)* to find an equation for r_1, the value of r where $P_{10}(r)$ has its maximum value. Does the result agree with the value seen in Fig. (4.2) and with that calculated from Eq. (4.48)? What is the physical significance of the value of r_1?

4.9 REFERENCES

1. Symon KR. *Mechanics*. 3rd ed. Reading, MA: Addison-Wesley Publ. Co.; 1971.
2. National Institute of Standards and Technology (NIST). Data Tables. http://www.nist.gov/pml/data/comp.cfm. Accessed March 8, 2018.
3. Einstein A. Zür Elektrodynamik bewegter Körper. *Annalen der Physik*. 1905;17:891-921.
4. Khan FM. *The Physics of Radiation Therapy*. 4th ed. Philadelphia: Lippincott Williams & Wilkins; 2010.
5. Bomford CK, Kunkler IH. *Walter and Miller's Textbook of Radiotherapy: Radiation Physics, Therapy and Oncology*. 6th ed. Edinburgh: Churchill Livingstone; 2003.
6. Hendee WR, Ibbott GS. *Radiation Therapy Physics*. 2nd ed. St. Louis: Mosby-Year Book, Inc.; 1996.
7. Washington C, Leaver D. *Principles and Practice of Radiation Therapy*. 3rd ed. St. Louis: Mosby; 2010.
8. Woodgate GK. *Elementary Atomic Structure*. 2nd ed. New York: Oxford University Press; 1983

CHAPTER 5

Atomic Physics II: Multielectron Atoms

CONTENTS

As was mentioned previously, the majority of atoms in the human body are hydrogen atoms. Therefore, in order for us to understand the formation of an image when x-rays are incident on a human body, we will certainly have to understand how x-rays can interact with hydrogen atoms, which means that it is important for us to understand the structure and possible energy states of these atoms. On the other hand, as we'll see later in this book, x-rays are produced in a clinical linear accelerator (or *linac*) by means of interactions between incident high-energy electrons and the atoms in a tungsten target. It will therefore also be very important for us to understand the structure and possible energy states of atoms such as tungsten if we wish to understand the interactions between the incident electrons and the tungsten atoms. But an understanding of more complex atoms such as tungsten is based on an understanding of hydrogen, which explains why we spent all of Chapter 4 building up our understanding of the energy states of hydrogen atoms. Having worked through the last chapter, we are now ready to move on to the complications that arise when there are more than one electron orbiting the nucleus in a multielectron atom.

5.1   AN INTRODUCTION TO MULTIELECTRON ATOMS

Recall from the previous chapter that the solution of the relativistic wave equation in quantum mechanics—the Dirac equation—leads naturally to four quantum numbers: n (the *principal quantum number*), ℓ (the *orbital angular momentum quantum number*), m_ℓ (the *z-component of orbital angular momentum quantum number*, or the *magnetic quantum number*), and m_s (the *z-component of spin angular momentum*

DOI: 10.1201/9781003477457-5

quantum number, often just called the *spin quantum number*). The possible values of these quantum numbers are given again below in Table (5.1) for convenience.

TABLE 5.1: The hydrogenic quantum numbers

Symbol	Possible Values
n	$1, 2, 3, \ldots$
ℓ	$0, 1, 2, 3, \ldots, n-1$
m_ℓ	$-\ell, -\ell+1, \ldots, 0, \ldots, \ell-1, \ell$
m_s	$-\frac{1}{2}, +\frac{1}{2}$

Atoms are complicated systems, and it's a non-trivial task to solve the Dirac equation for even the simplest of atoms, hydrogen. The solution to the Dirac equation for hydrogen gives us the wavefunctions for hydrogen corresponding to the different allowed states of the atom—as specified by the quantum numbers—along with the corresponding energies of these states. As was mentioned in the last chapter, adding even one more electron to the system—shifting from hydrogen to helium in the periodic table—renders the equations of quantum mechanics analytically unsolvable.

The Results for Multielectron Atoms are Approximations

So we now have a bit of a problem. We have the periodic table spread out before us, and we have just come to the realization that the only atom whose quantum mechanical equations can be solved analytically is hydrogen—the first, and the simplest in the entire table. What do we do now? How can we possibly understand the structure and behaviors of the rest of the elements if we can't solve the quantum mechanical equations describing them?

The answer is that we must make *approximations*. If you can't solve an equation exactly, then you make reasonable approximations that allow you to find an approximate solution. Then you analyze the approximate answers that you obtain. If the answers that you get with your approximate model of the system are valid—that is, if they agree reasonably well with experimental results—then the approximations were good ones, and you can move forward with your model. If the results are not good, on the other hand, then your approximation must be abandoned or revised.

Since the only atom whose quantum mechanical equations can be solved exactly is hydrogen, we make the approximation that the solutions (the possible wavefunctions and energies) for other, more complicated atoms have the same forms as the hydrogenic solutions. This means that, in our approximate model for multielectron atoms, we assume that the wavefunctions are characterized by a set of four quantum numbers, just as in hydrogen, and we assume that they have the same relations as those given in Table (5.1).

Comparison between the predictions resulting from this approximate model for multielectron atoms and the corresponding experimental findings shows that the approximate model works very well, assuming that appropriate revisions are taken into account for the interactions between the various electrons that do not exist in hydrogen. We will therefore adopt this model and move forward under the assumption that the quantum mechanical wavefunctions for multielectron atoms are very similar in basic structure to those of hydrogen. This means that we can adjust the results for the single-electron hydrogen atom in appropriate ways for our discussion of multielectron atoms.

The Pauli Exclusion Principle

Since our understanding of multielectron atoms comes in part from our assuming that the electrons in a multielectron atom occupy hydrogen-like orbitals, we can envision determining the electron configuration of a multielectron atom in its ground state by simply placing the electrons into the available hydrogen-like quantum states. Before attempting to do so, however, we must discuss the Pauli Exclusion Principle.

The *Pauli Exclusion Principle* states that no two electrons within a single system (atom) can occupy the same quantum state at the same time. Since a quantum state can be specified by the values of its quantum numbers, we can see that the Pauli Exclusion Principle is telling us that no two electrons in the same atom can have the same set of four quantum numbers at the same time—at least *one* of the quantum numbers must be different.

An electron belongs to a broad class of particles in physics called *fermions*. All fermions have spin quantum numbers $m_s = \pm\frac{1}{2}$. Electrons, protons, and neutrons are all fermions. The Pauli Exclusion Principle applies to all fermions, not just to electrons. Thus, we could restate the Pauli Exclusion Principle to say that no two identical fermions in the same quantum system can occupy the same quantum state at the same time. The fact that protons and neutrons must also satisfy the Pauli Exclusion Principle will play an important role in our discussion of nuclear physics in the next two chapters.

As a result of the allowed values for the four quantum numbers as given in Table (5.1), we introduce the following terminology:

- An *orbital* consists of all quantum states having the same values of n, ℓ, and m_ℓ. There are therefore 2 quantum states per orbital (one for each spin direction).

- A *subshell* consists of all quantum states having the same values of n and ℓ. There are therefore $2(2\ell + 1)$ quantum states per subshell.

- A *shell* consists of all quantum states having the same value of n. There are therefore $2n^2$ quantum states per shell.

These statements, along with the Pauli Exclusion Principle, tell us how many electrons can be added into a given *shell* (given value of n), *subshell* (given values of n and ℓ), or *orbital* (given values of n, ℓ, and m_ℓ).

The first statement above is easy enough to understand: for given values of n, ℓ, and m_ℓ—for example, for $n = 3$, $\ell = 1$, and $m_\ell = -1$—we could have $m_s = +\frac{1}{2}$ or $m_s = -\frac{1}{2}$, giving us *two* possible quantum states corresponding to the given values of n, ℓ, and m_ℓ. See if you can understand the reasoning for the second statement above. (You will be asked to prove the second and third statements in the homework.) As an example (*not a proof!*) of the third statement, refer back to Eq. (4.44) in the previous chapter in which all of the possible states for the $n = 3$ shell were listed (except for the two possible m_s values). Note that there are $2n^2 = 2 \cdot 3^2 = 18$ possible states.

Using Letters to Specify a Subshell

Things would get very tedious when specifying the quantum states of all of the electrons in an atom if we had to list the values of all four quantum numbers for each electron in the atom. To avoid having to do this, a shorthand spectroscopic notation is commonly used. An important part of this notation is the use of a *letter* to represent the value of the orbital angular momentum quantum number ℓ. This assignment of letters is given in Table (5.2) for the four lowest values of ℓ.

TABLE 5.2: Letters used to represent values of ℓ

Value	Letter	Historical Interpretation
$\ell = 0$	s	sharp
$\ell = 1$	p	principal
$\ell = 2$	d	diffuse
$\ell = 3$	f	fine

Table (5.2) shows the historical interpretations of the values of ℓ that came from a study of atomic spectra—that is, from a study of the various colored "lines" in the light given off by atoms after it passed through a diffraction grating. Each "line" corresponds to a different transition between the possible energy states of the atoms. (We'll discuss atomic spectra later in this chapter.) The lines in the spectra were described as looking "sharp", or "diffuse", *etc.* While these interpretations are no longer used, the letters play a fundamental role in spectroscopic notation and the specification of electron configurations in atoms.

We have already seen that there are $2(2\ell + 1)$ quantum states corresponding to a given value of ℓ (and n), which means that in a subshell with a given value of ℓ we can have up to $2(2\ell + 1)$ electrons. Table (5.3) shows the maximum number of electrons that can be in the given subshells, while Table (5.4) shows the maximum number of electrons allowed in a given shell for $n = 1$ through $n = 4$.

TABLE 5.3: Maximum number of electrons per subshell, $2(2\ell + 1)$

Letter	Value	Maximum Number of Electrons
s	$\ell = 0$	$2(2 \cdot 0 + 1) = 2$
p	$\ell = 1$	$2(2 \cdot 1 + 1) = 6$
d	$\ell = 2$	$2(2 \cdot 2 + 1) = 10$
f	$\ell = 3$	$2(2 \cdot 3 + 1) = 14$

Specifying Electron Configurations

We are now in a position to see how to build the configuration of, and the corresponding spectroscopic notation for, the states of the electrons for the ground state of a given atom. We start with the lowest energy levels, which tend to be the states

TABLE 5.4: Maximum number of electrons per shell, $2n^2$

Shell	Maximum Number of Electrons
$n = 1$	$2 \cdot 1^2 = 2$
$n = 2$	$2 \cdot 2^2 = 8$
$n = 3$	$2 \cdot 3^2 = 18$
$n = 4$	$2 \cdot 4^2 = 32$

having the lowest values of n and ℓ, although the energy of a state does not always increase if the value of n or ℓ is increased, especially for $n > 3$.

To start off, we write the *numerical* value of n, followed by the *letter* representing the value of ℓ. This letter is then followed by a *superscript* that represents the number of electrons in that subshell. If there is only one electron in the subshell, then the 1 superscript tends to be suppressed. (The values of m_ℓ and m_s are typically not included in spectroscopic notation.) For example, $3p^4$ would mean that there are four electrons in the $n = 3$, $\ell = 1$ subshell; we would say that there are four electrons in the $3p$ state.

Since the hydrogen atom in its ground state has one electron in the $n = 1$, $\ell = 0$ state, it follows that the electron configuration for the ground state of hydrogen could be represented by $1s^1$, or simply $1s$. Helium, with its two $n = 1$, $\ell = 0$ electrons, would then have an electron configuration given by $1s^2$.

Noting from Table (5.3) that an s-subshell can contain at most two electrons, and from Table (5.4) that the maximum number of electrons in the $n = 1$ shell is also 2, we can see that the third electron in lithium will have to go into the next shell ($n = 2$). Thus, the electron configuration for lithium is written $1s^2\,2s$. Noting that the configuration for helium comprises a filled shell (the $n = 1$ shell), we can look at the lithium configuration as consisting of a helium core (He $= 1s^2$) with a single $2s$ electron outside of it, so we could write the electron configuration for lithium using the following slightly more concise notation: [He]$2s$.

Table (5.5) was generated for the elements from hydrogen through aluminum ($Z = 13$) using these ideas of building the electron configuration for ground-state atoms. Note the shorthand notation as a given shell or subshell fills up. This shorthand is typically used to denote an especially stable core, such as a noble gas (helium, neon, argon, *etc.*), with extra electrons orbiting about it. We can appreciate from Table (5.5) how the shorthand notation can really be beneficial in the case of large-Z atoms.

This Method for Electron Configurations Does Not Always Work

This scheme for filling electron quantum states proceeds up through argon (Ar; $Z = 18$), after which the subshells start filling in different orders than expected based on our discussions above—typically as a result of the deep penetration of outer-lying s-subshells into the electron clouds of inner-shell electrons. (We'll discuss the penetrating property of outer-lying s-subshells later in this chapter.)

TABLE 5.5: List of electron configurations for the ground-state atoms through Z = 13

Element	Z	Spectroscopic Notation	Shorthand
H (hydrogen)	1	$1s$	
He (helium)	2	$1s^2$	
Li (lithium)	3	$1s^22s$	$[He]2s$
Be (beryllium)	4	$1s^22s^2$	$[He]2s^2$
B (boron)	5	$1s^22s^22p$	$[He]2s^22p$
C (carbon)	6	$1s^22s^22p^2$	$[He]2s^22p^2$
N (nitrogen)	7	$1s^22s^22p^3$	$[He]2s^22p^3$
O (oxygen)	8	$1s^22s^22p^4$	$[He]2s^22p^4$
F (fluorine)	9	$1s^22s^22p^5$	$[He]2s^22p^5$
Ne (neon)	10	$1s^22s^22p^6$	$[He]2s^22p^6$
Na (sodium)	11	$1s^22s^22p^63s$	$[Ne]3s$
Mg (magnesium)	12	$1s^22s^22p^63s^2$	$[Ne]3s^2$
Al (aluminum)	13	$1s^22s^22p^63s^23p$	$[Ne]3s^23p$

Example 5.1: The Electron Configuration of Potassium

As discussed at the end of Chapter 2, radiation can be used for imaging purposes or to kill cancer cells in tumors, but we must remember that it can also be the cause of cancer. As a result, exposure to various forms of radiation, from medical x-rays to sun exposure, should be minimized whenever possible. But even if we were to somehow completely shield ourselves from external sources of radiation, our bodies would still be susceptible to radiation damage. This is a result of the fact that there are sources of radiation *inside* our bodies. About 0.18% of all of the atoms in our body are potassium (chemical symbol = K; $Z = 19$).[1] Most of these are the stable K-39 isotope. But a small percentage (about 0.011 7%) are the radioactive isotope K-40, which emits radiation (electrons and high-energy photons) when it decays.[2] (We'll learn about radioactive decay in the next chapter.) Discuss the electron configuration of potassium.

Solution:
Before we discuss the electron configuration of potassium, let's talk about the electron configuration of argon (Ar: $Z = 18$). As we can see in Table (5.5), the last electron in aluminum ($Z = 13$) is starting to fill the $3p$ subshell. Since the p subshell corresponds to $\ell = 1$, we know that there are $2(2\ell + 1) = 6$ quantum states available in this subshell. Thus, we would expect to be filling up the $3p$ subshell as we proceed from $Z = 13$ through $Z = 18$, which is argon. This is indeed what happens, so the electron configuration of argon is $[Ne]3s^23p^6$, exactly as we would expect.

Now let's move on to potassium. We've seen that the last electron in argon completed the $3p$ subshell. But the maximum value of ℓ for the $n = 3$ shell is $\ell_{max} = n - 1 = 2$, which, according to Table (5.2), is a d-subshell. We would therefore expect the extra electron in potassium to go into the $3d$ subshell, resulting in an electron configuration for potassium of [Ar]$3d$. But this is not the case. The electron configuration of potassium is actually found to be given by [Ar]$4s$.

Why does the last electron in potassium go into the $4s$ subshell instead of the $3d$ subshell, as we would expect? The answer lies in the differences between the probability density distributions for an s subshell and for a d subshell. The (classical) orbit of an s electron in a multi-electron atom penetrates through the electron clouds of the other electrons all the way into the nucleus. Because of this, the deeply penetrating s orbits correspond to electrons that are more tightly bound to the nucleus than even d electrons in a shell having a smaller value of n—especially for higher-n electrons. The deeply penetrating characteristic of s electrons is a result of the fact that s-electron states have zero angular momentum. This will be discussed in much more detail in §5.3 of this chapter.

$\boxed{\textit{End of solution to Example 5.1.}}$

Building off of the previous example, we end this section by mentioning that the electron configuration of calcium (Ca: $Z = 20$) is [Ar]$4s^2$, and that for scandium (Sc: $Z = 21$) is [Ar]$3d4s^2$. We thus see that the $3d$ subshell does not start getting filled until after the $4s$ subshell has been completely filled, as suggested by the discussion above.

5.2 ELECTRON-ELECTRON AND ELECTRON-NUCLEUS INTERACTIONS

Hydrogen is the only atom that we really understand in the sense that it is the only atom whose wavefunction can be solved for exactly from the Schrödinger equation or from the relativistic Dirac equation. No other atom can be solved analytically without making some serious assumptions and simplifications. As a result, everything that we do in trying to understand other atoms ends up being based on hydrogen. Thus, as we saw previously, we treat all of the quantum states to be filled by successive electrons in multielectron atoms as being hydrogen-like states to the extent that they are described by the same set of four quantum numbers. This is apparently not a bad approximation, since we get results that compare well with experimental results.[a]

The Problem with More Than One Electron
Let's consider the simplest multielectron atom—a two-electron helium-like atom (that is, any atom with $Z \geq 2$ having only two electrons). With only one electron, we have true hydrogenic states. The electron sees the point-like bare nucleus and, in its ground state, orbits that nucleus in a $1s$ orbital. When a second electron is added, it also goes into a $1s$ orbital for the ground state configuration, except that its (z-component of) spin is opposite to that of the first electron. (Remember that the two available s-states correspond to $m_s = \pm\frac{1}{2}$.) While we might be tempted to think of each of

---

[a]Some types of approximations involving angular momentum coupling can result in different angular momentum quantum numbers, but there are still four quantum numbers in total.

these electrons as being in two regular hydrogenic $1s$ states corresponding to the given value of Z, this would be quite wrong. Let's see why.

The Orbit-Orbit Interaction

We first make an obvious observation—namely, that the two (negative) electrons in a helium-like atom repel one another due to the Coulomb force. Thus, for the sake of this discussion, if we were to consider the two electrons to be moving in classical orbits, we would see that, as one electron moves to one side of the nucleus, the other electron is most likely to be found on the opposite side. The orbit of one electron therefore effectively dictates the orbit of the other electron in the sense that the two electrons are most likely to be found on opposite sides of the nucleus at all times. Since the orbit dictates the orbital angular momentum for the electrons, we say that the orbital angular momentum of one electron is *coupled* to the orbital angular momentum of the other electron. This is the so-called *orbit-orbit interaction* between the two electrons in a helium-like ion.

The Spin-Orbit Interaction

There is also an important interaction between each of the electrons in the atom and the nucleus, other than the obvious attractive Coulomb interaction. Let's consider the interaction between a single electron and the nucleus. We can understand the fundamentals of this interaction by again invoking a classical view of the orbit. The electron orbits the nucleus from the point of view of the nucleus. However, in the electron's frame of reference, the electron is stationary while the nucleus orbits around it in the opposite direction. (See Fig. 5.1.) But the motion of the nucleus about the electron acts like a current loop around the electron, where the direction of the current flow is the direction of motion of the nucleus as seen by the electron. We further know that this effective nuclear current flow will result in a magnetic field in the region of the electron.

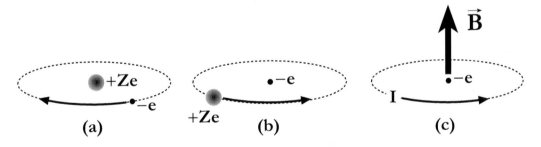

FIGURE 5.1: The origin of spin-orbit coupling. (a) The electron orbits the nucleus from the point-of-view of the nucleus. (b) The nucleus orbits the electron from the point-of-view of the electron. (c) The motion of the positive nucleus constitutes a current, I, which creates a magnetic field $\vec{B}$ at the position of the electron.

The electron has a magnetic dipole moment as a result of its spin, which means that it acts like a little bar magnet—or compass needle—in the magnetic field caused by the nucleus. Thus, the electron will experience a torque trying to align its magnetic dipole moment with the nuclear magnetic field. This torque results in a coupling between the spin magnetic dipole moment of the electron and the orbit of the nucleus as viewed by the electron. But the orbit of the nucleus around the electron is really just the orbit of the electron around the nucleus viewed from the electron's reference frame. The torque is therefore really the result of a coupling between the electron's spin magnetic dipole moment and its own orbit about the nucleus. We can thus view this as a coupling between the spin magnetic dipole moment and the orbital angular momentum of the electron itself, sometimes referred to as *LS coupling*, or the *spin-orbit interaction* between the electron and the nucleus.

Other Interactions

There are still other perhaps more subtle interactions going on, too. For example, the orbit of one electron around the nucleus causes a current loop and associated magnetic field with which the spin magnetic dipole moment of the other electron can interact; this is the so-called *spin-other orbit interaction*. Also, since the electron spin magnetic dipole moments act like little bar magnets, they also produce their own magnetic fields, so we can have a *spin-spin interaction* in which the spin of one electron interacts with the magnetic field resulting from the spin of the other electron. In addition, the nucleus itself can also sometimes have a spin magnetic dipole moment, in which case we can also have a *spin-nuclear spin interaction*.

Of the interactions just discussed, the orbit-orbit interaction, the spin-other orbit interaction, and the spin-spin interaction are all a result of there being two electrons in the helium-like atom. (The spin-orbit interaction also occurs in hydrogenic atoms since it is an electron-nucleus interaction.) The result of all of this is that, with even just two electrons in the atom, the picture is significantly more complex than in single-electron hydrogenic atoms—imagine the interactions that are taking place in the tungsten atom in which there are 74 electrons!

There is no way that we can think of the two $1s$ electron states in helium-like atoms as being just two single hydrogenic $1s$ states. Indeed, one could argue that we really have no business even using the notation for hydrogenic states in multielectron atoms—the states in multielectron atoms are simply much more complicated. Nevertheless, we find that, by using the hydrogen atom states as a beginning model, we can come to a good understanding of the structure and behavior of the significantly more complicated multielectron atoms. It is always important to keep in mind, however, that whatever descriptions of the multielectron energy states we use, they are always an *approximation*—there is simply no way that we can take all of the interactions into account when trying to understand these atoms.[b]

Since our discussion has centered around the picture of an electron orbiting a nucleus, all of our discussions above of the various interactions have relied on a simple

---

[b]Different so-called *coupling schemes* in atomic physics or theoretical chemistry take into account just some of these coupling interactions while neglecting others that are less dominant in the atom under study. These coupling schemes can then result in a variety of hybrid electron orbitals that can differ as a result of which interactions were taken into account. Which of these are correct? *None* of them—they are all approximations! But these approximations can nevertheless help elucidate some aspects of the atomic structure that result from the interactions incorporated into the coupling schemes.

classical (that is, not quantum mechanical) description of the atom. Nevertheless, we can still get a good understanding of some of the interactions between the electrons and nuclei from such a picture. However, there is another effect that is related to the orbit-orbit interaction that results from a quantum mechanical picture of the electrons—the so-called *nuclear screening* effect. We will discuss this effect after the next section, which discusses the classical view of electron orbits for quantum mechanical states.

5.3 CLASSICAL ORBITS AND QUANTUM STATES

In the next section, we will discuss the screening of the nucleus by inner-shell electrons in multielectron atoms. In order for us to be able to understand and apply the ideas of nuclear screening to electronic energy levels, however, it will be important for us to have a basic understanding of electronic orbits about the nucleus for different quantum states—in particular, we must understand the significance of the angular momentum quantum number ℓ as far as the orbits are concerned. That is the purpose of this section.

The very concept of an "electron orbit" in an atom is a classical one, since the quantum mechanical picture of an electronic orbital is a stationary electron cloud surrounding the nucleus. Our discussion in this section is therefore going to be within the realm of classical mechanics. In the next section we will see how these classical ideas of angular momentum and orbits apply to the quantum mechanical picture of electron clouds.

Classical Angular Momentum
Recall from introductory physics that the *angular momentum* of an object is given by the equation

$$L = I\omega, \tag{5.1}$$

where L is the angular momentum, I is the moment of inertia of the object as it rotates or revolves about a given axis, and ω is the angular frequency of rotation or revolution.[c] The moment of inertia is a measure of not only how much mass is in the object, but it is also a measure of how far that mass is distributed away from the axis of rotation or revolution. Thus, in our classical picture of the electron orbiting the nucleus, the farther the electron is, on average, from the nucleus, the greater will be its corresponding moment of inertia about an axis through the nucleus, which will then tend to increase the electron's orbital angular momentum.

But this is only half of the picture of the orbital angular momentum—we must also consider the angular frequency, ω. For this, we will move on to another simplification: let's consider the case of circular orbits, just to help us get a feel for how the angular frequency of the orbit varies with distance from the nucleus.

Consider an electron in a circular orbit of radius r about the nucleus, as shown in Fig. (5.2). The electron moves with speed v; the charge on the electron is $-e$, while

---

[c]Recall that an object *rotates* about an axis that passes through that object and that it *revolves* about an axis that is external to the object.

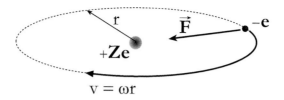

FIGURE 5.2: An electron of charge $-e$ orbits a nucleus of charge $+Ze$ in a circular orbit of radius r. The Coulomb electrical force $\vec{F}$ supplies the centripetal force required to hold the electron in its circular motion.

the charge on the nucleus is $+Ze$. As a result, there is a Coulomb force of attraction between the electron and the nucleus.

The magnitude of the force of attraction supplies the centripetal force that is needed to keep the electron moving in its (assumed) circular orbit:

$$k\frac{(e)(Ze)}{r^2} = m_e\frac{v^2}{r}, \tag{5.2}$$

where m_e is the mass of the electron and k is the Coulomb's law constant ($k = 8.99 \times 10^9 \ N \cdot m^2/C^2$). But, for a circular orbit,

$$v = \frac{2\pi r}{T} = 2\pi\nu r = \omega r, \tag{5.3}$$

where T is the period of the orbit, ν is the orbital linear frequency, and ω is the desired angular frequency. Substituting Eq. (5.3) for v in terms of ω into Eq. (5.2) and solving for the angular frequency yields

$$\omega = \sqrt{\frac{kZe^2}{m_e r^3}}. \tag{5.4}$$

Also, the moment of inertia of an electron of mass m_e moving in a circular orbit of radius r is given by

$$I = m_e r^2. \tag{5.5}$$

Using Eqs.(5.4) and (5.5) in Eq. (5.1) then gives us the following result for the orbital angular momentum, L:

$$L = \sqrt{kZe^2 m_e r}. \tag{5.6}$$

This shows the important result that, as the distance of the electron from the nucleus *increases*, the orbital angular momentum also *increases*. As we've seen, this follows from the fact that the moment of inertia increases more strongly with r than the angular frequency decreases with r.

Zero Angular Momentum States

We can get a little more insight into the orbital angular momentum of the electron by considering an alternate equation[d] for L:

$$L = m_e vr \sin\theta, \tag{5.7}$$

where θ is the angle between the electron's position vector $\vec{r}$ (the vector from the nucleus to the electron) and its velocity vector $\vec{v}$, as shown in Fig. (5.3a). This equation is true whether the electron's orbit is circular or not. For the special case of a circular orbit, we can show that we get exactly the same result for the orbital angular momentum L using Eq. (5.7) as we did using Eq. (5.1).

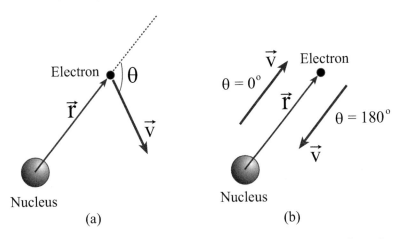

FIGURE 5.3: (a) The set-up for computing the angular momentum of an electron about a nucleus as given by Eq. (5.7). (b) The special case of an s-electron orbit. The electron's velocity would either have to point in the same direction as the electron's position $\vec{r}$ relative to the nucleus ($\theta = 0°$), or opposite to it ($\theta = 180°$).

We have repeatedly stated that the ground state of a hydrogen atom is specified by the quantum numbers $n = 1$ and $\ell = 0$—a so-called $1s$ state. The value $\ell = 0$ means that the angular momentum of the electron must be zero (see Eq. 5.8). What does it mean physically for an electron's orbit to have *zero angular momentum*?

From Eq. (5.1), we see that angular momentum of the electron can be zero if $I = 0$ or if $\omega = 0$. If $I = 0$, then the electron would be inside the nucleus (since r would have to be 0). If $\omega = 0$, it would follow that the electron would not orbit the nucleus at all. In addition, from Eq. (5.7), we see that $L = 0$ if $v = 0$, if $r = 0$, or if $\sin\theta = 0$. Is it possible for us to understand within the confines of our classical model the physical significance of an electronic s-state in which, by definition, the orbital angular momentum is equal to zero? The answer is *yes*.

Within our classical model, if the electron moves along a straight-line path back and forth directly through the nucleus, then that orbit would have zero angular momentum since the electron would not be going *around* the nucleus, and the angular

---

[d]This equation comes from the vector product equation $\vec{L} = \vec{r} \times \vec{p}$, where $\vec{p}$ is the linear momentum of the electron, $\vec{p} = m\vec{v}$.

frequency of its motion about the nucleus, ω, would also have to be *zero*. Alternatively, if the electron were moving back-and-forth along a straight-line path directly through the nucleus, then the angle θ in Eq. (5.7) would either equal 0°, corresponding to motion away from the nucleus, or 180°, for motion toward the nucleus, as shown in Fig. (5.3b). We also note that, for such a path, there would be times at which $v = 0$ as well as times at which $r = 0$—that is, there would be times at which the electron would stop (to turn around), and there would be times at which the electron would be found *inside the nucleus*!

Thus, when thinking of an s-state within our classical model, we will think of the electron moving along a straight-line path directly through the nucleus. As the value of the orbital angular momentum quantum number *increases* above zero, the corresponding value of the orbital angular momentum increases, and the orbit starts becoming elliptical, and then more and more circular. When the orbital angular momentum quantum number reaches its *largest* value ($\ell_{max} = n - 1$), the orbit will be the most circular.

It should be pointed out that, despite the fact that the quantum number ℓ is called the *orbital angular momentum quantum number*, its value in general does not equal the magnitude of the orbital angular momentum of the electron, L. Rather, the two are related by the quantum mechanical equation

$$L = \sqrt{\ell (\ell + 1)}\hbar. \tag{5.8}$$

We note that ℓ and L will only have the same value when $\ell = 0$—that is, for s states.

Comparing the Classical and Quantum Mechanical Pictures

Just to make some connection between the (incorrect) classical model and the (correct) quantum mechanical model, let's consider the s state. From the previous discussion, we know that the s state is a zero angular momentum state and thus represents a linear trajectory through the nucleus. Fig. (5.4a) shows an electron in a classical s orbit, moving back-and-forth along the trajectory shown, straight into and back out of the nucleus. In contrast, the p state represents a more circular orbit, as shown in Fig. (5.4b).

Quantum mechanically, we do not speak of specific trajectories, but rather of probabilities of finding the electron at various positions around the nucleus. The probability of finding the electron in the $1s$ state, for example, is represented pictorially as a fuzzy cloud around the nucleus, as shown in Fig. (5.5), rather than as a well-defined trajectory as shown in the classical case of Fig. (5.4a).

So how can we reconcile the classical and quantum mechanical s states shown in Figs. (5.4a) and (5.5)? We must keep in mind that the quantum mechanical distribution shows the probability of finding the electron in any direction and at any distance from the nucleus. Unless there are other forces around causing the electron to shift toward one side or another, it must have an equal probability of being found in any direction from the nucleus. This explains the spherically symmetric nature of the electron cloud in the $1s$ state.

The classical s orbit shown in Fig. (5.4a), however, is just one possible s orbit—it happens to be drawn heading toward the upper-right from the nucleus. It could just

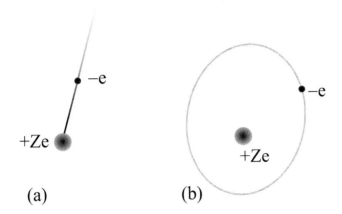

FIGURE 5.4: Classical electron orbits. (a) A classical *s* orbit. (b) A classical *p* orbit.

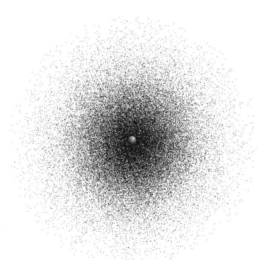

FIGURE 5.5: The quantum mechanical probability cloud corresponding to the 1*s* state of hydrogen. The small sphere at the center is the nucleus.

as well have been drawn toward the left of the nucleus, or heading down toward the lower-right. In order to really compare the classical and quantum representations of an s state, we need to show a representation of all possible classical s states, not just one random one. We should therefore grab the lower end of the s orbit shown in Fig. (5.4a) and swing it about the nucleus in all possible directions. If we could somehow take a time-lapse photograph of this swinging-around motion, we would see a representation very much like the quantum distribution shown in Fig. (5.5).[e]

This comparison between the classical and quantum representations of an s state has given us some insight into the (correct) quantum mechanical probability cloud representing an s state: the density of dots in Fig. (5.5) represents the probability of finding the electron at that location—the greater the density (the darker the cloud), the greater the probability—but we must also keep in mind that this s state represents an electron orbit that dives deep into the center of the atom toward (and possibly into!) the nucleus. This understanding will be very important in the next section.

5.4 NUCLEAR SCREENING AND THE EFFECTIVE ATOMIC NUMBER

Let's consider the two electrons in a helium atom, so that the atomic number is $Z = 2$. We have already discussed a number of the extra interactions that do not occur in hydrogen but do occur in helium because of the presence of the second electron. We are now in a position to appreciate another type of interaction that is related to the orbit-orbit interaction in that it also deals with the repulsive electrical Coulomb force between the two electrons.

Let's imagine labeling the two electrons in the helium atom 1 and 2. Electron 1 is in the $1s$ state, and therefore has a probability distribution like that shown in Fig. (5.5). Electron 2 is in a state that may be a $1s$ state, but it may also be in a higher energy excited state. Whatever the state of electron 2, the energy of this state is dictated not only by the charge on the nucleus (because of the Coulomb force acting between electron 2 and the nucleus) but also by any interactions with electron 1 or any other interactions with the nucleus. (By "interactions" we mean *forces*, which can have *potential energies* associated with them. Any extra interactions undergone by electron 2 can therefore change its total energy.)

Figure (5.6a) represents this situation from the viewpoint of electron 2, which sees the nucleus of charge $+Ze$ (at the center) as well as the probability distribution for electron 1, which is in the $1s$ state. Electron 2 is at some distance r from the nucleus. We can therefore see that the (negatively charged) probability cloud due to electron 1 partially screens electron 2 from the (positively charged) nucleus. Put another way, the pull that electron 2 feels toward the nucleus is diminished by the repulsive negative charge that is close to the nucleus. This means that the probability density cloud of electron 1 effectively reduces the nuclear charge seen by electron 2 by some amount.

It shouldn't come as too much of a surprise to find out that the amount of reduction in the nuclear charge $+Ze$ seen by electron 2 is simply equal to the magnitude

---

[e]It should be pointed out that reconciling the classical orbits with the quantum mechanical probability distributions gets significantly more difficult as the values of n and ℓ increase.

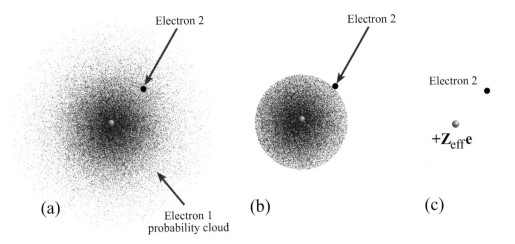

FIGURE 5.6: Modeling of a multielectron atom with an effective nuclear charge. (a) Electron 2 is within the probability density cloud of electron 1. (b) As seen by electron 2, the nucleus is screened only by the charge in that portion of the electron 1 probability distribution that is closer to the nucleus than the distance from the nucleus to electron 2. (c) The net result is that electron 2 sees a nucleus of reduced charge, as represented by the effective nuclear charge $+Z_{\text{eff}}\,e$, with no other electron cloud around it.

of the charge due to the probability cloud of electron 1 that lies within a sphere whose radius is r—the distance from the nucleus to electron 2—as represented in Fig. (5.6b).[f] This reduced nuclear charge seen by electron 2 is expressed in the form $+Z_{\text{eff}}\,e$, where Z_{eff} is the *effective atomic number* for the nucleus as seen by electron 2: $Z_{\text{eff}} < Z$. This effective nuclear charge takes into account the presence of electron 1 as far as the electrical force is concerned, and allows us to view the two-electron helium atom as simply a nucleus of charge $+Z_{\text{eff}}\,e$ with the single electron 2 orbiting about it, as shown in Fig. (5.6c).

Of course, if electron 2 is also in a $1s$ state, then the effective nuclear charge seen by electron 1 as a result of the electron cloud representing the probability density of electron 2 is also given by $+Z_{\text{eff}}\,e$. (If the two electrons are in different states, then they will see different effective nuclear charges.) For example, for each of the two $1s$ electrons in the ground state of helium, we would probably conclude that $Z_{\text{eff}} = Z - 1 = 1$ would be too much of a reduction in the nuclear charge due to the shielding from the other electron—all of the charge from one electron would not screen the second electron from the nucleus, on average. Perhaps $Z_{\text{eff}} = Z - 0.5 = 1.5$ would be more appropriate. The only way to tell for sure is to compare the results of calculations with experimental results.

Since the value of Z_{eff} already takes into account a major interaction between the two electrons in the atom, we could then say that, if we have chosen the value of

---

[f]If you are familiar with Gauss' law for the electric field, then this argument should be reminiscent of your calculations of electric field within a spherically symmetric distribution of charge—this is exactly the same idea.

Z_{eff} wisely, the energy of an electron in a multielectron atom would be given by the hydrogenic equation Eq. (4.52), with Z replaced by Z_{eff}:

$$E_n = E_1^{(H)} \frac{Z_{\text{eff}}^2}{n^2}, \tag{5.9}$$

where Z_{eff} is the effective atomic number of the nucleus as seen by the electron, $E_1^{(H)} = -13.6\,eV$ is the ground-state energy of the electron in atomic hydrogen, as defined previously in Chapter 4, and n is the principal quantum number of the electron that sees the screened nuclear charge and whose energy is being computed.

In the previous discussion we combined both quantum mechanical (the probability density function) and classical (a definite position for electron 2) ideas to form a model of a multielectron atom. Such a model is said to be a *semi-classical* model, since it involves both classical and quantum ideas. Semi-classical models are often used in research to help elucidate interactions within a system and to help aid the researcher in understanding the quantum phenomena being studied.

Example 5.2: The Effective Atomic Number for Helium

The ionization energy for an electron in the ground-state helium atom is found experimentally to be $24.5874\,eV$.[3] Find the effective atomic number for the two $1s$ electrons in helium and comment on your answer.

Solution:

Since the helium atom is in its ground state, both of the electrons must in the $1s$ state. This means that each electron must be shielded from the nucleus by the same amount due to the electron cloud from the other electron, so Z_{eff} must be the same for both electrons.

Since we are using the effective nuclear charge seen by one of the electrons, the atom that we are considering is effectively a one-electron atom with nuclear charge $+Z_{\text{eff}}\,e$—in other words, we are working with a hydrogenic atom. Since the ionization energy of the atom is $E_I = 24.5868\,eV$, it follows that the energy of each electron in the $1s$ state must be $E_{1s}^{(He)} = -E_I = -24.5868\,eV$.[g] From Eq. (5.9), we thus have that

$$E_{1s}^{(He)} = E_1^{(H)} \frac{Z_{\text{eff}}^2}{n^2} = E_1^{(H)} Z_{\text{eff}}^2, \tag{5.10}$$

where $n = 1$ for the $1s$ state. Using the value for the ground state energy of hydrogen given in Eq. (4.51) of Chapter 4 ($E_1^{(H)} = -13.6\,eV$), we get that

$$Z_{\text{eff}} = \sqrt{\frac{E_{1s}^{(He)}}{E_1^{(H)}}} = \sqrt{\frac{-24.5874\,eV}{-13.5984\,eV}} = \boxed{1.34}. \tag{5.11}$$

---

[g]This follows from the fact that the ionization energy for a given state is that energy required to *just* ionize the electron—that is, to raise its energy up to $E = 0$.

Since $Z = 2$ for helium, the effective nuclear screening of one $1s$ electron by the other $1s$ electron is equal to $Z - Z_{\text{eff}} = 0.66$, which is not far from our guess of 0.5 stated earlier. Therefore, this result seems reasonable.

> End of solution to Example 5.2.

5.5 ATOMIC SPECTRA AND ELECTRON TRANSITIONS

There are two types of electromagnetic atomic spectra: *emission* spectra and *absorption* spectra. Both of these types of spectra arise from the fact that the electrons in atoms (and molecules) can only have discrete energies.

Stationary States

The theory of the hydrogenic atom discussed in Chapter 4 was proposed by Niels Bohr in 1913. It is known from electromagnetic theory that accelerated charges emit electromagnetic radiation. If the charge's acceleration is simple harmonic with frequency ν, then the emitted radiation will also have frequency ν. This emission of energy from an accelerated charge caused problems in Bohr's classical model of the atom since the electron is constantly accelerating in its orbit about the nucleus. This means that the electron would constantly lose energy due to the emitted radiation, and would, therefore, readily spiral into the nucleus. This is not found to happen in nature, however, so there must be something fundamentally wrong with the physics— at least in the way it was applied to atoms. The problem, of course, was that *classical* physics was used in Bohr's model of the atom.

In Chapter 4 and in the previous sections in this chapter, we discussed the energy levels available to electrons in atoms. The quantum states corresponding to these energy levels, as specified by the set of four quantum numbers and the associated wavefunctions, are called *stationary states*. The reason for this is that the quantum electron probability distributions (the *electron clouds*) do not change with time as long as the electron remains in a stationary state. This stationary cloud of charge does not move, which means that it does not accelerate, which means that it does not emit electromagnetic radiation. All of this means that Bohr's problem of the atom constantly emitting radiation is gone in a quantum mechanical treatment of the atom, as long as the electrons in the atom remain in stationary states.

Absorption Spectra

An electromagnetic wave is a traveling wave of electric and magnetic fields. These fields exert forces on charges in the region of the wave. Therefore, if an electromagnetic wave passes by an electron cloud in an atom, it will be capable of causing the electron cloud to oscillate with a frequency equal to the characteristic frequency of the electromagnetic wave. However, the electron cloud in a given atom only has certain characteristic frequencies—called *resonant frequencies*—at which it will oscillate as it undergoes a transition from an initial stationary state of principal quantum number n_i to a final stationary state of principal quantum number n_f. These resonant frequencies are given by the equation

$$\nu_{if} = \frac{|E_f - E_i|}{h} = \frac{|\Delta E_{if}|}{h}, \tag{5.12}$$

where E_i is the energy of the initial stationary state, E_f is the energy of the final stationary state, and h is Planck's constant. Frequencies of electromagnetic radiation not equal to one of the resonant frequencies of the electron clouds will not typically affect them, and will therefore simply pass by the atom.

However, if an electromagnetic wave with a frequency ν that is equal to one of the resonant frequencies ν_{ij} of the atom's electron cloud passes by the atom, the electron cloud will start to oscillate with that same frequency ν. This oscillation of the electron cloud can then result in two different outcomes. First, the oscillating cloud can itself radiate electromagnetic radiation at the same frequency ν. From our viewpoint outside of the atom, we simply see the atom scattering the incident radiation, either in the same direction or in a different direction. (This can also happen with incident electromagnetic radiation at a frequency not equal to ν_{ij}, but with a reduced probability.) This type of interaction between the incident radiation and the atom is called *elastic scattering*.

The second possibility is for the electron cloud to absorb energy from the incident electromagnetic wave, in which case the electron ends up in the stationary quantum state having the *higher* energy E_f. From Eq. (5.12), we see that this new energy must be

$$E_f = E_i + \Delta E_{if} = E_i + h\nu_{if} \,. \tag{5.13}$$

In terms of the particle nature of light, we say that the electron in an initial stationary state of energy E_i has absorbed a photon of energy $h\nu_{if} = hc/\lambda = \Delta E_{if}$ and made a transition to a stationary state of higher energy, $E_f = E_i + h\nu_{if}$. The various frequencies or wavelengths of photons that can be absorbed by the electrons in the atom, and which therefore correspond to the various possible transitions between initial and final stationary states of the electrons in the atom, make up what is called the *absorption spectrum* of that atom.

Stimulated Emission

In the case of emission, an electron in an atom that is not in its ground state (the atom is in a higher-energy excited state) starts off in a stationary state of principal quantum number n_i having energy E_i. If there is a stationary quantum state having principal quantum number n_f and energy $E_f < E_i$ that is unoccupied by another electron, then the electron can be induced to make a transition down to the lower available energy state by a photon of frequency

$$\nu = \frac{|\Delta E_{if}|}{h} = \frac{|E_f - E_i|}{h} = \frac{E_i - E_f}{h} = \nu_{if} \tag{5.14}$$

(since $E_i > E_f$). In this case, we have the same scenario as in the case of absorption, except that now the final stationary state involved in the transition has a *lower* energy than that of the initial quantum state. Nevertheless, the incident electromagnetic wave causes the electron cloud to oscillate in a resonant mode. As a result of this oscillation (meaning that the electron cloud is accelerating), radiation of frequency ν_{if} is *emitted* by the electron cloud, resulting in a *decrease* in the energy of the electron to the final energy $E_f = E_i - h\nu_{if}$. That is, the electron has made a transition from an initial state of (higher) energy E_i to a final state of (lower) energy E_f with the emission of a photon of energy $|\Delta E_{if}|$ and frequency $\nu_{if} = |\Delta E_{if}|/h$. This is referred to as the *stimulated emission of radiation* by the atom. (This is the idea behind the LASER—Light Amplification by the *Stimulated Emission* of Radiation.)

Spontaneous Emission

There is another scenario that we must mention at this point—a scenario in which the electron still makes a transition down to an available lower-energy stationary state, but there is not a wave of photons incident on the atom to stimulate the transition.

Let's again consider the excited-state atom with an electron in a higher-energy state of principal quantum number n_i. It is found experimentally that there is a finite probability per unit time—called the *transition probability* or *transition rate*—that the electron will spontaneously make a transition to the available lower energy state. The problem is, however, that the electron is in a stationary state, which we can think of as a kind of equilibrium state—if an electromagnetic wave is not incident on the electron cloud to cause it to oscillate, then the electron will remain in that state indefinitely. So why would the electron cloud possibly undergo oscillations followed by a transition to a lower energy level and the resulting emission of radiation without an electromagnetic wave to encourage it to do so?

The answer is that it wouldn't—and it doesn't. But we can experimentally detect atoms emitting radiation in the absence of an incident electromagnetic wave all of the time. What's going on?

The answer to this apparent paradox lies within the realm of *quantum field theory*, in which the electromagnetic field is quantized to support the existence of packets of light energy, or *photons*—something that does not exist within the classical theory of electromagnetism. To avoid jumping into a discussion of quantum field theory, we will instead endeavor to understand what's going on within the context of the energy-time form of the Heisenberg Uncertainty Principle:

$$\Delta E \, \delta t \geq \frac{\hbar}{2}. \tag{5.15}$$

This form of the uncertainty principle tells us that a change in the energy of a system, ΔE, can take place over a time interval, δt, given by

$$\delta t \geq \frac{\hbar}{2\Delta E}. \tag{5.16}$$

One way to look at this form of the uncertainty principle is to say that it allows the energy of a system to deviate by a small amount ΔE for an interval of time δt no greater than that specified by Eq. (5.16). That is, an extra amount of energy up to the value of ΔE can apparently appear out of nowhere—out of a vacuum—within a time interval δt, and then disappear back into the vacuum by the end of that time interval. Equation (5.16) shows that, the larger the energy deviation, the shorter the time interval over which the deviation may exist. In other words, mass-energy is only conserved to within an energy ΔE and time interval δt as given by the uncertainty relation shown in Eq. (5.15).

One consequence of this interpretation of the Heisenberg uncertainty principle is the prediction of *vacuum fluctuations*, which we can think of as small fluctuations in the energy contained within a region of space. These fluctuations can take place whether the region in question contains energy and particles or not—hence the word *vacuum* in the name of the phenomenon. These fluctuations in energy can manifest themselves as particles and antiparticles, or as photons (electromagnetic waves), apparently appearing out of nowhere (the vacuum) and then, within a short time δt later, disappearing. In these cases, the energy ΔE in Eq. (5.16) is the total rest energy plus kinetic energy of the particles, or the energy $h\nu$ of the photons.[h]

An electron sitting in a stationary state of an atom would stay in that state forever if it were not acted upon by any external influences, such as electromagnetic waves. However, even if we tried to completely isolate the atom to keep it away from any external influences, our attempts at isolation would be futile, since the vacuum fluctuations in the region of space around the atom can result in the creation of electromagnetic waves that can interact with the probability cloud of the electron—albeit for only very short periods of time, as governed by Eq. (5.16). More to the point, such fluctuations can cause the electron cloud to oscillate in a resonant mode with a lower energy state if they have an appropriate frequency, as given by Eq. (5.14). This can then result in the emission of a photon, just as in the case of stimulated emission, except that in this case, the photon that induced the transition is gone by the time the transition is complete. This process is called the *spontaneous emission of radiation*. It's called *spontaneous* since we don't see the photons corresponding to the vacuum fluctuations, and so the atom appears to undergo a transition to a lower energy state on its own—*spontaneously*.

In general, atoms are continuously absorbing, scattering, or emitting photons. The wavelengths or frequencies of the various photons that are absorbed and emitted by an atom comprise what are called the *absorption* and *emission spectra* of the atom. These spectra can be used to identify the type of atom (that is, the *element*) since the characteristic energies or frequencies of the photons that are absorbed and emitted are a reflection of the discrete energies of the stationary states of the electrons in the atom—they act as fingerprints for each element.

5.6 X-RAY SPECTRA

In traditional physics disciplines, the words *x-rays* and *gamma-rays* (γ-rays) both refer to high-energy photons, the distinction between the two usually being their energy: γ-rays have higher energies than x-rays. The cut-off between when a photon is called an *x-ray* photon and when it is called a γ-ray photon is something not well defined, but is typically on the order of several hundred keV.

In radiation oncology physics the distinction is more clear-cut: *x-rays* are high-energy photons that result from *atomic* processes (electron transitions in atoms),

---

[h]It is important to note that, even though mass-energy is not strictly conserved, momentum and total charge *are* strictly conserved in vacuum fluctuations.

whereas *γ-rays* result from *nuclear* processes (transitions between stationary states of protons and neutrons in the nucleus, or the conversion of mass into energy according to $E = mc^2$—we'll discuss this in Chapter 7). This distinction is independent of the energy of the photon. Of course, we will adhere to the radiation oncology physics definition of these terms in this book.

As stated above, when we speak of *x-ray spectra*, we will typically mean the variety of wavelengths of high-energy electromagnetic radiation emitted from atoms as a result of electron transitions within those atoms. We will discuss this method of x-ray generation below. X-rays can also be produced by Coulomb-force interactions between high-speed electrons and high-Z nuclei in tissue or other media that result in accelerations of the electrons. These accelerations will result in the emission of radiation called *Bremsstrahlung*. This will be discussed further in §9.3.

We have seen that photons can be emitted from atoms when an electron in the atom makes a transition from a higher energy state to a lower energy state. But this often does not result in the emission of a *high*-energy photon. By a "high-energy photon" we will mean a photon that has an energy that is significantly greater than the ionization energy of a hydrogen atom in its ground state, $13.6\,eV$. Thus, for example, a 100 eV photon could be considered a high-energy photon, and certainly a 10 keV photon would be considered a high-energy photon. On the other hand, a $10.2\,eV$ photon that can be emitted by a hydrogen atom is clearly not something that we will call a *high*-energy photon. But there is no strict cut-off for what is considered *high* energy.

So how can atoms emit high energy photons?

Let's reconsider a *hydrogenic* atom. Recall that the energy of such an atom with its electron in a stationary state with principal quantum number n is given by

$$E_n = E_1^{(H)} \frac{Z^2}{n^2}, \tag{5.17}$$

where $E_1^{(H)} = -13.6\,eV$ is the ground-state energy for the electron in atomic hydrogen and Z is the atomic number of the atom. Thus, the lowest two energy levels in hydrogen have energies $E_1^{(H)} = -13.6\,eV$ and $E_2^{(H)} = E_1^{(H)}/2^2 = -3.40\,eV$, with an associated energy difference of $\Delta E_{1,2}^{(H)} = 10.2\,eV$.

We then note that, for example, if $Z = 10$ (for *neon*), then the ground-state energy in a hydrogenic neon atom is equal to $E_1^{(Ne)} = 100\,E_1^{(H)} = -1,360\,eV = -1.36\,keV$, with a first-excited-state energy of $E_2^{(Ne)} = -0.340\,keV$ and energy difference $\Delta E_{1,2}^{(Ne)} = 1.02\,keV$. Clearly, the energies associated with transitions in neon are significantly greater than the energies associated with transitions in hydrogen.

Let's keep going and take a look at mercury (*Hg*: $Z = 80$). In this case, we get that $E_1^{(Hg)} = 6,400\,E_1^{(H)} = -87.0\,keV$, $E_2^{(Hg)} = -21.8\,keV$, and $\Delta E_{1,2}^{(Hg)} = 65.2\,keV$.

It should be very clear at this point that high-energy photons can readily be emitted in transitions associated with high-Z atoms. In particular, transitions between low-lying energy levels (small values of n) in high-Z atoms will readily involve high-energy photons, or x-rays.

Since x-rays will be emitted from high-Z atoms when electrons make transitions down to low-lying energy levels, there is a special notation introduced for x-rays that indicates the stationary states involved in the transition that generates an x-ray photon. Table (5.6) shows the special notation used for referring to the low-lying energy levels in atoms.

TABLE 5.6: Energy-level designations for x-rays

Shell	$n = 1$	$n = 2$	$n = 3$	$n = 4$	$n = 5$
Designation	K	L	M	N	O

For example, a K-shell electron simply means an electron having principal quantum number $n = 1$. Noting that the wavelength of the photon associated with a transition of an atomic electron from a state of energy E_i to a state with energy E_f is given by (remember that $E_{photon} = hc/\lambda$)

$$\lambda = \frac{hc}{|\Delta E_{if}|}, \tag{5.18}$$

we can see that the *smaller* the energy difference ΔE_{if}, the *larger* will be the wavelength λ.

When discussing electron transitions from some initial state down to the $n = 1$ state, for example, we refer to K *x-rays*, and list them in the order of largest wavelength (smallest energy) to smaller and smaller wavelengths (increasing energy), using the letters of the Greek alphabet. In particular, K_α (*K-alpha*) refers to the largest wavelength x-ray emitted when an electron makes a transition down to the $n = 1$ energy level, meaning that this must correspond to the $n = 2$ to $n = 1$ transition. Likewise, K_β refers to the next largest wavelength x-ray emitted, corresponding to the $n = 3$ to $n = 1$ transition, *etc.* Table (5.7) summarizes this special notation for x-rays. The energy-level designations and x-ray photon notations are also shown in the energy-level diagrams of Fig. (5.7).

Of course, emitted x-rays do not tend to come from hydrogenic atoms, as this discussion has implied, but they do tend to come from transitions between low-n stationary states in high-Z multielectron atoms. Since inner-shell electrons in high-Z atoms feel a very strong pull from the nucleus, the effects of electron interactions with the other electrons in the atom will be minimal. As a result, we would expect the energy levels to be reasonably well approximated by hydrogenic energy relations, as given by Eq. (5.9).

5.7 AUGER ELECTRON TRANSITIONS

When an inner-shell electron is removed from an atom by, for example, an incoming high-energy electron or photon, the resulting inner-shell vacancy can be filled by the transition of a higher-energy electron in the atom making a transition down to the vacated energy state. In the process, either an x-ray photon can be emitted or an *Auger electron* can be emitted.

TABLE 5.7: X-ray notation used to specify the transitions associated with the emission of the given x-ray photon

Transition	Notation	Comment
$n = 2$ to $n = 1$	K_α	*largest wavelength*
$n = 3$ to $n = 1$	K_β	*next largest wavelength*
$n = 4$ to $n = 1$	K_γ	$\ldots$
$n = 5$ to $n = 1$	K_δ	*etc.*
$n = 3$ to $n = 2$	L_α	*largest wavelength*
$n = 4$ to $n = 2$	L_β	*next largest wavelength*
$n = 5$ to $n = 2$	L_γ	$\ldots$
$n = 6$ to $n = 2$	L_δ	*etc.*
$n = 4$ to $n = 3$	M_α	*largest wavelength*
$n = 5$ to $n = 3$	M_β	*next largest wavelength*
$n = 6$ to $n = 3$	M_γ	$\ldots$
$n = 7$ to $n = 3$	M_δ	*etc.*

Figure (5.8a) shows the lowest three energy levels in a multielectron atom, the K, L, and M shells, using the x-ray notation (which is also used to describe Auger electron emission). The small arrows in the figure represent electrons, and the directions of the arrows represent the spins of the electrons—spin up or spin down. Recalling that each shell of principal quantum number n can hold up to $2n^2$ electrons with spins up and down, we can see that each of the levels shown in Fig. (5.8a) is filled. (This is not necessary for the Auger process to take place.) There may be electrons occupying higher-energy shells than those shown in the figure—that is irrelevant for the present discussion.

Now, as mentioned above, we assume that an inner-shell electron has been ionized by an incoming charged or uncharged particle. In the case shown in Fig. (5.8b), the electron that was removed from the atom was a spin-down K electron. This inner-shell vacancy means that a higher-energy electron can make a spontaneous transition down to fill the vacancy. In the example shown in Fig. (5.8b), it is a spin-down M-shell electron that makes this transition. The energy lost by the M-shell electron as it makes the transition down to the K shell is $|\Delta E_{13}| = E_3 - E_1$. This energy could be released from the atom in the form of a photon—a process known as *x-ray fluorescence*—but in the Auger process the energy is given instead to another electron in the atom—an L-shell electron in this example.

The L-shell electron has an ionization energy equal to $E_{I,L} = |\Delta E_{2\infty}| = E_\infty - E_2 = -E_2 > 0$. If $|\Delta E_{13}| > E_{I,L}$, then it is possible for the transition energy to go into ionizing an L electron, which would be emitted with the excess energy in the form of kinetic energy $E_{k,L} = |\Delta E_{13}| - E_{I,L}$. (Note that these energy expressions are all approximate, as the energies involved all depend on the locations of vacancies in the various shells.)

The specific Auger process that is undergone by an atom can be designated with the use of three letters. These letters correspond to the x-ray designations of the three

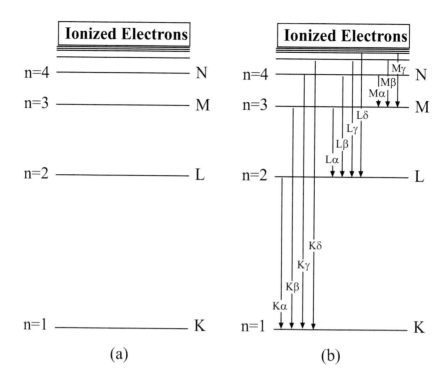

FIGURE 5.7: The generation of x-ray photons. (a) Energy levels for a hydrogenic atom showing the special x-ray designations. (b) Various transitions with the x-ray notation shown. The boxed-in region labeled *Ionized Electrons* is the region for which $E_{electron} \geq 0$.

shells involved in the process, listed in the following order: the shell corresponding to the location of the original vacated electron state, the shell from which the electron made a transition to fill the vacated state, and the shell from which the Auger electron was emitted. For example, the Auger process that is shown in Fig. (5.8b) can be designated *KML*.

Consider a beam of high-energy particles traveling through a medium. These particles can ionize inner-shell electrons, leaving behind inner-shell vacancies. These vacancies can then be filled by electron transitions from higher energy levels down to the vacated state, resulting in the emission of x-ray photons in the case of x-ray fluorescence, or in the emission of Auger electrons. Let N_{ion} represent the number of inner-shell ionizations caused by the incident particles, and let N_{Auger} represent the resulting number of Auger electrons emitted within the material. The *Auger-electron yield*, denoted η_{Auger}, is then defined to be[i]

$$\eta_{Auger} = \frac{N_{Auger}}{N_{ion}}. \tag{5.19}$$

A similar definition gives the x-ray fluorescence yield, η_{x-ray}.

The two processes of x-ray fluorescence and Auger electron emission compete with one another. Auger electron emission dominates for low-Z atoms (typically for

---

[i]η is the Greek letter "eta".

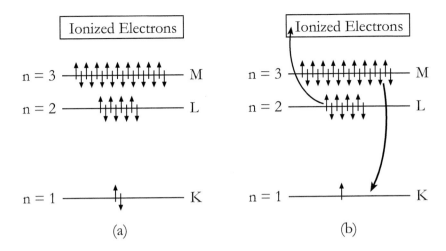

FIGURE 5.8: The Auger electron process. (a) The lowest three energy levels of a multi-electron atom, showing the electron populations in the three filled shells. Note the pairing of spin-up and spin-down electrons. (b) Auger-electron emission results from a vacancy appearing in a lower-shell orbital—in this case, a K ($n = 1$) electron has been ejected from the atom, leaving behind a vacancy. The vacancy is filled with a spin-down electron from the M shell ($n = 3$). Instead of going into a photon, the energy in the transition goes into ionizing an L-shell ($n = 2$) electron—the Auger electron.

$Z < 30$), while x-ray emission dominates for higher-Z atoms. This behavior is clearly displayed in Fig. (5.9),[4] which shows the x-ray (fluorescence) and Auger-electron yields resulting from a vacancy in the K-shell.

Auger Electrons in Radiation Therapy

There is much interest in Auger-electron emitting isotopes within the medical physics community. In particular, isotopes such as iodine-125 (I-125) emit low-energy Auger electrons[j] (about $20 - 500$ eV) that have small ranges of up to about $10\,nm$.[5] These low energies mean that the electrons readily give up their energies to their immediate surroundings. Within tissue, this often means that the electrons deliver their energy within subcellular distances. Thus, if Auger-emitters such as I-125 can be incorporated into cancer-cell DNA, the energy delivered by the emitted Auger electrons can result in death to the cell within which the Auger emitter was situated without any damage to surrounding cells. This is a result of the fact that the emitted low-energy Auger electrons appear to very efficiently cause double strand breaks in DNA molecules.[6]

The emitted Auger electrons seem to have a surprisingly high linear energy transfer (LET), putting them on par with high-LET alpha particles.[7] There appear to be several factors contributing to this, one of which is the cascade of Auger-electron emission that follows the initial Auger emission from an atom.[5] This cascade of Auger

---

[j]The reason why I-125 routinely undergoes Auger-electron emission is because of a process called *electron capture*. We'll study this process in §7.3.

electrons emitted from the same atom results in a higher ionization state of the atom while shifting the electron vacancies to higher energy levels.[8]

It was stated above that Auger electrons are very effective at killing cells as long as they are within very small distances of the DNA—this is because they deposit their energy into tissue within cellular dimensions. The problem is, how are the Auger-electron emitting atoms delivered to the cellular DNA—specifically to the DNA of tumor cells? This is the job of the pharmaceutical agents.[9] Pharmaceutical agents are molecules that are selectively absorbed in certain organs or tissues. Therefore, if an atom that radiates (emits particles) is attached to an appropriate pharmaceutical agent, it will deliver the radiating atom to the desired site. The combination of a pharmaceutical agent with a radiating atom is called a *radiopharmaceutical*.

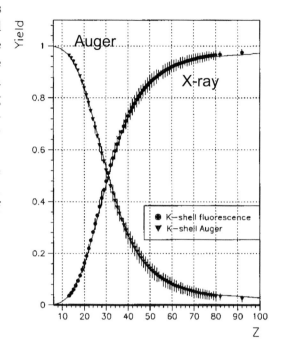

FIGURE 5.9: X-ray (fluorescence) and Auger-electron yields as a function of atomic number, Z, associated with K-shell vacancies. (Revised from Stepanek, with permission.)

A radiopharmaceutical that has attracted much clinical interest is I-UdR (an Auger-electron-emitting I-125 atom attached to 5-iodo-2′-deoxyuridine, which is a thymidine analog).[10] Since thymidine is used in the S phase of the cell cycle in preparation for DNA synthesis, it (and its analogs) is selectively pulled into the region of the cellular DNA.[6] Therefore, I-UdR will deliver the Auger-emitting I-125 atoms to the DNA, which is just what we wanted! A problem, however, is that it will be pulled in toward the DNA of *all* cells, not just tumor cells. Fortunately, I-UdR does not last long in a biological system,[10] so if it is deposited locally to the tumor cells it will be pulled into those cells, but will not last long enough to diffuse to neighboring healthy tissue.

This process has been used clinically for the treatment of glioblastoma in rats. Glioblastoma is a common malignant type of brain tumor that has resisted the standard treatment consisting of surgery, chemotherapy, and radiation therapy in humans. However, clinical trials on rats using the I-UdR radiopharaceuticals have shown very promising results,[10] meaning that Auger-electron emitting radiopharmaceuticals could play an important role in future treatments of cancer in humans.

Chapter 23 will discuss the important topic of radiopharmaceutical therapy.

Example 5.3: Auger Electrons from Gold Shielding

Uveal melanoma is a cancer of the eye originating from the cells that give the iris its color. The standard procedure for treating tumors associated with uveal melanoma is to insert radioactive seeds (small, radioactive sources about the size of a grain of rice)—typically iodine-125—into a silicon plaque. The plaque is then inserted into a gold-alloy backing.[11,12] The entire assembly is then attached to the eye above the tumor. Radiation from the radioactive seeds is then incident on the region of the tumor, while the gold backing keeps radiation from interacting with neighboring healthy tissue. Figure (5.10) shows the components of this treatment modality. (Note the grooves in the silicon plaque into which the radioactive seeds are inserted.)

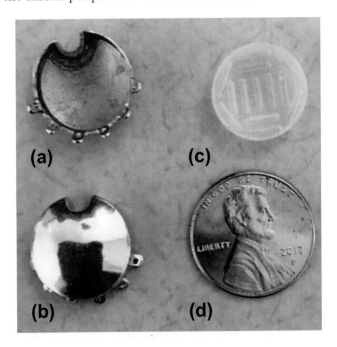

FIGURE 5.10: Plaque and shielding for brachytherapy treatment of uveal melanoma of the eye. (a) The underneath side of the gold shielding. (b) The top of the gold shielding. (c) The silicon plaque that is used to hold the radioactive I-125 seeds. (d) A penny for size comparison. (Photo courtesy of Manuel Morales.)

In addition to Auger electrons, I-125 also emits x-ray photons having energies in the range from 27 to 36 keV.[13] These photons can travel through the silicon plaque and interact with gold atoms in the backing.

The electrons in gold ($Z = 79$) have the following ionization energies (E_I): K-shell ($n = 1$) $E_{I,K} = 80{,}720\,eV$; L-shell ($n = 2$) $E_{I,L} = 14{,}350\,eV$; and M-shell ($n = 3$) $E_{I,M} = 3{,}420\,eV$.[14] Remember that the energies of the electrons in these shells are negative the ionization energies. Thus, for example, $E_1 = -E_{I,K} = -80{,}720\,eV$.

Let's say that an x-ray photon from an I-125 seed ionizes an L-shell electron in a gold atom in the gold-alloy backing. The vacancy thereby formed is then immediately filled by an M-shell electron in the gold atom; an M-shell Auger electron is released during this process.

Find the kinetic energy of the ejected Auger electron.

Solution:

We first note that the x-rays emitted by the I-125 seed could not ionize a K-shell electron in a gold atom, so an L-shell electron is the lowest-energy electron that could be ionized. We also note that the designation for this process is an LMM Auger process.

To find the kinetic energy, $E_{k,M}$, of the Auger electron ejected from the M shell, we must carefully follow where energy is going in this Auger-electron process.[k] We start with the L-shell electron having been ejected. This leaves a vacancy in the L shell. We are told that an electron in the M shell makes a transition down to fill the L-shell vacancy. This means that the M-shell electron has lost an amount of energy during the transition equal to $|\Delta E_{32}| = E_3 - E_2 = (-3{,}420\,eV) - (-14{,}350\,eV) = 10{,}930\,eV$. This energy lost by the M electron must first of all ionize the other M-shell electron; any energy left over must then supply the kinetic energy of the M Auger electron. Thus, $|\Delta E_{32}| = E_{I,M} + E_{k,M}$. It therefore follows that $E_{k,M} = |\Delta E_{32}| - E_{I,M} = 10{,}930\,eV - 3{,}420\,eV = 7{,}510\,eV = \boxed{7.51\,keV}$.

$$\boxed{\textit{End of solution to Example 5.3.}}$$

We should note some approximations implicitly made in the previous example solution. First of all, we have treated the energy levels as if they were hydrogenic, which they are not. Electron-electron interactions, such as the spin-orbit interaction, cause the different states within the L and M shells to have slightly different energies. Also, when an electron is ionized leaving behind a vacancy, the shielding of the nucleus by other electrons will change, as will the electron-electron interactions within the atom, all of which will change the energy levels from the values given (which were for a ground state, neutral gold atom). Our result is therefore an approximate result.

All of this points out the complexity of multielectron atoms. Nevertheless, a fundamental understanding of these complicated systems is important for an appreciation of various treatment modalities in radiation therapy.

5.8 QUESTIONS, EXERCISES, & PROBLEMS

5-1. (a) Prove that the maximum number of electrons that can occupy a subshell is $2(2\ell + 1)$. (b) Prove that the maximum number of electrons that can occupy a shell is $2n^2$. *Hint:* Note that

$$\sum_{i=0}^{N} i = \frac{N(N+1)}{2}. \tag{5.20}$$

5-2. In Ex.(5.1) we discussed the specification of the electron configuration for potassium (K). The electron configuration for gold $(Z = 79)$ is listed as $[Xe]\,4f^{14}fd^{10}6s$.

---

[k]Be very careful of the notation being used here: $E_{I,K}$ is the ionization energy of the K shell, while $E_{k,M}$ is the kinetic energy of the M-Auger electron.

(a) What is meant by [Xe]? (b) Xenon ($Z = 54$) is a noble gas, meaning that all of its occupied subshells are *completely* occupied. (Recall that a shell is all electrons having the same n value; electrons in the same subshell have the same n and ℓ values. If a subshell is filled, then all of the electrons in that subshell must be paired—spin up with spin down.) Look up and write down the explicit electron configuration for xenon. (That is, do not exploit shorthand notation like [Kr] in the configuration!) (c) Explain in terms of electron orbitals and energies why it is reasonable for the $5s$ and $5p$ subshells to be occupied before the $4f$ subshell contains *any* electrons, as is the case with xenon.

5-3. Just below Eq. (5.7) it is stated that, "For the special case of a circular orbit, we can show that we get exactly the same result for the orbital angular momentum L using Eq. (5.7) as we did using Eq. (5.1)". Show that this is, indeed, the case.

5-4. (a) Explain the difference between *stimulated emission* and *spontaneous emission*. (b) The *transition probability* for a given pair of quantum states in an atom is the probability that an electron in the upper-energy state will make a transition down to the lower-energy state per unit time (unit: s^{-1}). The *lifetime* of an excited state is defined as the average time spent by an electron in that state before making a transition down to a specific (unoccupied) lower-energy state (unit: s). Explain why it is reasonable that the transition probability and the lifetime are reciprocals of one another for a given pair of states. (Your explanation should be more involved than simply referring to the units.) (c) The average lifetime of an atomic state is on the order of $10^{-8}\, s$. What is the corresponding transition probability for such a state? (d) A *metastable state* is an electronic state that has a (relatively) long lifetime of up to $10^{-3}\, s$. What is the transition probability of such a metastable state?

5-5. In the discussion of Fig. (5.6), the following statement was made: "For example, for each of the two $1s$ electrons in the ground state of helium, we would probably conclude that $Z_{\text{eff}} = Z - 1 = 1$ would be too much of a reduction in the nuclear charge due to the shielding from the other electron—all of the charge from one electron would not screen the second electron from the nucleus, on average. Perhaps $Z_{\text{eff}} = Z - 0.5 = 1.5$ would be more appropriate". Clearly explain in your own words why $Z_{\text{eff}} = 1.5$ would be more appropriate for a ground-state helium atom than $Z_{\text{eff}} = 1$.

5-6. In Ex.(5.3) we computed the kinetic energy of an Auger electron in an LMM Auger process. Within the statement of that example, we were given the ionization energies for electrons in the K, L, and M shells for the ground-state, neutral gold atom. Compute the effective atomic numbers, Z_{eff}, for electrons in each of these shells, and comment on your answers.

5-7. *Brachytherapy* is a cancer-treatment modality in which radioactive *seeds* are implanted, either temporarily or permanently, into or next to the tumor being treated. (Brachytherapy will be discussed in Chapter 22.) One of the radioactive nuclides used in brachytherapy is palladium-103 (^{103}Pd). ^{103}Pd decays by means of electron capture, which means that the nucleus actually captures and holds onto an electron that was orbiting the nucleus. (a) Explain how the nucleus can capture an orbiting electron. *Hint:* The most likely electrons to be captured are s electrons. (b) After capturing a K-shell electron, the ^{103}Pd atom tends to emit x-rays with energies in the range from 20 to 23 keV, along with some Auger electrons. This all primarily results from an initial transition of an L-shell electron down to fill the K-shell vacancy left after the electron capture. Estimate (*make an educated guess*) the values of Z_{eff} for the single K electron and the L electrons before the L-electron transition. Then use these values to compute the expected energy of an x-ray that would be emitted as a result of the $L - K$ transition. How does your answer compare with the x-ray energy range given above? (c) Is palladium more likely to emit x-rays or Auger electrons in the $L - K$ transition after K-electron capture? Why? (d) If an Auger electron were emitted in the $L - K$ transition, what approximate kinetic energy would you expect it to have? Assume a KLL Auger process.

5-8. The energy differences between the lowest two hydrogenic energy levels in hydrogen, neon, and mercury were computed in §5.6. Verify these calculations, and then compute the wavelengths of the photons emitted in the transitions from $n_i = 2$ to $n_f = 1$ in these three hydrogenic atoms.

5-9. *"The Auger process is a three-electron process that leaves behind a doubly ionized atom"*. Describe the Auger process in your own words, and, in light of your description, explain the statement above. (A good diagram will help your description.)

5-10. The process of Auger emission is often followed by the emission of photons of various wavelengths.[15] Explain why this is the case. What also could be emitted other than photons?

5-11. (a) In addition to an atom often emitting a series of photons after Auger emission, it is also possible for it to emit a series, or *cascade*, of Auger electrons.[8] Explain why. (b) The following statement is given in the text: "This cascade of Auger electrons emitted from the same atom results in a higher ionization state of the atom while shifting the electron vacancies to higher energy levels". Explain this statement. (Good diagrams will help your explanation.)

5-12. Sketch an energy-level diagram similar to that shown in Fig. (5.8b) for each of the following Auger processes. (a) KLL (b) KLM (c) LMM

5-13. What would you expect the cell survival curve for Auger-electron induced damage to DNA to look like after Auger-electron-emitting I-125 atoms have been deposited in the vicinity of DNA by radiopharmaceuticals such as I-UdR? Why? (*Hint:* See §3.3.)

5.9 REFERENCES

1. United Nations Scientific Committee on the Effects of Atomic Radiation. *Sources and Effects of Ionizing Radiation, UNSCEAR 2000 Report to the General Assembly, Vol. 1.* (p. 94) New York: United Nations; 2000.

2. de Laeter JR, Böhlke JK, de Bièvre P, et al. Atomic Weights of the Elements: Review 2000 (IUPAC Technical Report). *Pure Appl. Chem.* 2003;75(6):747-748.

3. Kramida, A., Ralchenko, Yu., Reader, J., and NIST ASD Team. NIST Atomic Spectra Database (ver. 5.2). http://physics.nist.gov/asd. Accessed July 12, 2017.

4. Stepanek J. Methods to determine the fluorescence and Auger spectra due to decay of radionuclides or due to a single atomic-subshell ionization and comparisons with experiments. *Med. Phys.* 2000;27(7):1544-1554. doi: 10.1118/1.599020. PMID: 10947257.

5. Sastry KS. Biological effects of the Auger emitter iodine-125: A review. Report No. 1 of AAPM Nuclear Medicine Task Group No. 6. *Med. Phys.* 1992;19(6):1361-1370. doi: 10.1118/1.596926. PMID: 1461198.

6. Bodei L, Kasses AI, Adelstein SJ, and Mariani G. Radionuclide Therapy with Iodine-125 and Other Auger-Electron-Emitting Radionuclides: Experimental Models and Clinical Applications. *Cancer Biotherapy & Radiopharmaceuticals.* 2003;18(6):861-877. doi: 10.1089/108497803322702833. PMID: 14969599.

7. Booz J, Paretzke HG, Pomplun E, Olko P. Auger-electron cascades, charge potential and microdosimetry of iodine-125. *Radiat Environ Biophys.* 1987; 26(2): 151-162. doi: 10.1007/BF01211409. PMID: 3615808.

8. Partanen L. *Auger Cascade Processes in Xenon and Krypton Studied by Electron and Ion Spectroscopy. Report Series in Physical Sciences, Report No. 46.* Oulu, Finland: University of Oulu; 2007.

9. Knapp FF, Dash A. *Radiopharmaceuticals for Therapy.* New Delhi: Springer India; 2016.

10. Thisgaard H, Halle B, Aaberg-Jessen C, et al. Highly Effective Auger-Electron Therapy in an Orthotopic Glioblastoma Xenograft Model using Convection-Enhanced Delivery. *Theranostics.* 2016;6(12):2278-2291. doi:10.7150/thno.15898.

11. Washington C, Leaver D. *Principles and Practice of Radiation Therapy.* 3rd ed. St. Louis: Mosby; 2010.

12. Chiu-Tsao ST, Astrahan MA, Finger PT, et al. Dosimetry of ^{125}I and ^{125}Pd COMS eye plaques for intraocular tumors: Report of Task Group 129 by the AAPM and ABS. *Med. Phys.* 2012;39(10):6161-6184.

13. Bomford CK, Kunkler IH. *Walter and Miller's Textbook of Radiotherapy: Radiation Physics, Therapy and Oncology.* 6th ed. Edinburgh: Churchill Livingstone; 2003.

14. Bearden JA, Burr AF. Reevaluation of X-Ray Atomic Energy Levels. *Rev. Mod. Phys.* 1967;39(1):125-142.

15. Shapiro PR, Bahcall JN. X-ray Absorption and the Post-Auger Decay Spectrum of Multielectron Atoms. *Astrophysical Journal.* 1981;245:335-349.

CHAPTER 6

Nuclear Physics I: Structure and Stability

CONTENTS

It would not be too misleading to say that the *Physics* part of *Medical Physics* is the physics involving nuclei. Whether it's high-energy photons or charged particles interacting with nuclei (Chapters 8 and 9), or nuclei emitting high-energy photons and charged particles (Chapter 7), nuclei are at the heart of the most important clinical applications of physics within the field of Medical Physics. The purpose of this chapter is to lay the foundation upon which our understanding of nuclear interactions and emissions will be built.

6.1 STRUCTURE AND SIZE OF THE NUCLEUS

Recall that a neutral atom consists of a positively charged nucleus surrounded by a negatively charged cloud of electrons. As we have already seen, the size of an atom depends greatly on the states occupied by its electrons, but in general we can think of an atom as being on the order of $10^{-10}\,m$ in diameter.

Recall that the mass number A tells us the total number of protons plus neutrons in the nucleus—that is, it tells us the total number of *nucleons* in the nucleus. We have seen that the isotopic notation for a specific nucleus, or *nuclide*, can be written in several forms: $^{A}_{Z}X$, ^{A}X, or simply X–A. We therefore know that the nucleus of an atom whose isotopic notation is $^{A}_{Z}X$ contains A nucleons. The number of protons in the nucleus is the *atomic number*, Z, which is also the number of electrons orbiting the nucleus in the neutral atom. As mentioned previously, the atomic number specifies the *element*. While, for a given element, the value of Z cannot change, the value of A—and, therefore, the neutron number $N = A - Z$—*can* change. Nuclei of the same

DOI: 10.1201/9781003477457-6

element but differing in the value of their neutron numbers, N, are said to be different *isotopes* of that element.

The size of the nucleus is, of course, determined by the number of nucleons it contains. The radius of a nuclide, R, is found from experiment to be given approximately by

$$R \cong r_o A^{1/3}, \tag{6.1}$$

where $r_o = 1.2 \times 10^{-15}\, m$. Noting that one *femto-meter*, $1\, fm$, also called one *fermi*, is defined to be

$$1\, fm \equiv 1 \times 10^{-15}\, m, \tag{6.2}$$

we can write that $r_o = 1.2\, fm$. From this we see that the smallest nucleus is the ^1_1H isotope of hydrogen, which has a radius of

$$R\left(^1\text{H}\right) \cong r_o\left(1\right)^{1/3} = 1.2\, fm, \tag{6.3}$$

while a large isotope such as the uranium isotope $^{239}_{92}\text{U}$, for example, has a radius approximately equal to

$$R\left(^{239}\text{U}\right) \cong r_o\left(239\right)^{1/3} = 7.4\, fm. \tag{6.4}$$

An average-size nucleus—for example, the isotope $^{65}_{29}\text{Cu}$—has a radius

$$R\left(^{65}\text{Cu}\right) \cong r_o\left(65\right)^{1/3} = 4.8\, fm. \tag{6.5}$$

We can note two things from these simple calculations. First, that the size of the nucleus does not vary very much, despite the fact that the number of nucleons can change by a factor of over 200, and second, that the radius of an average nucleus is on the order of $10^{-15}\, m$.

The Quantum Fuzziness of Nuclei

As with atoms, it may at first be tempting to think of nuclei as small, hard spheres—especially since so many nucleons can be crammed into such a small volume. But this is not true. Quantum particles are known for their "fuzziness" due to their associated probabilistic nature, and nuclei are no exception. We know that nuclei are made up of protons and neutrons—positively charged and neutral quantum particles, respectively. So would it be more reasonable to consider these constituents of nuclei as hard spheres? Since electrons are much smaller than protons or neutrons, they can be used to probe for signs of an inner structure to these larger particles. In particular, the extent to which very fast electrons are deflected, or scattered, by the inner structure of nucleons and nuclei gives us hints of that inner structure.

Consider Fig. (6.1),[1] which shows a very interesting and, perhaps, surprising graph. This plot is a result of neutron experiments performed at various labs around the world using the technique of fast-electron scattering, as described above.[1] It

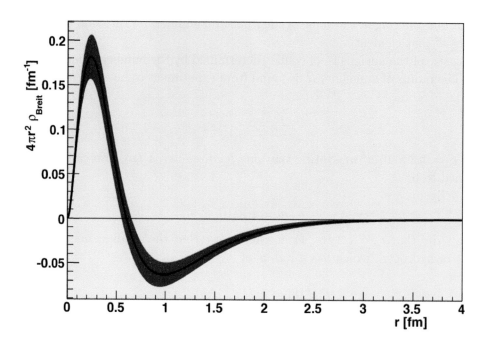

FIGURE 6.1: A plot of the charge per unit distance within a thin spherical shell of radius r as a function of the distance r from the center of a neutron. The shaded region around the solid curve denotes the uncertainties in the measurements. (Open Access: DOE/NSF Nuclear Science Advisory Committee.)

basically shows the charge contained within thin spherical shells of varying radii r within the neutron, with $r = 0$ taken to be at the center of the neutron.[a]

The first thing that's surprising about this graph is that there is any charge at all—a neutron is supposed to be neutral! The graph shows that there is *positive* charge within the neutron up to a distance of about $0.6\,fm$, with a charge density maximum at about $0.2\,fm$. So far this looks like what we might expect for the charge distribution inside a *proton*, not a neutron. But then, at about $0.6\,fm$, the charge distribution becomes *negative*, with the largest (magnitude) negative charge density at a distance of just beyond $0.9\,fm$ from the center of the neutron. The negative charge then fades out as r reaches $3\,fm$ and beyond. Note that there is no definite cut-off in the charge distribution of the neutron—it just gradually fades away. This is a sign of the quantum fuzziness, and the fact that there are both positive and negative regions inside the neutron implies that the neutron is made up of other things—it has an internal structure. We now know that those other things are *quarks*.

---

[a]Just to be clear, the thin spherical shell is taken to have a radius r, a thickness dr, and a volume $dV = 4\pi r^2\, dr$. (If the thin spherical shell were a soap bubble, the volume dV would be the volume of the soapy water forming the bubble.) If the charge-per-unit-volume of the neutron at a distance r from the center is $\rho = dQ/dV = dQ/(4\pi r^2\, dr)$, then the plot in Fig. (6.1) is a plot of $dQ/dr = 4\pi r^2 \rho$ vs. r.

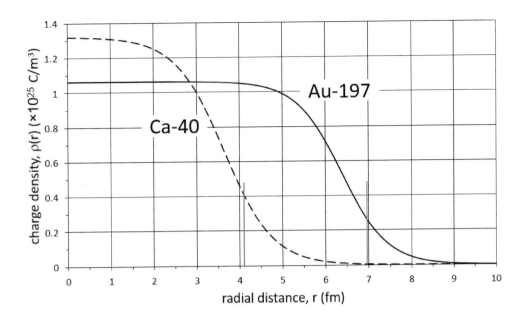

FIGURE 6.2: Charge density (in units of $10^{25}\,C/m^3$) as a function of distance from the center of the nucleus for calcium $\left(^{40}_{20}Ca\right)$ and gold $\left(^{197}_{79}Au\right)$. The data for these curves were obtained from the Fermi model with parameters to fit data from scattering experiments of high-energy electrons aimed at the nuclei. (Hofstadter; ref. 2.) The short vertical lines show the nuclear radii, R, for Ca-40 and Au-197 from Eq. (6.1).

Likewise, if we use fast electrons to map out the charge distribution in nuclei as a function of distance from the center, we find a similar quantum fuzziness. Figure (6.2) shows plots of volume charge density, ρ (*charge-per-unit-volume*; C/m^3) as a function of radial distance, r, for two different nuclei: the smaller calcium nucleus $^{40}_{20}Ca$, and the larger gold nucleus $^{197}_{79}Au$. (These plots were created using the Fermi model for nuclear charge densities with parameters given in Hofstadter[2] and Srivastava[3].) Note the region of near constant charge density toward the center of the nucleus followed by the gradual drop-off into the "quantum fuzziness". It is also interesting to note that the smaller, lower-Z nucleus has the larger central charge density.

We saw in Eq. (6.1) how to compute the radius of a given nuclide. The question now is, what does this radius even mean in light of Fig. (6.2), which clearly shows that the nucleus doesn't have a definite size, but rather just fizzles out? The answer is that the value of R given in Eq. (6.1) does give us some useful information—it tells us basically the extent of the charge and mass distribution within the nucleus. The short, vertical line segments shown in Fig. (6.2) at around 4 and 7 fm show the locations of the R values for the calcium and gold nuclei, respectively. We can see that these locations are the positions of the charge density reaching roughly 20–30% of its maximum value for a given nuclide.

6.2 NUCLEON ENERGIES

We saw in our discussion of quantum mechanics in Chapter 4 that any confined particle will have discrete energy levels characterized by one or more quantum numbers, depending on the dimensionality of the space associated with the confinement. For electrons in atoms, we found that there were four quantum numbers (corresponding to the four dimensions of relativistic spacetime) that were needed to specify the quantum states of the electrons. Different values of the quantum numbers specified different quantum states that, in general, had different energies associated with them. We also saw that any electron in an excited state could make a transition down to an available lower-energy state with the associated emission of a photon or electron of appropriate energy. In this sense, we may think of these photons and electrons as *atomic emissions.*

To get a very rough idea of the amount of energy associated with these atomic emissions (and thus of the associated electron transitions), we can exploit the position-momentum form of the *Heisenberg Uncertainty Principle*, which states that

$$\Delta r \Delta p_r \geq \frac{\hbar}{2}, \tag{6.6}$$

where the quantity $\hbar$ is the reduced Planck constant, $\hbar = h/2\pi = 1.05 \times 10^{-34} \, J \cdot s$. We are using the symbol r to denote the radial distance out from the center of the nucleus. In this equation, Δr represents the uncertainty inherent in the radial coordinate of an electron confined in the atom (due to its "quantum fuzziness"—the quantum mechanical probability distribution), and Δp_r represents the uncertainty inherent in the radial component of the electron's momentum—that is, its component of momentum directly toward or away from the nucleus.

We really don't know much more about the electron's position other than that it's somewhere in the atom, so we can say that, very roughly, $\Delta r \sim 10^{-10} \, m$. It then follows that

$$\Delta p_r \sim \frac{\hbar}{2 \, \Delta r} = 5 \times 10^{-25} \, kg \, \frac{m}{s}. \tag{6.7}$$

The electron's kinetic energy is given by

$$E_k = \frac{1}{2} m_e v^2 = \frac{1}{2m_e} \left(m_e v \right)^2 = \frac{p^2}{2m_e}, \tag{6.8}$$

where m_e is the electron's mass: $m_e = 9.11 \times 10^{-31} \, kg \cong 10^{-30} \, kg$. The electron's kinetic energy gives us a rough idea of the size of its total energy, $E_{atomic\,electron}$. If we use the uncertainty in p_r as a rough estimate of the magnitude of the momentum itself (the momentum will have to be *at least* this big in order to have that uncertainty), then we get from Eq. (6.8) that

$$E_{atomic\,electron} \sim \frac{\Delta p_r^2}{2m_e} \cong 1 \times 10^{-19} \, J \cong 0.6 \, eV. \tag{6.9}$$

(Recall that $1.0\,eV = 1.6 \times 10^{-19}\,J$.) This tells us that the energy of the electrons—and thus the energy associated with transitions between the allowed states of the electrons in the atom—will be on the order of *electron-volts*, eV.[b]

Now, let's do the same type of calculation for a nucleon in the nucleus. Since the radius of a typical nucleus is about $10^{-15}\,m$, we use $\Delta r \sim 10^{-15}\,m$, so that

$$\Delta p_r \sim \frac{\hbar}{2\Delta r} \cong 5 \times 10^{-20}\,kg\frac{m}{s}\,. \tag{6.10}$$

This then leads to energies on the order of

$$E_{nucleon} \sim \frac{\Delta p_r^2}{2m_n} \cong 6 \times 10^{-13}\,J \cong 4 \times 10^6\,eV = 4\,MeV\,, \tag{6.11}$$

where we have used the mass of a nucleon to be about $m_n \cong 2 \times 10^{-27}\,kg$.

This *very* approximate argument has led us to some useful information—namely, that we expect energies of atomic emissions to be on the order of *electron-volts* (which we saw in Chapter 4), and that the energies associated with the nucleons within the nucleus will be more on the order of *mega-electron volts*, *MeV*—a huge difference! Thus, if there are nuclear emissions, we expect the associated energies to be significantly larger than the energies of atomic emissions.

6.3   THE STABILITY OF NUCLEI

Many nuclei that are useful in the field of medical physics are not stable, and many of the unstable nuclei that are useful are not naturally occurring. We will address the ideas of stable and unstable nuclei in the remainder of this chapter. The topic of how to produce useful nuclei that are unstable and not naturally occurring will be addressed in the next chapter.

A plot of N *vs.* Z (*neutron number vs. atomic number*) for all the stable nuclei is shown in Fig. (6.3). (Data for this plot were taken from Audi and Wapstra.[4,5]) The line corresponding to $N = Z$—for nuclei having the same number of neutrons as protons—is added for reference.

There are two characteristics of this curve that are worth noting. The first is that the stable nuclides form a well-defined path through the graph of N *vs.* Z, called the *line of stability*. The second is that this path clearly bends away from the $N = Z$ line—the greater the value of Z, the more it bends away into the region of $N > Z$.

Those Amazing Stable Nuclei

That there even exists any stable nuclei other than the hydrogen nucleus with only one proton is amazing. To get an idea of just how amazing this is, let's first consider the two protons confined within a helium nucleus, He-4. Since $A = 4$, we get from Eq. (6.1) that $R \cong 1.9\,fm$, so that the two protons are about $2\,fm$ apart.

---

[b]This very "hand-wavy" argument using the Heisenberg Uncertainty Principle gives us, at best, a very rough idea of the sizes of things, but it can nevertheless provide useful information when all that is needed is an order-of-magnitude estimate, such as in this discussion.

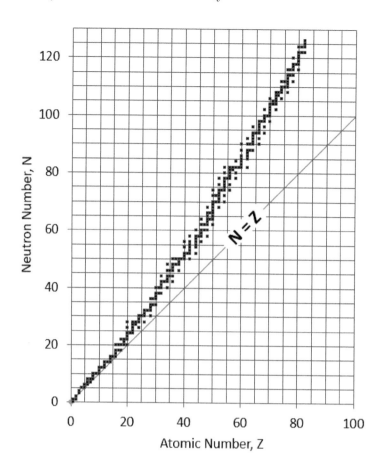

FIGURE 6.3: A plot of Neutron Number (N) vs. Atomic Number (Z) for the stable nuclides. The $N = Z$ line is drawn in for reference.

The electrical (Coulomb) force of repulsion trying to push the two protons away from each other and out of the nucleus is thus

$$F_E = \frac{k\,(e)\,(e)}{R^2} \cong 58\,N\,, \tag{6.12}$$

where $k = 9.0 \times 10^9\,Nm^2/C^2$ is the Coulomb's law constant. OK—this result may not seem very amazing, but let's think about this a bit more. A force of 58 N is a very *macroscopic* force—it corresponds to a weight of about 13 lbs. All of this force trying to push apart the two halves of a fuzzy ball that is about 10^5 times smaller than the smallest thing visible with an electron microscope! *Still* not impressed?—OK, we'll take this a step further. Let's consider a uranium nucleus.

Uranium-238 ($^{238}_{92}U$) is a nearly stable nucleus (it typically takes on the order of a billion years to decay)[6] that has a radius of about 7 fm. To simplify our calculations, let's say that we split the uranium nucleus into two halves, each of charge $+46e$, and separated by a distance of about 7 fm. The force trying to push these two halves apart is then approximately equal to

$$F_E = \frac{k\,(46e)\,(46e)}{R^2} \cong 9,950\,N\,,\qquad(6.13)$$

which corresponds to a weight of over one *ton* at the Earth's surface. It really is amazing that the nucleus doesn't just blow apart! Which begs the question, "So why doesn't the nucleus blow apart?"

The Strong Nuclear Force

There are two mechanisms responsible for the stability of the nucleus—two mechanisms that are like the two sides of the same coin. One is the attractive *strong nuclear force*, which is one of the four fundamental forces of nature.[c] The other is the nuclear binding energy.

The strong nuclear force acts only between nucleons, pulling them toward one another independent of whether they are charged (protons) or uncharged (neutrons). This force has a magnitude that is about 100 times that of the electrical force.[7] It also has a very short range—the strong nuclear force between two nucleons very quickly goes to zero as the two nucleons get further apart than about 2.5 fm. This has important consequences as far as the stability of the nucleus is concerned in that it means that the strong nuclear force is a *saturated* force. Let's see what this means.

We discussed above the electrical forces pushing the protons apart within the nuclei for the cases of helium and uranium. Note that the electrical force depends on the product of the two charges involved and on the distance-squared between the two charges: as the number of proton charges increases the force increases, and as the distance increases the force continuously and gradually decreases.

This is not the case with the strong nuclear force. The strong nuclear force drops off quickly to zero as the distance between two nucleons increases beyond 2 fm to about 3 fm, so that only nucleons that are *nearest neighbors* can interact via the strong nuclear force. Since this is the case, as more nucleons are added to form larger nuclei, the strength of the strong nuclear force does not increase for many nucleons within the nucleus. This is a result of the fact that nucleons that are not nearest neighbors to the added nucleons do not even know that more nucleons are around, as far as the strong nuclear force is concerned—the nuclear force that they feel remains constant. In this sense, we say that the strong nuclear force has become *saturated*.

One more comment about the strong nuclear force is in order before we move on. If the strong nuclear force is such a strong force pulling neighboring nucleons together, and if the nucleons are fuzzy balls as a result of being quantum particles, why doesn't the strong nuclear force pull the nucleons into one another? The answer is that the strong nuclear force is only a strong attractive force as long as the distance between the nucleons is between about 1 fm and 2.5 fm. Beyond 2.5 fm the force rapidly decreases until it is effectively zero beyond 3 fm. The interesting thing, however, is that the force becomes very strongly *repulsive* for distances less than about 0.5 fm.[7] This means that the nucleons effectively have a hard core that will only allow them

---

[c]In order of decreasing strength, the four fundamental forces of nature are the *strong nuclear force*, the *electromagnetic force*, the *weak nuclear force*, and the *gravitational force*.

to be squeezed together to a certain extent—beyond that point, the strong nuclear force keeps them from being compressed any further.

Now that we have discussed the basic properties of the strong nuclear force, we are in a position to understand, at least in part, the tendency of the N vs. Z graph of stable isotopes to bend above the $N = Z$ line—that is, the tendency for larger nuclei to have more neutrons than protons. Since the protons tend to push the nucleus apart and make it more unstable, adding more neutrons will add more "nuclear glue" by means of the strong nuclear force without adding more of the repulsive electronic force, thereby increasing the stability of the nucleus.

Assembling a He–4 Nucleus

To gain an understanding of the other mechanism for stabilizing nuclei, let's consider the stable helium-4 isotope as an example. He–4 ($^{4}_{2}$He) has 2 protons and therefore $4 - 2 = 2$ neutrons in its nucleus. If we were to add the mass of 2 protons to the mass of 2 neutrons, we would get a mass that is *greater than* the mass of the $^{4}_{2}$He nucleus! *How can this be?*

The explanation is straight-forward and related to our discussion of the strong nuclear force. Let's start with the constituent nucleons that make up the nucleus far apart from one another, and let's assemble the nucleus one nucleon at a time. We are interested in the energy that it takes for us to assemble the He–4 nucleus.

We bring in the first proton and place it at what we'll call the origin, where it remains fixed. Assuming the absence of any external fields, it takes us no work to accomplish this. We then move the second proton in toward the origin with a constant velocity. This proton is, of course, repelled by the first proton, so it takes us some positive amount of work to push the second proton with a constant velocity closer and closer to the first proton. Then, as we get the second proton to within about 3 fm from the first proton, the attractive strong nuclear force starts contributing to the net force acting on the second proton. This means that the net force trying to push the second proton away from the first is reduced. As we continue to push the second proton closer to the first, the strong nuclear force gets even stronger, but still not strong enough to overpower the $1/r^2$-behavior of the Coulomb repulsion between the two protons. By the time the second proton is in position at about 1 fm from the first proton, the net work that we have had to do—W$_{first\,proton}$ + W$_{second\,proton}$—is *positive*, meaning that we had to *add energy* to the system to get these two protons together; the energy of the system has *increased*. That means that this system is *unstable*, since the energy of the combined two-proton system is greater than the energy of the isolated protons, which was *zero*. Systems always tend toward configurations of *lower energy*. Thus, the protons want to be as far away from one another as possible. But, for the sake of this discussion, we imagine fixing the second proton in position while we continue to assemble the He–4 nucleus.

Now we bring in the first neutron. It has no net charge, so there is no Coulomb force acting on it, and it takes us no work to bring it in close to the two protons, until we get to within reach of the strong nuclear force, which then grabs it and starts pulling it in. This means that we have to pull back on the neutron to keep it from rushing into the two protons—we have to do a significant amount of *negative* work to move the neutron into position in the nucleus. It turns out that the *total* amount of work that we have to do up to this point, $W_{first\,proton} + W_{second\,proton} + W_{first\,neutron}$, is *negative*. The fact that we have to do net *negative* work to assemble what is at this point a $^3_2$He nucleus means that the energy of this system is *less than* the energy of the isolated protons and neutron, so the $^3_2$He nucleus is *stable*.

Finally, let's bring in the last neutron. Again, no work is required on our part until the second neutron gets to within about 3 fm of the other nucleons already in place, at which point the strong force starts taking over. Again, it takes negative work for us to move the second and last neutron into place, resulting in an even larger magnitude of negative work for us to assemble the entire $^4_2$He nucleus. This means that the energy of the assembled He–4 nucleus is significantly *lower* than the (zero) energy that the components of the system had when they were far apart from one another. Energy had to be *released* from the system by the time it was fully assembled.

Nuclear Binding Energy

We are now in a position to understand why the mass of the constituent nucleons is always greater than the mass of the assembled stable nucleus: since the assembled nucleus is stable, its energy must be less than the total energy of the separated constituent nucleons. Recall Einstein's famous mass-energy relation $E = mc^2$, showing the equivalence of mass and energy. We can therefore see that, if the energy of the system *decreases* as the system is assembled, then its associated mass must also decrease. This is always true for any kind of bound system, but the associated missing mass is typically negligible.—Not so for nuclei.

The result of all of this is that, in order for us to separate a stable nucleus into its well-separated constituent nucleons, we must do *positive* work—we have to give energy to the system. This energy is therefore called the *binding energy* of the system, E_B, and accounts for the "missing" mass. This missing mass—the difference in mass between the total mass of the constituent nucleons and the mass of the assembled nucleus—is called the *mass defect*, denoted μ. It is related to the binding energy by the equation $E_B = \mu c^2$.

Example 6.1: The Binding Energy of Boron-11

A recent type of treatment for high-grade gliomas (malignant brain tumors), head and neck, and liver cancers is called Boron Neutron Capture Therapy (BNCT).[8] This type of therapy involves attaching a boron-10 atom to a delivery agent that transports the atom to the tumor cells. Incident slow neutrons are then absorbed by the B-10 nuclei, which then transform to excited B-11 nuclei, and subsequently decay into helium nuclei (alpha particles) and other particles. The high LET characteristics of the emitted alpha particles result in significant DNA double-strand breaks and the subsequent death of the cancer cells. Clinical trials using BNCT have taken place in the United States, Japan, and in Europe; the future use of this type of therapy hinges on the development of more effective delivery agents for the B-10 atoms.[8]

Consider the boron isotope $^{11}_5$B. This isotope has a relative atomic mass of $A_r(^{11}_5\text{B}) = 11.009\,305\,55$.[9]

Data: (obtained from the NIST website[10])

$$m_{electron} = 5.485\,799\,090\,7 \times 10^{-4}\,u \quad m_{proton} = 1.007\,276\,466\,88\,u$$
$$m_{neutron} = 1.008\,664\,915\,88\,u \qquad\qquad 1\,u = 931.494\,095\,MeV/c^2$$
$$c = 299\,792\,458\,m/s$$

(a) Find the value of the mass defect, μ, for the nuclide ^{11}B. (b) Find the value of the binding energy, E_B, for ^{11}B. (c) Find the *average binding energy per nucleon* for the nucleons in the ^{11}B nucleus.

Solution:

(a) The mass defect is the difference in mass between the theoretical mass—the mass computed as the sum of the masses of the constituent nucleons—and the experimental mass—the mass of the nucleus measured in the laboratory. The experimental atomic mass of the B-11 atom is given to be $m_{exp} = 11.009\,305\,55\,u$. Note that this is the *atomic* mass—the mass of the neutral boron atom—so we must watch out for the electron masses. The theoretical mass is therefore, since there are 5 protons, 5 electrons and 6 neutrons: $m_{theo} = 5\,(m_{proton} + m_{electron}) + 6\,(m_{neutron}) = 11.091\,114\,72\,u$. The mass defect is therefore $\mu = m_{theo} - m_{exp} = \boxed{0.081\,809\,18\,u}$. Note that the electron masses cancel out, so that all we're left with is the difference between the constituent nucleon and assembled nucleus masses, as desired. (b) The binding energy for the B-11 nucleus is now simply given by $E_B = \mu c^2$. While this is simply an exercise in plugging in numbers, we must be very careful of units. Since the speed of light, c, is in SI units, we could start this solution by first converting the mass defect from atomic mass units (u) into kilograms (kg). Multiplying μ by c^2 would then give us the correct answer. But note that we are given a conversion for the atomic mass unit: $1\,u = 931.494\,095\,MeV/c^2$. The c^2 in the denominator means that we don't even need the value for c—the factors of c cancel out in the equation. Thus:

$$E_B = \mu c^2 = (0.081\,809\,18\,u) \cdot c^2 \left(\frac{931.494\,095\,MeV/c^2}{u} \right), \qquad (6.14)$$

or,

$$E_B = 76.204\,77\,MeV. \qquad (6.15)$$

This is the energy that would have to be added to the system (via work done by external forces) in order to separate the nucleus into its constituent nucleons. (c) The average binding energy per nucleon is simply the total binding energy divided by the number of nucleons in the nucleus—in this case, $A = 11$. Thus, $E_B/A = 76.204\,768\,MeV/11 = \boxed{6.927\,706\,MeV/nucleon}$.

Note the precision of the data and answers in this example, and the resulting care that was taken about significant figures. This is important in problems involving quantities like the mass defect, which may require that a relatively large number of significant figures be kept in order to end up with a meaningful result (since we are taking the difference of two numbers that are very close to one another).

$$\boxed{\textit{End of solution to Example 6.1.}}$$

Average Binding Energy per Nucleon

Following the procedure in the previous example, we can compute the value of the average binding energy per nucleon (E_B/A) of the various naturally occurring stable nuclides. A plot could then be constructed showing E_B/A vs. A. The result of such a plot is shown in Fig. (6.4). (Mass data for this plot were taken from Audi and Wapstra.[11,12]) The greater the average binding energy per nucleon, the greater the work that has to be done to remove each nucleon and therefore the more stable the nucleus.

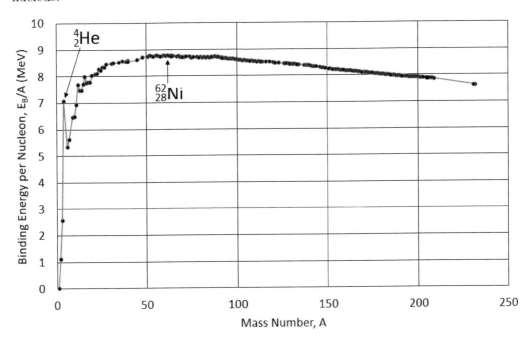

FIGURE 6.4: Plot of the average *Binding Energy per Nucleon* for the stable nuclides. The maximum of this curve occurs at Ni–62, with a local maximum at He–4.

We can see that the resulting plot rises steeply as A increases from 1 and reaches a maximum at the point corresponding to the nickel isotope $^{62}_{28}\text{Ni}$, after which the curve slowly decreases, with an average binding energy per nucleon value of about $8\,MeV$ per nucleon for large-A nuclei. We also note a sharp peak at $A = 4$, corresponding to the He–4 nuclide. This means that the He–4 nucleus is more stable than any of the nuclides in its vicinity (it has the largest E_B/A value of any nuclide with A from 1 through 11). We will return to this important point when we discuss alpha decay in the next chapter.

Looking back to Fig. (6.3), we can see that there exists at least one stable nuclide for each of the elements with $Z < 83$. In these nuclei, the energies of the bound nucleons are not sufficient to cause nuclear emissions, and the isotope remains unchanged and stable. However, for *some* isotopes with $Z < 83$ and for *all* isotopes with $Z \geq 83$, the energies are such that nuclear emissions can occur. Exactly *when* such emissions will occur is dictated purely by chance, although a given nucleus has a definite probability for emitting a particle (a nuclear emission) per unit time, as dictated by quantum mechanics. When a nucleus undergoes a change of state that results in a nuclear emission, we say that it has undergone a *radioactive decay*. We will discuss radioactive decay in Chapter 7.

6.4   NUCLEAR SPIN AND MAGNETIC DIPOLES

The Case of Electrons

Recall the discussion of the hydrogenic quantum numbers in Chapter 4, and the fact that four quantum numbers emerge from the relativistic quantum formulation of Dirac: n, ℓ m_ℓ, and m_s. It is the last quantum number—the spin quantum number, m_s—that is a result of special relativity being incorporated into quantum theory (the other quantum numbers appear exactly the same in non-relativistic quantum mechanics). The possible values of the spin quantum number are $m_s = \pm\frac{1}{2}$, and the corresponding values of the electron's (z-component of) spin angular momentum are given by $S_z = m_s\hbar = \pm\frac{1}{2}\hbar$.

Associated with the spin quantum number of the electron is a magnetic dipole moment. This means that the electron acts like a tiny bar magnet: it has an associated dipole magnetic field pattern, and it experiences an alignment torque when placed in an external magnetic field, trying to align the electron's magnetic field with the external field. (This is basically saying the same thing as *opposite poles attract and like poles repel* when discussing the north and south poles of a bar magnet.)

Also, recall from our discussion of multielectron atoms in Chapter 5, that electrons are *fermions*, and therefore must satisfy the *Pauli exclusion principle*, which states that no two identical fermions can occupy the same quantum state within the same quantum system. It is the Pauli exclusion principle that only allowed two electrons to occupy the $n = 1$ state in atoms, for example: both electrons having $n = 1, \ell = 0$, and $m_\ell = 0$, but one electron having spin *up* $(m_s = +\frac{1}{2}\hbar)$, and the other having spin *down* $(m_s = -\frac{1}{2}\hbar)$.

The Case of Nucleons

It turns out that protons and neutrons are also fermions, and therefore must also satisfy the Pauli exclusion principle. However, since protons and neutrons are not identical particles, a proton and a neutron can be in the same quantum state within the same nucleus—but two protons or two neutrons cannot.

In Chapter 4 we discussed the fact that it is the confinement of the electrons in the atom to the region around the nucleus that resulted in the quantum numbers. Since the quantum numbers specify the allowed energy states for the electrons, it follows that it is the confinement of the electrons to the region around the nucleus that dictates that the electrons must have discrete energy levels available to them as long as they are a part of the atom (that is, as long as they have not been ionized). When electrons having different sets of quantum numbers have filled the first shell $(n = 1)$, then the next electron added to the atom must move up to the next shell.

All of these ideas apply as well to nucleons within a nucleus. Since nucleons are confined to the nucleus, they will also be characterized by quantum numbers. In addition, they must have corresponding discrete energy levels that are much higher than electron energies in the atoms, as discussed earlier in this chapter. Protons and neutrons are also spin-$\frac{1}{2}$ fermions, so identical nucleons can be paired spin-up and spin-down, as with electrons. The Pauli exclusion principle will therefore be used to dictate how many protons and neutrons can occupy the various nuclear "shells".

It turns out that the strength of the strong nuclear force also depends on the spin of the nucleons interacting via this force: two nucleons having their spins in the same direction (both spin up or both spin down) feel a stronger force of attraction than two nucleons having opposite spins.

These characteristics resulting from the fermion nature of nucleons will be needed in the next section as we discuss the stability of various nuclides.

6.5   NUCLEON ENERGY LEVELS AND STABILITY

We know that the confinement of nucleons to the region inside the nucleus—a space on the order of $10^{-14}\,m$ in width—results in a discrete set of energy levels that the nucleons must occupy. We also know that these energy levels are described by quantum numbers. In addition, nucleons are spin-$\frac{1}{2}$ fermions, so the Pauli Exclusion Principle applies, meaning that no two protons and no two neutrons can be in the same quantum state at the same time. (A proton and a neutron *can* be in the same quantum state at the same time, however, since they are so-called *distinguishable particles*—they are not identical.) A nucleus will always try to minimize its energy in order to be as stable a nucleus as possible.

A Model for Nucleons in a Nucleus

Before discussing how nucleons can occupy the various energy levels available to them, we must first come up with a model to represent the system of nucleons under consideration. In the case of an electron in an atom, our model was the electrical Coulomb force that held the electron in orbit around the nucleus. The corresponding Coulomb potential energy was then fed into the Schrödinger equation, the solution of which gave us the allowed energies and wavefunctions for the electron in a hydrogenic atom. Our model for multielectron atoms was then based on our knowledge of hydrogen.

We can't do this for the case of nucleons in a nucleus, however, since the force holding the nucleons inside the nucleus—the strong nuclear force—is still basically an unknown quantity. We know some characteristics of the strong nuclear force—those that we've already discussed—but physicists have not yet determined an equation that describes the strong nuclear force, like the Coulomb equation describes the electrical force. Since we don't have an equation describing the strong nuclear force, we can't solve any equations for the resulting energy levels or wavefunctions. We can, however, make some approximations and come up with a model that can give us some insight into what is going on inside the nucleus.

In particular, we assume that the nucleons confined inside the nucleus experience an average force holding them in the nucleus—an average strong nuclear force. We further assume that there is associated with this force an average negative potential energy function experienced by the bound nucleons. We take the minimum of the potential energy function to be the *zero* energy level for the nucleons. (This is analogous to choosing the zero level for the gravitational potential energy of a ball to be at the level of the ground in your studies of introductory physics.) The various allowed energy levels for the nucleons in the nucleus are then energy levels above $E = 0$. The question then is, what are the allowed energies?

To help us with this, we will use an important result from quantum mechanics—a result that comes from a model for particles confined to a region of space of width w. This model is called the *square-well potential* model. Without going into the details of the model, we will simply state the results. Namely, the allowed energies for a particle of mass m confined to a region of space of width w are given by

$$E_n = \frac{n^2 \pi^2 \hbar^2}{2mw^2} = n^2 E_1 , \tag{6.16}$$

where n is the principal quantum number that has allowed values $n = \{1, 2, 3, \ldots\}$, $\hbar = 1.055 \times 10^{-34} J \cdot s$, and E_n is the energy of the allowed quantum state having principal quantum number n. Note that $E_1 = \pi^2 \hbar^2/(2mw^2)$ is the ground-state energy, which allows us to write that $E_n = n^2 E_1$, as stated above in Eq. (6.16).

As a quick check, we note that, using standard values for the width of an average nucleus and the approximate mass of a nucleon, we get that $E_1 \cong 3 MeV$, which is in agreement with our earlier discussion about expected energy levels in nuclei being on the order of MeV.

We now have a model for the allowed energies of nucleons inside a nucleus. Each energy level corresponds to a single value of the quantum number n, which means that we can have at most two nucleons in a single energy level—one with spin up, and one with spin down. Let's take a look at some specific nuclei and see if we can gain some insight into their stability or instability.

Example: The Isotopes of Boron

Consider the boron nucleus ($Z = 5$). The naturally occurring isotopes of boron are ^{10}B (19.9%) and ^{11}B (80.1%). Schematic energy level diagrams for these isotopes are shown in Fig. (6.5). Let's take a look at these diagrams one at a time.

Figure (6.5a) shows the energy levels for the 5 protons in boron. Let's first look at the energy levels available to the protons. The designated zero level of energy is shown, along with the levels for $n = 1, 2, 3$, and 4. Note also that we are following the square-well model in using $E_n = n^2 E_1$, as given in Eq. (6.16), so the energy levels are more widely spaced as the quantum number n increases.

The fact that we are considering a boron nucleus means that we must add 5 protons into the energy-level diagram. Note that our nucleons are described by only two quantum numbers within the square-well model: the principal quantum number, n, and the spin quantum number, m_s. We add the first proton, which is spin-up, into the E_1 energy level; the second proton must then be a spin-down proton in the same level. If we were to add one more proton into the $n = 1$ level, we would be violating the Pauli exclusion principle, since there would then be two protons having the same value of the principal quantum number $n = 1$ and the same value of m_s. So, we have

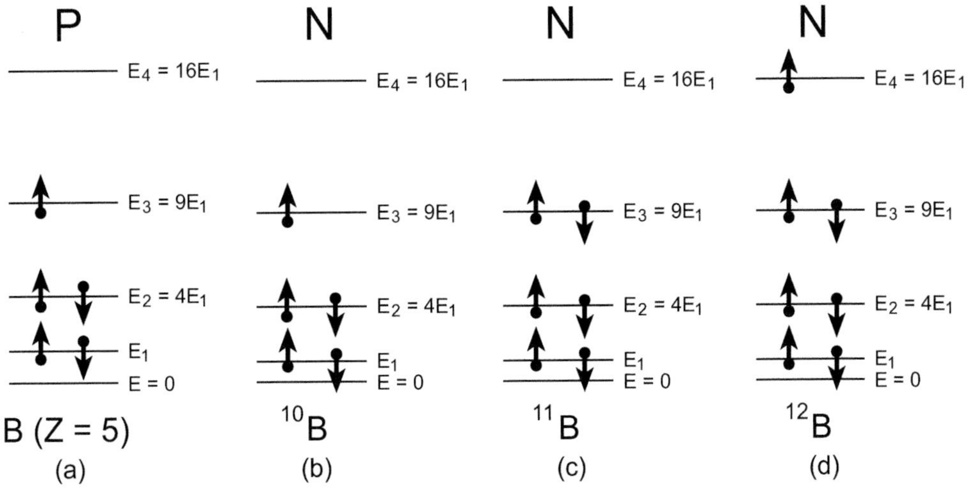

FIGURE 6.5: Schematic diagrams of nucleon energy levels in boron. (*Not drawn to scale.*) (a) Energy level diagram for the protons in the boron nucleus. (b) Energy level diagram for the neutrons in ^{10}B. (c) Energy levels for the neutrons in ^{11}B. (d) Neutron energy-level diagram to help explain why ^{12}B is an unstable isotope.

no choice but to add the third proton into the $n = 2$ level. Continuing in this fashion gives us the proton energy-level diagram shown in Fig. (6.5a).

Let's move on now to the neutron energy level diagram for the isotope ^{10}B shown in Fig. (6.5b). Again, let's first look at the available energy levels shown—in particular, let's compare the neutron energy levels to the proton energy levels. We can see that the $E = 0$ energy levels are the same, resulting from the minimum of the potential energy function corresponding to the strong nuclear force, which does not care if the nucleon is a proton or a neutron. However, the other energy levels are higher for the protons than they are for the neutrons. The reason for this is that the protons also experience the Coulomb repulsive force that has a corresponding positive potential energy contribution. It is this positive energy contribution that results in the upward shift of the proton energy levels relative to the neutron energy levels.

We now start filling the neutrons into the available energy levels according to the Pauli exclusion principle, as discussed for the case of the protons. We end up with the final neutron added into the $n = 3$ shell. Figures (6.5) (a) and (b) together show the complete energy level diagram for $^{10}_{5}$B, a stable isotope of boron. Note that $N = Z$ for this isotope and that it lies on the line of stability in Fig. (6.3).

Moving on to ^{11}B, we end up adding just one more neutron—spin down—into the $n = 3$ level. The energy level diagram for the $^{11}_{5}$B nuclide is thus as shown in Figs. (6.5) (a) and (c). We note that the highest occupied neutron energy level is a filled shell. $^{11}_{5}$B is also a stable isotope of boron.

Finally, let's consider the isotope ^{12}B. This isotope of boron was not listed as one of the naturally occurring isotopes at the beginning of this section. Let's find out why.

To construct the energy level diagram for ^{12}B, we need to add one more neutron to the neutron energy level diagram shown in Fig. (6.5c). Since the $n = 3$ level is filled, this means that we are placing a neutron into the E_4 energy level, as shown in Fig. (6.5d). Now, let's compare Figs. (6.5) (a), (c) and (d). Adding the extra neutron into the B-11 neutron diagram to obtain the B-12 diagram came at the expense of a good bit of energy—the single neutron in the $n = 4$ state added an amount of energy equal to $16\,E_1$. Meanwhile, the proton energy level diagram in Fig. (6.5a) shows a half-filled $n = 3$ shell. As far as constructing stable nuclei is concerned, it would be much more energetically favorable—and, therefore, more stable—to add a proton into the $n = 3$ level, costing an extra $9\,E_1$ amount of energy, than to add a neutron into the $n = 4$ level.

As a result, the B-12 isotope is energetically unstable—it is energetically favorable for the $^{12}_{5}$B isotope to somehow decay into a $^{12}_{6}$C isotope. It turns out that this decay can readily take place, since the neutron can decay into a proton plus an electron. We will discuss this type of decay, called *beta decay*, in the next chapter. For our purposes at this point, it is simply important for us to understand that the $^{12}_{5}$B isotope is unstable due to the available lower-energy proton state, and will therefore not be found in nature.

Example: The Isotopes of Carbon

Now let's add another proton to our discussion, and talk about the isotopes of carbon ($Z = 6$). The proton and neutron energy levels for the stable carbon isotopes ^{12}C, ^{13}C, and ^{14}C are shown in Fig. (6.6).

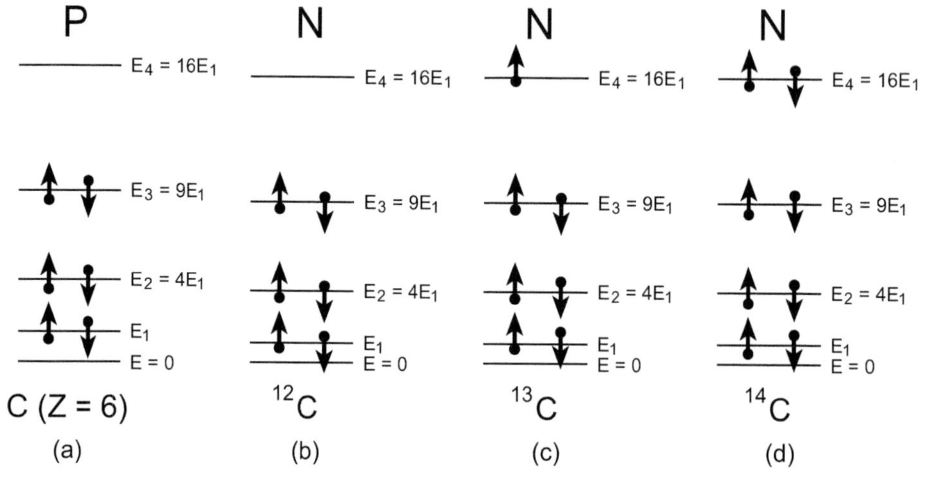

FIGURE 6.6: Schematic diagrams of nucleon energy levels in carbon. (*Not drawn to scale.*) (a) Energy level diagram for the protons in the carbon nucleus. (b) Energy level diagram for the neutrons in ^{12}C. (c) Energy levels for the neutrons in ^{13}C. (d) Neutron energy-level diagram for ^{14}C. All of these are stable isotopes of carbon.

Note in Figs. (6.6) (a) and (b) that, for C-12, $N = Z$—another entry for the line of stability in Fig. (6.3). (This is the isotope of carbon that results when we try to add another neutron to B-11 in an attempt to form B-12, as discussed previously.)

Adding another neutron to form C-13 gives us the neutron diagram shown in Fig. (6.6c). Since there is not an available spot in the proton $n = 3$ shell of Fig. (6.6a), this isotope is also stable, as is the isotope C-14. From our discussion of B-12, however, we expect C-15 to be unstable, as it is.

Example: The Isotopes of Beryllium

Despite its success in our discussions thus far, this simplified square-well potential model for the energy levels of nuclei has a limited applicability. Consider, for example, the proton and neutron energy level diagrams for the beryllium isotopes $^{8}_{4}\text{Be}$ and $^{9}_{4}\text{Be}$, shown in Fig. (6.7).

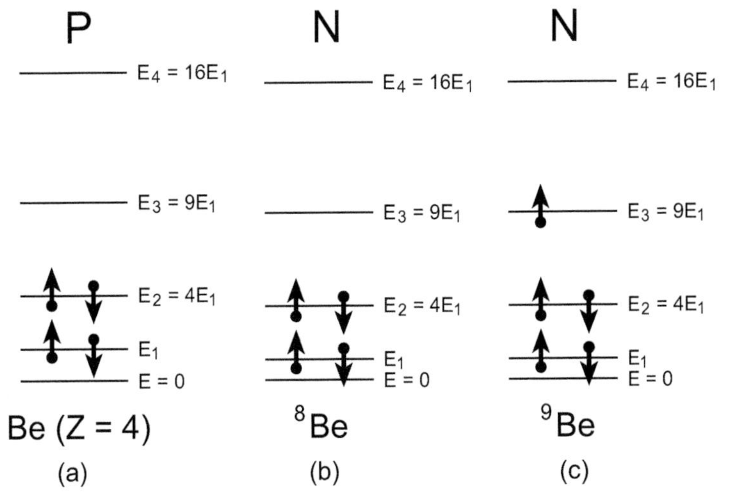

FIGURE 6.7: Schematic diagrams of nucleon energy levels in beryllium. (*Not drawn to scale.*) (a) Energy level diagram for the protons in the beryllium nucleus. (b) Energy level diagram for the neutrons in ^{8}Be. (c) Energy level diagram for the neutrons in ^{9}Be.

Looking at Figs. (6.7) (a) and (b), we see that the Be-8 isotope is not only an isotope on the line of stability, but it also has filled shells—we would expect it to definitely be a stable isotope. Further, from our previous discussions and from an inspection of Figs. (6.7) (a) and (c), we would also expect the Be-9 isotope to be stable. It will probably come as a surprise, therefore, to find out that only the Be-9 isotope is stable! The beryllium-8 isotope, which seemed to have guaranteed stability (*it's on the N = Z line for low Z!; it has filled shells!*) is *unstable*. We noted something previously that is the key to understanding this somewhat shocking claim of instability; let's dig into this a bit further.

Look back at the binding energy per nucleon discussion earlier in this chapter, and the associated plot shown in Fig. (6.4). The plot shown in Fig. (6.8) shows the *BE/A vs. A* plot of Fig. (6.4) zoomed in, to enable us to look more closely at the region of small *A* values.

We noted previously the relatively high value of binding-energy-per-nucleon for the helium isotope $^{4}_{2}\text{He}$. Moving toward the right in Fig. (6.8), we can see that even

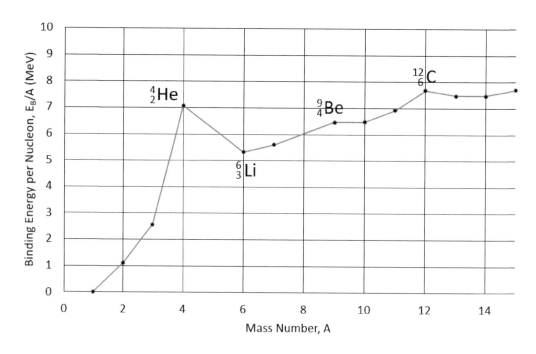

FIGURE 6.8: Plot of the average *Binding Energy per Nucleon* for the stable nuclides having small mass numbers.

Be-9 has a lower BE/A value than He-4. The He-4 isotope is simply a very tightly bound nucleus. If we were to put two He-4 nuclei together to form a larger nucleus, we would get—you guessed it—Be-8. Looking at the position corresponding to Be-9 in Fig. (6.8) gives us an idea of what the binding energy per nucleon for Be-8 would be like—definitely lower than the extremely stable He-4 nucleus. Remembering that systems always tend toward configurations of greater stability, or lower energy, it makes sense that the (less-tightly bound) Be-8 nucleus would simply break apart into two (more tightly bound) He-4 nuclei.

The He-4 isotopes are so stable that, when nuclei decay into lower-energy configurations, a remnant of the decay is often these He-4 nuclei. As a result, these nuclei are given a special name: *alpha particles*. We discussed the high LET properties of alpha particles and their damaging effects on DNA nuclei in Chapter 2—see, for example, Table (2.1) for the dramatic LET values of high-energy alpha particles.

Our discussion of nucleon energy levels and the associated stability of the isotopes of various elements have demonstrated the utility of the simple square-well potential model—and some of its limitations. Nevertheless, this simplified scheme allows us to gain useful insight into some important properties of nuclei. Our discussion has also led us to the mention of two types of decay that result from combinations of nucleons transforming into more energetically favorable configurations: *beta decay* and *alpha decay*. The topic of radioactive decay dominates the discussion in the next chapter.

6.6 QUESTIONS, EXERCISES, & PROBLEMS

6-1. (a) Find the radii of the Ca-40 and Au-197 nuclei using Eq. (6.1), and verify the locations of the short vertical lines shown in Fig. (6.2). (b) Using the radii values from part (a), compute the corresponding nuclear charge densities, ρ (in C/m^3), assuming that the nuclei are solid spheres with constant charge density. Compare your answers with the charge density distributions shown in Fig. (6.2).

6-2. The plots in Fig. (6.2) show the nuclear charge density as a function of radial distance from the center of the nucleus, $\rho(r)$ *vs.* r, for Ca-40 and Au-197. The values at the center of the nucleus, $\rho(0)$, for calcium and gold, are $1.32 \times 10^{25}\,C/m^3$ and $1.06 \times 10^{25}\,C/m^3$, respectively. Find the corresponding radii that the calcium and gold nuclei would have if they had a constant nuclear charge density equal to $\rho(0)$.

6-3. It was shown in this chapter using the Heisenberg uncertainty principle (HUP) that emissions from atoms due to electron transitions should have energies on the order of eV. However, in our discussion of x-ray and Auger-electron emission from atoms in Chapter 5, we were talking about energies on the order of keV. The purpose of this problem is to lead you through a HUP argument to see why keV energies might be reasonable. We will approach this argument by considering a tungsten atom, W ($Z = 74$). (a) Use Eq. (4.48) in Chapter 4 to find the approximate radius of a classical $1s$ electron orbit in a tungsten atom. (b) Do you think that the shielding of the nucleus by other inner-shell s-electrons will change your answer in (a) by much, relative to the nuclear charge? Why or why not? (c) Use the HUP to find a rough value for the radial component of momentum of the electron in the $1s$ state. (d) Use the momentum value from (c) to find a rough estimate of energies associated with this confinement of the $1s$ electron around the nucleus. (e) Does it seem reasonable that keV-energy x-rays could be emitted in electron transitions in high-Z atoms?

6-4. Compute (a) the mass defect, (b) the binding energy, and (c) the binding energy per nucleon for an alpha particle. The mass of a neutral He-4 atom can be found in the table of relative atomic masses on the NIST (*National Institute of Standards and Technology*) website.[13]

6-5. Compute (a) the mass defect, (b) the binding energy, and (c) the binding energy per nucleon for the nickel isotope $^{62}_{28}\text{Ni}$. The mass of a neutral Ni–62 atom can be found in the table of relative atomic masses on the NIST (*National Institute of Standards and Technology*) website.[13]

6-6. We discussed the stability of nuclei as far as the strong nuclear force and the binding energy are concerned, but we neglected the fact that nucleons have mass, and therefore also interact via the attractive gravitational force, which would further add to the stability of the nucleus. Why did we not discuss this contribution to the stability of nuclei? To answer this question, recall that the universal gravitational force is given by $F_G = Gm_1m_2/r^2$, where $G = 6.67 \times 10^{-11}\,N \cdot m^2/kg^2$. Provide arguments for helium–4 and uranium–238 as far as the attractive gravitational force is concerned, that mirror the approximate arguments given in the text for the repulsive electrical force in those nuclei. (*Hint:* Divide the nucleus up into two parts, each with $A/2$ nucleons and $Z/2$ protons, separated by a distance R.)

6-7. The text states the following: "We can therefore see that, if the energy of the system *decreases* as the system is assembled, then its associated mass must also decrease. This is always true for any kind of bound system, but the associated missing mass is typically negligible". Compute the "missing mass" for a simple hydrogen atom ($_1^1H$) in its ground state. Express your answer as a fraction of the electron mass. (*Big hint:* What is the binding energy for a ground-state electron in hydrogen?)

6-8. Look at the general shape of the *BE/A vs. A* curve shown in Fig. (6.4): it is lower at the two ends with a maximum in the middle. Explain why we should expect this general shape from the characteristics of the strong nuclear force and the Coulomb force. (*Hints:* Consider a deuterium nucleus, $_1^2H$. There are two nucleons with one strong-nuclear-force bond between them. Thus, there is *one-half* of a bond per nucleon. In tritium, $_1^3H$, there are three nucleons and three bonds, and so *one* bond per nucleon. For a four-nucleon system, like an alpha particle, there are four nucleons and six bonds, so *one-and-a-half* bonds per nucleon. Does this trend continue as we consider nuclei with larger and larger values of *A*? What does it mean when we say that the strong nuclear force is a saturated force? How does the Coulomb force contribute to this discussion?)

6-9. In the text it is stated that Eq. (6.16) yields a ground-state energy of $E_1 \cong 3\,MeV$. Show that this is the case.

6-10. It is stated in the text that the carbon isotope $_6^{15}C$ is unstable. Explain why this is so. What would you expect the $_6^{15}C$ nucleus to decay into? Support your answers with nuclear energy level diagrams.

6-11. The nitrogen isotopes N-14 and N-15 are stable, but the isotope N-16 is unstable. Explain why this is so. You should use both words and energy level diagrams in your explanation.

6-12. All of the oxygen isotopes O-16, O-17, and O-18 are stable. Explain why this is so. You should use both words and energy level diagrams in your explanation.

6-13. In the discussion of the Be-8 isotope, it is stated that this isotope is unstable because it readily splits into two He-4 nuclei—that is, two alpha particles. The text states that this is due to the fact that "... systems always tend toward configurations of greater stability, or lower energy...". But looking at Fig. (6.8), it looks like He-4 has a *higher* energy than Be-8 would have, not lower. Explain this apparent discrepancy.

6.7 REFERENCES

1. The DOE/NSF Nuclear Science Advisory Committee. The Frontiers of Science: A Long Range Plan. https://www.osti.gov/servlets/purl/1375323. Accessed July 11, 2017.
2. Hofstadter R. Nuclear and Nucleon Scattering of High-Energy Electrons. *Annu. Rev. Nucl. Sci.* 1957; 7: 231-316.
3. Srivastava BB. *Fundamentals of Nuclear Physics.* New Delhi, India: Rastogi Publ.; 2006.
4. Audi G, Wapstra AH. The 1993 atomic mass evaluation: (I) Atomic mass table. *Nuc. Phys. A.* 1993; 565(1): 1-65.
5. Audi G, Wapstra AH. The 1995 update to the atomic mass evaluation. *Nuc. Phys. A.* 1995; 595(4): 409-480.
6. National Nuclear Data Center. NuDat 2.7β. https://www.nndc.bnl.gov/nudat3/. Accessed July 13, 2017.
7. Harris R. *Modern Physics.* 2nd ed. San Francisco: Pearson Education, Inc.; 2008.
8. Barth RF, Coderre JA, Vincente MGH, and Blue TE. Boron Neutron Capture Therapy of Cancer: Current Status and Future Prospects. *Clin. Cancer Res.* 11(11): 3987-4002.

9. de Laeter JR, Böhlke JK, de Bièvre P, et al. Atomic Weights of the Elements: Review 2000 (IUPAC Technical Report). *Pure Appl. Chem.* 2003; 75(6): 683-800.

10. National Institute of Standards and Technology. https://physics.nist.gov/cuu/Constants/. The NIST Reference on Constants, Units, and Uncertainty. Accessed July 13, 2017.

11. Audi G, Wapstra AH. The 1993 atomic mass evaluation: (I) Atomic mass table. *Nuclear Physics A.* 565(1): 1-65.

12. Audi G, and Wapstra AH. The 1995 update to the atomic mass evaluation. *Nuclear Physics A.* 595(4): 409-480.

13. National Institute of Standards and Technology. Atomic Weights and Isotopic Compositions with Relative Atomic Masses. https://www.nist.gov/pml/atomic-weights-and-isotopic-compositions-relative-atomic-masses. Accessed July 17, 2017.

CHAPTER 7

Nuclear Physics II: Nuclear Reactions and Radioactive Decay

CONTENTS

In the last chapter we saw that nucleons confined to a small region of space about the size of one fermi $(1\,F = 10^{-15}\,m)$ occupy discrete nuclear energy levels, just as electrons confined to a region about the size of one ångstrom $(1\,\text{Å} = 10^{-10}\,m)$ occupy discrete atomic energy levels. Likewise, just as atoms in excited states can make transitions to lower energy levels with the emission of particles (photons or electrons), so, too, can nuclei in higher energy states emit particles. However, as we'll see in this chapter, the particles emitted by nuclei are a bit more varied than those emitted by atoms, and the processes involved are a bit more complicated. The spontaneous emission of these particles by nuclei is called *radioactive decay*. But before we can discuss radioactive decay, we must first understand the idea of nuclear reactions and the conservation principles that constrain them.

7.1 NUCLEAR REACTIONS

By a *nuclear reaction*, we mean a transition from an initial configuration of one or more nuclei, to a final configuration of possibly different nuclei and particles. Thus, for our purposes, we can represent the generic nuclear reaction as follows:

$$^{A_1}_{Z_1}X_1 + {}^{A_2}_{Z_2}X_2 \rightarrow {}^{A_3}_{Z_3}X_3 + (other\,particles) + Q\,, \qquad (7.1)$$

DOI: 10.1201/9781003477457-7

where Q is called the *Q-value* of the reaction and is equal to the energy equivalent of the missing mass (the mass of the initial reacting nuclei minus the mass of all of the final product nuclei and particles).[a] In Eq. (7.1), the "other particles" may include photons, fundamental particles, or additional nuclei. We'll be working with various forms of this generic equation throughout this chapter.

Conservation Principles

All nuclear reactions are constrained by six conservation principles.[1] Of these, we shall only be interested in three: the conservation of relativistic mass-energy, the conservation of charge, and the conservation of mass number (that is, the number of nucleons).[b] We have already touched on the conservation of relativistic mass-energy in our discussion of the Q-value above.

Since any amount of charge can be represented as some number of proton charges, Ze, we can restate the conservation of charge as the *conservation of atomic number*, as long as we acknowledge that negative charges will have a corresponding negative value of Z. We can therefore express the conservation of charge (or atomic number) in Eq. (7.1) as

$$Z_1 + Z_2 = Z_3 + \ldots , \tag{7.2}$$

where the sum on the right-hand side of Eq. (7.2) covers all of the particles in the final configuration of the system.

Likewise, since the number of nucleons is simply given by the mass number, A, we can express the *conservation of mass number* in Eq. (7.1) as

$$A_1 + A_2 = A_3 + \ldots . \tag{7.3}$$

Example 7.1: The Production of Co-60

All naturally occurring cobalt is in the form of the stable isotope Co-59. But the radioactive isotope Co-60 has a long history of use in radiation therapy and in brachytherapy. Another very important current use of Co-60 is for sterilization (of medical equipment, for example).[2] A sample of the useful isotope Co-60 is produced by bombarding a pellet of Co-59 with low-energy neutrons (referred to as *thermal neutrons*) inside a nuclear reactor.[3] Extra energy and momentum are carried off by a photon in this reaction. Write the reaction equation for the production of Co-60 from Co-59 using full isotopic notation, and then check that both charge and nucleon number are conserved.

Solution:

In the production of Co-60 from Co-59, a slow neutron is incident on a Co-59 nucleus. Looking up the atomic number of cobalt, we find that $Z = 27$, so we can write the reaction as follows:

$$^{59}_{27}\text{Co} + \text{n} \rightarrow {}^{60}_{27}\text{Co} + \gamma . \tag{7.4}$$

---

[a] By the "energy equivalent of the missing mass", we simply mean the relativistic energy, as given by Einstein's equation $E = (missing\,mass)\,c^2$.

[b] The other three quantities that are conserved in nuclear reactions are linear momentum, angular momentum, and parity.

This equation shows the neutron combining with the Co-59 nucleus to form a Co-60 nucleus with the emission of a photon (a gamma particle, γ), as described above. In order to check whether charge and nucleon number are conserved in this reaction, we must find the mass number and the atomic number for the neutron and the photon. Since a neutron is a nucleon ($A = 1$) but has no charge ($Z = 0$), and since a photon is not a nucleon ($A = 0$) and also has no charge ($Z = 0$), we can write the reaction equation as follows:

$$^{59}_{27}\text{Co} + ^{1}_{0}\text{n} \rightarrow ^{60}_{27}\text{Co} + ^{0}_{0}\gamma. \tag{7.5}$$

It then becomes a trivial matter to add up the A-values on the left and right sides of this equation to see that $59 + 1 = 60 + 0$, thereby verifying the conservation of nucleon number. Likewise, adding the atomic numbers on the left and right sides of Eq. (7.5) gives us that $27 + 0 = 27 + 0$, which verifies the conservation of charge.

> *End of solution to Example 7.1.*

In comparing Eqs.(7.5) and (7.1), we can see that, for the case of the production of Co-60, the second particle involved in the reaction was not a nucleus, but rather simply a neutron, and the production of the Co-60 nucleus was accompanied by the emission of a photon. Nevertheless, every term in Eq. (7.5) could be expressed using full isotopic notation, as suggested in the generic Eq. (7.1). This can be done with all nuclear reaction equations, making it very easy to check the conservation of nucleon number and charge, as was demonstrated in Ex.(7.1).

7.2 NUCLEAR FISSION AND NUCLEAR FUSION

In the previous chapter, we discussed the energy levels associated with the protons and neutrons within the nucleus. We also pointed out that some nuclei are unstable and will undergo transformations into a more stable configuration. We also discussed the binding energies, E_B, and binding energies-per-nucleon, E_B/A, associated with various nuclei.

Figure (7.1) is copied from Chapter 6—it shows a plot of E_B/A vs. A for stable nuclei. The dominant features pointed out previously in this plot are the initial sharp rise, the maximum at the nickel isotope $^{62}_{28}\text{Ni}$, and the gradual decline, hovering around $8\,MeV$. Let's focus our attention on the maximum at Ni-62.

Remember that the binding energy refers to the energy that is effectively holding the nucleus together—the component nucleons cannot be separated without supplying this energy to the nucleus. Therefore, the greater the binding energy per nucleon, the more stable the nucleus. Systems tend toward configurations of greater stability. These simple ideas lead us to some very fundamental and important conclusions.

Nuclear Fusion
First, Fig. (7.1) shows that small-A nuclei have smaller E_B/A values than nuclei that have A values closer to but less than 62. This means that it may well be energetically

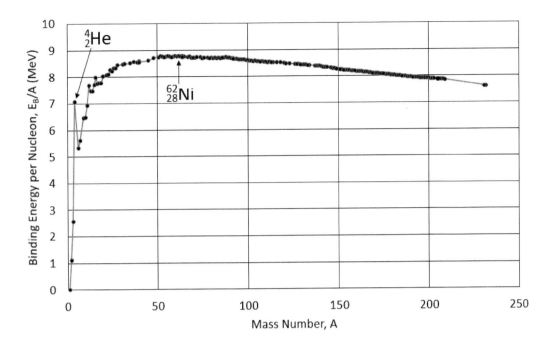

FIGURE 7.1: Plot of the average *Binding Energy per Nucleon* for the stable nuclides. The maximum of this curve occurs at Ni-62, with a local maximum at He-4.

favorable for two smaller nuclei to combine into a larger, more stable nucleus having $A \leq 62$. This process is known as *nuclear fusion*.

Nuclear Fission
Second, it is energetically favorable for some large-A nuclei to split into two different medium-mass nuclei, each having $A \geq 62$. Again, this is a result of the fact that, for large-A nuclei, E_B/A increases as the mass number approaches $A = 62$. This process of breaking up large nuclei into smaller, more stable nuclei is called *nuclear fission*. It should be pointed out that fission is accompanied by the emission of 2 to 3 neutrons, depending on the reaction.

Application: Reactors
The purpose of nuclear reactors in nuclear power plants is to produce thermal energy. Once the thermal energy is produced, that energy is used in traditional ways—for example, to heat up water, which then generates steam, which can then be used in turbine generators to produce electricity. The difference between fusion and fission reactors is how the thermal energy is produced—that, and the fact that working fusion reactors don't exist yet!

Fission Reactors   Nuclear fission involves a large-mass nucleus splitting into two medium-mass fragment nuclei. These two fragment nuclei have relatively large charges so that, after the original nucleus splits, there is a very large Coulomb repulsive force pushing the two fragments away from each other. This results in large kinetic energies of the fragment nuclei. These large energies can then be transferred to the materials in the reactor via collisions, resulting in the heating of the reactor core. This results in the desired thermal energy production.

In general, nuclei will be in an unstable excited state after absorbing a neutron. Nuclei in excited states tend to vibrate. The vibrating nucleus may then transition to a lower-energy state by emitting a high-energy photon (a *gamma ray*) or by emitting a neutron. If the absorbed neutron has a sufficiently high energy, then the resulting nucleus may be vibrating violently enough to result in fission.[1] A nuclide is said to be *fissionable* if it can undergo fission after absorbing a high-energy neutron. Uranium-238 is a fissionable isotope of uranium.

Some nuclides, on the other hand, can undergo nuclear fission if they absorb a neutron of any energy—even low-energy thermal neutrons. Such nuclides are said to be *fissile*. Uranium-235 is an example of a fissile nuclide. Naturally occurring uranium is 99.28% U-238 and 0.72% U-235.

Fission reactors use fuel pellets containing uranium—typically enriched so that U-235 comprises about 3 to 5% of the uranium isotopes present[4]—arranged into long tubes to produce thermal energy. U-235 can split into many different combinations of fragment nuclei, each having roughly half the mass of the original U-235 nucleus. For example, one such fission reaction that is exploited in fission reactors is as follows:

$$^{235}_{92}\text{U} + n \rightarrow {}^{92}_{36}\text{Kr} + {}^{142}_{56}\text{Ba} + 2n + 179.4\,\text{MeV}\,. \tag{7.6}$$

Note the two fission fragments, Kr-92 and Ba-142, and the two neutrons emitted in the U-235 reaction above. Immediately after the fission, the fission fragments tend to have more neutrons than stable nuclei having the same Z value. As a result, the fragments give off neutrons as a part of the fission process, which accounts for the two neutrons given off in the fission reaction shown above. In addition, both of the fission fragments Kr-92 and Ba-142 are radioactive.

On average, the fission of U-235 produces 2.5 neutrons per fission reaction.[5] These emitted neutrons could then go on to produce additional U-235 fission reactions, which would produce even more neutrons that could result in even more fission reactions, and so on, resulting in a chain reaction—which could mean an explosion. This is clearly not the desired result. To keep this from happening, *control rods* made of materials containing nuclides such as $^{113}_{48}\text{Cd}$, which is a nonfissionable nuclide that has a high probability of absorbing neutrons,[1] are inserted into the region around the fuel tubes.

The neutrons released in the fission of U-235 are high-energy neutrons, with kinetic energies on the order of several MeV. The very abundant U-238 nuclides are fissionable nuclides that will undergo fission if they absorb neutrons having kinetic energies around 1 MeV or greater. It is therefore possible for the neutrons released in the fission of U-235 to cause fission in the significantly more abundant U-238 nuclides in the fuel pellets, which could again lead to an undesired runaway effect.

To eliminate this possibility, low-mass materials are placed around the tubes of fuel pellets to serve as *moderators*. When the high-energy neutrons collide with the light nuclei in the moderator material, they give up a significant amount of their energy to the moderator, thereby putting them into the realm of thermal neutrons that can readily cause fission in U-235 nuclei but not in U-238 nuclei. The most common moderator materials are graphite, water, and deuterium-oxide (*heavy water*: D_2O, where D is a deuterium atom, ^2_1H).

The fact that moderators can be used in fission reactors to change the energy of the neutrons emitted in the fission processes, and that control rods can be used to control the number of neutrons moving through the core of the reactor, turn out to be very important for the production of radionuclides that are needed for the diagnosis and treatment of cancer. Reactors that are used to produce such radionuclides are referred to as *research reactors*. We will discuss more details associated with research reactors and radionuclide production later in this chapter.

Fusion Reactors Billions of dollars are being spent annually around the world on fusion research, all in the hope of being able to produce continuous, controlled, and self-sustaining fusion reactions. The fusion reaction that is most likely to be used in fusion reactors is that for the fusion of deuterium and tritium:

$$^2_1H + ^3_1H \rightarrow ^4_2He + n + 17.6\,\text{MeV}. \tag{7.7}$$

Comparing the fusion reaction most likely to be used in fusion reactors, Eq. (7.7), with a representative fission reaction that is characteristic of fission reactors, Eq. (7.6), we can see that the reasons for the billions of dollars spent annually on fusion research are simple and are directly related to the disadvantages of nuclear fission:

1. Whereas the fuel and the waste of fission reactors contain heavy, radioactive nuclei, the fuel and waste of nuclear fusion reactors would be light and stable.

2. Whereas the fuel for fission reactors (U-235) is very rare and hard to obtain in large quantities, the fuel for fusion reactors—deuterium, ^2_1H, and tritium, ^3_1H— is almost limitless. Deuterium is found in ocean water. Tritium, a radioactive isotope of hydrogen, is produced in trace amounts in the upper atmosphere by cosmic rays, and then falls down to earth in rain drops.[6] In addition, tritium is also very easy to produce in conventional nuclear fission reactors, and could also be produced within the nuclear fusion reactor itself and then used as fuel.[7]

Of course, using nuclear fusion in reactors is not without its problems—thus far, nearly insurmountable problems—which explains why we do not yet have fusion reactors. Consider the following.

In the fusion reaction shown in Eq. (7.7), the deuterium and tritium nuclei have to get to within nuclear dimensions ($10^{-15}\,m$) in order for the strong nuclear force to pull the two nuclei together, resulting in fusion. But until the strong nuclear force takes over, there is a strong electromagnetic force trying to push the two nuclei apart. The way we get these two nuclei close enough for fusion to take place is to have them move very quickly toward one another.

The average speed of particles in a gas is dictated by the absolute temperature of the gas, so the speeds of particles in a gas are often described in terms of the temperature of the gas. At a temperature of about $10^5\,K$, a gas of hydrogen atoms will become completely ionized, forming a gas of nuclei and electrons. However, the nuclei do not have enough energy to overcome the repulsion of the Coulomb force and undergo fusion until the temperature reaches about $10^7\,K$.[1] This is the temperature of the interior of the sun, which explains how the sun uses nuclear fusion to produce its energy. In order for nuclear fusion to proceed within a nuclear reactor, we have to produce conditions that simulate the extreme temperatures inside stars.

On 5 December, 2022, researchers at the U.S. National Ignition Facility (NIF) achieved what had never been done before: they created a nuclear fusion reaction that produced more energy than it consumed.[8] This nuclear fusion phenomenon is called *ignition*. Exploiting the reaction given in Eq. (7.7), the NIF researchers used 192 lasers to deliver over 2 MJ (mega-joules) of energy to a pea-sized gold cylinder containing the deuterium and tritium fuel. The resulting fusion reaction delivered a reported 3.15 MJ of energy. Although the NIF reaction did produce more energy than it consumed, it did not even get close to the 322 MJ of energy it took to power the lasers that produced it.[9] While this was a huge accomplishment in the efforts to produce a nuclear fusion reactor, the reality of such reactors is still a long way off.

Needless to say, the production of sustained and controlled nuclear fusion reactions that generate more energy than is used to produce them will be a huge scientific and engineering accomplishment; the payoffs will be immense if such fusion reactions can be produced within a reactor.

7.3 ALPHA, BETA, AND GAMMA DECAY

Radioactive nuclides are nuclides that spontaneously undergo transitions, emitting particles as a result. This process involving the spontaneous emission of particles is called *radioactive decay*. In radioactive decay it is possible for the atomic number of the radioactive isotope to change, or for the atomic number and the mass number to change, or for neither to change. The types of radioactive decay corresponding to these three scenarios are, respectively, *beta decay*, *alpha decay*, and *gamma decay*. Alpha, beta, and gamma particles can penetrate matter with increasing ability: alpha particles have the least penetrating ability (they can be stopped by a piece of cardboard), beta particles are more penetrating (they can be stopped by a sheet of aluminum), and gamma particles have the greatest penetrating ability (they can penetrate a slab of lead). All of these penetrating abilities depend on the energies of the particles. We will describe each of these types of decay in this section, starting with gamma decay.

Gamma Decay (γ-decay)

Gamma decay is a type of radioactive decay in which a high-energy photon, or *gamma ray*, is emitted from the nucleus. Why would a nucleus emit a photon? Basically for the same reason that an atom emits a photon. Recall that an atom will emit a photon if the atom is in an excited state. An electron in the excited atom will undergo a (stimulated or spontaneous) transition to a lower-energy level accompanied by the emission of a photon whose energy matches the energy difference between the two electron quantum states involved in the transition.

Likewise for the nucleus. As discussed in Chapter 6, nucleons within the nucleus can have discrete energy levels just like the electrons around the nucleus. If a nucleus is in an excited state, then it can undergo a transition to a lower-energy state accompanied by the emission of a photon whose energy equals the energy difference between the two nuclear quantum states involved in the transition. A high-energy photon emitted by an atom is called an *x-ray*, while a high-energy photon emitted by the nucleus is called a *gamma ray*.

A nuclide $_Z^A X$ that is in an excited state is denoted by a star: $_Z^A X^*$. This excited-state isotope can decay down to either another excited state or else to the ground state, in either case with the emission of a γ-particle of the appropriate energy. Symbolically, we can express this decay as

$$_Z^A X^* \longrightarrow {}_Z^A X + \gamma. \tag{7.8}$$

Many excited nuclear states decay by means of gamma decay within very short times—on the order of 10^{-11} s or shorter. An excited state is said to be a *metastable state* if it lasts for significantly longer times—from milliseconds up to several hours or even up to a number of years. An isotope in a metastable state is denoted $_Z^A X^m$:

$$_Z^A X^m \longrightarrow {}_Z^A X + \gamma. \tag{7.9}$$

If the decay goes from one metastable state to another, and then finally to the ground state, then this series of decays could be represented as

$$\begin{aligned}
_Z^A X^{m_1} &\longrightarrow {}_Z^A X^{m_2} + \gamma_1 \\
_Z^A X^{m_2} &\longrightarrow {}_Z^A X + \gamma_2.
\end{aligned} \tag{7.10}$$

An isotope in a metastable state is said to be an *isomer* of the original isotope. For this reason, gamma decay is also sometimes called an *isomeric transition*. Gamma decay always follows a different type of decay process in which the daughter nucleus in the decay is left in an excited state.

In a related process called *internal conversion,* the transition of the nucleus between isomers (different metastable states of the same isotope) results in the energy that would otherwise be released in the form of a γ particle being instead used to eject an inner-shell electron (K, L, ...) orbiting the nucleus. This process is then, of course, followed by the emission of x-rays or Auger electrons from the atom, as was discussed in Chapter 5.

Alpha Decay (α-decay)

Compared to other isotopes with close values of Z or A, the $_2^4 \text{He}$ isotope has a relatively large binding energy per nucleon, as shown in Fig. (7.1). As a result, particularly in heavier nuclei, it is possible for a nucleus to spontaneously emit a helium-4 nucleus, which is also called an *alpha particle*, sometimes written α or $_2^4 \alpha$. (Excess energy in the transition can be carried away by the alpha particle in the form of kinetic energy.) The resulting daughter nucleus is often left in an excited state, so it is common for the alpha decay of a given isotope to be followed by the gamma decay of the (excited-state) daughter isotope.

The generic alpha decay process can be written as

$$_Z^A X \longrightarrow {}_{Z-2}^{A-4}Y + {}_2^4He\,, \tag{7.11}$$

or, for a daughter nucleus in an excited state,

$$_Z^A X \longrightarrow {}_{Z-2}^{A-4}Y^* + {}_2^4He$$
$$_{Z-2}^{A-4}Y^* \longrightarrow {}_{Z-2}^{A-4}Y + \gamma\,. \tag{7.12}$$

Note that, in all of the equations in (7.11) and (7.12), the sums of the mass numbers on both sides of the arrows are the same, as are the sums of the atomic numbers on both sides of the arrows. This is *always* the case in any type of nuclear process and is a consequence of the fundamental principles of the *conservation of mass number* and the *conservation of charge*, respectively, as discussed at the beginning of this chapter.

Beta Decay (β-decay)

An electron is also historically called a *beta particle*. In beta decay a nucleus emits an electron. This of course immediately prompts the question, "*What was an electron doing in the nucleus in the first place?*"

It turns out that a neutron (n) will spontaneously decay into a proton (p) with the emission of an electron (e) and an *anti-neutrino* ($\bar{\nu}$):

$$n \longrightarrow p + e + \bar{\nu}\,. \tag{7.13}$$

The half-life of this decay process is about 610.1 s—a little over 10 minutes—when the neutron is outside of a nucleus.[10] (The half-life when the neutron is inside a nucleus is dictated by the nucleus.) A *neutrino*, ν (the Greek letter, "*nu*"), is a neutral particle having a very small mass[c] along with energy and momentum, so its contributions are important in the dynamics of any nuclear process involving neutrinos. *Antiparticles* have the same mass but opposite charge as their associated particle. They are typically denoted with a *bar* over the symbol for the particle. Therefore the *anti-electron*, or *positron*, denoted $\bar{e}$, has a charge $+e$, while the *anti-proton*, $\bar{p}$, has a charge $-e$. As with the neutrino ν, the anti-neutrino $\bar{\nu}$ is chargeless.

As a result of the decay of the neutron as given in Eq. (7.13), it is possible for one element to decay into another with the emission of an electron from its nucleus (as a result of the decay of one of its neutrons). For example, the beta decay of the gold isotope Au-198 is given by

$$^{198}\text{Au} \longrightarrow {}^{198}\text{Hg} + e + \bar{\nu}\,. \tag{7.14}$$

---

[c]The neutrino mass appears to be about $1.5\,eV/c^2$. This can be compared to the electron mass of $0.5\,MeV/c^2$.

To see why the product of this decay is the given isotope of mercury (Hg) we must note that $Z = 1$ corresponds to one proton charge, so that $Z = -1$ would correspond to *negative* the charge of a proton—in other words, the charge of the electron. We can therefore rewrite Eq. (7.14) using full isotopic notation as follows:

$$^{198}_{79}\text{Au} \longrightarrow {}^{198}_{80}\text{Hg} + {}^{0}_{-1}e + {}^{0}_{0}\bar{\nu}. \qquad (7.15)$$

Note in this equation that the mass number of the electron and anti-neutrino are both zero (neither one is a nucleon), and the atomic number of the anti-neutrino is zero (it has no charge). Again, note the conservation of mass number (A) and atomic number (Z) on both sides of the arrow.

The generic beta-decay equation is therefore given by

$$^{A}_{Z}X \longrightarrow {}^{A}_{Z+1}Y + {}^{0}_{-1}e + {}^{0}_{0}\bar{\nu}. \qquad (7.16)$$

Note that we can use the atomic number of the given parent isotope, Z, to calculate the atomic number of the daughter isotope, $Z + 1$, which we can then use (perhaps along with a periodic table) to determine the element for the daughter isitope (Y).

Related to beta decay are two other processes: *positron decay* and *electron capture* (sometimes called *inverse-beta decay*). These processes are defined in the generic equations given below.

Positron Decay

$$^{A}_{Z}X \longrightarrow {}^{A}_{Z-1}Y + {}^{0}_{1}\bar{e} + {}^{0}_{0}\nu \qquad (7.17)$$

Electron Capture

$$^{A}_{Z}X + {}^{0}_{-1}e \longrightarrow {}^{A}_{Z-1}Y + {}^{0}_{0}\nu \qquad (7.18)$$

7.4   RADIOACTIVE DECAY SERIES

Recall that α-, β-, and γ-decay are a means for an isotope to reduce its energy by the emission of one or more particles. These decay processes may be summarized as shown below.

α**-decay:**

$$^{A}_{Z}X \longrightarrow {}^{A-4}_{Z-2}Y + {}^{4}_{2}He \qquad (7.19)$$

β**-decay:**

$$^{A}_{Z}X \longrightarrow {}^{A}_{Z+1}Y + e + \bar{\nu} \qquad (7.20)$$

γ**-decay:**

$$^{A}_{Z}X^{*} \longrightarrow {}^{A}_{Z}X + \gamma \qquad (7.21)$$

There are 92 naturally occurring elements on Earth. Those elements with low Z tend to be stable, while those with higher values of Z tend to be radioactive. *All elements with $Z > 83$ are radioactive.*

In general, when one radioactive nuclide decays it produces another nuclide, which itself might be radioactive, leading to a decay into another possibly radioactive nuclide, and so on. Such a sequence of successive decays leads to the concept of a *decay series*. All naturally occurring radioactive nuclides are a part of a decay series.

Let's say that a certain decay series starts with the radioactive nuclide $^{A_o}_{Z_o}X$. After some number of α-decays, N_α, and some number of β-decays, N_β, we end up with the nuclide $^A_Z Y$, where

$$A = A_o - 4N_\alpha \tag{7.22}$$

and

$$Z = Z_o - 2N_\alpha + N_\beta . \tag{7.23}$$

Equations (7.22) and (7.23) follow from the fact that each α-decay reduces the mass number (A) of the parent nuclide by 4 and reduces the atomic number (Z) by 2, while each β-decay does not change the mass number, but increases the atomic number by 1. We can then see that all nuclides in a given decay series will have their mass numbers differing by some multiple of 4. This implies that there are *four* possible decay series in nature. Each of these decay series can be represented mathematically by one of the following schemes representing the values of the mass number A of each nuclide in the series: $4n$, $4n + 1$, $4n + 2$, or $4n + 3$, where n is a positive integer. Note that, if we had written a fifth series, represented by $4n + 4$, then we could have written this as $4(n + 1) = 4n'$, where n' is another integer, so that this would really be just another nuclide in the $4n$ series and not an independent fifth series at all.

The four series mentioned above can be written out in terms of the possible A values in the series, starting with $A = 1, 2, 3$, or 4, as follows (remember that only α-decay affects the value of the mass number A, and that each α-decay changes the A value by 4):

Series 1: $A = 1 \leftarrow 5 \leftarrow 9 \leftarrow 13 \leftarrow 17 \leftarrow 21 \leftarrow 25 \leftarrow \ldots$

Series 2: $A = 2 \leftarrow 6 \leftarrow 10 \leftarrow 14 \leftarrow 18 \leftarrow 22 \leftarrow 26 \leftarrow \ldots$

Series 3: $A = 3 \leftarrow 7 \leftarrow 11 \leftarrow 15 \leftarrow 19 \leftarrow 23 \leftarrow 27 \leftarrow \ldots$

Series 4: $A = 4 \leftarrow 8 \leftarrow 12 \leftarrow 16 \leftarrow 20 \leftarrow 24 \leftarrow 28 \leftarrow \ldots$

We can see that if we tried another series we would just get back to where we started (series 1), as discussed above:

Series 5: $A = 5 \leftarrow 9 \leftarrow 13 \leftarrow 17 \leftarrow 21 \leftarrow 25 \leftarrow 29 \leftarrow \ldots$

Note that *Series 4* listed above must correspond to the $4n$ series since each of the A-values in the series equals 4 times an integer. It then follows that *Series 1* corresponds to the $4n+1$ series, *Series 2* corresponds to $4n+2$, and *Series 3* corresponds to $4n+3$.

All naturally occurring radioactive nuclides are found to fall into one of the three series $4n$, $4n+2$, or $4n+3$; the series represented by $4n+1$ (*Series 1* above) is found only in artificially produced nuclides.[d] These three naturally occurring series and the one artificially produced series, along with their parent nuclides, the half-lives of the parents, and the stable nuclide at the end of the series, are listed in Table (7.1). (See Ex. 7.2 for a discussion of radioactive half-life.) Note that each of the naturally occurring decay series ends in an isotope of lead (*Pb*).

TABLE 7.1: The four possible decay series

Series	Series Name	Parent Nuclide	$T_{1/2}$ (years)	End Nuclide
$4n$	Thorium	Th-232	1.39×10^{10}	Pb-208
$(4n+1)$	Neptunium	Np-237	2.25×10^6	Bi-209
$4n+2$	Uranium	U-238	4.51×10^9	Pb-206
$4n+3$	Actinium	U-235	7.07×10^8	Pb-207

7.5 RADIOACTIVE DECAY: GENERAL THEORY

Consider a generic nuclide $^A_Z X$ that has a certain probability per unit time of undergoing radioactive decay. In such a decay it is possible for the atomic number Z to change, or for the atomic number and the mass number A to change, or for *neither* of these quantities to change. The original nuclide before the decay takes place is called the *parent* nuclide. The nuclide that remains after the decay takes place is called the *daughter* nuclide. If the daughter nuclide decays into another nuclide with the emission of a particle or photon, then the resulting nuclide is called the *granddaughter* nuclide.

In practice, it is very difficult for us to measure directly how many radioactive nuclei are present in a given sample. (In general, samples are not pure, and can contain many different nuclei of different elements, or even a "pure" sample of a single element can contain different isotopes of that element.) What we *can* measure, however, is the *rate* at which radioactive decays are taking place, since it is often relatively easy to detect the nuclear emissions from the decaying nuclei. This rate of decay is called the *activity* of the sample and is denoted $\mathscr{A}$. The *SI* unit of activity is the *becquerel*, *Bq*: $1\,Bq = 1\,decay/s$. An older but still commonly used unit of activity is the *curie*, *Ci*, equal to the activity of one gram of pure radium: $1\,Ci = 3.7 \times 10^{10}\,Bq$.

Let's consider a sample that contains some number $\mathscr{N}$ of a specific radioactive nuclide $^A_Z X$. (The sample may contain other nuclides than this one, but we are assuming

---

[d]This can be understood by inspection of Table (7.1) and noting that the age of the Earth is about 4.5×10^9 years.

that none of them are radioactive.) This nuclide decays into a daughter nuclide that we assume is not radioactive.

The (*differential*) number $d\mathcal{N}$ stands for the (*very small*) change in the number of radioactive nuclei in the sample during the (*very small*) time interval dt. Since the number of radioactive nuclei in the sample *decreases* as the nuclei decay (they change from parent nuclides into daughter nuclides, thereby decreasing the number of parent nuclides $^A_Z X$), we see that the *change* in the number $\mathcal{N}$ is *negative*, $d\mathcal{N} < 0$, so that $|d\mathcal{N}| = -d\mathcal{N}$. The *rate* of decay of parent nuclides in the sample—that is, the number of decays per second—is then given by

$$\mathcal{A} = \frac{\#decays}{time} = \frac{|d\mathcal{N}|}{dt} = -\frac{d\mathcal{N}}{dt} . \tag{7.24}$$

Note that, despite the minus sign, the activity $\mathcal{A}$ is a *positive* quantity (since $d\mathcal{N} < 0$).

The activity of a radioactive sample is proportional to the number of radioactive nuclei in the sample. This should make sense to us since, if there are twice as many radioactive nuclei in the sample, then there will be twice as many decays per second. We can thus write that $\mathcal{A} \propto \mathcal{N}$. We can change any proportionality to an equality by the introduction of a *constant of proportionality*. In this case, we give the constant of proportionality the symbol λ and call it the *decay constant*. We can then write that

$$\mathcal{A} = \lambda \mathcal{N} . \tag{7.25}$$

Note that the units of the decay constant λ must be s^{-1} since the units of $\mathcal{A}$ are s^{-1}, and $\mathcal{N}$ is a unitless number. Combining equations (7.24) and (7.25) then give us the result

$$\mathcal{A} = -\frac{d\mathcal{N}}{dt} = \lambda \mathcal{N} . \tag{7.26}$$

Separating variables and integrating then yields:

$$d\mathcal{N} = -\lambda \mathcal{N} dt \tag{7.27}$$

$$\int_{\mathcal{N}_o}^{\mathcal{N}(t)} \frac{d\mathcal{N}}{\mathcal{N}} = -\int_0^t \lambda dt , \tag{7.28}$$

or

$$\mathcal{N}(t) = \mathcal{N}_o e^{-\lambda t} . \tag{7.29}$$

Here, $\mathcal{N}_o$ is the number of radioactive nuclei present at the time $t = 0$, and $\mathcal{N}(t)$ is the number present at some later time t. It then follows from Eqs. (7.25) and (7.29) that the activity at the time t is given by

$$\mathcal{A}(t) = \lambda \mathcal{N}(t) = \lambda \mathcal{N}_o e^{-\lambda t} = \mathcal{A}_o e^{-\lambda t} , \tag{7.30}$$

where $\mathcal{A}_o \equiv \lambda \mathcal{N}_o$ is the activity of the sample at the initial time $t = 0$.

Before proceeding with our discussion of radioactive decay, let's take a minute to dig a bit more deeply into the significance of the decay constant, λ. Rearranging Eq. (7.26) slightly gives us that

$$\lambda = \frac{(-d\mathcal{N}/\mathcal{N})}{dt}. \tag{7.31}$$

Noting that $-d\mathcal{N}$ is the number of parent nuclei at the time t that decayed within the small time interval dt out of a total number of parent nuclei $\mathcal{N}$, we can see that the quantity $-d\mathcal{N}/\mathcal{N}$ gives us the *probability* that any given nucleus would decay during this time interval. It then follows that λ tells us the probability of decay for any nucleus per unit time.

For example, if, at some time t, there are $\mathcal{N} = 100$ parent nuclides, and during the following second (so that $dt = 1\,s$) 3 of those parent nuclei decay (so that the change in the number of parent nuclides is $d\mathcal{N} = -3$), then it follows that the probability that any nucleus would have decayed during that second was 3 out of 100, or $-d\mathcal{N}/\mathcal{N} = 3/100 = 0.03$. The probability of decay per unit time would then be $0.03\,s^{-1}$, which would be the value of the decay constant, λ. Since λ is a constant for a given decay, it follows that the probability of decay per unit time for any given parent nucleus is a constant. This says that, even if a parent nucleus has lasted a very long time without decaying, and all of the other parent nuclei around it have decayed into daughter nuclei, the probability of it decaying in the next second is exactly the same as it was at $t = 0$ before any decays had taken place.

7.6 IMPORTANT RESULTS FROM THE GENERAL THEORY OF RADIOACTIVE DECAY

We will here first summarize the important results from the previous section and then we will show how they can be used to derive some very important equations in the theory of radioactive decay.

First, the activity of a sample, $\mathscr{A}$, containing some number $\mathcal{N}$ of identical radioactive parent nuclei is defined to be the number of decays per second of the parent nuclei. If the sample contained twice the number of radioactive parent nuclei, then we would expect to get twice the number of decays in one second—and, hence, twice the activity. This means that the activity must be proportional to the number of radioactive parent nuclei in the sample at any instant of time. But, if two quantities are proportional, then one quantity must equal a constant (called the *constant of proportionality*) times the other quantity. We thus must have that

$$\mathscr{A} = \lambda \mathcal{N}, \tag{7.32}$$

where λ (*lambda*) is the symbol used to represent the proportionality constant. As a result of the radioactive decays, the number of parent nuclei in the sample must decrease with time. The equation describing the number of radioactive parent nuclei as a function of time is given by

$$\mathcal{N}(t) = \mathcal{N}_o\, e^{-\lambda t}, \tag{7.33}$$

where $\mathcal{N}_o$ is the number of parent nuclei in the sample at the time $t = 0$, and $e^{-\lambda t} = exp(-\lambda t)$ is the exponential function evaluated at $-\lambda t$. ("e" is the base of the natural logarithm, and has a value approximately equal to 2.718.) Substituting Eq. (7.33) into Eq. (7.32) then gives us the equation for the activity of the radioactive sample as a function of time:

$$\mathcal{A}(t) = \lambda \mathcal{N}(t) = \lambda \mathcal{N}_o \, e^{-\lambda t} = \mathcal{A}_o \, e^{-\lambda t} \,. \tag{7.34}$$

In this equation, we have defined $\mathcal{A}_o \equiv \lambda \mathcal{N}_o$ to be the activity of the sample at the initial time $t = 0$.

Example 7.2: Radioactive Half-life

Consider a sample containing a large number of a single type of radioactive nuclide. We define the *half-life* of that radioactive nuclide to be the average amount of time for one half of the radioactive nuclei present in the sample to undergo radioactive decay—that is, the half-life is the average amount of time for the number of parent nuclei remaining to drop to *one half* of its initial value. Find an expression for the half-life in terms of the decay constant, λ.

Solution:

Letting $T_{1/2}$ denote the half-life, we then have by definition that

$$\mathcal{N}(T_{1/2}) = \frac{1}{2}\mathcal{N}_o \,. \tag{7.35}$$

Combining equations (7.35) and (7.33) then gives us that, at the time $t = T_{1/2}$,

$$\frac{1}{2}\mathcal{N}_o = \mathcal{N}_o \, e^{-\lambda T_{1/2}} \tag{7.36}$$

or

$$e^{\lambda T_{1/2}} = 2 \,. \tag{7.37}$$

Taking the natural log (logarithm base e) of both sides then gives us that

$$\lambda T_{1/2} = \ln(2) \tag{7.38}$$

or, finally,

$$\boxed{T_{1/2} = \frac{\ln(2)}{\lambda}} \,. \tag{7.39}$$

End of solution to Example 7.2.

Example 7.3: Radioactive Mean-life

Consider a particular radioactive nuclide, or *radionuclide*, and a sample containing many such nuclei. The *mean-life* of the radionuclide, denoted T_{ave}, is defined to be the average amount of time after $t = 0$ before a nucleus in the sample decays. Stated another way, T_{ave} is the average time of survival for a nucleus in the sample. Find an expression for the mean life of a radionuclide whose decay constant is λ.

Solution:

As explained in the example statement, the mean-life is the average amount of time for a given nucleus to decay. Let's say that we start off with some number $\mathcal{N}_o$ of parent nuclides, and that it takes a time T_{total} for all $\mathcal{N}_o$ of the nuclides to decay. The average time for each decay must therefore be

$$T_{ave} = \frac{T_{total}}{\mathcal{N}_o}. \tag{7.40}$$

The number of decays during a time interval dt at the time t is given from Eq. (7.26) by

$$-d\mathcal{N} = \mathcal{A}\,dt = \lambda\mathcal{N}(t)\,dt. \tag{7.41}$$

Since these $-d\mathcal{N}$ parent nuclei survived a time t before they decayed, the (tiny) contribution to the total decay time T_{total} from these $-d\mathcal{N}$ nucleir must be

$$dT_{total} = t\,(-d\mathcal{N}) = t\lambda\mathcal{N}(t)dt. \tag{7.42}$$

Using Eq. (7.33) in Eq. (7.42), and then integrating over all times t, will give us the total time T_{total}:

$$T_{total} = \int dT_{total} = \int_0^\infty t\lambda\mathcal{N}(t)dt = \lambda\mathcal{N}_o \int_0^\infty t\,e^{-\lambda t}\,dt. \tag{7.43}$$

Using integration by parts (letting $u = t$ and $dv = e^{-\lambda t}\,dt$), we get that this integral becomes

$$\begin{aligned}
T_{total} &= \lambda\mathcal{N}_o \left(\left[-\frac{t}{\lambda}\,e^{-\lambda t} \right]_0^\infty + \frac{1}{\lambda}\int_0^\infty e^{-\lambda t}\,dt \right) \\
&= \lambda\mathcal{N}_o \left([0] + \frac{1}{\lambda}\left(-\frac{1}{\lambda} \right)\left[e^{-\lambda t} \right]_0^\infty \right) \\
&= -\frac{\mathcal{N}_o}{\lambda}\,(0 - 1) \\
&= \frac{\mathcal{N}_o}{\lambda}.
\end{aligned} \tag{7.44}$$

It then immediately follows from Eq. (7.40) that

$$\boxed{T_{ave} = \frac{1}{\lambda}}. \tag{7.45}$$

$$\boxed{\textit{End of solution to Example 7.3.}}$$

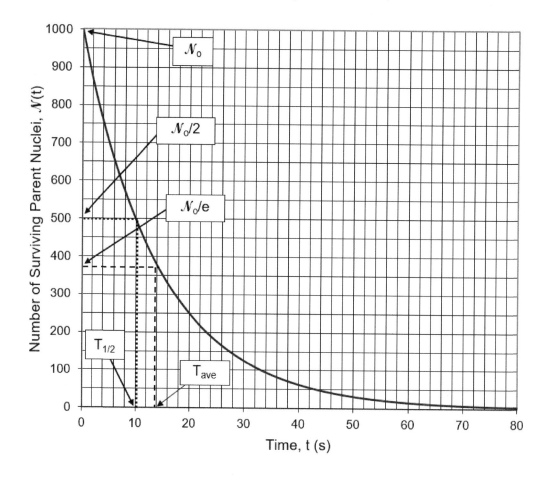

FIGURE 7.2: Plot of the number of radioactive parent nuclei surviving after a time t, $\mathcal{N}(t)$, as a function of t. Shown on the graph are the *half-life*, $T_{1/2}$, and the *mean-life*, T_{ave}. Note that the initial number of parent isotopes is $\mathcal{N}_o = 1000$.

Note that, since

$$T_{1/2} = \frac{\ln 2}{\lambda} = \ln 2 \cdot T_{ave}, \tag{7.46}$$

and $\ln 2 \cong 0.693$, we have that $T_{1/2} < T_{ave}$, which means that the average time it takes for half of the initial population a given radioactive nucleus to decay is less than the average time it takes for any given nucleus to decay. We can also note that, at the time $t = T_{ave} = 1/\lambda$,

$$\mathcal{N}(T_{ave}) = \mathcal{N}_o \, e^{-\lambda T_{ave}} = \mathcal{N}_o \, e^{-\lambda(1/\lambda)} = \frac{\mathcal{N}_o}{e}. \tag{7.47}$$

Since $e \cong 2.718$, we can see that T_{ave} is the time at which the number of radioactive nuclei has dropped to just over *one third* of its initial population $\mathcal{N}_o$. Fig. (7.2) shows the exponential-decay behavior of a sample of radioactive nuclides having an initial population $\mathcal{N}_o = 1000$ along with the half-life and mean life for the decay.

Example 7.4: Treating Liver Cancer with Y-90

Brachytherapy is a short-range form of radiation therapy in which radioactive elements are placed within the region to be treated. (Chapter 22 covers cancer treatment with brachytherapy.) In order to treat liver cancer, yttrium-90 is embedded inside glass microspheres that have a diameter of about 25 μm. Y-90 is a strong beta-emitter that has a half-life of 64.1 hours. The electrons emitted in the beta decay have an average kinetic energy of 0.937 MeV, and penetrate tissue with an average penetration depth of 2.5 mm. A dose of 50 Gy is provided to 1 kg of tissue by 1 GBq of Y-90.[11] To treat the liver tumor, millions of the radioactive beads are injected into the arteries that supply blood to the tumor. This is done by means of a catheter that is threaded into the liver from an artery in the groin.[12] Once injected, the microbeads irradiate the tumor from within.

Consider a 0.145 GBq sample of Y-90 that is being used to treat a 145-gram tumor in the liver. (a) Write out the decay equation for the decay of yttrium-90 using full isotopic notation. (b) Find the value of the decay constant for this decay. (c) What is the value of the mean-life? (d) How many moles of Y-90 are present in the sample at time $t = 0$? (e) How many radioactive yttrium-90 nuclei are present 24 hours after injection? (f) What is the activity of the sample after 24 hours? (g) How long after $t = 0$ does it take for the activity of the sample to drop by 90%?

Solution:

(a) The generic equation for beta decay is shown in Eq. (7.16). A quick glance at a Periodic Table of the Elements (or online search) tells us that $Z = 39$ for yttrium. Applying the conservation of charge (Z values) then tells us that the atomic number of the daughter nucleus must be $39 + 1 = 40$, which corresponds to an isotope of zirconium (Zr). Conservation of nucleon number (A values) then tells us that the daughter nuclide must be $^{90}_{40}Zr$. Putting this into the beta-decay equation then gives us the following:

$$\boxed{^{90}_{39}Y \longrightarrow \, ^{90}_{40}Zr + \, ^{0}_{-1}e + \, ^{0}_{0}\overline{\nu}}. \tag{7.48}$$

(b) Since, from Eq. (7.39), $T_{1/2} = 64.1 hr = ln(2)/\lambda$, it follows that $\lambda = ln(2)/T_{1/2} = \boxed{0.0108 \, hr^{-1}}$.

(c) From Eq. (7.45), $T_{ave} = 1/\lambda = \boxed{92.5 \, hr}$.

(d) We can find the number of moles of Y-90 if we know the number of Y-90 nuclei in the sample, since the number of nuclei in one mole is given by Avogadro's number, $N_A = 6.02 \times 10^{23} mol^{-1}$. Since, from Eq. (7.32) evaluated at $t = 0$, $\mathscr{A}_o \equiv \lambda \mathscr{N}_o$, where $\mathscr{A}_o = 0.145 \, GBq = 0.145 \times 10^9 \, Bq$, it follows that $\mathscr{N}_o = \mathscr{A}_o/\lambda = 1.34 \times 10^{10} = nN_A$, where n is the number of moles of Y-90. We thus get that $n = \mathscr{N}_o/N_A = \boxed{2.23 \times 10^{-14} \, moles}$.

(e) **Method 1.** (In this first method we will use the full power of the equation for the number of nuclei as a function of time. In the second method we will use the meaning of the half-life.) The number of Y-90 nuclei present after 24 hr is given by Eq. (7.33): $\mathcal{N}(t) = \mathcal{N}_o e^{-\lambda t}$. Inserting in the values of $\mathcal{N}_o$, λ, and t and evaluating then gives us that $\mathcal{N}(t = 24\,hr) = \boxed{1.03 \times 10^{10}\,\text{nuclei}}$. **Method 2.** We know that the half-life is equal to $T_{1/2} = 64.1\,hr$. We are interested in the number of nuclei after a time $t = 24\,hr$, given that the initial number of nuclei is $\mathcal{N}_o = 1.34 \times 10^{10}$, from part *(d)*. The important thing here is to express the time t as some multiple of the half-life: $t = NT_{1/2}$. This is easy: simply divide the time by the half-life to get $N = t/T_{1/2} = 24\,hr/64.1\,hr = 0.3744$. But, remember the meaning of the half-life: after every half-life the number of nuclei decreases by a factor of $1/2$. Therefore, after N half-lives, the number of nuclei must decrease by a factor of $(1/2)^N$. We thus must have that, after 24 hr, $\mathcal{N} = \mathcal{N}_o(1/2)^N = \boxed{1.03 \times 10^{10}\,\text{nuclei}}$.

(f) From Eq. (7.32) we have that the activity at time $t = 24\,hr$ is equal to $\mathcal{A}(t) = \lambda \mathcal{N}(t) = \boxed{0.112\,GBq}$. (Or, you can use Eq. 7.34.)

(g) We wish to find the time t such that the activity has decreased *by* 90%. This means that the activity at time t must be 10% of its initial activity: $\mathcal{A}(t) = \frac{1}{10}\mathcal{A}_o$. From Eq. (7.34) it then follows that $\frac{1}{10}\mathcal{A}_o = \mathcal{A}_o e^{-\lambda t}$, or, solving for the exponential term, $e^{+\lambda t} = 10$. To solve for a quantity in an exponent, we need to exploit the properties of a logarithm. Since we have the base of the natural logarithm e in our equation, we will take the *natural* logarithm of both sides, which then gives us that $\lambda t = ln(10)$. Finally, solving for t yields $t = ln(10)/\lambda = \boxed{213\,hr}$.

$$\boxed{\textit{End of solution to Example 7.4.}}$$

7.7 COUPLED RADIOACTIVE DECAYS

In §7.4 we discussed decay series in which a parent nuclide decays into another possibly radioactive nuclide, which itself may decay into yet another possibly radioactive nuclide, *etc.* In this section, we will consider the relationship between radioactive nuclei in a decay series in a more mathematical fashion.

When a radioactive parent nuclide decays, it produces a daughter nuclide, along with other products of the radioactive decay. The daughter nucleus itself may or may not be radioactive. Equation (7.29) tells us that the number of parent nuclei as a function of time is given by

$$\mathcal{N}_p(t) = \mathcal{N}_{po}\, e^{-\lambda_p t}, \tag{7.49}$$

where $\mathcal{N}_{po}$ is the number of radioactive parent nuclei present at the time $t = 0$ and λ_p is the decay constant for the decay of the parent nuclide. In obtaining this equation (see the discussion leading up to Eq. 7.29) we used two different equations for the activity:

$$\mathcal{A}(t) = \lambda \mathcal{N}(t), \tag{7.50}$$

and

$$\mathcal{A}(t) = -\frac{d\mathcal{N}}{dt}. \tag{7.51}$$

This last equation shows us that the differential change in the population under consideration, $d\mathcal{N}$, is given by

$$d\mathcal{N} = -\mathcal{A}(t)dt \ . \tag{7.52}$$

Use of Eq. (7.50) then yields

$$d\mathcal{N} = -\lambda\mathcal{N}(t)\,dt \ . \tag{7.53}$$

The minus signs in Eqs.(7.51), (7.52) and (7.53) tell us that the number of radioactive nuclei undergoing the radioactive decay *decreases* with time, meaning of course that the *change* in the number of radioactive nuclei $d\mathcal{N}$ is negative. While Eq. (7.50) for the activity is *always* true, Eq. (7.51) and the equations that come from it, Eqs.(7.52) and (7.53), are *not* always true. Let's find out why.

Let's consider a hypothetical situation in which a parent nuclide decays into a stable daughter nuclide. This decay process takes place with a half-life $T_{1/2,\,p}$ and corresponding decay constant $\lambda_p = \ln 2/T_{1/2,\,p}$ and is represented schematically in Fig. (7.3). We denote the populations of the parent and daughter nuclides at the time $t = 0$ by $\mathcal{N}_{po}$ and $\mathcal{N}_{do}$, respectively. Since the parent nuclides are simply decaying into the daughter nuclides with the decay constant λ_p, the parent population as a function of time must be given by Eq. (7.49), and the change in the number of parent nuclei within a differential time interval dt at the time t must be given by Eq. (7.53), which we rewrite here for the parent nuclide population:

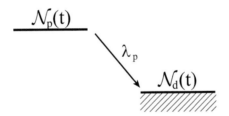

FIGURE 7.3: Schematic representation of a radioactive parent nucleus decaying into a stable daughter nucleus. (The hatched box beneath the daughter nucleus level is intended to indicate that the daughter nucleus is stable against radioactive decay.)

$$d\mathcal{N}_p = -\lambda_p\,\mathcal{N}_p(t)\,dt \ . \tag{7.54}$$

Again, the change in the number of parent nuclei given in Eq. (7.54) is negative, representing a *decrease* in the number of parent nuclei during the tiny time interval dt. This decrease in the number of parent nuclei represents an *increase* in the number of daughter nuclei since all of the parents decay into daughter nuclei. Since the daughter nuclides are stable against radioactive decay, this increase in the number of daughter nuclei during the time interval dt is the *total* change in the number of daughter nuclei during that interval, $d\mathcal{N}_d$, so we must have that

$$d\mathcal{N}_d = |d\mathcal{N}_p| = +\lambda_p\,\mathcal{N}_p(t)\,dt \ . \tag{7.55}$$

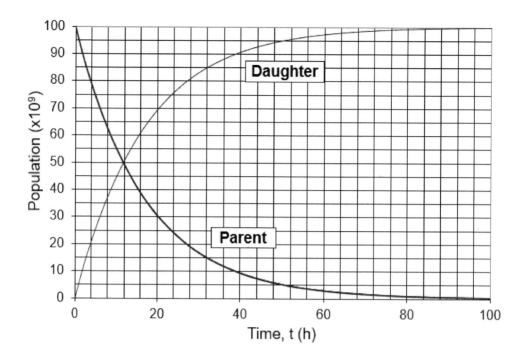

FIGURE 7.4: Plot of parent and daughter nuclide populations as a function of time for the case of a stable daughter nuclide. See Eqs.(7.49) and (7.59). For the generation of these plots, it was assumed that $\mathcal{N}_{po} = 100 \times 10^9$ and that $\mathcal{N}_{do} = 0$.

Use of Eq. (7.49) then gives us that

$$d\mathcal{N}_d = +\lambda_p \mathcal{N}_{po} e^{-\lambda_p t} dt . \tag{7.56}$$

This equation can be directly integrated. Recalling that the number of daughter isotopes at time $t = 0$ is $\mathcal{N}_{do}$, we get that

$$\int_{\mathcal{N}_{do}}^{\mathcal{N}_d(t)} d\mathcal{N}_d = +\lambda_p \mathcal{N}_{po} \int_0^t e^{-\lambda_p t} dt , \tag{7.57}$$

from which it follows that

$$\mathcal{N}_d(t) - \mathcal{N}_{do} = \frac{\lambda_p \mathcal{N}_{po}}{-\lambda_p} \left(e^{-\lambda_p t} - 1 \right) , \tag{7.58}$$

or

$$\mathcal{N}_d(t) = \mathcal{N}_{do} + \mathcal{N}_{po} \left(1 - e^{-\lambda_p t} \right) . \tag{7.59}$$

This equation describes the variation in the population of the daughter isotopes as a function of time for the case of a stable daughter isotope. This variation is shown in Fig. (7.4) for the special case in which $\mathcal{N}_{do} = 0$. Also shown is the parent population $\mathcal{N}_p(t)$, as given by Eq. (7.49).

We note in passing that the sum of the parent and daughter populations is given by:

$$\mathscr{N}_p(t) + \mathscr{N}_d(t) = \mathscr{N}_{po}\, e^{-\lambda_p t} + \mathscr{N}_{do} + \mathscr{N}_{po}\left(1 - e^{-\lambda_p t}\right), \qquad (7.60)$$

or

$$\mathscr{N}_p(t) + \mathscr{N}_d(t) = \mathscr{N}_{po} + \mathscr{N}_{do} = constant. \qquad (7.61)$$

Of course—since the daughter nuclides are stable and the parent nuclides can only decay into the daughter nuclides, the total number of parent plus daughter nuclei cannot change. The total number of parent plus daughter nuclei at any time must be the same as the total initial sum of the parent and daughter nuclei.

Let's return now to a consideration of Eqs.(7.50) and (7.53). Equation (7.50), $\mathscr{A}(t) = \lambda \mathscr{N}(t)$, tells us that the activity of a given sample of radioactive nuclei at any time is proportional to the number of nuclei present at that same time—so if you have twice as many identical nuclei in sample A as in sample B, you will find that sample A has twice the activity as sample B. This is simply a result of the probabilistic nature of radioactive decay.[e] On the other hand, Eq. (7.53), $d\mathscr{N} = -\lambda \mathscr{N}(t)\, dt$, tells us that the change in population of a given sample within a time interval dt is dictated by the activity of that sample (decays per second) as given by Eq. (7.50). Let's look at this within the context of the stable daughter population in the discussion above.

We saw in Eq. (7.59) that the population of daughter nuclei is certainly *not* constant—it changes with time as is seen in Fig. (7.4). It therefore follows that $d\mathscr{N}_d \neq 0$. However, since the daughter nuclides are *stable* (that is, the are *not* radioactive), it follows that there can be no activity associated with the decay of the daughter nuclei—that is, $\mathscr{A}_d(t) = 0$ (or, equivalently, $\lambda_d = 0$). Thus, the left-hand side of Eq. (7.52) (or 7.53) is *not* equal to zero while, at the same time, the right-hand side *must* equal zero. Clearly something is wrong here!

You have probably already figured out that what's wrong is that the change in population $d\mathscr{N}$ isn't only due to the decay of the nuclide under consideration (in our case, the daughter nuclide), but that a change in population will also occur if the decay of another (parent) nuclide feeds into the given population. In the case of the parent nuclide decaying into a stable daughter nuclide, the decay of the parent population feeds into the daughter population, so that the daughter population changes with time despite the fact that the daughter nuclides themselves do not decay. Therefore, if we wish to use an equation like Eq. (7.53), we must be very careful to check whether the decay of another nuclide feeds into the population we're interested in.

We are now ready to move to a more general discussion—namely, one in which the daughter nuclide is also radioactive. To this end, let's consider a case in which the parent nuclide decays into a daughter nuclide that is also unstable. That is, the daughter nuclide can decay into a granddaughter nuclide, which may or may not be unstable.[f] We assume that the parent nuclide decays with a half-life $T_{1/2,p}$ and decay

---

[e]Given a sample of a certain type of radioactive nuclide, the probability of undergoing decay within a given time interval is a constant, independent of the time. That is, a nucleus that has survived for ten half lives has the same probability of decay per unit time as it did after only one half life—its probability of decay does not build up over time.

[f]Whether the granddaughter nuclide is stable or not has no bearing on the current discussion.

constant $\lambda_p = \ln 2/T_{1/2,\,p}$, while the daughter nuclide decays with a half-life $T_{1/2,\,d}$ and decay constant $\lambda_d = \ln 2/T_{1/2,\,d}$. These coupled decays of the parent and daughter nuclides are represented schematically in Fig. (7.5). As before, the populations of the parent and daughter nuclei at the time $t = 0$ are denoted $\mathcal{N}_{po}$ and $\mathcal{N}_{do}$.

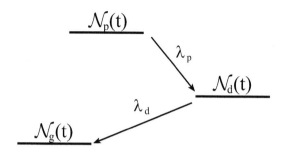

FIGURE 7.5: Schematic representation of a radioactive parent nuclide decaying into a radioactive daughter nuclide, which subsequently decays into a granddaughter nuclide.

Since the parent nuclides are simply decaying into the daughter nuclides with the decay constant λ_p, the parent population as a function of time must still be given by Eq. (7.49): $\mathcal{N}_p(t) = \mathcal{N}_{po}\, e^{-\lambda_p t}$. Also as before, this decay of the parent nuclei feeds into the population of the daughter nuclides. But now we must be very careful since, at the same time, the daughter nuclei are decaying into granddaughter nuclei. We thus have two competing processes: one trying to *increase* the daughter population and the other trying to *decrease* it.

Since the decay of parent nuclei contributes to an *increase* in the population of the daughter nuclei, we denote the differential change in the daughter population due to the decay of the parent nuclides during a time interval dt by $d\mathcal{N}^{(+)}$ and write, in analogy with Eqs.(7.55) and (7.56),

$$d\mathcal{N}_d^{(+)} = |d\mathcal{N}_p| = +\lambda_p\, \mathcal{N}_{po}\, e^{-\lambda_p t} dt\,. \qquad (7.62)$$

But, at the same time, the daughter population is decaying into granddaughter nuclei, contributing to a *decrease* in the daughter population according to Eq. (7.53). We denote this change in the daughter population due to the decay of the daughter nuclei by $d\mathcal{N}_d^{(-)}$, and write:

$$d\mathcal{N}_d^{(-)} = -\mathcal{A}_d(t)\, dt\,, \qquad (7.63)$$

or

$$d\mathcal{N}_d^{(-)} = -\lambda_d \mathcal{N}_d(t)\, dt\,. \qquad (7.64)$$

The *net* change in the daughter population during the differential time interval dt is therefore given by

$$d\mathcal{N}_d = d\mathcal{N}_d^{(+)} + d\mathcal{N}_d^{(-)} = +\lambda_p\, \mathcal{N}_{po}\, e^{-\lambda_p t} dt - \lambda_d \mathcal{N}_d(t)\, dt\,, \qquad (7.65)$$

or, dividing both sides by dt to get the rate of change in the number of daughter nuclei:

$$\frac{d\mathcal{N}_d}{dt} = +\lambda_p \, \mathcal{N}_{po} \, e^{-\lambda_p t} - \lambda_d \mathcal{N}_d(t) \, . \tag{7.66}$$

We wish to solve Eq. (7.66) for the unknown function $\mathcal{N}_d(t)$, the daughter population as a function of time. When we did this previously for the case of the *stable* daughter nucleus in Eq. (7.56) we were able to simply integrate both sides of the equation. However, we cannot simply integrate Eq. (7.66) as we did Eq. (7.56). Equations such as Eq. (7.56) and (7.66) are called *differential equations* and cannot always be solved as simply as we solved Eq. (7.56).[g] We therefore simply state that the solution to Eq. (7.66) is given by

$$\mathcal{N}_d(t) = \mathcal{N}_{do} \, e^{-\lambda_d t} + \left(\frac{\lambda_p}{\lambda_d - \lambda_p} \right) \mathcal{N}_{po} \left(e^{-\lambda_p t} - e^{-\lambda_d t} \right) \, . \tag{7.67}$$

Note that, when Eq. (7.67) is evaluated at $t = 0$, we get that $\mathcal{N}_d(0) = \mathcal{N}_{do}$, as required. Figure (7.6) shows the resulting behavior of the daughter population $\mathcal{N}_d(t)$ as a function of time as described by Eq. (7.67) under the condition that the initial daughter population is zero, $\mathcal{N}_{do} = 0$. We can see that, when the daughter population is small for small values of t, the positive contribution to the daughter population from the decay of the parent nuclei outweighs the negative contribution to the daughter population from the decay of the daughter nuclei into granddaughter nuclei. This is because $\mathcal{N}_d(t)$ is small for small times in Eq. (7.64), resulting in a small value of the population change $d\mathcal{N}_d^{(-)}$. However, as time progresses and the daughter population builds, so does the daughter population decay term $d\mathcal{N}_d^{(-)}$, resulting in an eventual decline of the population growth until the growth stops, and the daughter population starts declining.

We note in Fig. (7.6) that the daughter population eventually starts decaying along with the parent population—that is, the two populations seem to be the same with the same rate of decay, or the same *activity*. This condition is not always found in coupled radioactive decays, so the conditions under which it does occur are very special and worthy of some attention. This condition of *radioactive equilibrium* is the topic of the next section.

7.8 TRANSIENT AND SECULAR EQUILIBRIUM

Let's consider once more a radioactive parent nuclide that decays into a radioactive daughter nuclide, as is schematically represented in Fig. (7.5). In our discussion of that system, we found that the parent population varies with time according to the equation

$$\mathcal{N}_p(t) = \mathcal{N}_{po} \, e^{-\lambda_p t} \, , \tag{7.68}$$

---

[g]Equation (7.56) is a particularly simple form of differential equation—one that can be solved using a technique called the *separation of variables*, which is the method we applied in Eqs.(7.57) through (7.59). We must use more complicated methods to solve differential equations such as Eq. (7.66).

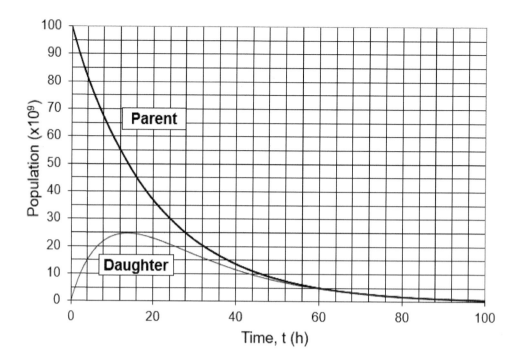

FIGURE 7.6: Plot of parent and daughter nuclide populations as a function of time for the case of an unstable daughter nuclide.

while the daughter population varies according to

$$\mathcal{N}_d(t) = \left(\frac{\lambda_p}{\lambda_d - \lambda_p}\right) \mathcal{N}_{po} \left(e^{-\lambda_p t} - e^{-\lambda_d t}\right), \qquad (7.69)$$

where we have taken the initial daughter population to be zero at time $t = 0$, $\mathcal{N}_{do} = 0$.

We say that two nuclear species are in *equilibrium* or *ideal equilibrium* when their activities (*decays per second*) are equal. In particular, the parent and daughter populations are said to be in equilibrium at some time t_E when

$$\mathcal{A}_d(t_E) = \mathcal{A}_p(t_E). \qquad (7.70)$$

For the daughter population, this means that, at the time t_E, the rate at which new daughter nuclei are being formed from the decay of the parent nuclei is equal to the rate at which daughter nuclei are decaying into granddaughter nuclei. This condition lasts for only an instant, but it is a necessary condition between the parent and daughter populations if the system is to be in *ideal* equilibrium.

We are interested in conditions of *approximate* equilibrium. In particular, there are two types of (*non-ideal*) equilibrium for us to consider: *transient equilibrium*, in which the parent and daughter activities are close for an extended period of time, and *secular equilibrium*, in which the equilibrium condition is more persistent. Both of these types of equilibrium take place after several half-lives of the daughter nuclide.

Transient Equilibrium

We assume that the parent-nuclide half-life is *greater than* the daughter half-life,

$$T_{1/2,p} > T_{1/2,d}, \tag{7.71}$$

from which it follows that, since $\lambda = \ln 2/T_{1/2}$,

$$\lambda_p < \lambda_d. \tag{7.72}$$

From Eqs.(7.68) and (7.69), we have that

$$\mathscr{A}_p(t) = \lambda_p \mathscr{N}_p(t) = \lambda_p \mathscr{N}_{po} e^{-\lambda_p t} \tag{7.73}$$

and

$$\mathscr{A}_d(t) = \lambda_d \mathscr{N}_d(t) = \lambda_d \left(\frac{\lambda_p}{\lambda_d - \lambda_p}\right) \mathscr{N}_{po} \left(e^{-\lambda_p t} - e^{-\lambda_d t}\right). \tag{7.74}$$

Taking the ratio of the daughter to the parent activities, we then get that

$$\frac{\mathscr{A}_d(t)}{\mathscr{A}_p(t)} = \frac{\left(\frac{\lambda_d \lambda_p}{\lambda_d - \lambda_p}\right) \mathscr{N}_{po} \left(e^{-\lambda_p t} - e^{-\lambda_d t}\right)}{\lambda_p \mathscr{N}_{po} e^{-\lambda_p t}}, \tag{7.75}$$

or

$$\frac{\mathscr{A}_d(t)}{\mathscr{A}_p(t)} = \frac{\lambda_d}{\lambda_d - \lambda_p} \left(1 - e^{-(\lambda_d - \lambda_p)t}\right). \tag{7.76}$$

After a sufficiently long time, the exponential term in Eq. (7.76) gets small compared to 1, and we get approximately that

$$\frac{\mathscr{A}_d(t)}{\mathscr{A}_p(t)} \cong \frac{\lambda_d}{\lambda_d - \lambda_p} = \text{constant} > 1. \tag{7.77}$$

Thus, after sufficient time, the ratio of the daughter to the parent activities becomes approximately a constant, with

$$\mathscr{A}_d(\text{large } t) > \mathscr{A}_p(\text{large } t). \tag{7.78}$$

Since the initial daughter population was assumed to be zero ($\mathscr{N}_{do} = 0$), and since $\mathscr{A}_d(t) = \lambda_d \mathscr{N}_d(t)$, it follows that the activity of the daughter nuclide was $\mathscr{A}_d = 0$ at $t = 0$. Thus, at $t = 0$, we must have that

$$\mathscr{A}_d(t = 0) < \mathscr{A}_p(t = 0). \tag{7.79}$$

Comparison of Eqs.(7.78) and (7.79) then shows that, at some time after $t = 0$, the daughter and parent activities must have been equal as the daughter activity increased past the parent activity. We will again call this time the *equilibrium time*, denoted t_E. Thus, at time $t = t_E$,

$$\mathscr{A}_d(t_E) = \mathscr{A}_p(t_E). \tag{7.80}$$

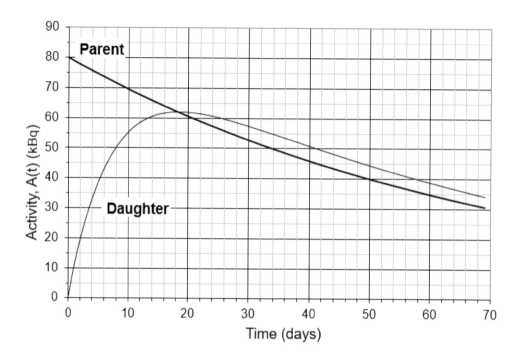

FIGURE 7.7: Plot of parent and daughter activities as a function of time for the case of transient equilibrium ($\lambda_p < \lambda_d$). For this plot, $\lambda_d = 10\lambda_p$.

This is the condition for ideal equilibrium as given in Eq. (7.70) and is only true for a short period of time (officially only for an *instant!*). This is the condition of *transient equilibrium*. As the system passes the condition of transient equilibrium, it shifts into a realm in which the ratio of daughter to parent activities is approximately a constant, as given in Eq. (7.77). Systems exhibiting transient equilibrium typically have[13]

$$\text{Transient Equilibrium: } T_{1/2,p} \simeq 10\, T_{1/2,d}. \tag{7.81}$$

The behavior for transient equilibrium is shown in Fig. (7.7), which shows a plot of parent and daughter activities as a function of time for the case of $\lambda_d = 10\lambda_p$, or $T_{1/2,p} = 10\, T_{1/2,d}$.

Secular Equilibrium

Let's now consider the special case in which the half-life of the parent isotopes is *much greater* than that of the daughter isotopes:

$$T_{1/2,d} \ll T_{1/2,p}, \tag{7.82}$$

from which it follows that

$$\lambda_p \ll \lambda_d . \tag{7.83}$$

This means that the parent isotopes will decay at a much slower rate than the daughter isotopes, so that, relatively speaking, the parent population will remain very nearly constant over at least several half-lives of the daughter isotopes. We can thus write that

$$\lambda_d - \lambda_p \cong \lambda_d . \tag{7.84}$$

This approximation then allows us to rewrite Eq. (7.69) in a more convenient form, as follows:

$$\mathcal{N}_d(t) = \frac{\lambda_p}{\lambda_d - \lambda_p} \, \mathcal{N}_{po} e^{-\lambda_p t} \left(1 - e^{-(\lambda_d - \lambda_p)t}\right)$$

$$\cong \frac{\lambda_p}{\lambda_d} \, \mathcal{N}_{po} e^{-\lambda_p t} \left(1 - e^{-\lambda_d t}\right) , \tag{7.85}$$

or, using Eq. (7.68),

$$\mathcal{N}_d(t) \cong \frac{\lambda_p}{\lambda_d} \, \mathcal{N}_p(t) \left(1 - e^{-\lambda_d t}\right) . \tag{7.86}$$

Multiplying both sides of the equation by λ_d and recalling from Eq. (7.50) that $\mathcal{A} = \lambda \mathcal{N}$, we then get that

$$\mathcal{A}_d(t) \cong \mathcal{A}_p(t) \left(1 - e^{-\lambda_d t}\right) . \tag{7.87}$$

From this equation we can see that, after a sufficient amount of time has passed (at least several daughter half-lives), the exponential term $e^{-\lambda_d t}$ dies out and becomes negligible compared to 1, so that

$$\mathcal{A}_d(t) \cong \mathcal{A}_p(t). \tag{7.88}$$

Thus, once a sufficiently long time has passed, the condition for equilibrium as specified by Eq. (7.70) is approximately satisfied. This form of equilibrium is called *secular equilibrium*. The behavior of coupled decays for the case in which $\lambda_d = 100 \, \lambda_p$, which is within the realm of secular equilibrium, is shown in Fig. (7.8). We say that a system of coupled decays will eventually (after several daughter half-lives) reach secular equilibrium if

$$\text{Secular Equilibrium: } T_{1/2,p} \gtrsim 100 \, T_{1/2,d} . \tag{7.89}$$

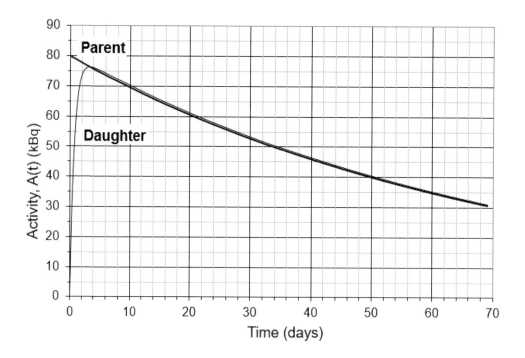

FIGURE 7.8: Plot of parent and daughter activities as a function of time for the case of secular equilibrium ($\lambda_p \ll \lambda_d$). For this plot, $\lambda_d = 100\lambda_p$.

7.9 THE PRODUCTION OF RADIONUCLIDES FOR NUCLEAR MEDICINE AND RADIATION THERAPY

Radioactive nuclei are of fundamental clinical importance in nuclear medicine and in radiation therapy. The field of *nuclear medicine* uses unsealed radio-pharmaceuticals—radioactive nuclides (or *radionuclides*) attached to organic molecules that are selectively absorbed by specific organs, tissues, or cells—for the diagnosis or treatment of disease. (See Chapter 23 for much more detail on cancer treatment with radiopharmaceuticals.) The field of *radiation therapy* sometimes uses sealed radionuclides to irradiate diseased tissue from outside the body (*radiotherapy*) or from within the tumor (*brachytherapy*), in addition to other treatment modalities. Regardless of which treatment modality is exploiting their properties, radionuclides are crucial to the detection and treatment of cancer.[h]

Example (7.1) introduced us to the idea of producing a nuclide that is useful in radiation therapy by bombarding a stable nuclide with neutrons. Indeed, *all* radioactive nuclides used in nuclear medicine are produced using methods similar to those discussed in Ex.(7.1)—that is, by bombarding one nuclide with particles in order to produce a different, more clinically useful nuclide. The three primary means of producing these bombardments are with particle accelerators, within nuclear reactors,

---

[h]Chapter 23 will deal with radiopharmaceutical therapy, Chapters 18 through 21 will deal with radiation therapy, and Chapter 22 will deal with brachytherapy.

and in radionuclide generators.[13] In this section, we will briefly discuss these three methods used to produce these important radionuclides for clinical use.

The Use of Particle Accelerators to Produce Radionuclides

Particle accelerators use electric and magnetic fields to produce forces that accelerate charged particles—typically protons, deuterons, alpha particles, or H^- ions. Since magnetic fields can only turn charges—they can never speed them up or slow them down—it is always electric fields that are used to change the speeds of the charges. Magnetic fields are used to steer or focus the charged-particle beams.

Accelerators basically come in two forms: linear accelerators and circular accelerators. The accelerator that can speed up massive particles (protons and lead ions) to the highest energies—the LHC (Large Hadron Accelerator)—accomplishes this feat with a combination of both linear and circular accelerators.[14]

Cyclotron Basics

The accelerators used to produce the radioactive nuclides used in nuclear medicine tend to be circular accelerators or, more specifically, *cyclotrons*. A very basic schematic of a cyclotron is shown in Fig. (7.9).[15]

The small shaded circle toward the center of the figure represents a charged particle. The curved solid line extending from the particle represents the path of the particle. Note that the particle path passes back-and-forth through two unshaded mirror-image regions in the shape of a "D". (These regions are cleverly called "dees".) The symbol at the bottom of the figure represents the fact that the two dees have an alternating voltage applied to them, so that which dee is positive and which is negative continuously alternates at a set frequency called the *cyclotron frequency*.

For example, if the particle being accelerated is a positive ion, then, as the ion passes into the narrow (shaded) gap between the two dees at the top of its trajectory moving from right to left, the

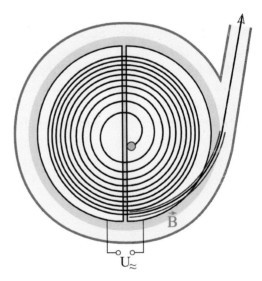

FIGURE 7.9: Schematic of a cyclotron. (Image created by Klaus Föhl: Wikimedia Commons.)

right dee would be positively charged and the left dee would be negatively charged. This would result in the *electric field* between the two dees accelerating the ion toward the left, thereby making it speed up. The region inside each dee contains an externally imposed *magnetic field* that simply serves to steer the ion in a circular path as long as it is inside the dee. Once the ion reaches the bottom of its trajectory, it moves again into the gap between the two dees, at which point the polarity of the two dees switches, making the left dee positive and the right dee negative. This again results in the ion being sped up in the region between the two dees. As the ion speeds up, the radius of its circular path inside each dee increases, as shown in the figure.

This process continues until the ion reaches the desired speed (or energy), at which point it is extracted from the cyclotron and is typically steered into an awaiting target. The collision between the incoming accelerated particle and a stationary target nucleus can result in the deflection or absorption of the incident particle, leaving the resulting target nucleus in an excited state. The excited-state nucleus then transitions to a lower energy state by emitting a photon or other particles.

For example, fluorine-18 (*F-18*) is used in 70−80% of all Positron-Emission Tomography (*PET*) scans.[13] PET is a diagnostic imaging modality that can show if a particular organ is functioning properly. (PET will be discussed in Chapter 12 of this book.) F-18 can be produced in a cyclotron by bombarding oxygen-18 nuclei with protons (hydrogen nuclei, $^1_1$H):

$$^{18}_8\text{O} + ^1_1\text{H} \rightarrow ^{18}_9\text{F} + ^1_0\text{n} \,. \tag{7.90}$$

Fluorine-18 then decays primarily by positron emission with a half-life of 109.8 minutes.[16]

The Use of Nuclear Reactors to Produce Radionuclides

As discussed previously, nuclear reactors are used to produce fission reactions. For example, the fission of uranium-235 is used in many nuclear reactors. One fission equation for U-235 was given earlier in this chapter, Eq. (7.6), in which the uranium nucleus absorbs a neutron and then splits into isotopes of krypton and barium with the emission of two neutrons. But the uranium-235 nucleus can produce several hundred different combinations of nuclei after fission.[17] We here give two more processes for the fission of U-235:

$$^{235}_{92}\text{U} + n \rightarrow ^{93}_{37}\text{Rb} + ^{141}_{55}\text{Cs} + 2n \,, \tag{7.91}$$

and

$$^{235}_{92}\text{U} + n \rightarrow ^{134}_{50}\text{Sn} + ^{99}_{42}\text{Mo} + 3n \,. \tag{7.92}$$

We pointed out previously that the neutrons emitted in the fission of uranium-235 (about 2.5 on average)[17] make it possible for a chain reaction to take place. It is this possibility of a chain reaction that allows us to control the rate of the fission reactions within the reactor, and to keep the reactor self-sustaining.

There are fundamentally two different ways to produce medical radionuclides: *nuclear fission* and *neutron activation*. Equations (7.6), (7.91), and (7.92) show how six of hundreds of radionuclides having mass numbers between 70 and 160 are produced in the fission of U-235 within a reactor,[13] all happening simultaneously with various probabilities. The desired nuclides are then chemically separated from the other fission products.

Neutron Activation

We will now focus on the fact that the 2.5 neutrons given off (on average) in each fission reaction of U-235 means that we have a surplus of neutrons for each reaction (accounting for the one neutron that is used to produce each fission reaction). This means that we will have a cloud of neutrons moving about within the core of reactor. (We discussed previously the use of moderators and control rods for controlling the energy distribution and number of neutrons within the reactor.) It is this cloud of neutrons that is exploited for producing radionuclides within reactors by means of neutron activation.

The idea of neutron activation is very simple, and was already discussed in Ex.(7.1). Neutron activation means that a stable nucleus absorbs a neutron, resulting in a radioactive nucleus—often accompanied by the emission of a gamma particle. In Ex.(7.1), we discussed the bombardment of the stable isotope Co-59 with neutrons in order to produce the radioactive isotope Co-60, which is used in radiation therapy for cancer treatment. The problem is, how do we bombard stable nuclides with neutrons in order to produce radionuclides given that neutrons have zero net charge and therefore cannot be accelerated and fired at targets as is done with charged particles in cyclotrons? The answer, of course, lies within nuclear reactors.

Research reactors are nuclear reactors that are used for research and for the production of radionuclides. These reactors have ports that lead into the core of the reactor where the nuclear fuel (U-235) is placed. Due to the excess of neutrons produced in the fission reactions, there is a constant cloud of neutrons swirling around the fuel pellets. The nuclei that we wish to bombard are simply inserted into the region around the fuel via the insertion ports. As a result, the stable nuclei will be bombarded by the neutrons produced during the nuclear fission reactions within the fuel pellets. Once a target nucleus absorbs a neutron, it tends to immediately emit a gamma particle, leaving behind a radionuclide that most often decays by means of beta emission.

For example, strontium-89 (Sr-89) is used for pain relief from tumors in bone resulting from the spread of cancer cells from the primary site of the cancer. (This spreading of cancer cells to different parts of the body is called *metastasis*.) Sr-89 is produced by neutron activation from the stable isotope Sr-88:

$$\ce{^{88}_{38}Sr} + n \rightarrow \ce{^{89}_{38}Sr} + \gamma. \tag{7.93}$$

The radioactive Sr-89 nucleus then undergoes beta decay with a half-life of 50.56 days.[18]

The Use of Radionuclide Generators to Produce Radionuclides

A number of radionuclides useful in nuclear medicine have very short half-lives, making any kind of transport or storage not feasible. However, it is possible to keep a ready supply of such radionuclides if we can exploit the phenomenon of radioactive equilibrium, as was discussed in §7.8. In particular, if the half-life of a parent radionuclide is longer than that of the daughter radionuclide, then, after a sufficiently long time, the daughter nuclide will effectively be produced with the half-life of the parent. This is the case of *transient equilibrium* that was discussed earlier. A storage device that stores the population of parent radionuclide and allows for the easy removal of the population of short-lived daughter radionuclide is called a *radionuclide generator*.

The parent radionuclide is produced either in a cyclotron or by neutron activation and is then placed in the generator for storage and production of the desired daughter radionuclide. In order for the radionuclide generator to be useful, the daughter nuclide must be chemically distinct from the parent nuclide so that it can be separated from the parent by simple chemical means. This tends not to be an issue, however, since, as already mentioned, the parent nuclides typically decay by beta emission, resulting in a nucleus having a different atomic number, and thus a different chemical nature.

The following example discusses the issues associated with the production of an extremely important radionuclide in nuclear medicine using a radionuclide generator.

Example 7.5: The Crisis of Molybdenum-99

Technetium-99m is probably the most important radionuclide in the world.[i] This is because it is the most widely used radioisotope in diagnostic imaging. Indeed, Tc-99m is used in about 30 million nuclear medicine procedures around the world annually.[19] Unfortunately, Tc-99m has the very short half-life of 6.01 hours,[18] making it very difficult to store for clinical use.

Discuss how Tc-99m is produced for clinical use and the issues associated with that production.

Solution:

Tc-99m is the daughter nuclide of molybdenum-99 (*Mo-99*), which is a radioactive nuclide having a half-life of 65.98 hours.[18] This means that Mo-99 can be stored in a radionuclide generator, which can be kept in the clinic and accessed as needed to retrieve the desired Tc-99m nuclides. The Mo-99/Tc-99m generator is often referred to as a "moly generator", or, even more colloquially, as a "cow". The extraction of the desired Tc-99m from the generator is achieved by flushing the system with oxygenated saline in a process referred to as "milking the cow".[13] While this bovine set-up is certainly advantageous for the clinic, it unfortunately introduces a number of issues.

Molybdenum-99 is produced by neutron activation in nuclear fission research reactors. According to the International Atomic Energy Agency,[19] there is a worldwide shortage of Mo-99. As of 2017 there were only six reactors worldwide used to produce Mo-99. These reactors were located in Belgium, the Netherlands, the Czech Republic, Poland, Australia, and South Africa. Canada stopped producing Mo-99 in October of 2016.[20,21] Since there was such a small number of reactors that produced Mo-99, a crisis in the supply of Mo-99 would result if anything were to happen to any of the reactors. Indeed, such a crisis occurred in 2007 when Canada had to unexpectedly shut down its production for repairs, followed by unrelated instances in other facilities that temporarily slowed or stopped production.[19] The short supply of Mo-99 was further exacerbated by the fact that the majority of reactors that were used to produce it used what is called *highly enriched uranium*.

---

[i]Recall that a nucleus that is in a relatively long-lived excited state is said to be in a *metastable* state. (This same terminology is used for electronic excited states in atoms.) The "m" in technetium-99m refers to the fact that the nuclide Tc-99 is in a metastable state.

Naturally occurring uranium ore contains about 99.27% U-238, and about 0.72% fissile U-235, along with trace amounts of U-234.[22] Mo-99 is produced in the fission of U-235 according to Eq. (7.92), which was given as an example of using nuclear fission to produce radionuclides. Since U-235 comprises such a small percentage of naturally occurring uranium ore, the uranium ore is put through a process of *enrichment*, meaning that it is processed so that the percentage of U-235 is increased.

Most uranium-enrichment facilities in the world produce *low enriched uranium (LEU)*, which is defined to be uranium enriched up to 20% U-235 by weight. The reason for this cut-off is that uranium fuel having less than 20% U-235 cannot be used for nuclear explosive devices without further enrichment.[23] However, as mentioned above, most research reactors that produce Mo-99 use *highly enriched uranium (HEU)*. As of 2016 there were only four countries producing HEU: India, Pakistan, Russia, and North Korea.[24,25]

For reasons that should be very clear, there has been a strong international push for the reduction in and eventual elimination of the production and civilian use of HEU. (The military does not only use HEU for making nuclear weapons—nuclear-powered ships and submarines also use HEU as fuel.) Indeed, the International Atomic Energy Agency (IAEA) developed a coordinated research project that involved the participation of fourteen IAEA Member States, the purpose of which was to develop alternate means of producing Mo-99 that did not involve HEU.[19] Engineering, financial, and political issues make the elimination of the civilian use of HEU highly unlikely, however—at least within the near future.

The National Nuclear Security Administration (NNSA) was established by the U.S. congress in 2000 for the purpose of enhancing national security through nuclear science.[26] Part of its mission is to minimize the use of HEU in civilian applications. As a result, the Office of Material Management and Minimization (M3) in the NNSA manages the Mo-99 Program. As a result of financial and technical assistance from the NNSA, all four major suppliers of Mo-99 for U.S. patients now use LEU in the production of Mo-99. [27]

In 2018, the NNSA funded opportunities for companies in the United States to work on producing Mo-99 without the use of HEU.[28] As a result, the NNSA currently manages three modes of Mo-99 production that are being developed at three U.S. companies: NorthStar Medical Radioisotopes proposes using neutron capture (using Mo-98) and accelerator-based (using Mo-100) technologies, SHINE Technologies proposes using accelerator/fission technology with an LEU solution, and Niowave proposes using LEU targets in a superconducting linear accelerator with fission technology.[29]

| *End of solution to Example 7.5.* |

Until alternate means of producing sufficient Mo-99 without the use of HEU are not only developed, but are also used to replace the Mo-99 production that currently uses HEU across the world, we will have to deal with the potential shortages of Mo-99 for use in nuclear medicine as well as with the dangers associated with increasing stockpiles of weapons-grade uranium.

7.10   QUESTIONS, EXERCISES, & PROBLEMS

7-1. Verify that the following nuclear reaction equations in this chapter satisfy the requirements of charge and nucleon number conservation. (a) Eq. (7.6) (b) Eq. (7.7) (c) Eq. (7.13) (d) Eq. (7.14) (e) Eq. (7.48) (f) Eq. (7.90) (g) Eq. (7.91) (h) Eq. (7.92) (i) Eq. (7.93)

7-2. Equation (7.13) shows what is going on inside the nucleus during the generic beta decay of a radionuclide, as given by Eq. (7.16). Similarly, write down the equations showing what must be going on inside the nucleus during positron decay and electron capture.

7-3. The bromine isotope Br-75 undergoes positron decay 71% of the time, and electron capture 29% of the time.[16] Write out the decay equations for each of these processes using full isotopic notation.

7-4. Write the decay equation for fluorine-18 using full isotopic notation, given the information surrounding Eq. (7.90).

7-5. Palladium-103 is used in brachytherapy seeds that are permanently implanted in the prostates of some early-stage prostate cancer patients. Pd-103 decays by electron capture with a half-life of 16.99 days. It is the soft x-rays emitted by Pd-103 after it undergoes electron capture that are used for treating the prostate. (a) Write out the electron capture decay equation for Pd-103 using full isotopic notation. (b) How long does it take for the activity of a Pd-103 seed to drop to 20% of its initial value? (c) Explain why the soft x-rays that are used for the prostate treatment are emitted as a part of the decay process of Pd-103.

7-6. In Ex.(7.1) we discussed the production of the radionuclide cobalt-60 by neutron activation. In the example statement, it was mentioned that Co-60 can be used for sterilization. Indeed, Co-60 is often used for the sterilization of medical equipment, pharmaceuticals, cosmetics, and toiletries, to name but a few examples. The "gamma sterilization process" is advertised as being capable of killing microorganisms on or in products, even when those products are already packaged.[2] Explain the ideas behind gamma sterilization.

7-7. In Eq. (7.6), both Kr-92 and Ba-142 are radioactive—they both undergo beta decay. Write out the decay equations for these two fission fragments using full isotopic notation.

7-8. The isotope magnesium-27 undergoes beta decay with a half-life of 9.46 minutes. A sample of pure magnesium-27 has an activity of 6.25×10^{18} Bq at the time $t = 0$. (a) Write out the decay equation for the decay of magnesium-27 using full isotopic notation. (b) Find the value of the decay constant for this decay. (c) What is the value of the mean-life? (d) How many moles of magnesium-27 are present in the sample at time $t = 0$? (e) How many radioactive magnesium-27 nuclei are present after one hour? (f) What is the activity of the sample after one hour? (g) How long after $t = 0$ does it take for the activity of the sample to drop by 65%?

7-9. Lutetium-177 is a beta emitter that is used for brachytherapy treatment of small tumors.[31] It is produced by the neutron activation of Lu-176 targets, and undergoes beta decay with a half-life of 6.65 days.[18] Write out the equations showing the neutron activation of Lu-176 and the beta decay of Lu-177 using full isotopic notation.

7-10. In Ex.(7.1), we discussed the production of the radioactive nuclide Co-60 by the neutron activation of the stable nuclide Co-59. As mentioned in that example, Co-60 is a very important radionuclide for both radiotherapy and for brachytherapy. The utility of Co-60 stems from the fact that it undergoes beta decay to an excited state of nickel. This excited-state nucleus quickly decays by gamma emission ($\gamma_1 = 1.17\,\text{MeV}$) to another excited state of the same nuclide, which immediately decays to the ground state with the emission of a second gamma ray ($\gamma_2 = 1.33\,\text{MeV}$). Starting with the Co-60 nuclide, write out the decay equations leading to the production of the ground-state nickel nuclide. (It is the two gamma rays, and not the emitted electron, that provide the useful radiation in Co-60 decay.[30])

7-11. (a) Find the value of the decay constant λ corresponding to the exponential behavior shown in Fig. (7.2). Do this three different ways. (All three ways involve taking data from the graph.) (b) In which of your three values from part (a) do you have the most confidence? Why?

7-12. Rubidium-82 undergoes positron emission with a half-life of 1.2575 minutes.[18] It is used as an imaging agent for PET scans in myocardial perfusion imaging[31]— a so-called nuclear stress test for the heart. Rb-82 is the daughter nucleus in the positron decay of Strontium-82. (a) Write out the decay equation for Sr-82 using full isotopic notation. (b) Write out the decay equation for Rb-82 using full isotopic notation. (c) Rb-82 has such a short half-life that it would be hard to store for use in the clinic. Explain how this storage can take place. Is this exploiting transient or secular equilibrium? How do you know?

7-13. After Eq. (7.46) it is concluded using mathematics that the half-life must be less than the mean-life. Explain conceptually (without using mathematics) why this must be true. Hint: Examine the exponential behavior shown in Fig. (7.2).

7-14. Explain why the $4n+1$ decay series is not a naturally occurring series on Earth.

7-15. The half-life of the parent nuclide in the Actinium ($4n+3$) series, U-235, is less than the age of the Earth, and yet the fissile nuclide U-235 is still found in naturally occurring uranium ore, as discussed in this chapter. Explain this observation.

7-16. In Example 7.3, we showed that the mean-life is given by $1/\lambda$, where λ is the decay constant for the radioactive decay under consideration. Show that the mean-life can also be thought of as the time within which all of the radioactive nuclei would decay if the activity remained constant at its initial value, $\mathscr{A}_o = \lambda \mathscr{N}_o$.

7-17. (*This problem involves calculus.*) The differential equation describing the rate of change of the daughter population in a system of coupled decays was found to be given by Eq. (7.66). The solution for the daughter population as a function of time was then stated to be given by Eq. (7.67), assuming that the initial daughter population is zero. (a) Show that the solution given in Eq. (7.67) gives the expected value when evaluated at $t = 0$. (b) Prove that the given function for the daughter population, Eq. (7.67), really is a solution to the differential equation given by Eq. (7.66) by substituting the solution into the differential equation and showing that you get an identity. (That is, show that both sides of the equation that you end up with are obviously equal to one another.)

7-18. (*This problem involves calculus.*) The expression for the daughter population as a function of time in a radioactive decay series is given by Eq. (7.67). Use this equation to show that, for the case of zero initial daughter population, the daughter population reaches a maximum value when the condition for ideal equilibrium is reached.

7-19. Consider the alpha decay of U-238 ($T_{1/2}$ = 4.468 billion years) into thorium-234, and the subsequent beta decay of Th-234 ($T_{1/2}$ = 24.10 days) into the radioactive nuclide protactinium-234 (Pa-234). Pa-234 also undergoes beta decay, with a half-life of 6.70 hours. (a) Write out the decay equations for U-238, Th-234, and Pa-234 using full isotopic notation. These are the first three decays in the uranium decay series. (b) Discuss the expected relationships between the rates of decay of the U-238, Th-234, and Pa-234 nuclides in naturally occurring ore samples containing these nuclides found in the earth's crust. Explain your reasoning.

7-20. In the text it is stated that, "For reasons that should be very clear, there has been a strong international push for the reduction in and eventual elimination of the production and civilian use of HEU". Explain the reasons for this strong international push.

7-21. The use of radionuclide generators to produce the important radionuclide Tc-99m from Mo-99 was discussed at the end of this chapter. After a sufficiently long time (several half-lives of Tc-99m), is the Mo-99/Tc-99m system in transient or secular equilibrium? How do you know?

7-22. (a) Research and give your findings for the current status of the use of highly enriched uranium (HEU) in the production of Mo-99. (b) Research and explain as best as you can the alternate methods that are currently available for the production of Mo-99 that do not use HEU.

7.11 REFERENCES

1. Eisberg R, Resnick R. *Quantum Physics of Atoms, Molecules, Solids, Nuclei, and Particles.* 2nd ed. New York: John Wiley & Sons; 1985.
2. STERIS Applied Sterilization Technologies. *Gamma Irradiation Processing.* http://www.steris-ast.com/services/gamma-irradiation/. Accessed September 1, 2017.
3. International Atomic Energy Agency (IAEA). *Manual for Reactor Produced Radioisotopes.* Vienna, Austria: IAEA; 2003.
4. Nuclear Energy Institute (NEI). Nuclear Fuel Processes. https://www.nei.org/Knowledge-Center/Nuclear-Fuel-Processes. Accessed August 23, 2017.
5. Krane KS. *Introductory Nuclear Physics.* Hoboken, NJ: John Wiley & Sons; 1988.
6. Idaho State University Radiation Information Network. Tritium Information Section. https://shop.tarjomeplus.com/UploadFileEn/TPLUS_EN_2037.pdf. Accessed August 23, 2017.
7. World Nuclear Association. Nuclear Fusion Power. http://www.world-nuclear.org/information-library/current-and-future- generation/nuclear-fusion-power.aspx. Accessed August 23, 2017.
8. US Department of Energy. DOE National Laboratory Makes History by Achieving Fusion Ignition. https://www.energy.gov/articles/doe-national-laboratory-makes-history-achieving-fusion-ignition. Accessed February 4, 2023.
9. Tollefson J, Gibney E. Nuclear-fusion lab achieves 'ignition': what does it mean? https://www.nature.com/articles/d41586-022-04440-7. Accessed February 4, 2023.
10. Patrignani C. et al. (Particle Data Group). *Chin. Phys. C.* 2016 (2017 update); 40: 100001. http://pdg.lbl.gov/2017/tables/rpp2017-sum-baryons.pdf. Accessed August 28. 2017.
11. Al-Kalbani A, Kamel Y. Y-90 Microspheres in the Treatment of Unresectable Hepatocellular Carcinoma. *Saudi J. Gastroenterol.* 2008; 14(2): 90-92.
12. University of Washington Medical Center. Yttrium-90 Radiotherapy: Treatment for Liver Tumors. https://www.uwmedicine.org/sites/default/files/2019-07/IR-Yttrium-90-Radiotherapy.pdf. Accessed August 24, 2017.
13. Bushberg JT, Seibert JA, Leidholdt EM Jr, Boone JM. *The Essential Physics of Medical Imaging.* 3rd ed. Philadelphia: Lippincott Williams & Wilkins; 2012.
14. CERN. How an accelerator works. https://home.cern/about/how-accelerator-works. Accessed August 26, 2017.

15. KlausFoehl (https://commons.wikimedia.org/wiki/File:Zyklotron_Prinzipskizze02.svg), "Zyklotron Prinzipskizze02", marked as public domain, more details on Wikimedia Commons: https://commons.wikimedia.org/wiki/Template:PD-self. Accessed February 12, 2023.

16. International Atomic Energy Agency (IAEA). Cyclotron Produced Radionuclides: Physical Characteristics and Production Methods, Technical Reports Series No. 468. http://www-pub.iaea.org/MTCD/Publications/PDF/trs468_web.pdf. Accessed August 27, 2017.

17. World Nuclear Association (WNA). Physics of Uranium and Nuclear Energy. http://www.world-nuclear.org/information- library/nuclear-fuel-cycle/introduction/physics-of-nuclear-energy.aspx. Accessed August 27, 2017.

18. National Nuclear Data Center, Brookhaven National Laboratory. NuDat 2.7β: Levels and Gammas Search. https://www.nndc.bnl.gov/nudat2/. Accessed August 27, 2017.

19. International Atomic Energy Agency (IAEA). Feasibility of Producing Molybdenum-99 on a Small Scale Using Fission of Low Enriched Uranium or Neutron Activation of Natural Molybdenum, Technical Reports Series No. 478. http://www-pub.iaea.org/MTCD/Publications/PDF/trs478web-32777845.pdf. Accessed August 27, 2017.

20. The National Academies of Sciences, Engineering, and Medicine. Molybdenum-99 for Medical Imaging. Washington DC: The National Academies Press; 2016.

21. Tollefson J. Reactor shutdown threatens world's medical-isotope supply, http://www.nature.com/news/reactor-shutdown-threatens-world-s-medical- isotope-supply-1.20577. Accessed August 27, 2017.

22. National Institute of Standards and Technology (NIST). Atomic Weights and Isotopic Compositions for Uranium. https://physics.nist.gov/cgi-bin/Compositions/stand_alone.pl?ele=92. Accessed August 28, 2017.

23. Glaser A. About the Enrichment Limit for Research Reactor Conversion : Why 20%?. https://www.princeton.edu/~aglaser/2005aglaser_why20percent.pdf. Accessed August 28, 2017.

24. Lane E, American Association for the Advancement of Science (AAAS). New Report: Time to Ban All Production of Highly Enriched Uranium. https://www.aaas.org/news/new-report-time-ban-all-production-highly-enriched-uranium. Accessed August 28, 2017.

25. Hecker SS, Braun C, Lawrence C. North Korea's Stockpiles of Fissile Material. *Korea Observer*. 2016; 47(4): 721-749. http://www.iks.or.kr/rankup_module/rankup_board/attach/vol47no4/14833231665766.pdf. Accessed August 28, 2017.

26. US Department of Energy, National Nuclear Security Administration. About NNSA. https://www.energy.gov/nnsa/about-nnsa. Accessed February 12, 2023.

27. US Department of Energy, National Nuclear Security Administration. NNSA's Molybdenum-99 Program: Establishing a Reliable Domestic Supply of Mo-99 Produced Without Highly Enriched Uranium https://www.energy.gov/nnsa/nnsas-molybdenum-99-program-establishing-reliable-domestic-supply-mo-99-produced-without. Accessed February 12, 2023.

28. World Nuclear News. https://www.world-nuclear-news.org/Articles/Four-US-companies-chosen-for-Mo-99-production-fund. Accessed February 12, 2023.

29. US Department of Energy. Argonne National Laboratory: Mo-99 Technology Development. https://mo99.ne.anl.gov/. Accessed February 12, 2023.

30. Johns HE, Cunningham JR. *The Physics of Radiology.* 4th ed. Springfield: Charles C. Thomas Publ.; 1983.

31. World Nuclear Association. Radioisotopes in Medicine. http://www.world-nuclear.org/information-library/non-power-nuclear-applications/radioisotopes-research/radioisotopes-in-medicine.aspx. Accessed August 30, 2017.

CHAPTER 8

Interactions of High-Energy Photons with Matter

CONTENTS

The interaction of radiation with matter plays a fundamental role in radiation oncology physics, both from the diagnostic as well as the treatment points of view. In particular, beams of x-rays and γ-rays can cause ionizations as they pass through matter; *ionization* is the principal means of delivering dose to tissue, which can result in DNA damage and possible cell death, as discussed previously (see Chapter 2).

In this chapter, we will consider high-energy photons traversing matter. There are a number of ways in which these high-energy photons can interact with the atoms in the target material. Of these, we shall be primarily interested in only three: the *photoelectric effect, Compton scattering*, and *pair production*. These are the three most important types of photon interactions with matter as far as the clinical diagnosis and treatment of cancer are concerned.

This chapter and the next are somewhat more theoretical in nature than the preceding chapters as we will be delving into the fundamentals of particle interactions. As result, these chapters do not contain discussions that are directly associated with work in the clinic. But do not be misled—an understanding of the ideas in these two chapters is fundamental to understanding the physics behind the treatment plans

DOI: 10.1201/9781003477457-8

developed for cancer patients by the radiation oncologists and medical physicists in the clinic.

8.1 THE PHOTOELECTRIC EFFECT

The traditional experimental setup for the photoelectric effect involves a beam of light shining on a clean metal surface. As a result of the incident light, electrons may be emitted from the metal surface. The emitted electrons are called *photoelectrons* since their emission was caused by the absorption of the incident light. This effect, which had previously been discovered experimentally by Hertz, was explained theoretically by Einstein in 1905. (See Fig. 8.1.) Although the photoelectric effect was originally discovered in metals, it applies equally well to other atoms.

What is fundamentally happening in the photoelectric effect is easy for us to understand at this point given our previous discussions of atomic physics. An incoming high-energy photon of frequency ν and energy $h\nu$ is absorbed by a target atom, resulting in the ionization of an electron from the atom. (See Fig. 8.2.)

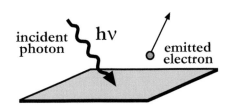

FIGURE 8.1: In the photoelectric effect, a photon incident on a clean metal surface may result in the ejection of an electron if the energy of the incident photon, $h\nu$, is greater than the work function of the metal.

If E_B represents the binding energy of the emitted electron, then the kinetic energy of that electron must be given by $E_k = h\nu - E_B$. If the atom is at or near the surface of the target, then the electron may exit the target surface with this energy. However, electrons emitted from atoms that are buried deeper within the target material will lose energy through interactions with other target electrons and nuclei as they work their way up to the target surface.[a] Such electrons will exit the target surface with an energy that is less than E_k. It therefore follows that the *maximum* kinetic energy of electrons emitted from the target surface is given by

$$E_{k,max} = h\nu - E_{B,min}\,, \tag{8.1}$$

where $E_{B,min}$ stands for the binding energy of the least-tightly bound electrons in the target atoms and is typically called the *work function* of the target.

After the emission of the photoelectrons, the target atom may have an inner-shell vacancy. In such a case, an electron in a higher energy level may make a transition down to the vacated state, resulting in the emission of a photon, or possibly an Auger electron. Since transition energies associated with typical atoms in biological tissue are on the order of keV or smaller, it follows that the energies of photons emitted after the emission of a photoelectron tend to be relatively low. Whereas high-energy

---

[a]Of course, not all of the emitted electrons will head toward the surface, but these are the only ones we'll be interested in, since these are the only ones that are detected.

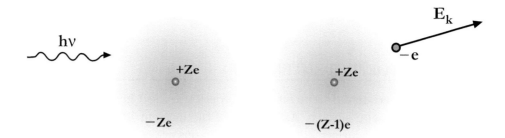

FIGURE 8.2: Schematic of the photoelectric effect process from the atomic point of view. The faint clouds surrounding the nuclei in this figure represent the electron distributions having the charges shown. The small balls at the center of the electron distributions represent the nuclei. *Left*: A high-energy photon approaches a target atom of nuclear charge $+Ze$ surrounded by an electron cloud of charge $-Ze$. *Right*: If the incident photon has enough energy, an electron may be ionized from the atom. The ejected electron leaves the newly created ion with some kinetic energy, E_k.

photons are able to traverse relatively large distances in tissue before being absorbed, low-energy photons tend to be absorbed in the vicinity of where they were emitted.

An incident photon is most likely to be absorbed for a photoelectric process when its energy is about the same size as the binding energy of the electron that it releases. As the energy of the incident photon, $E_{ph} = h\nu$, increases above the electron binding energy, it is found that the probability of photoelectric (*PE*) absorption tends to vary inversely with E_{ph}^3. The probability of a photoelectric absorption is also proportional to the cube of the atomic number Z of the target atom. As a result, we can write that the probability for an incident photon to undergo a photoelectric interaction with a target atom varies according to

$$\text{Prob(PE)} \propto \frac{Z^3}{E_{ph}^{\ 3}}. \tag{8.2}$$

The strong dependence of this probability on Z results from the fact that an isolated electron cannot fully absorb the energy of an incident photon while simultaneously conserving momentum. However, if the electron is bound to a nucleus within an atom, then it becomes possible for the atom to carry away some of the incident photon's momentum, and the absorption of the photon becomes possible. As the value of Z increases, the electron becomes more tightly bound to the atom, so that momentum can be more readily transferred to the atom, and momentum conservation becomes more easily achieved. Thus, a larger value of Z results in an increase in the probability of photon absorption and the subsequent emission of an electron.

The dependence of the photoelectric probability on $(Z/E_{ph})^3$ means that lower-energy photons will be preferentially absorbed by higher-Z atoms. Thus, for example, since bone has a relatively high average value of Z compared to tissue, the low-energy x-rays used in diagnostic imaging (compared to treatment energies) will be absorbed to a greater extent in bone than in tissue. This explains the contrast between bone and tissue in a good x-ray image.

8.2 COMPTON SCATTERING

Arthur Compton provided conclusive evidence for the particle-like nature of photons in 1922 when he observed that scattered x-rays from graphite emerged with slightly longer wavelengths (or slightly lower energies) than the incident x-rays.[b] This observation directly contradicted classical electromagnetic theory, which suggested that the electrons in the graphite atoms should oscillate as a result of the incoming electromagnetic wave (the x-rays) and then re-radiate energy in the form of another electromagnetic wave in a (possibly) different direction, but with the same wavelength.

To explain his observations, Compton treated the incoming light as particles, or *photons*, and applied the conservation of energy and the conservation of momentum to the collision between the incoming photon and an atomic electron. Let's try to follow in Compton's footsteps by analyzing the photon-electron collision.[c]

We start by making some assumptions that will result in a simplification of the mathematical description of the interaction between the incoming photon and the atomic electron. In particular, we assume that the electron in the target atom is initially at rest, and that it is not bound to the atom. While these assumptions are clearly false, they are nevertheless reasonable *if* the energy of the incident x-ray, $h\nu$, is significantly larger than the binding energy of the electron in the target atom:

$$\text{Assumption:} \quad h\nu \gg E_B . \tag{8.3}$$

After the incoming photon interacts with the electron, the electron emerges with a speed v, while the photon emerges with frequency ν' and energy $h\nu'$, where ν' is smaller than the incident frequency ν. It then follows that the change in frequency of the x-ray photon, $\Delta\nu$, is equal to:

$$\Delta\nu = \nu' - \nu , \tag{8.4}$$

so that $\Delta\nu < 0$. The Compton scattering process from an energy standpoint is shown schematically in Fig. (8.3).

The *conservation of energy* tells us that the energy of the incident photon must equal the energy of the outgoing photon plus the energy of the outgoing electron:

$$h\nu = h\nu' + \frac{1}{2} m_e v^2 , \tag{8.5}$$

---

[b]Compton received the Nobel Prize in Physics in 1927 for this work. He was also one of the leading scientists working on the Manhattan Project during the second world war.

[c]Compton performed a fully relativistic treatment of the collision between the incident x-ray photon and the atomic electron in the target. Since we have not had much of an introduction to special relativity, we shall do an approximate classical calculation. Nevertheless, our approximate result will turn out to be the same as that obtained by Compton using the correct relativistic equations.

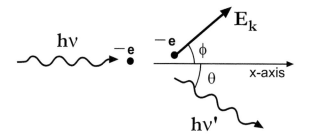

FIGURE 8.3: Schematic of the Compton scattering process from an energy standpoint. The positive x-axis is taken to be the direction of the incoming photon.

where m_e is the mass of the electron. Use of Eq. (8.4) then gives us that

$$\frac{1}{2} m_e v^2 = h\nu - h\nu' = -h\Delta\nu. \tag{8.6}$$

In order to apply the conservation of momentum, we must recall the expression for the momentum of the photon. We obtained this expression during our discussion of quantum mechanics and, more specifically, during the discussion of the deBroglie relation $p = h/\lambda$ in §4.4. From Eqs.(4.33) and (4.34), we have that the momentum of a photon, p_{ph}, is given by

$$p_{ph} = \frac{E_{ph}}{c} = \frac{h\nu}{c}. \tag{8.7}$$

The conservation of momentum (a *vector* equation) then tells us that, since the initial momentum of the electron is zero (it is assumed to be initially at rest), and since the atom carries away no momentum (the electron is assumed *not* to be bound to the atom),

$$\vec{p}_{\text{incoming photon}} = \vec{p}_{\text{outgoing photon}} + \vec{p}_{\text{outgoing electron}}. \tag{8.8}$$

To help us apply this equation, we draw a momentum diagram as shown in Fig. (8.4).

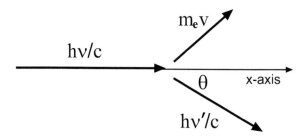

FIGURE 8.4: Schematic of the Compton scattering process from a momentum point of view. The positive x-axis is taken to be the direction of the incoming photon.

Equation (8.8) tells us that, if we add the vectors $\vec{p}_{\text{outgoing photon}}$ and $\vec{p}_{\text{outgoing electron}}$, we should get the vector $\vec{p}_{\text{incoming photon}}$. Drawing this vector addition graphically will therefore give us a vector triangle for momentum. This vector addition is shown in Fig. (8.5). Note that the angle θ gives the direction of the outgoing photon relative to the direction of motion of the incoming photon—that is, the angle θ is the *scattering angle* for the photon.

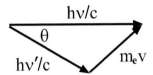

FIGURE 8.5: The vector-addition triangle corresponding to Eq. (8.8).

Applying the *Law of Cosines* from trigonometry to the vector triangle of momentum shown in Fig. (8.5) gives us that

$$(m_e v)^2 = \left(\frac{h\nu}{c}\right)^2 + \left(\frac{h\nu'}{c}\right)^2 - 2\frac{h\nu}{c}\frac{h\nu'}{c}\cos\theta. \tag{8.9}$$

Using Eq. (8.4) and simplifying then gives us that

$$
\begin{aligned}
(m_e v)^2 &= \left(\frac{h\nu}{c}\right)^2 + \left(\frac{h(\nu+\Delta\nu)}{c}\right)^2 - 2\frac{h\nu}{c}\frac{h(\nu+\Delta\nu)}{c}\cos\theta \\
&= \left(\frac{h\nu}{c}\right)^2 \left[1 + \left(1 + \frac{\Delta\nu}{\nu}\right)^2 - 2\left(1 + \frac{\Delta\nu}{\nu}\right)\cos\theta\right] \\
&= \left(\frac{h\nu}{c}\right)^2 \left[2 + 2\frac{\Delta\nu}{\nu} + \left(\frac{\Delta\nu}{\nu}\right)^2 - 2\left(1 + \frac{\Delta\nu}{\nu}\right)\cos\theta\right]. \tag{8.10}
\end{aligned}
$$

The change in frequency of the photon is assumed to be a small fraction of the frequency ν, so the ratio $\Delta\nu/\nu$ will be a small number compared to 1. But if the number $\Delta\nu/\nu$ is small compared to 1, then $(\Delta\nu/\nu)^2$ will be negligible compared to other terms in Eq. (8.10). (If a number is small compared to 1, then that number *squared* will be *tiny*!) We therefore get that

$$
\begin{aligned}
(m_e v)^2 &\cong \left(\frac{h\nu}{c}\right)^2 \left[2\left(1 + \frac{\Delta\nu}{\nu}\right) - 2\left(1 + \frac{\Delta\nu}{\nu}\right)\cos\theta\right] \\
&\cong \left(\frac{h\nu}{c}\right)^2 2\left(1 + \frac{\Delta\nu}{\nu}\right)(1 - \cos\theta). \tag{8.11}
\end{aligned}
$$

But from Eq. (8.6), $m_e v^2 = -2h\Delta\nu$, so that

$$(m_e v)^2 = m_e^2 v^2 = m_e\left(m_e v^2\right) = -m_e(2h\Delta\nu). \tag{8.12}$$

Equation (8.11) then becomes

$$-2m_e h\Delta\nu \cong \frac{h^2\nu^2}{c^2}2\left(1+\frac{\Delta\nu}{\nu}\right)(1-\cos\theta)\,, \tag{8.13}$$

or

$$\Delta\nu \cong \frac{-h\nu^2}{m_e c^2}\left(1+\frac{\Delta\nu}{\nu}\right)(1-\cos\theta)\,. \tag{8.14}$$

Then, using

$$1+\frac{\Delta\nu}{\nu}=\frac{\nu+\Delta\nu}{\nu}=\frac{\nu+(\nu'-\nu)}{\nu}=\frac{\nu'}{\nu}\,, \tag{8.15}$$

we see that Eq. (8.14) becomes

$$\frac{\Delta\nu}{\nu'}\simeq\frac{-h\nu}{m_e c^2}(1-\cos\theta)\,. \tag{8.16}$$

Given the frequency of the incoming x-ray and the angle of detection of the outgoing x-ray, Eq. (8.16) allows us to solve for the frequency ν' of the outgoing photon.

We can rework Eq. (8.16) into a more common form in terms of the *wavelengths* of the incoming and scattered photons as follows. Since $c=\lambda\nu$, so that $\nu=c/\lambda$, it follows that

$$\frac{\Delta\nu}{\nu'}=\frac{\nu'-\nu}{\nu'}=1-\frac{\nu}{\nu'}=1-\frac{c/\lambda}{c/\lambda'}=1-\frac{\lambda'}{\lambda}=\frac{\lambda-\lambda'}{\lambda}\equiv\frac{-\Delta\lambda}{\lambda}\,, \tag{8.17}$$

where we have used the change in wavelength $\Delta\lambda=\lambda'-\lambda>0$. Equation (8.16) then becomes

$$\frac{-\Delta\lambda}{\lambda}\simeq\frac{-h}{m_e c^2}\frac{c}{\lambda}(1-\cos\theta)\,, \tag{8.18}$$

or

$$\Delta\lambda\equiv\lambda'-\lambda=\lambda_C(1-\cos\theta)\,, \tag{8.19}$$

where

$$\lambda_C\equiv\frac{h}{m_e c}\cong 2.426\times10^{-12}\,m \tag{8.20}$$

is called the *Compton wavelength*. Note that the Compton wavelength gives the general size of the wavelength shift associated with Compton scattering. Equation (8.19) is the desired Compton scattering formula.

Since the Compton effect assumes that the binding energy of the electron in the target atom is negligible compared to the energy of the incident photon, and since the electron binding energy depends on the atomic number of the target atom, Z, it follows that the probability for Compton interactions is nearly independent of Z. On the other hand, a more careful analysis of Compton scattering shows that the probability of an incident photon undergoing Compton scattering with a target atom decreases as the incident photon energy increases significantly beyond the binding energies of the electrons in the target atoms.

Compton scattering is of fundamental importance in the treatment of cancer with radiation. Indeed, the dose delivered to tumors by radiation is predominantly delivered by means of the electrons emitted in Compton scattering events.

Example 8.1: Dose Delivery to Tumors via Compton Scattering

Compton scattering results in the emission of electrons that, once released, can deliver their energy to the surrounding tissue as *dose*. This is the dominant means of dose delivery to tumors by high-energy photons in the cancer clinic.

Consider a 1.7 MeV photon incident on atoms in tissue. The photon undergoes Compton scattering; the scattered photon is seen to emerge from the scattering event moving in a direction that is 22° from the original direction of the incoming photon. (a) What is the wavelength of the incident photon? (b) What is the wavelength of the scattered photon? (c) What energy does the emitted electron have available to contribute to dose in the surrounding tissue?

Solution:
(a) The incident photon energy is $E_{ph} = (1.7 \times 10^6 \, eV) \, (1.602 \times 10^{-19} \, J/eV) = 2.7 \times 10^{-13} \, J$. Since $E_{ph} = hc/\lambda$, it follows that $\lambda = hc/E_{ph} = \boxed{7.3 \times 10^{-13} \, m}$.
(b) The change in wavelength of the scattered photon relative to incident photon is given by Eq. (8.19). For $\theta = 22°$, we get that $\Delta\lambda = 1.7 \times 10^{-13} \, m = \lambda - \lambda'$. The wavelength of the scattered photon is therefore $\lambda' = \lambda + \Delta\lambda = \boxed{9.0 \times 10^{-13} \, m}$. (c) The energy available to the electron is its kinetic energy, which we can get from the conservation of energy applied to the Compton scattering event: $E_K = hc/\lambda - hc/\lambda' = \boxed{5.1 \times 10^{-14} \, J = 320 \, keV}$. Note that not all of this energy is necessarily deposited into the surrounding tissue as dose—some of it can be lost to radiation emitted by the electrons as they interact with other atoms in the surrounding tissue (*bremsstrahlung*—see §9.3).

End of solution to Example 8.1.

8.3 PAIR PRODUCTION

In the pair-production process, a high-energy photon interacts with a nucleus in the target medium, resulting in the production of an electron and its antiparticle, a position. The electron and positron form a so-called *electron-positron pair*. Recall that both the electron and the positron have the same mass, equal to

$m_e = 9.1095 \times 10^{-31}\,kg$, which has an energy equivalent of

$$
\begin{aligned}
E_{electron} &= E_{positron} = m_e c^2 \\
&= \left(9.1095 \times 10^{-31}\,kg\right)(299\,792\,458\,m/s)^2 \\
&\cong 8.187 \times 10^{-14}\,J \left(\frac{1\,eV}{1.602\,189 \times 10^{-19}\,J}\right) \\
&\cong 5.110 \times 10^5\,eV \\
&\cong 0.511\,MeV\,.
\end{aligned}
\tag{8.21}
$$

Clearly, in order for the photon to produce an electron and positron, it must have an energy at least equal to the sum of the electron and positron rest-mass energies:

$$
E_{ph} = h\nu \geq 2\,(0.511\,MeV) = 1.022\,MeV\,.
\tag{8.22}
$$

As the probability of Compton scattering decreases in the high-incident-photon-energy limit, the probability of the incident photon undergoing *pair production* increases.

In the process of pair production, the atomic nucleus that interacts with the incoming photon plays a secondary role in that its presence is necessary only to carry away some momentum and energy—without its presence, momentum and energy cannot be conserved and the pair-production process will not take place. To see why this is the case, let's consider a pair-production scenario in which the nucleus does not play a role.

Consider a high-energy photon of energy $E_{ph} = h\nu$ incident along the positive-x direction. The photon spontaneously decays into an electron-positron pair, assumed for simplicity to be moving with equal momentum magnitudes and with directions symmetrically placed to either side of the positive x-direction. This scenario is shown in Fig. (8.6).

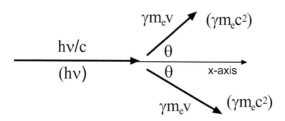

FIGURE 8.6: Schematic of the pair-production process from a momentum point of view. (The corresponding energies are shown in parentheses.)

We know from Eq. (8.22) that the incoming photon energy must be at least as great as the total rest-mass energy of the electron and positron, each of which has a mass m_e. Indeed, the conservation of energy in this set-up will tell us exactly what the energy of the incoming photon must equal. However, since the energy of the incoming photon, and therefore the kinetic energies of the outgoing particles, may be very large, we must be careful to do a proper relativistic treatment of the conservation of energy and of momentum for pair production. We have seen that the rest energy associated with a particle of mass m_e is given by m_ec^2. But, if the particle is moving and therefore has kinetic energy, its relativistic energy must be greater than the rest energy. The total relativistic energy of a particle of mass m_e moving with a speed v is given by

$$E = \gamma m_e c^2 \,, \tag{8.23}$$

where γ is a relativistic factor defined to be

$$\gamma \equiv \frac{1}{\sqrt{1 - v^2/c^2}} \,. \tag{8.24}$$

Note that $\gamma > 1$ since we must always have that, for any material particle, $v < c$. We therefore get from the conservation of energy that, for pair production without the presence of a nucleus,

$$\text{Conservation of Energy:} \quad h\nu = 2\gamma m_e c^2 \,. \tag{8.25}$$

Likewise, we know that momentum must be conserved by components in this process. The magnitude of the relativistic momentum of a particle of mass m_e and speed v is given by the expression

$$p = \gamma m_e v \,. \tag{8.26}$$

The conservation of momentum in the x-direction therefore gives us that

$$\text{Conservation of Momentum:} \quad \frac{h\nu}{c} = 2\gamma m_e v \cos\theta \,, \tag{8.27}$$

where $h\nu/c$ is the relativistic momentum of the incident photon, as given in Eq. (8.7). Substitution of Eq. (8.25) into Eq. (8.27) then gives us that

$$\frac{2\gamma m_e c^2}{c} = 2\gamma m_e v \cos\theta \,, \tag{8.28}$$

from which we get that

$$\cos\theta = \frac{c}{v} \,. \tag{8.29}$$

But since $v < c$, this says that $\cos\theta > 1$, which is not possible for any real value of θ. We therefore have a contradiction, which tells us that we *cannot* satisfy both the conservation of momentum and the conservation of energy if an isolated photon is to spontaneously change into an electron and a positron. This isolated process cannot (*and does not!*) occur. The conservation of momentum and energy *can* be simultaneously satisfied, however, if the electric fields of the electron and positron can interact with a third massive charged object such as a nucleus, which would subsequently carry away some momentum and energy.

The probability for an incident photon of energy E_{ph} to undergo a pair-production interaction with a target nucleus tends to increase with increasing photon energy as well as with increasing atomic number of the target nucleus, Z. In particular, the probability of a pair-production interaction of an incident high-energy photon with a target nucleus of atomic number Z is found to vary according to

$$\text{Prob(PP)} \propto Z^2 ln\left(E_{ph}\right) \tag{8.30}$$

for very high incident photon energies.[1] As with the photoelectric effect, the Z^2 dependence results from the requirement that the emitted charges interact strongly with the target nucleus, thereby allowing some of the momentum of the incident photon to be carried off by the nucleus.

8.4   SUMMARY OF PHOTON INTERACTIONS

In this chapter we have so far overviewed the three types of photon interactions with matter that are most significant for cancer diagnosis and treatment with radiation: the photoelectric effect, the Compton effect, and pair production.

In 1955, Robley D. Evans published a book on nuclear physics that contained a seminal plot showing the regions of dominance of these three important processes.[1] In 2009, Siebers and Hugo[2] published an updated Evans plot using data generated by the program XCOM, which is a photon cross sections database made available on the National Institute of Standards and Technology website.[3] Figure (8.7) shows a revised version of the Siebers and Hugo plot. The solid lines within the plot show the borders along which the probabilities of photoelectric and Compton effects are equal (left curve) and the Compton and pair-production probabilities are equal (right curve).

For convenience, we summarize in Table (8.1) the important characteristics of the photoelectric, Compton, and pair-production processes as discussed so far in this chapter.

8.5   THE ATTENUATION COEFFICIENT

Consider a beam of monoenergetic, high-energy photons, each of energy $E_{ph} = h\nu$, incident on a uniform target medium having density ρ. The surface of the medium is at $z = 0$, and the medium extends into the region $z > 0$. We are interested in finding out how the intensity of the radiation beam varies with depth z into the medium.

The intensity of a radiation beam, I, is defined to be the amount of energy, E, flowing per unit time, Δt, through a given area, A:

$$I = \frac{E}{A \cdot \Delta t}. \tag{8.31}$$

The units of intensity are W/m^2. We assume that the intensity of the radiation beam incident at the surface $z = 0$ of the material has a value $I(z = 0) \equiv I_o$. The intensity at the depth z is denoted $I(z)$.

Now consider a thin slab of material of cross-sectional area A and thickness Δz located at a depth z beneath the surface of the material, as shown in Fig. (8.8).

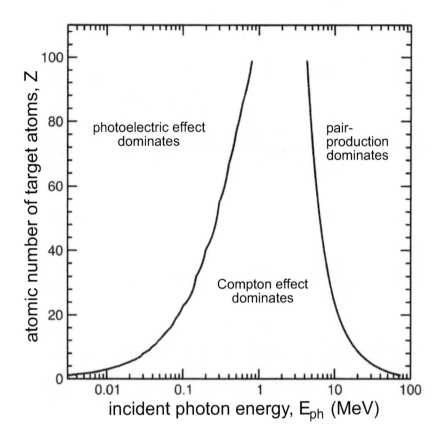

FIGURE 8.7: Regions of dominance of the photoelectric, Compton, and pair-production processes for high-energy photons incident on matter. The plot shows the dominance of the processes as a function of the atomic number of the target material, Z, as well as with the incident photon energy, E_{ph}. (Medical Physics Publishing, revised with permission.)

Certainly, the intensity of the radiation changes as we move from the depth z at the top of the slab to the depth $z + \Delta z$ at the bottom of the slab:

$$I(z + \Delta z) = I(z) + \Delta I. \tag{8.32}$$

For a uniform material, the change in intensity, ΔI, is proportional to the intensity incident on the slab, $I(z)$, and to the thickness of the slab, Δz: $\Delta I \propto I(z)\Delta z$. We can change the proportionality to an equality with the introduction of a proportionality constant. Since we expect the intensity of radiation to decrease as z increases, we must have that $\Delta I < 0$. Therefore, to keep the proportionality constant positive, we make the minus sign explicit, and write

$$\Delta I = -\mu I \Delta z, \tag{8.33}$$

where the positive quantity μ is the proportionality constant. This constant is called the *attenuation coefficient* and has SI units m^{-1}. The value of the attenuation

TABLE 8.1: Summary of high-energy photon interactions for photons of energy E_{ph} interacting with target atoms having atomic number Z. The ranges of dominance given below are taken from Fig. (8.7) using the effective atomic number for tissue, $Z_{tissue} = 7.64$. (See the homework for more information)

Process	Dominates in E_{ph} range	As Z increases, probability ...	As E_{ph} increases, probability ...
Photoelectric:	3 to 20 keV	increases as Z^3	generally decreases as $1/E_{ph}^{3}$
Compton:	20 keV to 20 MeV	remains nearly constant	decreases
Pair Production:	20 to 100 MeV	increases as Z^2	increases as $ln\,(E_{ph})$

coefficient depends on the physical characteristics of the absorbing medium (mass density, electron density, and average atomic number of atoms in the absorbing medium), as well as on the type of interaction undergone by the incident photons and on the photon energy, E_{ph}.

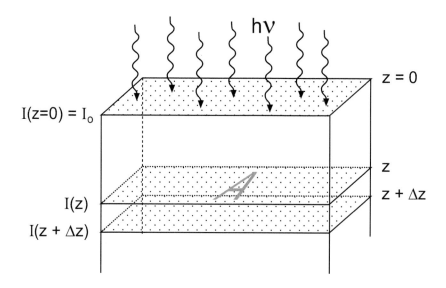

FIGURE 8.8: The intensity of photons passing through an area A of material having density ρ is an exponentially decreasing function of the depth z into the material.

In the limit as the thickness of the absorbing slab goes to zero, we can replace the deltas in Eq. (8.33) with differentials, and write

$$dI = -\mu I dz .\tag{8.34}$$

Separating variables and integrating from the surface of the material down to the depth z then gives us that

$$\int_{I_0}^{I(z)} \frac{dI}{I} = -\int_0^z \mu dz .\tag{8.35}$$

Evaluation of the integrals then yields, assuming that μ can be treated as a constant throughout the depth z of material,

$$\ln\left(\frac{I(z)}{I_0}\right) = -\mu z ,\tag{8.36}$$

or, exponentiating both sides,

$$I(z) = I_0 e^{-\mu z} .\tag{8.37}$$

Equation (8.37) gives the variation of the intensity of the incident radiation with depth into the absorbing medium. This is a very fundamental and important equation in radiation physics. Figure (8.9) shows the behavior of intensity with depth according to this equation, where $I/I_0 = e^{-\mu z}$.

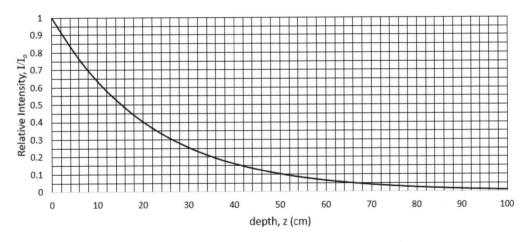

FIGURE 8.9: The variation of relative intensity, I/I_0, with depth as given by Eq. (8.37).

8.6   THE MASS ATTENUATION COEFFICIENT

In the previous section, we showed that the intensity of radiation, defined to be the energy per unit time passing through a given cross sectional area of an absorbing medium, varies with depth into the material, z, according to

$$I(z) = I_0 e^{-\mu z} ,\tag{8.38}$$

where I_o is the intensity of radiation at the surface of the medium, $z = 0$, and where μ is the *attenuation coefficient*, which is characteristic of the given material and of the incident radiation. The incident radiation was assumed to be monochromatic of energy $E_{ph} = h\nu$. It was pointed out that the attenuation coefficient depends on the physical characteristics of the medium, including the mass density of the medium, ρ.

To aid in comparing the absorbing properties of different materials, it is convenient to extract the density dependence from the attenuation coefficient, μ. To this end, we define the *mass attenuation coefficient*, κ, to be

$$\kappa \equiv \frac{\mu}{\rho} \, . \tag{8.39}$$

This definition then allows us to rewrite Eq. (8.39) in the form

$$I(z) = I_0 e^{-\kappa \rho z} \, . \tag{8.40}$$

Since μ must have the units of m^{-1} in SI units, we can see from Eq. (8.39) that κ must have SI units of m^2/kg. The quantity ρz in Eq. (8.39) is often referred to as the *absorber thickness*. The values of mass attenuation coefficient are tabulated for various materials of interest in radiation oncology.[d]

8.7   INTERACTION CROSS SECTIONS: THE GENERAL IDEA

A fundamental concept in discussions of particle interactions is the *cross section*. The cross section for a given interaction effectively tells us about the *probability* that the interaction will take place. A confusing aspect of the interaction cross section, however, is that it has units of *area*, so that in SI units, for example, the cross section would be expressed in m^2. The purpose of this section is to provide a basic understanding of the interaction cross section, and to understand how it gives us information about the probability of an event happening while having the units of an area.

Consider once more the set-up shown in Fig. (8.8). A monochromatic beam of photons having energy $E_{ph} = h\nu$ is incident on an absorbing medium of cross sectional area A. The *intensity* of the beam is the energy per unit time per unit area incident on the medium: $I = E/(A \cdot \Delta t)$. In this definition, the time interval Δt is the amount of time it takes for the total photon energy E to be incident on the area A of the absorbing medium. Since the incident radiation is monochromatic, all the photons must have the same energy E_{ph}, so we can write the total incident energy E as $E = N_{ph}E_{ph}$, where N_{ph} is the number of photons incident on the absorbing medium within the time interval Δt. The intensity of the incident radiation beam can therefore be written in the form

$$I = \frac{N_{ph}E_{ph}}{A \cdot \Delta t} \, . \tag{8.41}$$

---

[d]In tables, the mass attenuation coefficient is often simply denoted (μ/ρ). The units used in medical physics tables are typically *cgs* units, so that the mass attenuation coefficient is given in cm^2/g.

Since the unscattered photons in the incident beam have a constant energy E_{ph}, it follows that the decrease in intensity of the beam as it travels through the medium corresponds to a decrease in the number of the incident photons, N_{ph}. Let's consider this in more detail.

Following the arguments in the previous two sections on the attenuation coefficient, let's consider Fig. (8.10), which shows a monochromatic beam of photons of energy E_{ph} incident on an absorbing medium. (This figure is a slightly revised version of Fig. (8.8), and our discussion here will closely follow the discussion associated with that figure.)

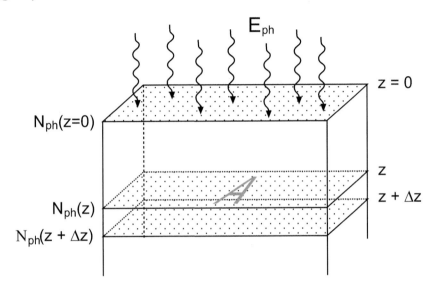

FIGURE 8.10: The number of incident photons N_{ph} passing through an area A of an absorbing medium. The photon number decreases with increasing depth z into the medium.

The number of the incident photons at a depth z beneath the surface of the medium is given by $N_{ph}(z)$, and that at a slightly larger depth $z + \Delta z$ is given by $N_{ph}(z + \Delta z)$. Since the medium will absorb some of the incident photons within the slab of thickness Δz, it must follow that there will be a change in photon number, ΔN_{ph}, as a result of the interactions between the incident photons and the atoms in the absorbing medium. Note that, since the medium is *absorbing* photons, ΔN_{ph} must be *negative*. As a result, the intensity of the incident beam photons must decrease as the beam travels from the depth z to the depth $z + \Delta z$:

$$I(z + \Delta z) = I(z) + \Delta I,\qquad(8.42)$$

where, from Eq. (8.41),

$$\Delta I = \frac{\Delta N_{ph} E_{ph}}{A \cdot \Delta t},\qquad(8.43)$$

which must be negative since ΔN_{ph} is negative.

In what follows, we will assume that one photon is absorbed per interaction of the incident photon beam with atoms within the absorbing medium. (This is the case with the interactions of interest: the photoelectric effect, Compton scattering, and pair production.)

Since each interaction of an incident photon with a target medium atom results in the removal of one beam photon, it follows that

$$N_{int} = -\Delta N_{ph} \,, \tag{8.44}$$

where N_{int} is the number of interactions taking place within the slab of thickness Δz at the depth z.

Let $N_{ph}(z)$ represent the number of incident photons remaining at the depth z. Since N_{int} represents the number of interactions within the slab of thickness Δz at the depth z, if follows that the probability that an incident photon will undergo an interaction within the slab at depth z is given by

$$p_{int} = \frac{N_{int}}{N_{ph}(z)} \,. \tag{8.45}$$

We can then define the *interaction area*, A_{int}, such that

$$p_{int} = \frac{N_{int}}{N_{ph}(z)} = \frac{A_{int}}{A} \,. \tag{8.46}$$

Thus, the size of A_{int} relative to the size of A tells us about the probability that an interaction will take place between an incident photon and a target-medium atom within the slab of thickness Δz at the depth z. See Fig. (8.11).

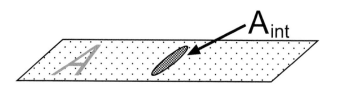

FIGURE 8.11: The size of the interaction area A_{int} relative to the cross-sectional area of the slab, A, gives the probability of an incident photon interaction with an atom in the absorbing medium within the slab of thickness Δz at the depth z.

It therefore follows that

$$N_{int} = \frac{A_{int}}{A} N_{ph}(z) \,, \tag{8.47}$$

so that, from Eq. (8.44),

$$\Delta N_{ph} = -N_{int} = -\frac{A_{int}}{A} N_{ph} \,, \tag{8.48}$$

where N_{ph} is the number of incident photons surviving at depth z.

We now make an additional assumption in this discussion. Namely, we now assume that all of the atoms within the target medium are the same. This assumption is for the sole purpose of simplifying our discussion. If this assumption is not true, then the following argument should be applied to each type of atom within the target medium.

Let the *atomic number density*, ρ_a, be the number of target atoms per unit volume (so that the units of ρ_a are cm^{-3}). It then follows that the number of target atoms, N_a, within the slab of thickness Δz at the depth z within the target medium, as shown in Fig. (8.10), is given by

$$N_a = \rho_a \cdot A \Delta z. \tag{8.49}$$

Let's now divide the interaction area, A_{int}, shown in Fig. (8.11), equally among the N_a atoms within the slab of thickness Δz. We will denote the resulting *interaction area per target atom* by σ (the lower case Greek letter *sigma*):

$$\sigma \equiv \frac{A_{int}}{N_a} = \frac{A_{int}}{\rho_a \cdot A \Delta z}. \tag{8.50}$$

The interaction area per target atom, σ, is called the *interaction cross section*, or simply the *cross section*.

Solving Eq. (8.50) for A_{int} and substituting the result into Eq. (8.48) and simplifying, we get that the change in the number of incident beam photons as the beam travels through the slab of thickness Δz at the depth z is given by

$$\Delta N_{ph} = -\sigma \rho_a N_{ph} \Delta z. \tag{8.51}$$

We can now use this result in Eq. (8.43) to show, using Eq. (8.41), that

$$\Delta I = \frac{-\sigma \rho_a N_{ph} \Delta z \cdot E_{ph}}{A \, \Delta t} = -\sigma \rho_a I \Delta z. \tag{8.52}$$

In order to relate this result to results that we obtained earlier, recall from our discussion of the attenuation coefficient, μ, that the change in beam intensity is also given by Eq. (8.33),

$$\Delta I = -\mu I \Delta z. \tag{8.53}$$

Comparison of Eq. (8.53) with the latter part of Eq. (8.52) shows us the fundamental relationship between the attenuation coefficient and the interaction cross section:

$$\mu = \sigma \rho_a. \tag{8.54}$$

It should make complete sense that the attenuation coefficient is directly related to the cross section, which represents the probability that an incident photon will interact with a target atom as it traverses the target medium.

8.8   PHOTOELECTRIC EFFECT CROSS SECTIONS

Recall that the photoelectric effect involves the emission of an atomic electron after an incident photon has been absorbed by a target atom. It is important to note that the emitted electron must be bound in an atom in order for the photoelectric effect to take place—that is, it is impossible for an unbound electron to completely absorb an incident photon. As discussed previously, the reason for this is that momentum and energy cannot simultaneously be conserved if the electron is not interacting (by means of the electric field) with the more massive nucleus of the atom. (This is why it is more correct to speak of the *atom* absorbing the photon instead of just the electron.) Indeed, the more tightly bound an electron is in an atom, the more readily the atom will be able to absorb the photon and eject the electron. About 80% of photoelectrons emitted from atoms are K-shell electrons ($n = 1$), assuming of course that the incident photons have sufficient energy to emit the K-electrons.

We shall denote the photoelectric cross section by σ_{PE}.[e] The variation of σ_{PE} with target-atom atomic number and with incident energy is rather complicated, although the dependence of σ_{PE} on Z is a power law given approximately as

$$\sigma_{PE} \cong (constant)\, Z^n \,, \tag{8.55}$$

where n varies from about 4.0 to 4.6 as the incident photon energy ranges from about 0.1 MeV to 3 MeV.[1]

The variation of σ_{PE} with incident photon energy E_{ph} is even more complicated. Above about 0.1 MeV, the variation of σ_{PE} with E_{ph} depends on both the values of Z and E_{ph}. In particular, for a given value of Z, the dependence of σ_{PE} on E_{ph} changes continuously as the value of E_{ph} is increased. In addition, for a given energy range, σ_{PE} tends to vary inversely with E_{ph} raised to a higher power (*e.g.*, $1/E_{ph}^3$) for low Z than it does for higher values of Z (*e.g.*, $1/E_{ph}^2$).[1]

No closed formula exists for the general dependence of σ_{PE} on Z and E_{ph}. This is a consequence of complications introduced by the fact that the incoming photon energy may be comparable to the binding energy of the electron ejected in the process, which leads to abrupt increases in σ_{PE} as the binding energy of each electron is reached. This results in jagged edges appearing in plots of σ_{PE} vs. E_{ph}. Nevertheless, neglecting the details associated with the absorption edges, order-of-magnitude estimates for σ_{PE} are given for low energies ($\sim 100\,\text{keV}$) and high energies ($\sim 10\,\text{MeV}$) as follows:[4]

$$\sigma_{PE} \sim \frac{Z^4}{E_{ph}^3} \qquad (low\ energy)\,, \tag{8.56}$$

and

$$\sigma_{PE} \sim \frac{Z^5}{E_{ph}} \qquad (high\ energy)\,. \tag{8.57}$$

8.9 COMPTON SCATTERING CROSS SECTIONS

For the Compton scattering process there exists a relationship[1] between the photon scattering angle θ and the electron scattering angle ϕ (see Fig. 8.3):

$$\cot\phi = (1 + \alpha)\tan\left(\frac{\theta}{2}\right)\,, \tag{8.58}$$

---

[e]The somewhat more cryptic symbol τ is traditionally used in medical physics to denote the photoelectric-effect scattering cross section.

where

$$\alpha \equiv \frac{h\nu}{m_e c^2}. \tag{8.59}$$

The parameter α specifies the incident photon energy in terms of a dimensionless quantity: the ratio of the photon energy, $E_{ph} = h\nu$, to the rest-mass energy of the electron, $E_{rel,0} = m_e c^2 = 0.511$ MeV (see Eq. 4.27).[f] The plot in Fig. (8.12) shows the relation between the electron scattering angle, ϕ, and the photon scattering angle, θ, for two values of the incident photon energy parameter, α.

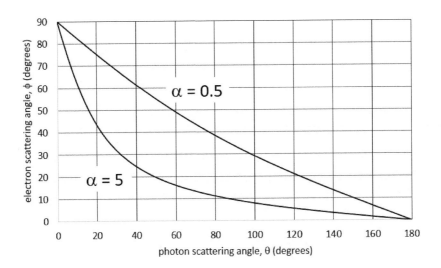

FIGURE 8.12: A plot showing the dependence of the electron scattering angle, ϕ, as a function of the photon scattering angle, θ, for two values of the incident photon energy parameter, α, in a Compton scattering event. See Fig. (8.3) for the meanings of the angles.

In general, as the photon scattering angle gets smaller (that is, the direction of the scattered photon becomes more aligned with the direction of the incoming photon), the electron scattering angle gets larger.

In 1928, Klein and Nishina applied the then new relativistic quantum theory that had been developed by Dirac to the process of Compton scattering. In contrast to the case of the photoelectric process in which a closed expression for the scattering cross section can not be obtained, a closed expression for the Compton scattering

---

[f]Dimensionless parameters are useful since they can give the value of a quantity—the incident photon energy in this case—in terms of a value that is independent of the system of units being used.

cross section σ_{CS}[g] was derived by Klein and Nishina.[h] The result they obtained, now called the *Klein-Nishina scattering cross section*, is given by[1]

$$\sigma_{CS} = 2\pi r_o^2 Z \left\{ \frac{1+\alpha}{\alpha^2} \left[\frac{2(1+\alpha)}{1+2\alpha} - \frac{1}{\alpha} \ln(1+2\alpha) \right] + \frac{1}{2\alpha} \ln(1+2\alpha) - \frac{1+3\alpha}{(1+2\alpha)^2} \right\}. \tag{8.60}$$

In this equation, α is again the dimensionless incident photon energy defined in Eq. (8.59), Z is the atomic number of the scattering atom, and r_o is the *classical electron radius*, given by

$$r_o = \frac{e^2}{4\pi\epsilon_o m_e c^2} \cong 2.82 \times 10^{-15}\, m. \tag{8.61}$$

A plot of σ_{CS} as a function of the dimensionless incident photon energy parameter α is shown in Fig. (8.13).

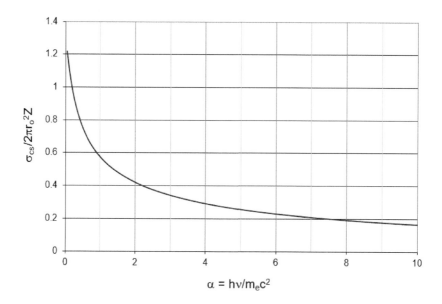

FIGURE 8.13: The dimensionless total Klein-Nishina Compton scattering cross section σ_{CS} per electron as a function of the dimensionless incident photon energy parameter α. The value $\alpha = 1$ corresponds to an incident photon energy equal to the rest-mass energy of an electron, 0.511 MeV.

[g]The Compton-scattering cross section is traditionally denoted by simply σ in the field of medical physics.

[h]The assumption that the incident photon energy is much greater than the binding energy of the emitted electron, so that the electron can be treated approximately as a free particle, resulted in sufficient simplification that Klein and Nishina were able to obtain a closed expression for the Compton scattering cross section.

Klein and Nishina also derived a *differential scattering cross section* for Compton scattering, $d\sigma_{CS}(\theta)/d\Omega$. Differential scattering cross sections are so common and useful in the description of scattering processes that it is worth taking a little time to discuss their significance.

8.10 DIFFERENTIAL CROSS SECTIONS

As discussed previously, the cross section basically tells us about the probability of a certain scattering process taking place. In the case of the Klein-Nishina scattering cross section σ_{CS}, the process is the Compton scattering of an incident photon, the result of which is the photon being scattered at some angle θ relative to the incident photon direction and an electron being emitted at a corresponding angle ϕ. For this (*total*) cross section, the emitted photon and electron directions can take on any values within the constraints dictated by Eq. (8.58).

However, if we were to study the Compton scattering process experimentally, it would be more useful to have an expression for the probability of the electron or photon scattering in the direction at which we place our electron or photon detector. This is important, since the probability of detecting, say, the photon at an angle θ actually depends on the value of the scattering angle θ. This angular dependence is not represented by the total cross section given in Eq. (8.60).

For this reason, we are often interested in the *differential scattering cross section*, which gives us just such angular information. In particular, the differential cross section, denoted $d\sigma_{CS}(\theta)/d\Omega$, tells us the probability of the *photon* being scattered into a small aperture in a photon detector placed some distance away at a photon scattering angle θ (we don't care exactly where the electron goes in this measurement). The size of the "small aperture" as viewed from the initial position of the target electron is represented by the *differential solid angle* $d\Omega$. (The explicit mathematical form of $d\Omega$ does not concern us here.) A schematic of this set-up is shown in Fig. (8.14).

If we could experimentally determine how many photons were incident on the target, and with our detector measure how many photons were scattered via the Compton process in the direction of the small aperture in the detector that was placed at the angle θ, then we could determine the probability of this particular type of scattering event taking place for the given value of θ, and thus experimentally test the theoretical results predicted by the Klein-Nishina expression for $d\sigma_{CS}(\theta)/d\Omega$.[i]

If we wished, we could similarly write down the expression for the differential *electron* scattering cross section $d\sigma_{CS}(\phi)/d\Omega$, and then test it by placing an *electron* detector with a small aperture at the angle ϕ. Measuring the number of electrons scattered into the differential solid angle $d\Omega$ at the angle ϕ for a given number of incident photons would then allow us to determine the probability of an electron being scattered at this angle into the detector.

---

[i]Note that the experimental value for $d\sigma_{CS}(\theta)/d\Omega$ would actually be obtained by summing the detector readings obtained as the detector is moved around the x-axis while keeping the angle θ a constant.

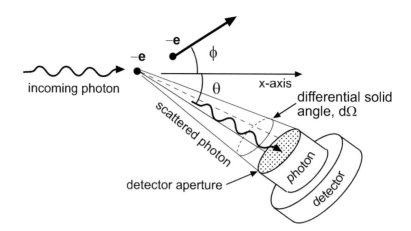

FIGURE 8.14: Schematic of the Compton scattering set-up for measuring the differential cross section. Left: a photon incident on the (approximately) free electron. Right: the Compton-scattered photon and electron. Shown is the photon detector positioned at the scattering angle θ, and the associated differential solid angle $d\Omega$. This solid angle is associated with the differential scattering cross section $d\sigma_{\text{CS}}(\theta)/d\Omega$, as given in Eq. (8.62).

Furthermore, if we followed this same procedure, but placed *both* our photon detector at some angle θ *and* our electron detector at an angle ϕ, and then checked to see when a Compton scattering process resulted in an electron being scattered at the given angle ϕ *and* the photon simultaneously being scattered at the angle θ, then we would be experimentally determining what is called the *doubly differential scattering cross section*. This differential scattering cross section is often denoted $d^2\sigma_{CS}/d\theta d\phi$, or more simply by $\sigma_{\text{CS}}(\theta, \phi)$.

The point is that scattering cross sections give us information about the probability of a particular kind of scattering event taking place. *Differential* cross sections give us more detailed information about those probabilities.

The Klein-Nishina result for the differential Compton scattering cross section for a photon to be scattered into the angle θ is given by[1]

$$\frac{d\sigma_{\text{CS}}(\theta)}{d\Omega} = Zr_o^2 \left[\frac{1}{1+\alpha(1-\cos\theta)}\right]^3 \left(\frac{1+\cos^2\theta}{2}\right) \left(1 + \frac{\alpha^2(1-\cos\theta)^2}{(1+\cos^2\theta)[1+\alpha(1-\cos\theta)]}\right). \tag{8.62}$$

Figure (8.15) shows two polar plots of the Klein-Nishina Compton scattering differential cross section as a function of photon scattering angle θ. The upper plot corresponds to an incident photon energy $E_{ph} = 0.50\,keV$ ($\alpha = 0.001$), and the lower plot corresponds to an incident photon energy $E_{ph} = 4.0\,MeV$ ($\alpha = 7.8$). These plots suggest two things. First of all, that the probability of an incident photon undergoing a Compton scattering event (the area inside the curve) decreases with increasing

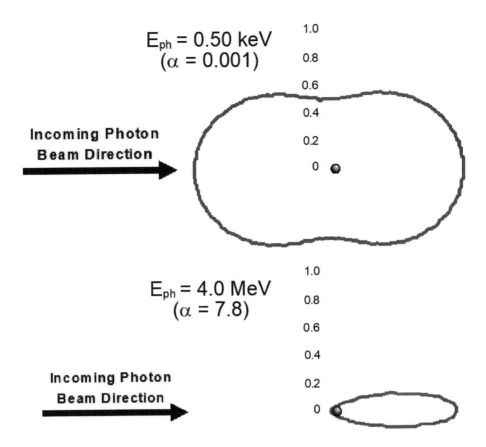

FIGURE 8.15: Polar plots of the Klein-Nishina scattering differential cross section as given in Eq. (8.62). The plots show the results for two different incident photon energies. The scales in the two plots are shown for comparison purposes. The small ball to the right of the zero in the scale is the position of the atom with which the incident photon interacts; it is at the origin of the plots. The forward direction toward the right is taken to be $\theta = 0°$. For any given value of θ, the greater the distance from the origin to the curve, the greater the probability of the photon being emitted in that direction. The total area inside the curve represents the total probability of a Compton scattering event with the incident photon.

photon energy—this behavior is also shown clearly in Fig. (8.13). Second, these plots show that the scattered photon will be preferentially scattered forward at smaller angles θ as the incident photon energy increases. Therefore, higher-energy incident photons are less likely to be scattered and, when they are scattered, they tend to be more *forward-scattered* than lower-energy photons.[j]

---

[j] These results will lead to the clinically significant topic of beam hardening discussed at the end of this chapter.

8.11   PAIR PRODUCTION CROSS SECTIONS

The pair-production cross section σ_{PP} generally tends to increase with increasing photon energy $E_{ph} = h\nu$, and increases as Z^2 with increasing target atomic number:[k]

$$\sigma_{PP} = \sigma_o Z^2 \overline{P} , \tag{8.63}$$

where

$$\sigma_o = \frac{1}{137} \left(\frac{e^2}{m_e c^2} \right)^2 \cong 5.80 \times 10^{-28} \frac{cm^2}{atom} , \tag{8.64}$$

and where $\overline{P}$ is a complicated dimensionless function of E_{ph} and Z that varies from 0 up to about 20.[1] A closed expression for σ_{PP} does not exist.

8.12   THE TOTAL ATTENUATION COEFFICIENT

We found previously that the change in intensity of a photon beam incident on a target medium having an atomic number density ρ_a and thickness Δz at depth z is given by

$$\Delta I = -\sigma \rho_a I \Delta z , \tag{8.65}$$

where σ is the cross section for the process under consideration. If there is more than one process potentially taking place, then the total change in intensity as the incident photon beam goes into a target medium is given by the sum of the changes in intensity due to each of the processes potentially taking place. It therefore follows that we can write the net change in intensity as

$$\begin{aligned} \Delta I &= \Delta I_{PE} + \Delta I_{CS} + \Delta I_{PP} \\ &= -\sigma_{PE} \rho_a I \Delta z - \sigma_{CS} \rho_a I \Delta z - \sigma_{PP} \rho_a I \Delta z \\ &= -(\sigma_{PE} + \sigma_{CS} + \sigma_{PP}) \rho_a I \Delta z \\ &\equiv -\sigma_{tot} \rho_a I \Delta z , \end{aligned} \tag{8.66}$$

$$\tag{8.67}$$

where σ_{tot} is the *total interaction cross section*. Following the derivation leading up to Eq. (8.37), it can then be shown that

$$I(z) = I_o e^{-\sigma_{tot} \rho_a z} = I_o e^{-\mu_{tot} z} . \tag{8.68}$$

In this equation, μ_{tot} is the total attenuation coefficient for all applicable processes:

$$\mu_{tot} \equiv \sigma_{tot} \rho_a . \tag{8.69}$$

---

[k]The pair production scattering cross section is traditionally denoted by the symbol π in the field of medical physics.

It then follows that

$$\mu_{\text{tot}} = (\sigma_{\text{PE}} + \sigma_{\text{CS}} + \sigma_{\text{PP}})\,\rho_a \equiv \mu_{\text{PE}} + \mu_{\text{CS}} + \mu_{\text{PP}}\,. \tag{8.70}$$

That is, the total attenuation coefficient is simply the sum of the attenuation coefficients corresponding to scattering processes that play a significant role in the attenuation of the incident photon beam.

8.13 THE HALF-VALUE LAYER

As we have seen, the intensity of a photon beam that is incident on a target material will decrease as the beam travels into the material. This decrease in intensity is due to scattering events that take place between the photons in the incident beam and the target atoms. The variation of intensity with depth is given by the equation

$$I(z) = I_o\,e^{-\mu_{tot}z}\,, \tag{8.71}$$

where μ_{tot} is the total attenuation coefficient given in Eq. (8.70). The behavior of $I(z)$ as given in Eq. (8.71) is shown in the plot of Fig. (8.16).

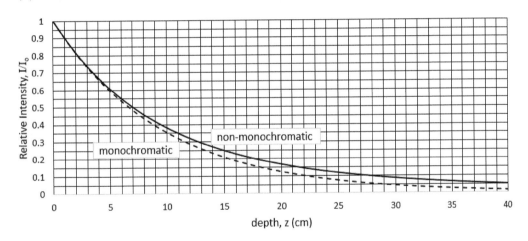

FIGURE 8.16: Plot of the intensity variation with depth as given in Eq. (8.71). This plot (solid line) represents the general intensity variation of a non-monochromatic incident beam of photons for which the HVL is a function of depth. For comparison, the dashed curve shows the exponential decay for a monochromatic beam having an attenuation coefficient equal to the value of the attenuation coefficient for the non-monochromatic beam at $z = 0$.

The *half-value layer*, denoted HVL, is defined to be that thickness of material beyond a given starting depth within which the beam intensity decreases by a factor of 2. That is, the HVL at the depth z within the target material is defined such that

$$I(z + \text{HVL}) = \frac{1}{2}\,I(z)\,. \tag{8.72}$$

In general, the HVL is a function of depth into the target material. (See the next section on beam hardening.) The HVL is often expressed in units of *cm*.

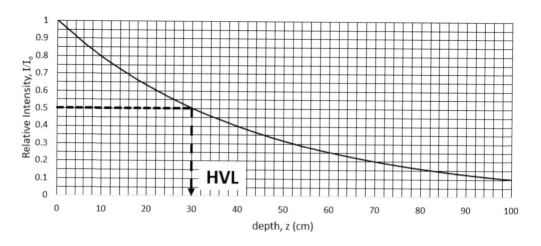

FIGURE 8.17: Plot of the intensity variation with depth for the case of a monoenergetic photon beam of energy $E_{ph} = 10$ MeV. The significance of the half-value layer (HVL) is shown.

For an incident *monoenergetic* photon beam, the value of HVL is constant with depth—that is, the HVL is not a function of z. In this case, we can simply think of the HVL as that thickness of material that the incident beam must traverse such that its intensity decreases by a factor of *2*:

$$I(\text{HVL}) = \frac{1}{2} I_o, \qquad (8.73)$$

where I_o is the intensity of radiation incident on the surface of the target material (that is, at $z = 0$). The definition of HVL for the case of a monoenergetic incident photon beam is shown in Fig. (8.17). You are asked in the homework to show that, in this case of a monoenergetic incident beam, the value of the HVL is determined by the total attenuation coefficient, according to

$$HVL = \frac{ln(2)}{\mu_{tot}}. \qquad (8.74)$$

8.14   BEAM HARDENING

It is important to note that most photon beams used in the treatment of cancer—in particular, those beams of high-energy photons produced by clinical linear electron accelerators (or *linacs*)—are not monoenergetic, but rather have a continuous spread of photon energies from very low energies up to a maximum photon energy dictated by the accelerating voltage of the accelerator. (This will be discussed in more detail in the next chapter and in Part III of this book, which discusses the treatment of cancer with photon beams.) Let's consider what happens as such a photon beam having a broad spectrum of photon energies is incident on a target material. We shall assume that the photon energies extend from very low energies up to typical clinical energies of about 10 or 20 MeV.

As noted in Table 8.1, photon interactions in such a beam will be dominated by the photoelectric and Compton processes. Also as noted in that table, the interaction cross sections (probabilities) *decrease* as the photon energy *increases*. In particular, the plot in Fig. (8.13) shows the characteristic decrease of the Compton scattering cross section with increasing photon energy. This is a very important characteristic. This means that lower energy photons are more likely to undergo a scattering interaction than higher energy photons. Let's consider an important consequence of this fact.

As a photon beam with a broad energy spectrum enters a target material, the photons at the lower energy end of the spectrum are selectively removed from the beam as a result of the correspondingly higher cross sections for photoelectric or Compton scattering processes. As the lower-energy photons are removed, the average energy of the beam is increased. This means that, on average, the photons in a beam traveling through a target medium will have a *lower* probability of undergoing a scattering interaction and being removed from the beam the *farther* the beam has traveled into the material.

A photon beam with a high average energy is referred to as a *hardened* beam, and the effect discussed above in which the average beam energy of an incident photon beam increases with depth into the material is called *beam hardening.*

The effect of beam hardening has an important consequence on the value of the HVL with depth. In particular, as the photon beam gets hardened with depth into the target material, the likelihood that photons will be removed from the beam decreases. This means that the photon beam will have to travel even farther before its intensity drops by a factor of 2. Therefore, the HVL will increase with depth into the material. Figure (8.16) demonstrates the case in which the HVL is a function of depth into the scattering medium corresponding to a non-monochromatic incident beam of photons. (See the homework for more information about the differences between the plots shown in Figs. 8.16 and 8.17.)

The effect of beam hardening and the associated increase in HVL with depth are direct consequences of the decrease in the photoelectric and Compton scattering cross sections with increasing photon energy.

8.15   QUESTIONS, EXERCISES, & PROBLEMS

8-1. In our discussion of the photoelectric effect, it is stated that an isolated electron cannot absorb the energy of an incident photon while conserving both energy and linear momentum. Show that this is the case. (Hint: Assume that the electron is nonrelativistic. If the photon is initially moving along the positive-x direction, then the electron must likewise move along the positive-x direction after it absorbs the photon. *Why?*)

8-2. The effective atomic numbers of muscle, fat, bone, and air are 7.64, 6.46, 12.3, and 7.78, respectively (taken from Table A.7 in Khan[6]). (a) Explain why an x-ray image can be used to study the anatomy of a patient in terms of the photoelectric effect. Approximately what range of x-ray photon energies could be used to form such an image? Why? (b) The effective atomic numbers of muscle and air are rather close to one another. According to Eq. (8.2), it would then be difficult to distinguish the lungs and the surrounding muscle in an x-ray image, since they would have close to the same chance of scattering incident photons of the same energy. Do you think that this argument makes sense? Do you think that it would be difficult to distinguish between the lungs and the surrounding tissue in an x-ray image? (Try looking up an x-ray image of the lungs online.) Explain.

8-3. X-ray images are often used to examine the bones within the body. Bones consist of 50% mineral and about 50% proteins, by volume. Of the mineral portion, approximately 64% is calcium.[5] The work function of calcium is 3.2 eV. Find the maximum kinetic energy of the electrons emitted from a calcium sample if the incident photons have a wavelength equal to (a) 1.2 nm; (b) 57 nm; (c) 270 nm; and (d) 440 nm. (Note that only the wavelength in part (a) officially corresponds to the x-ray region of the electromagnetic spectrum, which is often taken to extend from about 0.01 to 10 nm.)

8-4. At what angle in Compton scattering is the change in wavelength equal to one-half the Compton wavelength?

8-5. A 2.1 MeV photon undergoes Compton scattering in tissue. The scattered photon has a wavelength of 1.36×10^{-12} m. (a) What is the value of the scattering angle for the scattered photon? (b) How much energy does the emitted electron have to deliver to the surrounding tissue immediately after it is released in the scattering event?

8-6. Show that the Compton wavelength λ_C is equal to the wavelength that a photon would have if its energy were equal to the rest energy of an electron.

8-7. It is most probable for the electron and positron in pair production to have equal total relativistic energies after they are created. Show that, in this case, the scattering angles of the electron and positron *must* have the same value, as shown in Fig. (8.6).

8-8. Just as a photon can spontaneously be converted into an electron-positron pair, it is also possible for an electron and positron to combine and annihilate one another, resulting in so-called *annihilation radiation*. Explain why it is impossible for the annihilation radiation to consist of a single photon. (*Hint:* Consider the center-of-mass reference frame in which the electron and positron are moving toward one another with equal speeds, but in opposite directions.)

8-9. (a) Explain why the attenuation coefficient μ must have SI units of m^{-1}. (b) Explain why the SI units of the mass attenuation coefficient $\kappa = \mu/\rho$ must be m^2/kg. (c) What are the SI units of the so-called *absorber thickness, ρz*?

8-10. Determine the number density of carbon atoms in a sample of graphite, which has a density of $\rho = 2.23\,g/cm^3$.

8-11. Equation (8.58) gives the relation between the electron and photon scattering angles in Compton scattering. Show that, as the incident photon energy gets very small, the equation for the electron scattering angle, ϕ, in terms of the photon scattering angle, θ, becomes linear with a slope equal to $-1/2$ and a vertical intercept of $90°$. This behavior is suggested in the plots of Fig. (8.12).

8-12. The plot in Fig. (8.13) shows the "dimensionless total Klein-Nishina Compton scattering cross section" as a function of the "dimensionless incident photon energy". (a) Explain why the quantity shown on the vertical axis is called the "dimensionless total Klein-Nishina Compton scattering cross section". (b) Explain why the dimensionless quantities shown are plotted instead of simply plotting σ_{CS} as a function of photon energy $h\nu$. (c) What is the approximate value of the Compton scattering cross section σ_{CS} when the incident photon energy is equal to twice the rest-mass energy of the electron, as obtained from the graph shown in Fig. (8.13)?

8-13. Explain in your own words the difference between a cross section and a differential cross section.

8-14. (*This problem involves calculus.*) Work through arguments similar to those given in this chapter to show that the fluence of an incident beam of monochromatic photons varies with depth z into an absorbing medium according to

$$\Phi(z) = \Phi_o\, e^{-\mu z}, \tag{8.75}$$

where Φ_o is the fluence of the beam at the surface of the medium ($z = 0$), and μ is the attenuation coefficient of the medium.

8-15. Discuss the probability that an incident photon will be scattered by an atom via a Compton scattering event, and describe the probable directions (θ) of the scattered photon for low and high incident photon energies as displayed in the plots of Fig. (8.15). (In other words, interpret the plots shown.)

8-16. The data in Table (8.2), taken from Table A.7 in Khan[6], show the (total) mass attenuation coefficient, μ/ρ, and the density, ρ, for several absorbing media (and for various photon energies). (a) Use the data in Table (8.2) to determine the absorbing medium associated with the *intensity vs. depth* plot shown in Fig. (8.17). (b) Use the data in Table (8.2) to determine the absorbing medium associated with the *intensity vs. depth* plot shown in Fig. (8.9).

TABLE 8.2: Mass attenuation coefficients and densities

Medium	μ/ρ (m^2/kg)	ρ (kg/m^3)
fat	0.004963	920
water	0.003969	1000
air	0.004447	1.205
muscle	0.002195	1040
bone	0.004732	1850

8-17. Verify the approximate ranges of dominance listed in Table (8.1) for the photoelectric, Compton, and pair-production processes using Fig. (8.7), along with the fact that the effective atomic number of tissue (muscle) is $Z_{tissue} = 7.64$ (from Johns and Cunningham[7], Table A-3c).

8-18. (a) Verify the unique property of the decreasing exponential function, $f(x) = e^{-x}$—that it decreases by equal fractions within equal intervals of x, independent of the value of x—by showing that

$$Fraction = \frac{f(x + \Delta x)}{f(x)} \tag{8.76}$$

depends only on the value of Δx, not on the value of x. (b) Explain the relevance of this property of exponentials to the HVL of monocromatic photon beams traveling through an absorbing medium.

8-19. A photon of wavelength $6.9 \times 10^{-13}\,m$ emerges from a linac during the x-ray treatment of a patient in a cancer clinic. The photon is incident on bone, where it undergoes a Compton scattering event. The electron emitted during the scattering event effectively delivers all of its energy to the surrounding bone. The electron was emitted at an angle of $72°$ relative to the direction of the incident photon. (a) What was the energy of the scattered photon? (b) How much energy did the electron deliver to the bone?

8-20. Starting with Eq. (8.71), show that the HVL for a monochromatic photon beam incident on an absorbing medium is given by Eq. (8.74).

8-21. (a) What is meant by "beam hardening"? (b) Describe in your own words how the Klein-Nishina differential scattering cross section leads to the idea of beam hardening for a non-monochromatic beam of photons incident on a scattering medium.

8.16 REFERENCES

1. Evans RD. *The Atomic Nucleus.* New York: McGraw-Hill; 1955.
2. Siebers JV, Hugo GD. Basic Radiation Interactions, Definition of Dosimetric Quantities, and Data Sources. In: Rogers DWO, Cygler JE, eds. *Clinical Dosimetry Measurements in Radiotherapy.* Madison, WI: Medical Physics Publishing; 2009.
3. National Institute of Standards and Technology (NIST). XCOM: Photon Cross Sections Database. https://www.nist.gov/pml/xcom-photon-cross-sections-database. Accessed September 30, 2017.
4. Hirayama H. Lecture Note on Photon Interactions and Cross Sections. https://rcwww.kek.jp/research/shield/photon_r.pdf. Accessed February 19, 2023.
5. Anderson GD. Protein, Calcium and Bone Density, Part I, Dynamic Chiropractic. http://www.dynamicchiropractic.com/mpacms/dc/article.php?id=15392. Accessed January 4, 2018.
6. Khan FM. *The Physics of Radiation Therapy.* 4th ed. Philadelphia: Lippincott Williams & Wilkins; 2010.
7. Johns HE, Cunningham JR. *The Physics of Radiology.* 4th ed. Springfield: Charles C Thomas; 1983.

CHAPTER 9

Interactions of Charged Particles with Matter

CONTENTS

9.1 INTRODUCTION TO CHARGED-PARTICLE INTERACTIONS

A very important difference exists between the passage of electromagnetic radiation (*photons*) through matter and the passage of charged particles such as electrons and protons through matter. As high-energy photons pass through matter, the intensity of the radiation field decreases exponentially with distance traveled into the target medium according to

$$I(z) = I_o e^{-\mu z} , \qquad (9.1)$$

as we've seen previously (see §8.5). At clinical beam energies, this decrease in intensity is due to photons being removed from the beam as a result of photoelectric, Compton, or pair-production interactions with the target atoms. The photons that have not undergone interactions continue their journey forward with undiminished energy until they, too, undergo an interaction and are absorbed or scattered.

On the other hand, charged particles passing through matter are continuously being slowed down by the successive Coulomb interactions with the electrons and nuclei making up the atoms in the target. As we'll see, the change in energy of the charged particles in the particle beam as a result of these interactions is described in terms of the *stopping power* of the target medium. Thus, an incident beam of charged

DOI: 10.1201/9781003477457-9

particles will have not only diminished *numbers* of particles as it traverses the target medium, but the remaining particles in the beam will also experience a continuous decrease in energy. It therefore follows that the intensity (or number intensity) of electrons passing through matter does *not* decrease according to Eq. (9.1).

In general, charged particle interactions within the target material can be broken down into four distinct categories:

1. elastic collisions with atomic electrons;

2. elastic collisions with atomic nuclei;

3. inelastic collisions with atomic electrons, causing excitation and ionization of those electrons; and

4. inelastic collisions with nuclei, resulting in the emission of photons.

In an *elastic* collision, by definition, the total kinetic energy of the particles involved in the collision remains unchanged, although the energy may end up redistributed among those particles. If an electron beam is incident on a *low-Z* target material (such as tissue in the human body), then excitation and ionization of atomic electrons in the target tend to be the dominant modes of energy loss, while radiative energy loss due to inelastic collisions with target nuclei tends to dominate for *high-Z* materials such as lead and tungsten. The latter mode of energy loss in high-Z target materials forms the basis for the production of x-rays in modern electron accelerators used for cancer treatment.

9.2 THE DISCOVERY OF X-RAYS

In 1895 Wilhelm Röntgen, a professor of physics at Würzburg, was investigating the characteristics of electrical discharges through rarified gases. A photograph of the type of tube used by Röntgen in his experiments is shown in Fig. (9.1).[1] Labeled in the image are the anode and cathode. Also shown are possible paths followed by the electrons as they are accelerated from the cathode to the anode. Note that some of the electrons may miss the anode, thereby hitting the glass tube around the anode.

The entire glass tube in Röntgen's set-up was encased in a tight-fitting, black cardboard cover that had been treated with barium-platino-cyanide. At one point, when the room was completely dark, Röntgen discovered that the cardboard cover glowed due to fluorescence. Further investigation showed that it did not matter whether the treated side of the cardboard faced in toward the glass tube or outwards away from the tube—the cardboard glowed either way. Röntgen found that the position of the fluorescence was the position where the electron beam (the so-called "*cathode rays*") hit the side of the glass tube. Immediately after these findings, Röntgen dropped his previous research and began to work full-time on an investigation of these new, unknown rays, which he called "*x-rays*".

Röntgen investigated which substances produced x-rays along with the characteristics of the x-rays that were produced. In particular, Röntgen studied the penetrating power of the x-rays. He found that, "If the hand is held between the discharge tube

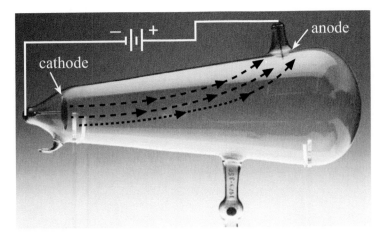

FIGURE 9.1: A photograph of an x-ray tube of the type used by Röntgen in his experiments leading to the discovery of x-rays. The dashed arrows show the paths of electrons accelerating from the cathode to the anode, some of which may miss the anode and hit the glass, thereby producing x-rays. (Open Access: Science Museum Group Collection.)

and the screen the dark shadow of the bones is visible within the slightly dark shadow of the hand".[2] This realization of the penetrating power of the x-rays and their ability to allow us to "see" the internal structure of the hand led to a very rapid application of x-rays to medicine. (See Fig. 11.3 and the associated discussion of radiography in Part III of this book.)

We will now examine the characteristics of x-ray spectra and work toward a fundamental understanding of the characteristics of these spectra.

9.3 BREMSSTRAHLUNG

As in Röntgen's original experiments, x-rays are easily produced by firing high-energy electrons into a solid target.[a] What comes out of the target depends on the energy of the incident electron beam, the composition of the target, and on the target thickness. As shown in Fig. (9.2), some electrons may emerge from the other side of the target in addition to the emitted x-rays if the target is not too thick.

In general, as the electrons move through the target, they interact via the electrical Coulomb force with the electrons and nuclei in the target atoms. Interactions of the beam electrons with the target electrons have very little effect on the motion of the electrons in the beam. However, interactions of the beam electrons with the target nuclei can result in quite dramatic changes in the motion of the beam electrons.

Interactions between the beam electrons and the target atoms can be either elastic or inelastic. In *elastic* collisions, the beam electrons can leave the interactions with the same energy with which they entered. *Inelastic* interactions, on the other hand, result

---

[a]Modern x-ray devices and their role in clinical accelerators for radiation therapy will be addressed in Part III of this text in which we discuss the production of x-rays for cancer treatment.

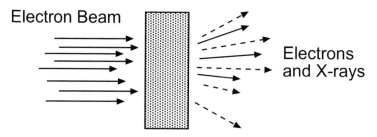

Electron Beam

Electrons and X-rays

FIGURE 9.2: A schematic diagram of the basic process of producing x-rays (dashed arrows) with an incident beam of high-energy electrons (solid arrows).

in a loss of energy of the beam electrons. In the remainder of this section, we will be primarily interested in what happens to the energy lost in inelastic interactions.

It is well known from classical electrodynamics that accelerated charges emit electromagnetic radiation. The wavelength, λ (or frequency, ν) of the emitted radiation is determined by the amount of energy that goes into a quantum (or photon) of the radiation according to the Einstein-Planck relation

$$E_{photon} = \frac{hc}{\lambda} = h\nu \,. \tag{9.2}$$

As electrons in the incident electron beam interact with the charges in the target atoms, they are pushed and pulled by the various electrical forces exerted by the target atoms. The beam electrons accelerate as a result of these interactions, and consequently emit electromagnetic radiation (photons). Sometimes the acceleration is very small, either resulting from interactions with target electrons or with distant target nuclei. These small accelerations result in the emission of photons having low energies, low frequencies, and large wavelengths.

On the other hand, if an electron in the incident beam travels very close to a nucleus, it can be suddenly deflected through a large angle in a fast and relatively violent interaction with the nucleus, resulting in the loss of a large fraction or even possibly all of its energy.[b] In this case, the emitted photon energy can be relatively large, resulting in a large frequency and small wavelength photon.

Is there a maximum energy for an emitted photon when a given beam of incident electrons is incident on a high-Z target? *Of course*—an incident electron cannot give up more energy in a Coulomb interaction than it possess in the form of kinetic energy. The most energetic photon that can be emitted by a beam of incident electrons interacting with target charges is thus a photon whose energy is equal to the kinetic energy of the most energetic incident electron.

The interactions of the electrons in the incident beam with the target nuclei are generically called "*braking* interactions". As a result, this radiation is sometimes called "*braking radiation*". However, it is more commonly known by its German name, "*Bremsstrahlung*".

---

[b]Remember that momentum and energy must always be conserved in any collision. In this case, the "collision" is the Coulomb interaction between the incident electron and the target nucleus.

Some typical Bremsstrahlung x-ray spectra are shown in Fig. (9.3).[3] Note the wide range of emitted wavelengths, the broad peak, and the abrupt, low-wavelength cut-off below which no radiation is emitted. These are all general characteristics of any Bremsstrahlung spectrum.

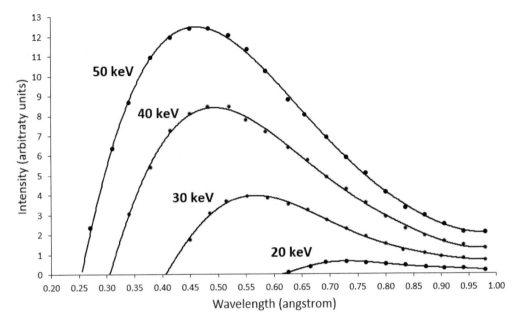

FIGURE 9.3: Bremsstrahlung spectra (*intensity vs. wavelength*) produced by electron beams of various energies (as labeled) incident on a tungsten target. The points are experimental data from Ulrey (1918); the solid lines are best-fit curves.

9.4 CHARACTERISTIC PEAKS IN X-RAY SPECTRA

Figure (9.4)[4] shows the x-ray spectra produced by a beam of 35 keV electrons incident on chromium, molybdenum, and tungsten targets. Even a cursory glance at these spectra shows a dramatic difference between the molybdenum spectrum and the other two spectra shown in the figure, let alone the spectra shown in Fig. (9.3): the appearance of high, sharp peaks superimposed on the otherwise continuous, broad Bremsstrahlung spectrum. (The tops of the peaks go beyond the range of the plot.) These peaks are characteristic of the target material and are therefore called "*characteristic peaks*". The high-energy photons associated with these peaks are correspondingly called "*characteristic x-rays*".

To understand the origin of these peaks, we must return to the atomic energy levels associated with multi-electron atoms that we discussed previously in Chapter 5.

Figure 9.5(a) shows the schematic energy-level diagram that we examined previously in Chapter 5. The figure shows the values of the principal quantum numbers n associated with several of the lowest energy levels. To the right of each energy level is also shown a letter: K for $n = 1$, L for $n = 2$, M for $n = 3$, and N for $n = 4$.

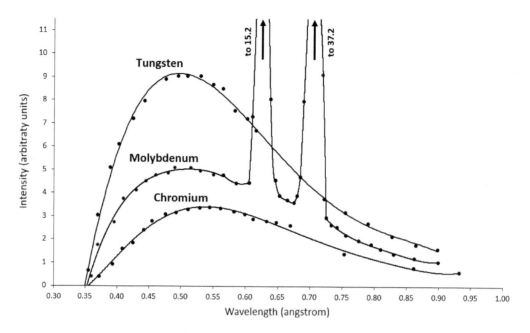

FIGURE 9.4: X-ray spectra (*intensity vs. wavelength*) of 35 keV electrons incident on the targets indicated. The sharp peaks in the molybdenum spectrum are called *characteristic peaks*. The points are experimental data from Ulrey (1918); the solid lines are best-fit curves.

(This convention continues: O for $n = 5$, *etc.*) As we have already seen (see §5.6), it is standard to use the letters K, L, M, *etc.*, when discussing x-ray spectra instead of giving the values of the principal quantum number n.

We first note that, when discussing x-ray spectra, we must be talking about the *lower* energy levels (that is, the inner-shell electron orbitals close to the nucleus) in *high-Z* atoms. This is because only the inner-shell orbitals of high-Z atoms have the sufficiently large energy differences between them that are needed to result in the emission of high-energy (x-ray) photons. (See §5.6 if you need a reminder of the production of x-ray photons.)

When an incident electron interacts with a high-Z target atom, it may supply sufficient energy to the atom so that an inner-shell electron is knocked out—that is, the incident electron may ionize an inner-shell electron from the atom. The ionized atom can then be thought of as being in an excited state, since energy had to be added to the atom in order to get it into this state. The "*state of excitation*" of the atom is described in terms of the state from which the electron was ejected. Thus, an *L excited state* means that an L-electron ($n = 2$) has been removed from the atom.

As a result of this excited state, higher-energy electrons in the atom may make a transition down to the lower-energy vacated state, possibly emitting one or more high-energy photons in the process. The energies of these emitted photons correspond to the differences in energy of the states involved in the transition(s). Since the energy levels are characteristic of the atomic number Z of the target atom, the energies of the photons emitted during transitions between these energy levels will also be

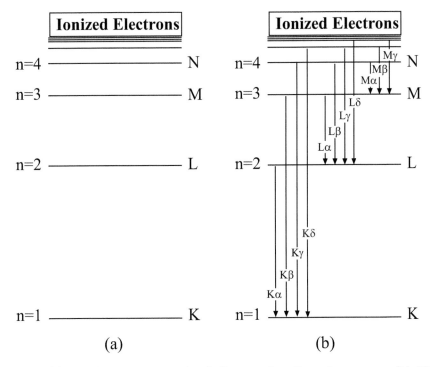

FIGURE 9.5: (a) A schematic energy-level diagram for discussing x-rays. (b) The x-ray energy level transitions showing the origin of the $K_\alpha, K_\beta, \ldots, L_\alpha, L_\beta$, etc., x-rays.

characteristic of the target atoms. It is the emission of these characteristic photons of specific energies and therefore of specific wavelengths that form peaks on top of the continuous Bremsstrahlung spectrum, such as those seen in the molybdenum spectrum of Fig. (9.4).

Example 9.1: The X-ray Spectrum of Molybdenum

Electrons of kinetic energy 35 keV are incident on various targets. The resulting spectra are shown in Fig. (9.4). (a) Quantitatively explain the low-wavelength cut-off seen in these spectra. (b) Quantitatively explain the two sharp peaks observed in the molybdenum spectrum. Molybdenum has an atomic number Z = 42. (c) Comment on your answers.

Solution:

(a) The first thing we notice about the low-wavelength cut-offs of the spectra shown in the figure is that they are basically the same for all three spectra. This makes perfect sense, since the low-wavelength, high-energy cut-off is the result of some of the incident-beam electrons giving up all of their energy to a single photon when they undergo a violent interaction with a target nucleus—this is a characteristic of the incident electron beam, not of the target material. Thus, since the incident electrons have an energy of 35 keV $= 5.6 \times 10^{-15}$ J, it follows that $E_{photon,max} = 5.6 \times 10^{-15}$ J. Then, from Eq. (9.2), it follows that

$$\lambda_{min} = \frac{hc}{E_{photon,max}} = 3.54 \times 10^{-11} \text{ m} = 0.354 \text{ Å}. \tag{9.3}$$

(b) The two sharp peaks in the molybdenum spectrum must come from transitions of the electrons in the molybdenum atom from one shell (or n value) to another. Thus, in order to compute the wavelengths of the photons emitted in the transitions, we must first compute the energies of the different shells. Not knowing which shells are involved, we will simply try the lowest energy levels. Starting with the K shell ($n = 1$), we estimate that there is minor screening of the bare nucleus by the other s-electrons in the atom, so we will assume that the effective atomic number for the K-shell is $Z_{eff,K} = 41.5$. (See §5.4 for a discussion of nuclear screening and the effective atomic number.) Likewise, we estimate that $Z_{eff,L} = 41$ and $Z_{eff,M} = 40.5$ for the L ($n = 2$) and M ($n = 3$) shells, respectively. (Note that these estimates are just that—*estimates*. Perhaps you would have come up with close but different estimates than those assumed here. That is to be expected!) With these values for the effective atomic numbers, we can then use Eq. (5.9) to find the corresponding approximate energies. Doing so yields $E_1 = E_K = -2.34 \times 10^4$ eV, $E_2 = E_L = -5.72 \times 10^3$ eV, and $E_3 = E_M = -2.48 \times 10^3$ eV. If we further assume that the observed peaks come from the K_α (*2 to 1*) and K_β (*3 to 1*) transitions, then the energy differences are $\Delta E_{K\alpha} = E_L - E_K = 1.77 \times 10^4$ eV and $\Delta E_{K\beta} = E_M - E_K = 2.09 \times 10^4$ eV. Using the Planck constant in the form $h = 4.136 \times 10^{-15}$ eV·s to simplify the calculations, so that $hc = 1.24 \times 10^{-6}$ eV·m, we then get from Eq. (9.2) that $\lambda_{K\alpha} = 7.01$ Å and $\lambda_{K\beta} = 5.94$ Å. (c) Comparing the results from (a) and (b) with the molybdenum spectrum shown in Fig. (9.4), we find that the result for λ_{min} is in excellent agreement with that shown in the figure. This excellent agreement is to be expected, however, since the value only depends on the energy of the incoming beam of electrons, which we knew. Examination of the wavelengths corresponding to the observed peaks in the spectrum, however, shows that our results for the two wavelengths are good, but not excellent. It is clear that the low-wavelength peak does indeed correspond to the K_β transition, and the higher-energy peak to the K_α transition. However, while our result for the K_α transition seems very good, the result for the K_β transition is somewhat off. This, of course, is a result of our guesses for the effective screening of the molybdenum nucleus by the other electrons in the atom. Nevertheless, it may be somewhat surprising that our results are as good as they are given the complex issues associated with the effective atomic number values.

End of solution to Example 9.1.

9.5 INTRODUCTION TO HEAVY CHARGED-PARTICLE INTERACTIONS

As photons travel through matter, they tend to give up their energy in discrete interactions with the target atoms. Indeed, some photons may travel through a given thickness of target matter without undergoing any interactions at all, resulting in those photons exiting the far side of the material with the same energy with which they entered the front. This scenario is fundamentally impossible for charged particles.

Charged particles undergo many interactions with the matter through which they are traveling—indeed, they are effectively undergoing continuous interactions with, in particular, the electrons in the target atoms. These interactions take place by means of the electric fields of the incident charged particles and the target atoms. An average incident electron, for example, will undergo about 10^5 interactions before losing all of its initial energy.[5]

In our discussion of incident charged particles interacting with matter, we shall make the *continuous slowing down approximation (CSDA)*, in which we shall assume that all of the energy lost in the many interactions of the incident charged particles with target atoms may be thought of as a continuous reduction in the energy of the incident particles as they traverse the target material.

The Continuous Slowing Down Approximation (CSDA)

Consider a heavy incident beam particle (B) of positive charge $Q_B = +Z_B e$, where Z_B is the atomic number of the incident beam particle. We further assume that the incident particles have mass M_B and (non-relativistic) kinetic energy $E_{k,B} = \frac{1}{2}M_B v^2$. As the beam particle traverses the target medium, it undergoes many interactions via the Coulomb force, primarily with the target electrons.

We start our analysis by considering the interaction of the beam particle with just one target-atom electron $(Q_T = -e; M_T = m_e)$. We assume that we can neglect any initial motion of the target electron in our analysis, so we treat the electron as being initially at rest. The perpendicular distance between the (initially stationary) target electron and the trajectory of the incident beam particle is called the *impact parameter* and is denoted b. See Fig. (9.6a).

The magnitude of the force acting on the electron due to the presence of the beam particle is given by

$$F = \frac{kZ_B e^2}{r^2}, \tag{9.4}$$

where k is the Coulomb's law constant and r is the distance between the target electron and the beam particle. Since we are considering the case of *heavy* incident beam particles, it is reasonable to assume that $M_B \gg m_e$, so the deflection of the beam particle will be very small. We therefore assume that the beam particle will follow a linear trajectory (along the positive z-axis in Fig. 9.6a).

Consider the beam particle at two positions that are symmetric about the origin, denoted *1* and *2*, as shown in Fig. (9.6a). As a result of the beam particle at these two positions, the electron will feel forces $\vec{F}_1$ and $\vec{F}_2$, shown in Fig. (9.6b). The net effect of these two forces acting on the electron is a force $\vec{F}_{net}$ that has the components

$$F_{net,z} = F_{1z} + F_{2z} = -F\sin\theta + F\sin\theta = 0, \tag{9.5}$$

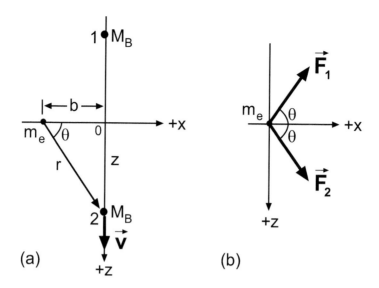

FIGURE 9.6: (a) An incident beam particle of mass M_B moves with velocity $\vec{v}$ along a linear trajectory past an atomic electron of mass m_e. The two symmetric positions about the origin, 1 and 2, are shown. Also shown is the impact parameter, b. (b) The forces $\vec{F_1}$ and $\vec{F_2}$ acting on the target electron resulting from the beam particle at positions 1 and 2, shown in (a).

and

$$F_{net,x} = F_{1x} + F_{2x} = +2F\cos\theta, \tag{9.6}$$

where F is given in Eq. (9.4). We can see that there will be a net force in the positive-x direction acting on the target electron as the beam particle passes by. We therefore need only consider the x-components of forces acting on the electron as the beam particle moves past it.

Let's now consider the beam particle at just one general position—say, position 2 shown in Fig. (9.6a). From Newton's second law, we know that the x-component of the force acting on the electron tells us how the x-component of the electron's momentum changes with time:

$$F_x = m_e a_x = m_e \frac{dv_x}{dt} = \frac{d(m_e v_x)}{dt} = \frac{dp_{e,x}}{dt}, \tag{9.7}$$

where $p_{e,x}$ is the x-component of the target electron's momentum. It then follows that $dp_{e,x} = F_x dt$, or, integrating both sides,

$$\Delta p_{e,x} = \int_{-\infty}^{+\infty} F_x dt. \tag{9.8}$$

The limits on the previous integral reflect the fact that we wish to find the total change in the target electron's momentum, or the total impulse delivered to the electron by the incident beam particle as it approaches, passes, and then leaves the region of the target atom. Since, with the beam particle at position 2, $F_x = F \cos \theta$, it follows that

$$\Delta p_{e,x} = \int_{-\infty}^{+\infty} F \cos \theta \, dt = k Z_B e^2 \int_{-\infty}^{+\infty} \frac{\cos \theta}{r^2} dt \,, \qquad (9.9)$$

where we have made use of Eq. (9.4). We note that both θ and r are functions of time.

We now consider the right triangle having legs b and z and hypotenuse r shown in Fig. (9.6a). Inspection of this triangle shows that $z = b \tan \theta$, so that

$$v = \frac{dz}{dt} = b \sec^2 \theta \frac{d\theta}{dt} \,, \qquad (9.10)$$

or,

$$dt = \frac{b}{v} \sec^2 \theta \, d\theta \,. \qquad (9.11)$$

We can also see from the right triangle that $r = b \sec \theta$. Using this result along with Eq. (9.11) in Eq. (9.9) then yields that

$$\Delta p_{e,x} = k Z_B e^2 \int_{-\pi/2}^{+\pi/2} \frac{\cos \theta}{b^2 \sec^2 \theta} \frac{b}{v} \sec^2 \theta \, d\theta \,. \qquad (9.12)$$

Assuming that the beam-particle speed v is constant, we see that the integral simplifies and becomes trivial:

$$\Delta p_{e,x} = \frac{k Z_B e^2}{bv} \int_{-\pi/2}^{+\pi/2} \cos \theta \, d\theta = \frac{k Z_B e^2}{bv} \left. \sin \theta \right]_{-\pi/2}^{+\pi/2} = \frac{2 k Z_B e^2}{bv} \,. \qquad (9.13)$$

This equation gives us the change in x-component of momentum of a target electron due to the passage of a massive, charged beam particle moving with a speed v. However, since there is no other component to the change in momentum of the target electron, this must also be the change in momentum magnitude, Δp_e. Furthermore, since we are assuming that the initial speed—and therefore the initial momentum—of the electron is zero, we must also have that the change in momentum of the electron is equal to the final momentum. It therefore follows that the change in the kinetic energy of the target electron is given by

$$\Delta E_{k,e} = \frac{1}{2} m_e v_{e,f}^2 = \frac{p_{e,f}^2}{2 m_e} = \frac{\Delta p_{e,x}^2}{2 m_e} \,. \qquad (9.14)$$

From Eq. (9.13), we thus have that

$$\Delta E_{k,e} = \frac{1}{2 m_e} \left(\frac{2 k Z_B e^2}{bv} \right)^2 = \frac{2 k^2 Z_B^2 e^4}{m_e b^2 v^2} \,. \qquad (9.15)$$

This is the change in the kinetic energy of the target electron due to the passage of the charged beam particle.

The increase in the electron's energy must come from somewhere—clearly, it must come at the expense of the energy of the incoming beam particle. A simple application of the conservation of energy shows us that

$$\Delta E_{k,e} = -\Delta E_{k,B} \,. \qquad (9.16)$$

Note that the change in kinetic energy of the beam particle, $\Delta E_{k,B}$, is negative, so that $-\Delta E_{k,B} = \Delta E_{loss}$, the amount of energy *lost* by the beam particle in its interaction with *one* target electron. We can thus write that

$$\Delta E_{k,e} = \frac{\Delta E_{loss}}{electron}. \tag{9.17}$$

We now address the fact that the incident beam particle interacts with *many* target electrons as it traverses the target medium.

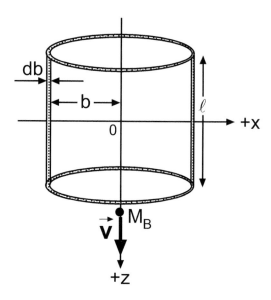

FIGURE 9.7: A differentially thin, cylindrical shell of radius b, thickness db, and length ℓ, whose axis coincides with the trajectory of a beam particle. The volume of the differential shell is $2\pi b\ell\, db$.

Let n_e represent the number density of electrons in the target medium (the number of target electrons per unit volume). We consider a differentially thin, cylindrical volume of radius b, thickness db, and length ℓ, whose axis is the z-axis, the direction of motion of the incident beam particles. See Fig. (9.7).

We note that the differential, cylindrical shell is like an empty tin can with its ends removed. If we were to cut the can along its length and lay it out flat, we would find that we have a rectangle of area $(2\pi b)(\ell)$ and thickness db. The volume of the shell (the volume of the metal making up the tin can) is then $(2\pi b)(\ell)\, db$. It then follows that the number of target electrons, dN_e, within the shell of thickness db is given by

$$dN_e = n_e \cdot 2\pi b\ell\, db. \tag{9.18}$$

As a result of its interactions with these dN_e electrons, each with an impact parameter b, the beam particle will lose an amount of energy given by

$$dE_{loss} = \left(\frac{\Delta E_{loss}}{electron} \right) \cdot dN_e = \left(\frac{2k^2 Z_B^2 e^4}{m_e b^2 v^2} \right) (n_e 2\pi b\ell \, db) , \qquad (9.19)$$

where we have used Eqs.(9.17) and (9.15). Simplifying then yields the result that the energy lost by an incident beam particle as it interacts with target electrons within a length ℓ of the target medium at an impact parameter b is given by

$$dE_{loss} = \left(\frac{4\pi k^2 Z_B^2 e^4 n_e \ell}{m_e v^2} \right) \frac{db}{b} . \qquad (9.20)$$

Not all target electrons will interact with an incoming beam particle. If we take the range of impact parameters within which there will be a significant interaction with a given beam particle to be $b_{min} \leq b \leq b_{max}$, then the total energy lost by the beam particle as it travels through a distance ℓ of target material is given by

$$E_{loss} = \int dE_{loss} = \left(\frac{4\pi k^2 Z_B^2 e^4 n_e \ell}{m_e v^2} \right) \int_{b_{min}}^{b_{max}} \frac{db}{b} , \qquad (9.21)$$

or,

$$E_{loss} = \left(\frac{4\pi k^2 Z_B^2 e^4 n_e \ell}{m_e v^2} \right) \ln \left(\frac{b_{max}}{b_{min}} \right) . \qquad (9.22)$$

Some Comments on the Limits b_max and b_min

An assumption made in the derivation of Eq. (9.22) was that the target electron was initially stationary. This is a reasonable assumption as long as the incident beam particle is moving much more quickly than the target electron. But we have also ignored the fact that the target electrons are bound to target nuclei, so that it will take a minimum amount of energy—the ionization energy, E_I—to release the electrons from the target atoms. From Eq. (9.15), we can see that the energy transferred to the electron varies inversely with the square of the impact parameter. Therefore, a minimum energy transferred corresponds to a maximum impact parameter. This is the origin of the upper limit on impact parameter, b_{max}. Let's look at this limit in a bit more detail.

We will include all ionization events in our range of impact parameters as long as b_{max} is chosen such that the energy transferred to the electron is equal to the minimum energy needed to ionize the target electron; any smaller impact parameter will then result in a larger energy transfer. Thus, we will include all ionization events in our range of impact parameters as long as $\Delta E_{k,e} \geq E_I$. From Eq. (9.14), it then follows that the minimum change in the electron's momentum that can result in ionization is given by

$$\Delta p_{e(min)} = \sqrt{2m_e E_I} . \qquad (9.23)$$

Since the minimum momentum transferred for ionization corresponds to the maximum impact parameter, Eq. (9.13) finally gives us that

$$b_{max} = \sqrt{\frac{2}{m_e E_I}} \left(\frac{k Z_B e^2}{v} \right) . \tag{9.24}$$

Our discussion of b_{min} will be a bit more involved. We consider a beam particle of mass M_B and speed v undergoing a collision with a stationary electron of mass m_e. The final speeds of the beam particle and electron are v_{Bf} and v_{ef}. (In the case under consideration, the collision takes place via the electrostatic Coulomb force.) We assume that the collision is a non-relativistic, classical collision. The maximum energy will be transferred to the electron when the collision is a *head-on* elastic collision, meaning that the collision is a 1-D collision. Both momentum and kinetic energy must be conserved in this simple collision:

$$M_B v_{Bf} + m_e v_{ef} = M_B v , \tag{9.25}$$

and

$$\frac{1}{2} M_B v_{Bf}^2 + \frac{1}{2} m_e v_{ef}^2 = \frac{1}{2} M_B v^2 . \tag{9.26}$$

Solving Eq. (9.25) for v_{Bf}, substituting into Eq. (9.26), and simplifying yields the following equation:

$$(m_e + M_B) v_{ef}^2 + (-2 M_B v) v_{ef} = 0 . \tag{9.27}$$

This equation has two solutions for the final speed of the electron. One solution is $v_{ef} = 0$, which corresponds to the projectile not interacting with the electron at all—in other words, a complete miss and no collision. The more interesting solution is the second, which says that

$$v_{ef} = \frac{2 M_B v}{m_e + M_B} . \tag{9.28}$$

If we rewrite this result in terms of the final kinetic energy of the electron and the initial kinetic energy of the beam particle, we get that

$$E_{k,e} = \left(\frac{4 m_e M_B}{(m_e + M_B)^2} \right) E_{k,B} . \tag{9.29}$$

This result shows us two interesting things. First, if the beam particle is much more massive than the electron (even a proton is almost 2000 times more massive than the electron!), then the kinetic energies are related by the approximate expression $E_{k,e} \cong (4 m_e / M_B) E_{k,B}$. Keeping in mind that this result comes from a head-on collision set-up in which the maximum energy will be transferred to the electron, this result shows that even a proton will only transfer at most about $1/500 = 0.002$ of its kinetic energy; a C-12 nucleus will transfer at most about $1/6000 = 0.00017$ of its kinetic energy. This result supports our constant-speed beam particle approximation in the derivation of Eq. (9.22). Second, Eq. (9.29) shows us that *all* the energy will be transferred if $M_B = m_e$—in other words, if the beam particle is an electron. We will discuss this interesting and clinically important case of incident electron beams later in this chapter.

Keeping in mind that Eq. (9.28) was derived assuming a maximum-energy-transfer scenario (a head-on collision), it then follows that the maximum change in the electron's momentum is given by

$$\Delta p_{e\,(max)} = m_e v_{ef\,(max)} = \frac{2m_e M_B v}{m_e + M_B}. \tag{9.30}$$

Equation (9.13) shows us that the maximum momentum transferred must correspond to the minimum impact parameter. Equating the two expressions for the change in electron momentum in Eqs.(9.13) and (9.30) then yields the following approximate result for the minimum impact parameter value:

$$b_{min} = \frac{kZ_B e^2}{v^2} \left(\frac{m_e + M_B}{m_e M_B} \right). \tag{9.31}$$

9.6   MASS STOPPING POWER FOR HEAVY CHARGED PARTICLES

In the last section we found that the amount of energy lost by an incident heavy beam particle as it interacts with target electrons within a linear distance ℓ inside the target material is given by Eq. (9.22). In this equation, Z_B is the atomic number of the beam particle, n_e is the number of target electrons per unit volume, m_e is the electron mass, and v is the speed of the beam particle (assumed constant). The perpendicular distance from the incoming beam-particle trajectory to the target electron is called the *impact parameter*, b. (See Fig. 9.6a.) The quantities b_{min} and b_{max} in Eq. (9.22) are the minimum and maximum values of the impact parameter that may result in a significant interaction between the beam particle and the target electrons. For the purposes of medical physics, "significant interaction" means an interaction in which the target electron could be ionized, resulting in possible DNA damage.

The rate at which energy is lost by an incident beam particle as it traverses a linear distance ℓ through the target material is called the *linear stopping power* of the target medium and is denoted S. The units of linear stopping power are typically given as J/m or MeV/cm. The stopping power that we computed in the previous section is called the *electronic ionization stopping power*, denoted S_{ion},[c] since it is the loss of beam-particle energy as a result of collisions between the incident beam particle and the target electrons that may result in the ionization of the target electrons.[6] We

---

[c]This quantity is traditionally called the *collisional stopping power*, S_{coll}, but ICRU Report No. 85 (2011) suggests that the *electronic* Coulomb interaction should be emphasized, resulting in the notation S_{el}. We shall use S_{ion}, however, emphasizing that it is the *ionization* of target electrons that is the result of interest from the interaction, even though S_{ion} may also include contributions from atomic excitation.

thus have from Eq. (9.22) that, for heavy charged incident beam particles,

$$S_{ion} = \frac{E_{loss}}{\ell} = \left(\frac{4\pi k^2 Z_B^2 e^4 n_e}{m_e v^2} \right) \ln \left(\frac{b_{max}}{b_{min}} \right). \tag{9.32}$$

A quantity related to the stopping power is the *mass stopping power*, which can be thought of as the stopping power per unit density of the target material. If ρ is the density of the target medium, then the mass stopping power is equal to S/ρ.[d]

If we divide the right-hand side of Eq. (9.32) above by ρ, we can see that we end up with two quantities in the equation that relate directly to the target material: the electron number density n_e and the mass density ρ. Noting that, if $A_g(T)$ stands for the gram atomic mass of the target material and N_A denotes Avogadro's number, then the quantity

$$\frac{N_A}{A_g(T)} = \frac{atoms/mole}{g/mole} = \frac{atoms}{g} \tag{9.33}$$

must be the number of target atoms per unit mass. Using centimeters for distance units and grams for mass units, it then follows that

$$\rho \frac{N_A}{A_g(T)} = \frac{g}{cm^3} \cdot \frac{atoms}{g} = \frac{atoms}{cm^3}. \tag{9.34}$$

Since the atomic number of the target material (Z_T) is the number of electrons per target atom, we have that

$$Z_T \frac{\rho N_A}{A_g(T)} = \frac{electrons}{atom} \cdot \frac{atoms}{cm^3} = \frac{electrons}{cm^3} \equiv n_e, \tag{9.35}$$

which is just the target electron number density. It therefore follows from Eqs.(9.32) and (9.35) that the mass electron stopping power for heavy charged particles is given by

$$\frac{S_{ion}}{\rho} = \frac{1}{\rho} \frac{E_{loss}}{\ell} = \left(\frac{4\pi k^2 Z_B^2 e^4}{m_e v^2} \right) \frac{N_A Z_T}{A_g(T)} \left[\ln \left(\frac{b_{max}}{b_{min}} \right) \right]. \tag{9.36}$$

It is important to remember that this equation was derived under very simplistic assumptions: high-energy but non-relativistic incident beam particles moving with a constant-velocity, and target electrons that are initially stationary.

A significantly more correct (and significantly more complicated) derivation was originally worked out by Bethe in 1930, who first used a weak scattering approximation in quantum mechanics called the Born approximation to derive an equation for the mass electron ionization stopping power.[7] Bethe then improved on his theory in 1932 by incorporating special relativity into the formalism.[8] Bethe's theory was further improved by removing some of the restrictions of the Born approximation in

---

[d]The mass stopping power is often also denoted by S, so care must be taken when reading the medical physics literature which definition of S is intended. Unfortunately, the mass stopping power is also sometimes simply referred to as the *stopping power*, so which stopping power is being discussed must be inferred from the discussion at hand or from the units.

1933 by Bloch,[9] and then much later (in 1956[10] and 1963[11]) by Barkas *et al.* The result was the following equation for the mass electron ionization stopping power,[12] which is known as the *Bethe-Bloch equation*:

$$\frac{S_{ion}}{\rho} = \left(\frac{4\pi k^2 Z_B^2 e^4}{m_e v^2}\right) \frac{N_A Z_T}{A_g(T)} \left[\mathscr{L}(v, Z_T)\right]. \tag{9.37}$$

We can see that the natural logarithm in Eq. (9.36) has been replaced by a function $\mathscr{L}(v, Z_T)$ in Eq. (9.37), which is a complicated, slowly increasing function of the energy of the incident beam particles.[5] The Z_T-dependence of the function $\mathscr{L}$ represents a dependence on the binding energies associated with the electrons orbiting the target nuclei.[13] The function $\mathscr{L}(v, Z_T)$ contains the various quantum mechanical and relativistic correction terms to the classical result of Eq. (9.36) that were derived by Bethe, Bloch, and Barkas.

But the exciting part about the result shown in Eq. (9.37) is that the entire expression in front of the square brackets is exactly the same as that in Eq. (9.36), which we obtained from our simple classical model! It is this part of the equations in front of the square brackets in both (9.36) and (9.37) that contains the strongest dependence of the mass electron ionization stopping power on the speed—and, therefore, the energy—of the beam particles.[5] This means that the dominant physics explaining the behavior of S_{ion}/ρ is contained within our classical model.

9.7   THE BRAGG PEAK

We note from Eq. (9.37) (as well as from Eq. (9.36)) that higher-Z target materials have a larger amount of energy deposited per *cm* than lower-Z materials, and that beam particles with a greater charge (larger value of Z_B) deposit more energy per *cm*. In addition, we can see from the $1/v^2$ term that, as the beam particles slow down, the amount of energy deposited per centimeter *increases*. This feedback loop of a slower particle causing a greater amount of energy deposition per *cm*, which in turn causes the particle to slow down even more, implies that heavy charged particles traversing matter tend to give up their energy in a sudden and final burst of energy loss before they come to a stop.

We also note the following. Since the (classical) kinetic energy of the beam particles is given by $E_{k,B} = (1/2) M_B v^2$, we can express the denominator of Eq. (9.36) in terms of the beam-particle kinetic energy and mass:

$$\frac{S_{ion}}{\rho} = \frac{1}{\rho}\frac{E_{loss}}{\ell} = \left(\frac{2\pi k^2 Z_B^2 e^4}{m_e}\right)\left(\frac{M_B}{E_{k,B}}\right)\frac{N_A Z_T}{A_g(T)}\left[\ln\left(\frac{b_{max}}{b_{min}}\right)\right]. \tag{9.38}$$

The mass stopping power equation written in this form shows us that, for beam particles of the same energy, higher-mass particles will transfer more energy to the target material per *cm*, especially after the beam particle has lost most of its energy so that $E_{k,B}$ is small.

We must be very cautious about using Eq. (9.36) to extrapolate the behavior of the mass electron ionization stopping power to the beam particles as they lose a significant fraction of their energy, however—remember that we assumed that the velocity of the beam particles was approximately constant as they lost energy. We made this assumption rationalizing that the energy lost per interaction with a target electron was a tiny fraction of the beam particle's energy. Nevertheless, as the particle moves through the target material, it interacts with many target electrons, meaning that its speed will eventually start to decrease significantly.

We could argue that, in this case, we could theoretically break the target material up into slabs such that the speed of the beam particle is approximately constant within each slab. We could then decrease the (assumed constant) speed in each slab to model the loss of beam-particle energy in the previous slab, for example. This would at least help improve the approximation. But even this approach could not be used with Eq. (9.36) to argue the sudden "end-of-life" behavior that we discussed above as the particle's energy runs out and it gives it all up in a "sudden and final burst" of energy deposition. The reason is that we also assumed that the beam particle is moving with speeds much larger than the orbital speeds of the various electrons in the target atoms, so that we could assume that the target electrons were initially at rest.

Even the more rigorous Eq. (9.37) has issues with the lower speeds of the beam particles. Although significantly more rigorous and certainly more applicable than our constant-velocity theory, the Bethe-Bloch equation nevertheless results in significant error when the beam particles reach low energies. In particular, as the incident nuclei reach low speeds, they can start capturing target-medium electrons and then, possibly, losing electrons, which means that the effective atomic number Z_B can change for low energies.[12] This further complicates an already complicated scenario.

As a result of these and other complexities at low energies, a semi-empirical approach is taken in the literature that combines behaviors from different theories in various energy regimes along with the results of experiment.[12] Interestingly, what is ultimately found from experiment is that the end-of-energy behavior of heavy charged particles that we inferred from Eq. (9.36) is actually what happens.

The plots in Fig. (9.8)[14] show the experimental behaviors of the linear energy transfer of high-energy proton and carbon-ion beams as a function of distance into a high-density target material.[e] The expected dramatic end-of-energy behavior can be seen as pronounced peaks in the experimental data. These peaks exemplify the sudden burst of energy deposition into the target just before the beam ions give up the last of their energy. These peaks are called *Bragg peaks* and are characteristic of mass electron ionization stopping powers for heavy charged ions traversing a target material.

Two comments concerning the mass of the beam particles are in order. First, look at the widths of the two Bragg peaks shown in Fig. (9.8), being careful to note the depth scales on the two curves. The peak for the carbon ions is significantly more narrow than that for the proton beam, as anticipated from Eq. (9.38).

---

[e]Remember that the linear energy transfer is the energy-restricted stopping power. See §2.5 if you need a reminder about linear energy transfer.

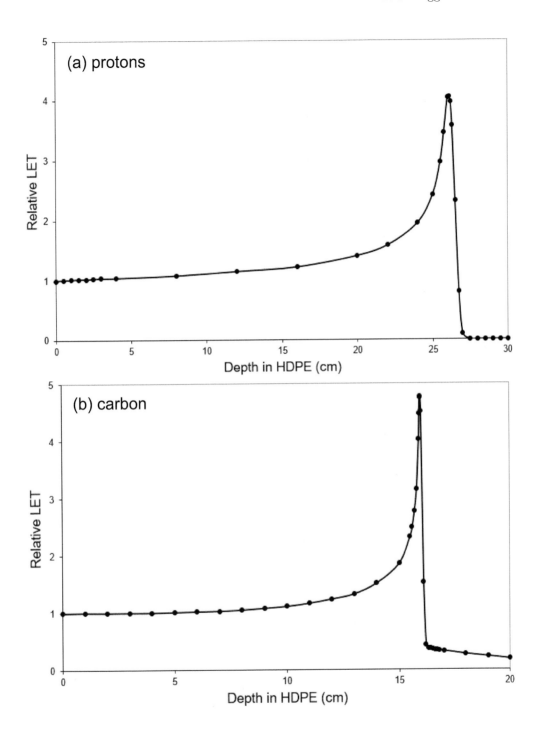

FIGURE 9.8: Linear energy transfer (LET; the restricted stopping power) as a function of distance into the target material, which is high density polyethylene (HDPE) having a density of $0.97\,g/cm^3$. The beam particles are (a) 205 MeV protons and (b) 292.7 MeV per nucleon carbon ions. The relative LET results from the experimental technique of comparing the readings of two ion chambers, one upstream and one downstream of the beam. The plots were created using data from Brookhaven National Laboratory.

The second comment concerns the drop-off of the two curves after the Bragg peak. The proton curve in (a) drops off to relative LET = 0 almost immediately after the peak, while the C-12 curve in (b) drops off to relative LET = 0.4 immediately after the peak, and then slowly decreases in a long tail. The reason for the long tail is an experimental one: it is possible to break up heavy nuclei into lighter nuclei as they travel through the high-density target material, which is called the *degrader*.[14] Since these lighter nuclei have smaller values for Z_B and M_B, it follows from Eq. (9.38) that the lighter nuclei will have significantly lower energy loss per *cm*, and therefore a significantly longer range.

The Bragg peak in the stopping power *vs.* depth behavior of heavy ions makes heavy charged particles the treatment modality of choice for the treatment of pediatric cancers with radiation and for well-localized tumors in adults (such as prostate cancer). Cancer treatment using charged particles will be discussed in Chapter 19.

9.8   MASS IONIZATION STOPPING POWER FOR ELECTRONS

Electrons undergo the same interactions when traversing matter as heavy charged particles. Indeed, as the interactions tend to be electrostatic in nature, the electrons undergo virtually the same interactions as protons traversing matter. It is the consequences of those interactions that differ so greatly for the cases of electron interactions and proton interactions. This is primarily due to the significantly smaller mass of the electron:

$$m_{proton} \cong 1836 \, m_{electron}. \tag{9.39}$$

This smaller mass means that the same interaction will result in a much greater acceleration for the electron than for the proton. Indeed, from Newton's second law,

$$a_{electron} \cong 1836 \, a_{proton}. \tag{9.40}$$

There are some very significant consequences of this difference in acceleration. One important consequence is the trajectory followed by the proton versus that followed by the electron. Recall that we assumed that the trajectory of the heavy charged particle was approximately a straight-line trajectory as the particle traversed matter. While this was a reasonable assumption for a heavy particle such as a proton or alpha particle, it is not a reasonable assumption at all for an electron—the electron's trajectory will tend to be quite chaotic as a result of its small mass.

A second consequence of the small mass and correspondingly large accelerations experienced by an electron traversing matter involves the radiation produced by charged particles as a result of their acceleration. This *radiative stopping power* will be addressed in the next section.

When special relativity and quantum mechanics are taken into account, the following result for the mass ionization stopping power for electrons is obtained:[5]

$$\frac{S_{ion}}{\rho} = \left(\frac{2\pi k^2 e^4}{m_e v^2} \right) \frac{N_A Z_T}{A_g(T)} \left[G\left(E_{k,B}, Z_T \right) \right] . \tag{9.41}$$

In the given equation, $G(E_{k,B}, Z_T)$ is a slowly increasing function of the incident electron beam kinetic energy $E_{k,B}$ for a given value of the target atomic number Z_T, and a slowly decreasing function of Z_T for a given value of $E_{k,B}$. Also, remember that $A_g(T)$ stands for the gram atomic mass of the target material.

For incident electron energies somewhat less than the electron rest-mass energy $(m_e c^2)$, Eq. (9.41) is dominated by the term in front of the square brackets, so the mass stopping power decreases with increasing electron energy (or electron speed, v) for a given target material. But, for higher incident electron energies, the function inside the square brackets dominates, and the mass stopping power then increases slightly with increasing beam energy. The result of all of this is that the mass stopping power must have a minimum, which turns out to occur at an incident electron energy of roughly 1 MeV, depending on the target material.[5]

A comparison of Eq. (9.41) for electrons with Eq. (9.37) for heavy charged particles shows striking similarities. The primary differences include the factor of 2 in Eq. (9.41) versus the factor of 4 in Eq. (9.37), which results from the electron-electron interaction in the former equation involving two equal masses interacting with one another instead of one very light mass interacting with a very heavy mass in the latter equation. The factor of Z_B^2 appears to be missing in Eq. (9.41), but has really only been replaced by its numerical value $Z_B^2 = 1$ (since $Z_B = -1$ for an electron). The function G in Eq. (9.41) is a slowly varying function of the beam energy and the target atomic number; basically the same is true of the function $\mathscr{L}$ in Eq. (9.37).

In light of the discussion above concerning the similar nature of the interactions of heavy charged particles in matter and those of electrons in matter, and the discussion about the stark differences in the results of those interactions as a result of the differences in mass, a further comment relating to Eq. (9.41) is warranted.

The great similarity between equations (9.37) and (9.41) is a result of the great similarity between the interactions experienced by the heavy charged particles and the light (charged) electrons. The interactions are electrostatic in nature and equivalent or nearly equivalent for electrons and heavy charged particles (depending on the heavy particle we're talking about). Electrons lose very close to the same amount of energy due to collisions per *cm* as protons. The difference is where that energy is delivered.

Whereas heavy charged particles such as protons keep moving in a relatively linear trajectory, leaving their trail of deposited energy as they move through the material, electrons tend to undergo many large accelerations. These large accelerations result in a chaotic path, meaning that the electrons will not travel far from where they began their trajectory through the target material, especially for lower-energy electrons. This scenario is depicted schematically in Fig. (9.9). A consequence of this difference is that, although the energy lost per *cm* is very similar in the two cases, the volume of target material within which the electron deposits its energy tends to be much smaller than that for a heavy charged particle. This means that electrons tend to deposit a greater average dose (energy per unit mass) to the target material than do protons of the same energy.

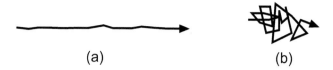

(a)   (b)

FIGURE 9.9: (a) A schematic of the path followed by a heavy charged particle through matter. (b) The path followed by an electron through matter. The electron deposits its energy locally compared to a heavy charged particle.

9.9   MASS RADIATIVE STOPPING POWER FOR ELECTRONS

As was just discussed, the significantly smaller mass of the electron as compared to that of the proton or other heavy charged particles results in the electron experiencing significantly larger accelerations. It is well-known from electromagnetic theory that an accelerated charge radiates electromagnetic energy (*photons*) at a rate that is proportional to the square of the acceleration of the charge.

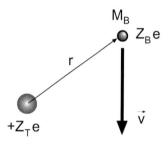

FIGURE 9.10: A charged beam particle of mass M_B and charge $Z_B e$ moving past a target nucleus of charge $+Z_T e$ with velocity $\vec{v}$.

Consider the set-up shown in Fig. (9.10) in which a beam particle of mass M_B moves past and interacts with a target nucleus. The target nucleus has a charge $+Z_T e$ and the beam particle has a charge $Z_B e$ ($Z_B = -1$ if the beam particle is an electron). The magnitude of the electrostatic force exerted by the target nucleus on the beam particle is, from Coulomb's law and Newton's second law,

$$F_B = \frac{k|Z_B e||Z_T e|}{r^2} = \frac{k|Z_B|Z_T e^2}{r^2} = M_B a_B, \qquad (9.42)$$

from which we get that the acceleration magnitude of the beam particle is given by

$$a_B = \frac{k|Z_B|Z_T e^2}{M_B r^2}. \qquad (9.43)$$

Since the rate at which an accelerated charge emits electromagnetic radiation is proportional to the square of its acceleration, it follows that the beam particle will emit radiation with a power

$$P \propto \frac{Z_B^2 Z_T^2}{M_B^2}. \qquad (9.44)$$

We note from this result that the radiated power will increase as Z_T increases and as $|Z_B|$ increases. But we also see that P increases as (Z_B^2/M_B^2) increases. While the charge on the electron ($Z_B = -1$) is comparable to that of a proton ($Z_B = +1$) or even an alpha particle ($Z_B = +2$), the value of (Z_B^2/M_B^2), and hence the radiated power, will be significantly greater for an incident electron than it would be for an incident proton or alpha particle due to the very small mass of the electron. Indeed, the energy loss due to electromagnetic radiation by heavy charged particles is negligible compared to their ionization energy loss. Such is certainly not the case for electrons.

The result of a careful calculation of the mass radiative stopping power for an incident beam of electrons, including relativistic and quantum mechanical effects, is given as follows:[5]

$$\frac{S_{rad}}{\rho} = \frac{4k^2 e^4}{m_e^2 c^4} \frac{E_{k,B}}{137} \frac{N_A Z_T^2}{A_g(T)} \left[\ln \left(\frac{2 \left(E_{k,B} + m_e c^2 \right)}{m_e c^2} \right) - \frac{1}{3} \right], \tag{9.45}$$

where, as before, $E_{k,B}$ is the kinetic energy of the incident electron beam, and $A_g(T)$ is the gram atomic mass of the target material. (The result in Eq. (9.45) is only valid as long as the incident electron energy is below $100\,MeV$—a limit well beyond clinical electron-beam energies.) Note the strong (Z_T^2) dependence of S_{rad}/ρ on the target atomic number. This means that high-Z target materials will produce a significant amount of x-rays when bombarded with high-energy electrons.

The electromagnetic radiation produced as a result of the acceleration of the incident beam electron is what we introduced earlier as *Bremsstrahlung*—x-rays emitted as a result of the "braking" of the incident electrons. We note from Eq. (9.45) that the production of this Bremsstrahlung radiation increases dramatically with increasing target atomic number Z_T, and increases somewhat more slowly with increasing incident electron kinetic energy $E_{k,B}$.

9.10   THE TOTAL MASS STOPPING POWER

In general, the total mass stopping power for charged particles traversing matter is a sum of the contributions to the energy loss per unit distance through the target material due to ionization and excitation, S_{ion}/ρ, and due to a loss of energy due to Bremsstrahlung radiation, S_{rad}/ρ:

$$\frac{S_{tot}}{\rho} = \frac{S_{ion}}{\rho} + \frac{S_{rad}}{\rho}. \tag{9.46}$$

Since energy loss due to radiation by heavy charged particles is negligible, the total mass stopping power in that case is simply equal to the contribution from ionization and excitation. As already mentioned, however, the contribution from radiation loss for an incident beam of electrons can be significant, even at clinical energies.

The ratio of the mass stopping power for radiation to that for ionization for a beam of electrons traveling through a target material of atomic number Z_T is given approximately by

$$\frac{S_{rad}}{S_{ion}} \cong \frac{E_{k,B} Z_T}{\kappa}, \tag{9.47}$$

where $E_{k,B}$ is the kinetic energy of the incident beam electrons expressed in MeV, Z_T is the atomic number of the target element, and κ is a number that depends on $E_{k,B}$ and is typically taken to be in the range $600\,MeV \leq \kappa \leq 800\,MeV$ for common clinical energy ranges of about $1\,MeV$ to $10\,MeV$.[13]

Table (9.1) lists values of S_{ion}/ρ, S_{rad}/ρ, S_{tot}/ρ, and S_{rad}/S_{ion} for various materials and electron-beam energies. (All tabulated data are from ICRU Report No. 37.[15]) Note that all mass stopping powers are given in units of $MeV \cdot cm^2/g$.

TABLE 9.1: Mass stopping powers in units of $MeV \cdot cm^2/g$ for $0.100\,MeV$, $1.00\,MeV$, and $10.0\,MeV$ electron beams traveling through hydrogen, oxygen, water, tungsten, gold, and lead. All data are from ICRU Report 37 (1984)

$E_{k,B}\,(MeV)$	S_{ion}/ρ	S_{rad}/ρ	S_{tot}/ρ	$(S_{rad}/S_{ion}) \times 1000$
Hydrogen (H_2)				
0.100	8.737	0.001216	8.738	0.139
1.00	3.816	0.005152	3.821	1.350
10.0	4.391	0.08809	4.479	20.06
Oxygen (O_2)				
0.100	3.586	0.004607	3.591	1.285
1.00	3.586	0.004607	3.591	1.285
10.0	1.967	0.1932	2.160	98.22
Water				
0.100	4.115	0.004228	4.119	1.027
1.00	1.849	0.01280	1.862	6.923
10.0	1.968	0.1814	2.149	92.18
Tungsten (W)				
0.100	2.047	0.04084	2.088	19.95
1.00	1.016	0.1159	1.132	114.1
10.0	1.203	1.132	2.335	941.0
Gold (Au)				
0.100	2.006	0.04348	2.049	21.68
1.00	1.004	0.1249	1.129	124.4
10.0	1.196	1.188	2.385	993.3
Lead (Pb)				
0.100	1.964	0.04454	2.008	22.68
1.00	0.9939	0.1290	1.123	129.8
10.0	1.201	1.206	2.407	1004

| **Example 9.2: X-ray Production in Tungsten** |

X-rays are produced in clinical *linacs* (linear accelerators) by sending a beam of high-energy electrons into a block of tungsten. Consider a beam of 10.0 MeV electrons incident on a tungsten block. The beam has a diameter of 1.00 cm and delivers a total energy of $4.47 \times 10^5 \, MeV$ to the block. The density of tungsten is $19.3 \, g/cm^3$. (a) How many electrons collide with the block? (b) What is the fluence of the incident electrons? (c) What total energy is released to the top $0.500 \, mm$ of the block as a result of ionization and excitation? (d) What total energy is released to the top $0.500 \, mm$ of the block as a result of Bremsstrahlung emission? (e) What value of κ corresponds to this electron beam in tungsten?

Solution:

(a) Since the energy per incident electron is $E_{k,B} = 10.0 \, MeV$, and the total energy delivered to the block by the incident electrons is $E = 4.47 \times 10^5 \, MeV$, it follows that the total number of incident electrons is

$$N = \frac{E}{E_{k,B}} = \boxed{4.47 \times 10^4 \, electrons}. \tag{9.48}$$

(b) From the definition of fluence in Eq. (2.5), it follows that, since the radius of the electron beam is $r = 0.500 \, cm$,

$$\Phi = \frac{N}{A} = \frac{N}{\pi r^2} = \boxed{5.70 \times 10^4 \, \frac{electrons}{cm^2}}. \tag{9.49}$$

(c) To find the total energy released from ionization and excitation within a distance of $\Delta z = 0.0500 \, cm$ from the surface of the tungsten, we first need to compute the stopping power S_{ion}. Since the density of tungsten is $\rho = 19.3 \, g/cm^3$, and since the mass ionization stopping power for $10.0 \, MeV$ electrons in tungsten is, from Table (9.1), $S_{ion}/\rho = 1.203 \, MeV \cdot cm^2/g$, it follows that

$$S_{ion} = \left(\frac{S_{ion}}{\rho}\right) \cdot \rho = 23.2 \, MeV. \tag{9.50}$$

The energy delivered by all N incident electrons as a result of ionization and excitation within a distance Δz of the tungsten surface is then

$$\Delta E_{ion} = N S_{ion} \Delta z = \boxed{2.08 \times 10^5 \, MeV}. \tag{9.51}$$

(d) Similarly,
$$\Delta E_{rad} = N \left(\frac{S_{rad}}{\rho}\right) \cdot \rho \Delta z = \boxed{1.95 \times 10^5 \, MeV}. \tag{9.52}$$

Since the atomic number of tungsten is $Z_T = 74$, we get from Eq. (9.47) that

$$\kappa = E_{k,B} Z_T \left(\frac{S_{ion}}{S_{rad}}\right) = \boxed{788}. \tag{9.53}$$

This falls within the typical range for this variable, as given in the discussion following Eq. (9.47).

End of solution to Example 9.2.

The Total Mass Stopping Power in Compounds

Equation (9.46) tells us that the mass stopping powers are additive—that is, the total mass stopping power is simply the sum of the constituent stopping powers. This is true no matter the composition of the target material.

But Eqs.(9.41) and (9.45) for S_{ion}/ρ and S_{rad}/ρ require the value of the atomic number Z_T of the target material, meaning that these equations are only valid for pure materials (*copper, lead, tungsten*), not for compounds (*water*). How are the values for the mass stopping powers of compounds computed?

Consider a compound consisting of atoms of some number of elements. Let j represent a particular element in the compound. (For example, for water, $j = \{hydrogen, oxygen\}$.) It then follows that the mass stopping power of the compound is approximately given by the weighted sum of the mass stopping powers of the constituent atoms in the compound.[15] That is,

$$\frac{S}{\rho} = \sum_j w_j \cdot \left(\frac{S}{\rho}\right)_j, \tag{9.54}$$

where the weighting factor w_j is the fraction by weight of the atomic constituent j in the compound. It therefore must follow that

$$\sum_j w_j = 1. \tag{9.55}$$

Equation (9.54) holds true for both the ionization and radiative mass stopping powers. Once they are known for a given compound, the total mass stopping power for that compound is then computed from Eq. (9.46).

9.11   THE RANGE OF CHARGED PARTICLES IN MATTER

The *range* of a beam of charged particles incident on the surface of a target material is defined to be the distance within which all incident particles come to rest. As opposed to photons whose intensity decreases exponentially with depth into the target material and thus have, at least theoretically, an infinite range, the range of charged particles is finite.

The range of heavy charged particles is easy to find—the energy deposited by the beam as a function of depth simply drops off to zero at a certain depth into the target material. This depth is the range. Finding the range is not so clear-cut for electrons, however. The chaotic path followed by the electrons as they travel through the target medium results in a behavior of energy deposited as a function of depth that is not as easy to understand as far as range is concerned. As a result, there are a number of ways to compute the range of electrons incident on a target material—we will discuss two of them.

The easiest range that we will discuss is the range denoted R_{50}, which is simply the depth at which the relative energy deposited into the target material as a function of depth[f] reaches 50% of the maximum value. The second range that we will discuss is called the *practical range*, denoted R_p. The practical range is also computed from a plot of the relative energy deposited as a function of depth, z, into the material. Figure (9.11) shows such a plot, along with the ranges R_{50} and R_p.

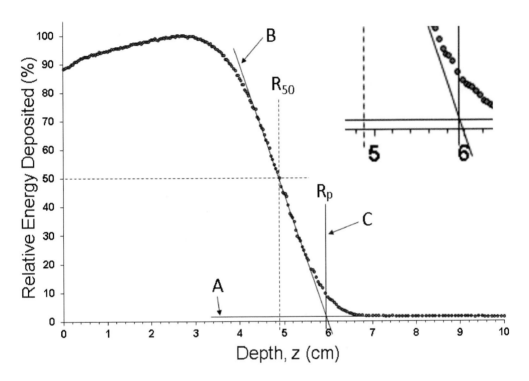

FIGURE 9.11: Finding R_{50} and the practical range, R_p for a $12\,MeV$ electron beam incident on water. The vertical axis gives the percent of the maximum dose (energy per unit mass) deposited into the target material; the horizontal axis gives the depth into the target material ($z = 0$ is at the target surface). The insert at the upper right shows a zoomed-in view of the depth axis at the positions of R_{50} and R_p. See the text for an explanation of the lines drawn on the plot.

It is easy enough to see how to find the range R_{50} in Fig. (9.11): simply draw a horizontal line at the position where the relative energy deposited equals 50%. Then draw a vertical line where the horizontal line reaches the data. The position of the vertical line on the depth axis gives the value of R_{50}. These two lines are drawn as

[f]More specifically, this is a plot of the percent of maximum dose (energy deposited per unit mass of the target material) as a function of depth into the target material. This plot is referred to as a *percent depth dose* (PDD) plot, and plays a fundamental role in clinical treatment planning. The PDD plot will be discussed in much more detail in Chapter 18.

dashed lines in Fig. (9.11). We can see from the figure that the value of R_{50} is just below 4.9 cm.

The procedure to compute R_p is a bit more complicated. We first note that the data in Fig. (9.11) show a large value at the surface (about 88%) with a gradual rise up to the maximum at 100%. The data then display a steep decrease during which they exhibit a nearly linear behavior. The data then level off at a small value of relative energy deposited—somewhere around 2%. This behavior should be really confusing if you remember our discussion of *range* at the beginning of this section: the range of charged particles should be finite, meaning that the curve shown in Fig. (9.11) should drop down to zero. Instead, the behavior displayed by the data appears to be horizontal, implying an *infinite* range!

The word "infinite" should give you a hint of what is going on. We stated that the range of photons is infinite since the intensity of photons decreases exponentially with depth into a medium, and an exponential function never (theoretically) reaches zero. This means that the horizontal behavior shown by the data for large depth values must be due to *photons*. Where do the photons come from?—They are, of course, Bremsstrahlung photons produced by interactions of the incident electrons with target nuclei! The long, horizontal tail shown by the data in the plot is called the *Bremsstrahlung tail*.

We therefore realize that the plot shown in Fig. (9.11) displays not only energy deposited into the target material by the incident electron beam but also energy deposited by the Bremsstrahlung photons resulting from the interactions of the electrons in the incident beam with the target nuclei. So how do we extract the electron range information from these complicated data?

Here is the procedure for finding the practical range corresponding to the data shown in Fig. (9.11):

1. Start by drawing a straight line through the horizontal Bremsstrahlung tail. Extend the line back toward smaller depth values. (This is line A in Fig. 9.11.)

2. Then draw a line along the linear portion of the data past the peak. This occurs along the portion where the data displays its steepest descent.[16] Extend this line to the depth axis. (This is line B in Fig. 9.11.)

3. Finally, draw a vertical line that passes through the point where the two previously drawn lines (A and B) intersect. (This is line C in Fig. 9.11.) The position of this line on the depth axis gives the value of R_p.

Following this procedure, we can see that the value of the practical range R_p for the data of a beam of 12 MeV electrons incident on water displayed in Fig. (9.11) is slightly greater than 5.9 cm.

It is interesting to note that the numerical value of the practical range expressed in *centimeters* from Fig. (9.11) (somewhat greater than 5.9 cm) is approximately equal to one half of the energy of the incident electron beam expressed in *MeV* (12 MeV). This is found by experiment to be approximately true in general for electron beams incident on water (or tissue, which is predominantly water):

$$R_p \ (in \ cm) \cong \frac{E_{k,B} \ (in \ MeV)}{2} .$$ (9.56)

This is a quick and easy *rule of thumb* that can be used to estimate the depth to which an electron beam will deposit its energy in a patient.

9.12 QUESTIONS, EXERCISES, & PROBLEMS

9-1. Quantitatively explain the sharp low-wavelength cut-off of each of the x-ray spectra shown in Fig. (9.3).

9-2. Figure (9.4) shows the x-ray spectra for three different target materials. The spectrum for molybdenum was explained in Ex.(9.1). In particular, the two dominant peaks in the molybdenum spectrum were discussed. Quantitatively explain the *absence* of such peaks in the tungsten and chromium spectra.

9-3. In Ex.(9.1) we assumed that the observed peaks came from the $2 \to 1$ and $3 \to 1$ transitions. Why did we not use the $3 \to 2$ transition (L_α) for the second peak instead of the $3 \to 1$ transition (K_β)? Answer this question by computing $\lambda_{L\alpha}$ and comparing your result with the observed wavelengths in Fig. (9.4).

9-4. In Ex.(9.1), we worked through finding the wavelengths of the two observed peaks in the molybdenum spectrum shown in Fig. (9.4). In that example, we had to guess the values of the effective atomic numbers associated with the K, L, and M levels in atomic molybdenum. We found that we obtained good, but not excellent, results. In this problem you are to reverse-engineer this process to find the best values for $Z_{eff,K}$, $Z_{eff,L}$, and $Z_{eff,M}$. That is, by estimating as precisely as you can the values of $\lambda_{K\alpha}$ and $\lambda_{K\beta}$ from Fig. (9.4), use these values to find good values for the associated effective atomic numbers. Comment on your results.

9-5. The discussion starting at Eq. (9.13) and ending at Eq. (9.15) is a bit tedious and becomes easily confusing. Work through the details, starting with Eq. (9.13) and ending with Eq. (9.15), showing explicitly all of the small but important details. Make sure that every step in the reasoning makes sense to you.

9-6. The CSDA was discussed in this chapter, and Eq. (9.36) was derived (making numerous approximations) for incident heavy beam particles interacting with target electrons. Show, using a similar derivation, that the mass electronic ionization stopping power for incident beam particles interacting with target *nuclei* is negligible compared to that for electrons. Assume that the target nuclei have atomic number Z_T and mass m_T.

9-7. Explain using your own words the presence of a sharp peak (the Bragg peak) that appears in a plot of stopping power *vs.* depth into a target medium for incident heavy charged particles.

9-8. Figure (9.8) shows plots of restricted stopping power *vs.* depth for incident beams of protons and carbon ions. Explain using your own words why the carbon plot displays a long tail at large depths into the target medium, but the proton plot does not.

9-9. The FWHM (*"full-width-half-max"*) is a means of specifying the width of a peak: simply measure the width of the peak at the height of half of the maximum height of the peak. (a) Find the FWHM for the proton and carbon Bragg peaks shown in Fig. (9.8). (b) Explain using your own words why the proton curve has a larger FWHM than the carbon curve. (c) What is a clinical advantage that one of these beams has over the other when treating tumors in patients with heavy charged particles? (The best beam for treatment is often not the beam that is used because of cost issues. There will be more discussion of treatment with heavy ions in Chapter 19.)

9-10. High energy protons are used in proton therapy, which is a treatment modality sometimes used for treating pediatric cancers and prostate cancer, for example. Proton therapy typically uses proton beams with kinetic energies from $70\,MeV$ up to $250\,MeV$. In order to come up with good treatment plans for patients, medical physicists must understand how radiation beams interact with tissue. When experimentally studying these interactions, however, it is clearly not feasible to use tissue as a target medium. Instead, a material that behaves like tissue as far as particle interactions is concerned must be used. Such a substitute material for the study of how beams of radiation would interact with tissue is called a *phantom*. One such phantom material is called A-150, which is a tissue-equivalent plastic. Consider a beam of protons of kinetic energy $150.0\,MeV$ incident on A-150, which has a density of $1.1270\,g/cm^3$. The total mass stopping power of $150.0\,MeV$ protons in A-150 is $5.479\,MeV \cdot cm^2/g$ (from ICRU Report No. 49).[12] In our derivation of the mass ionization stopping power for heavy charged particles in Eq. (9.36) we assumed, among other things, that the speed of the incident beam particles was constant. Let's check that assumption. (a) Compute the initial speed of the protons entering the A-150 phantom. (b) Then compute the amount of energy lost by the beam particles after traveling through $1.00\,cm$ of the A-150 target material. (c) Using this information, compute the final speed of the beam particles, along with the percent change in speed from its initial value. (d) Do you think that the constant-speed assumption was a good one for proton beams used in clinical settings? *Hint:* $150.0\,MeV$ protons are relativistic, so relativistic expressions for kinetic energy must be used. The equation for the relativistic kinetic energy of a particle of mass m traveling with speed v is $E_k = (\gamma - 1)mc^2$, where the relativistic gamma-factor is given by $\gamma = 1/\sqrt{1 - \beta^2}$, and $\beta = v/c$.

9-11. Clinical electron linear accelerators (*linacs*) accelerate electrons to high speeds in order to produce either electron beams or x-ray beams for patient treatment. In order to produce x-rays, the high-energy electrons within the linac are made incident on a block of tungsten. (a) Explain, in your own words, why sending the high-speed electrons into the tungsten block produces x-rays. (b) Look up the melting points of the elements. Also examine the mass stopping power values given in Table (9.1). Then explain why tungsten is used to produce x-rays in linacs instead of other dense, high-Z materials such as gold or lead.

9-12. Figure (9.12) shows a plot of relative energy deposited as a function of depth for a beam of electrons incident on water. Find the corresponding values of the ranges R_{50} and R_p, and determine an approximate value for the energy of the incident electrons.

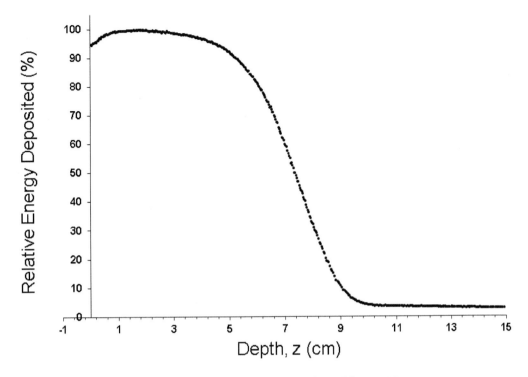

FIGURE 9.12: Plot for homework problem 9-12.

9-13. It was stated at the beginning of the last section in this chapter that, "As opposed to photons ... the range of charged particles is finite". Why must the range of charged particles traveling through matter be finite?

9-14. Medical physicists often use water as a substitute for tissue since tissue is mostly made up of water. The last section explained how to compute the approximate total mass stopping power for compounds. Let's see how well this method performs. (a) Using the values of mass ionization and radiation stopping powers for electrons incident on hydrogen and oxygen in Table (9.1), compute S_{ion}/ρ, S_{rad}/ρ, and S_{tot}/ρ for $0.100\,MeV$, $1.00\,MeV$, and $10.0\,MeV$ electrons incident on water. Compare your results with those listed for water in Table (9.1). What do you conclude about the applicability of Eq. (9.54)? (b) Note that Table (9.1) lists mass stopping powers for hydrogen gas (H_2) and oxygen gas (O_2). Does this mean that you should divide the values listed by 2 in order to get the corresponding values needed for your water calculations in part (a)? Explain.

9.13 REFERENCES

1. Science Museum Group Collection. The original figure was cropped and labels added. https://collection.sciencemuseumgroup.org.uk/objects/co32408/x-ray-tube-x-ray-tube. License: https://creativecommons.org/licenses/by-nc-sa/4.0/legalcode. Accessed October 25, 2017.
2. Röntgen. Sensational Worded Story. *Electrician*. 1896; 36: 334.
3. Data for this plot were taken from p. 407 of Ulrey, CT. An Experimental Investigation of the Energy in the Continuous X-Ray Spectra Of Certain Elements. *Phys Rev.* 1918; 11(5): 401-410.

4. Data for this plot were taken from p. 405 of Ulrey, CT. An Experimental Investigation of the Energy in the Continuous X-Ray Spectra Of Certain Elements. *Phys Rev.* 1918; 11(5): 401-410.
5. Johns HE, Cunningham JR. *The Physics of Radiology.* 4th ed. Springfield: Charles C Thomas; 1983.
6. The International Commission on Radiation Units and Measurements. *ICRU Report No. 85: Fundamental Quantities and Units for Ionizing Radiation (Revised).* Oxford University Press; 2011.
7. Bethe H. Zür Theorie des Durchgangs schneller Korpuskularstrahlen durch Materie. *Annalen der Physik.* 1930; 397: 325-400.
8. Bethe H. Bremsformel für Elektronen relativistischer Geschwindigkeit. *Zeitschrift für Physik.* 1932; 76: 293-299.
9. Bloch F. Zür Bremsung rasch bewegter Teilchen beim Durchgang durch die Materie. *Annalen der Physik.* 1933; 408: 285-320.
10. Barkas WH, Birnbaum W, Smith FM. Mass Ratio Method Applied to the Measurement of L-Meson Masses and the Energy Balance in Pion Decay. *Phys. Rev.* 1956; 101: 778-795.
11. Barkas WH, Dyer NJ, and Heckmann HH. Resolution of the Σ^--Mass Anomaly. *Phys. Rev. Lett.* 1963; 11(1): 26-28.
12. The International Commission on Radiation Units and Measurements. *ICRU Report No. 49: Stopping Powers and Ranges for Protons and Alpha Particles.* Bethesda, MD: ICRU; 1993.
13. Attix FH. *Introduction to Radiological Physics and Radiation Dosimetry.* New York: John Wiley & Sons; 1986.
14. NASA Space Radiation Laboratory, Brookhaven National Laboratory. NSRL User Guide: Bragg Curves and Peaks. https://www.bnl.gov/nsrl/userguide/bragg-curves-and-peaks.php. Accessed March 28, 2018.
15. The International Commission on Radiation Units and Measurements. *ICRU Report No. 37: Stopping Powers for Electrons and Positrons.* Bethesda, MD: ICRU; 1984.
16. Podgorsak EB. *Radiation Physics for Medical Physicists.* Switzerland: Springer International; 2016.

III

Application: Imaging and Therapy

Introduction to Medical Imaging

CONTENTS

In Part I of this book we discussed the cell cycle and how a malfunction of the growth inhibitors in the cycle can lead to cancer. We then went on to discuss the fundamentals of radiobiology, which deals with the effects of radiation on cells. We learned that double strand breaks in the DNA can most likely lead to cell death. That simple idea set out the motivation for treating cancer with radiation: if incident radiation can result in double strand breaks, then that radiation could be used to kill cancer cells and bring tumors at least under control. But how can radiation result in double strand breaks?

Part II of this book was dedicated to learning about how radiation incident on tissue can deposit energy into that tissue. If the radiation is ionizing radiation, then the electrons released from the target atoms will undergo many interactions with local atoms in the tissue, leading to further local energy deposition, more electron emission, and perhaps DNA damage. This combination of ionization and energy deposition can lead to molecular bond breaking and, possibly, to double strand breaks.

If the incident radiation consists of photons, then these photons can undergo interactions with target atoms in the tissue—typically by means of the Compton effect during cancer treatment—that can result in the emission of electrons and possible subsequent DNA damage. On the other hand, if the incident radiation consists of charged particles, then energy is continuously imparted to the surrounding medium (the tissue), which can then result in the direct ionization of electrons.

Part III of this book finally pulls together the ideas in Parts I and II to discuss the detection and treatment of cancer. Starting in Chapter 13, we will discuss the ideas of cancer treatment in the clinic: how are treatment plans developed by medical physicists and radiation oncologists? How are these treatment plans implemented?

But before treatment plans can be developed and before the physics that we've learned dealing with the interactions of radiation with matter can be exploited, we

DOI: 10.1201/9781003477457-10

have to first of all determine that there *is* disease to be treated and we have to determine the location and extent of that disease. This is the domain of *radiology* and *diagnostic medical physics*.

At the very foundation of radiology and diagnostic medical physics is medical imaging. How are images of the interior of the body obtained? What are the different types of imaging modalities and what are their characteristics and limitations? Are there any risks associated with these imaging modalities? Answering these questions is the purpose of the first three chapters in Part III of this book.

In this chapter we will introduce the topic of imaging with some basics: an historical overview and a brief discussion of topics associated with imaging, image quality and dose delivered to the patient during the imaging procedure. We will then close this chapter with a brief discussion of new imaging modalities on the horizon of diagnostic medical physics that will most likely play important roles in the clinic in the near future. Chapters 11 and 12 will then introduce the primary imaging modalities that are currently used in the clinic and that are of interest to us in this brief overview of medical imaging.

10.1 A BRIEF HISTORICAL OVERVIEW

The earliest "instrument" used for diagnostic medicine was the human eye, which focuses visible light onto the retina by means of refraction of the light at the surface of the eye (the cornea) and within the eye's lens.

The study of human *anatomy* is the study of the *structure* of the human body. On the other hand, *physiology* describes the *function* of the various parts of the anatomy—how the various parts work and interact with one another. By *medical imaging* we will mean that imaging of the anatomy and physiology of the body that goes beyond that which can be observed with the human eye—at least without opening up the body in a surgical procedure.

Many modern imaging modalities resulted from technologies and procedures developed in research labs that studied the properties of atoms and nuclei. These research efforts were organized and focused by the military during the second world war, resulting in technologies that led to the imaging modalities in clinical use today.

Medical imaging really began with the discovery of x-rays by Wilhelm Röntgen in 1895. As discussed in §1.1, Röntgen's discovery was quickly exploited for medical purposes, allowing physicians to view internal anatomy and to treat patients with the newly discovered rays. While much improvement in the technology and resulting images in x-ray radiographs have taken place since Röntgen's time, it is nevertheless amazing that the same fundamental physics discovered by Röntgen still underlies modern radiographs, which are the most frequently used mode of medical imaging today.

The First Nobel Prize

Alfred Nobel died on Thursday, December 10, 1896. In his last will and testament he stated that a significant portion of his assets were to be used "...to constitute a fund, the interest on which is to be distributed annually as prizes to those who, during the preceding year, have conferred the greatest benefit to humankind". The first prize mentioned in his will was for "...the person who made the most important discovery or invention in the field of physics".[1]

Correspondingly, the first Nobel prize ever awarded during the first Nobel Prize Award Ceremony on December 10, 1901—exactly five years after Nobel's death—was for physics.[2] That first prize was awarded to Wilhelm Röntgen, "...in recognition of the extraordinary services he has rendered by the discovery of the remarkable rays subsequently named after him".[3] In hindsight, we can say that the first Nobel prize ever awarded was for the discovery that began the field of modern medical imaging.

Imaging Advances

Other advances in medical imaging followed Röntgen's discovery. A brief summary of some of these advances is given below, starting with Röntgen's discovery.

1895: X-Rays Discovered Medical imaging applications are immediately recognized after Röntgen's discovery of x-rays, or "Röntgen-rays". Within one year x-rays are being used by doctors around the world.

1896: Fluoroscope Invented Thomas Edison displays his newly invented fluoroscope at an exhibition in New York City in which people are able to view their own bones.

1896: Radioactivity Discovered Henri Becquerel discovers radioactivity in a sample of uranium.

1942: Ultrasound Used for Diagnostic Purposes Karl Dussik, along with his brother Friederich, uses ultrasound to search for brain tumors. Image artifacts interfere with the image, but a later improvement in the ultrasound equipment enables successful diagnosis of brain tumors in 1947.

1946: NMR Discovered Nuclear Magnetic Resonance (NMR) is discovered independently by Edward Purcell and Felix Bloch; they receive the Nobel Prize in 1952 for this discovery. NMR is the foundation of Magnetic Resonance Imaging (MRI).

1950: First Positron Imaging Device Built Gordon Brownell and William Sweet at the Massachusetts General Hospital build the first imaging device that uses annihilation radiation following positron emission. The annihilation gamma rays are detected using two sodium iodide detectors placed on opposite sides of the patient. This device is then used to image patients with suspected brain tumors.[4,5]

1958: Gamma Camera Invented Hal Anger invents a camera that uses gamma rays emitted by radiopharaceuticals to image a patient's physiology.

1958: First Ultrasound Image of Fetus Published Along with Tom Brown and John MacVicar, Ian Donald develops an ultrasound scanner that is then used to diagnose an ovarian cyst. The publication of the first ultrasound image of a fetus in 1958 generates great interest in the gynecological use of ultrasound imaging.

1961: First PET Machine Built James Robertson builds a 32-crystal ring-shaped annihilation-radiation detector at Brookhaven National Lab. This machine, called the "head-shrinker", is the forerunner of modern positron-emission tomography (PET) machines.[6]

1971: Cancer Diagnosis Potential of NMR Suggested Raymond Damadian publishes a paper[7] in which he describes differences in the NMR signals between normal tissue and tumors, suggesting that these differences can be exploited to detect malignant tumors.

1971: Prototype CT Machine Built Godfrey Hounsfield and Allan Cormack install the first computerized tomography (CT) machine and use it to perform the first CT brain scan on a living person. (Hounsfield and Cormack were awarded the 1979 Nobel Prize in Physiology or Medicine for their work on computerized tomography.)

1973: First 2-D and 3-D MRI Images Produced Paul Lauterbur expands a 1-D technique to generate the first 2-D and 3-D MRI images.[8] (Lauterbur shared the 2003 Nobel Prize in Physiology or Medicine with Peter Mansfield for the development of MRI.)

1973: First PET Scanner Built Michael E. Phelps, Edward Hoffman and Michael M. Ter-Pogossian build the first PET scanner for human examination at the Washington University School of Medicine. This instrument employs mathematical algorithms to produce 3D images of the human brain, liver, and cardiovascular system.[9,6,10]

1977: MRI Significantly Improved Peter Mansfield improves on work by Lauterbur by improving the image quality and significantly decreasing the time for the image production. He does this by introducing line-scanning[11] and echo-planar imaging[12] techniques. Mansfield publishes the first cross sectional MRI image of *in vivo* human anatomy (a finger).[11] (Mansfield shared the 2003 Nobel Prize in Physiology or Medicine with Paul Lauterbur for the development of MRI.)

1998: PET-CT Scan Invented The combination PET-and-CT machine is invented by Ronald Nutt and David Townsend. This hybrid machine facilitates tumor location while reducing costs.

2018: First Total-Body PET/CT Scanner Built Simon Cherry and Ramsey Badawi at UC Davis design and create the first total-body PET/CT scanner. The scanner, called EXPLORER, can simultaneously scan all of the organs and tissues in the human body in as little as one second; the scan results in a 3D PET image. The first human images produced by EXPLORER are unveiled on 17 November 2018 at the IEEE Medical Imaging Conference in Australia.[13]

10.2 IMAGE QUALITY

Medical imaging has several purposes. First, medical imaging is used to help diagnose disease or other medical issues. This involves first of all determining whether medical issues are present and where, determining the extent of those issues, and possibly determining the cause of those issues. For these reasons, medical imaging is also referred to as *diagnostic imaging.* But medical imaging also serves purposes associated with the *treatment* of disease. For example, CT, fluoroscopy and ultrasound can be used during medical procedures or treatments to help guide the procedure or the course of the treatment, and various medical imaging modalities can be used after procedures or treatment to gauge the effectiveness of the procedure or treatment. In other words, the results of medical imaging can be exploited at all stages of the diagnosis and treatment of disease or other medical issues.

By the *quality* of a medical image we mean the extent to which the image serves its purpose, be it in helping to diagnose disease or evaluate the efficacy of treatment.

There are a number of factors that can reduce image quality. First of all, the image quality is certainly sacrificed if the appropriate imaging modality is not used for the given medical issue, or if the wrong region of the patient is imaged. But, barring basic mistakes such as these, the image quality can be thought of as the clarity of the image. By the image *clarity* we will mean the extent to which the image displays the desired information about the patient. Fundamentally, image clarity is influenced by five factors: blur, contrast, noise, distortion, and artifacts.[14]

Blur is exactly what it sounds like—the lack of clarity or sharpness of the image. Certainly, if light forming an image is not focused properly the image will be blurred. But blur also includes other effects. For example, if the patient moves during the image acquisition the image will certainly be blurred. Blur is also influenced by the spatial resolution of the image. The *spatial resolution* of an image can fundamentally be thought of as the smallest feature in the patient that can be imaged. The spatial resolution is limited by such factors as the size of a pixel in a digital image, the size of a grain in the emulsion of a photographic image, or it can be limited by diffraction due to the wavelength of radiation being used to produce the image.

Contrast in an image means being able to detect subtle changes in the image between adjacent anatomical regions within the patient where these two regions respond in almost the same way to whatever imaging modality is being used. For example, two adjacent parts of the anatomy that have nearly the same density may appear to have nearly the same grayscale in a radiographic image, thereby making it very difficult to distinguish where one part ends and the next starts. An image with a higher contrast will be able to distinguish the border between these two regions. Of course, contrast in the image can be primarily dictated by actual differences in the physical characteristics of the different parts of the anatomy being studied—mass density, effective atomic number, proton density, acoustic impedance, *etc.* Beyond that, contrast can be improved by the technique being used (choosing the proper modality to begin with, and then using an appropriate energy for the imaging beam, etc.), exploiting the properties of a contrast agent, or being able to improve the contrast after the image has been obtained—for example, numerical filtering techniques applied to digital images.

Noise is that contribution to the image that is not associated with the purpose of the image—in other words, noise is that part of the image that gets in the way of being able to extract the desired information about the patient. From this definition, noise can be something as simple as portions of the anatomy getting in the way of what is being imaged, or scattering of the image radiation from structures in the anatomy that are not of interest. But sources of noise can also be more subtle—for example, a non-uniformity in the radiation field being used to create the image, a non-uniformity in the detector characteristics across the face of the detector, or so-called *quantum mottle*, which is a spotted characteristic of the image resulting from the discrete nature of the photons or particles being used to create the image. Quantum mottle becomes an issue in very low-intensity images.

Distortion is the unequal magnification of different structures in the anatomy. For example, two parts of the anatomy having the same size can appear to have different sizes in the image if one part of the anatomy is closer to the detector system than the other part.

Artifacts are portions of the image that are not associated with the patient's anatomy. For example, non-uniformities in the magnetic fields in an MRI, a crinkling of the film in radiography, a misplacement of refracted sound waves in an ultrasound image, or the presence of metal fillings in teeth or pacemakers when forming an X-ray CT image can all cause image artifacts. Although many artifacts are easily recognized by experienced imaging practitioners, artifacts can cause difficulties when they are misinterpreted as a part of the patient's anatomy.

10.3   A CONCERN: DOSE IN IMAGING

Ionizing radiation is radiation—charged or uncharged particles or photons—that has sufficient energy to ionize atoms in tissue. The electrons thereby released can then result in energy deposition within the tissue. The energy deposited per unit mass is called the *absorbed dose*, or simply dose, to the tissue: when 1 J of energy has been deposited into 1 kg of tissue, we say that the tissue has received a dose of *one gray (1 Gy)*. But 1 Gy of one type of radiation can produce a very different biological result than 1 Gy of a different type of radiation, so the dose is often multiplied by a unitless *radiation weighting factor* to produce a more biologically meaningful quantity. This more meaningful quantity is called the *equivalent dose* and is measured in units of *sieverts (Sv)*.

As discussed in Part I of this book, dose to tissue can result in the killing of cancer cells, which is the topic of the latter part of this book on cancer treatment with radiation starting in Chapter 13. It is important to point out, however, that ionizing radiation can also *cause* cancer. For this reason, it is very important for us to keep track of the radiation exposure of a typical person in today's modern society. The most recent report of the National Council on Radiation Protection and Measurements (NCRP) that outlines the average annual dose to citizens of the United States is Report No. 160, which gives the results of data obtained in the year 2006.[15]

According to Report 160, the average equivalent dose received per person in the United States per year is about 6.25 mSv *(milli-sieverts)*. To put this amount of dose in perspective, the NCRP has pulled together available data to come up with an estimate of the excess risk of dying from cancer that results from various doses of ionizing radiation.[16] There is general agreement that, below 10 mSv, there are no data to suggest an increased risk of cancer. Likewise, it is readily accepted that there is clear evidence of cancer risk for doses above 100 mSv.[17] Where the interpretation of the data is more controversial, however, is for doses in the range 10–100 mSv.

From its review of the available data, the NCRP suggests a total detriment toward dying from cancer of 0.05 Sv^{-1}. This means, for example, that if a patient receives four PET/CT scans with an average effective dose of 25 mSv each, then their risk of dying from cancer is increased by $4 \times 25\,mSv \times 0.05\,Sv^{-1} = 0.005$, or 0.5%. This result is to be compared with the natural lifetime risk of dying from cancer, which is about 22% for men and 19% for women.[18]

The average annual effective dose of 6.25 mSv can be divided into three parts. The first part, contributing 3.11 mSv (49.8%), is due to radiation exposure obtained from natural sources, including radioactive minerals in the ground, radon gas that seeps through cracks in the ground and often collects in basements, radiation emitted by stars that travels through space and makes its way to the Earth's surface (so-called *cosmic rays*), and even radiation emitted by our own bodies. (Exposure from minerals and radon gas can vary greatly with location.) The second part, which contributes 0.14 mSv (2.2%) to the total annual average, results from human activities: consumer goods and occupational and industrial sources—sources that can be thought of as man-made environmental sources.

The two parts of our annual radiation dose mentioned above account for 52.0% of that dose. The remaining 48.0%—3.00 mSv—is due to medical imaging. Of that dose, nearly half comes from x-ray CT scans. The remainder comes from nuclear medicine, interventional fluoroscopy, and conventional radiography and fluoroscopy.[19] (A patient receiving radiation for cancer treatment would receive significantly more dose than 3 mSv.)

Diagnostic medical imaging plays not only a fundamental role in cancer care but also in many other types of medical procedures, including routine dental exams. Indeed, medical imaging has become so ubiquitous that we often don't even think about it when our doctor recommends some sort of "scan". But rising health-care costs and an increasing awareness of annual dose have both the public and medical practitioners thinking more carefully about automatically relying on medical imaging for the answers to many medical questions.

10.4   ANATOMICAL VS. FUNCTIONAL IMAGES

This chapter has presented a brief overview of some of the major advances made in imaging since Röntgen's discovery of x-rays in 1895, a discussion of what is meant by image quality, and pointed out the potential risks in the form of dose delivered to tissue by the radiation being used to form the image. What we have not discussed in this chapter are the types of images that can be formed and their characteristics.

In particular, different imaging modalities exploit the properties of different types of radiation in different ways. Why would one imaging modality be used over another for a given patient? The following two chapters introduce the various ways that images can be formed along with some of the properties of those images. But, given that there are two chapters in which to do this, it means that the various imaging modalities have to be split into two categories. What categories can be used to divide the various imaging modalities that we'll be discussing?

One way to do this is to divide the various imaging modalities into the two categories of *anatomical imaging* and *functional imaging*. As the name implies, an anatomical image shows the patient anatomy—what is located where. This is probably the type of image that you think of when you think of a medical image.

On the other hand, a functional image gives information about how various parts of the anatomy are functioning, which means that a functional image gives information about the patient's physiology. This is accomplished by exploiting the properties of radiopharmaceuticals. A *radiopharmaceutical* consists of a radioactive isotope bound to an organic molecule. Which radioisotope is used is based on its half life and on the characteristics of the radiation that it emits—often gamma- or x-rays. The organic molecule is chosen for the regions of anatomy into which it tends to be selectively absorbed or deposited. The radiopharmaceutical is useful when healthy tissue accumulates different amounts of the organic molecule than the corresponding diseased tissue. Given that this is the case, more or less radiation coming from a given region of the anatomy in a functional image shows whether that region is functioning properly or not. Since this type of imaging technique exploits the properties of radioactive nuclei, it is often referred to as a *nuclear medicine image*.

As we describe the various imaging modalities in the following two chapters, you should be able to explain why the image produced is an anatomical image or a nuclear medicine, or functional, image.

But that is not how we are going to divide the imaging modalities. Instead, we will discuss *projection images* in Chapter 11 and then *reconstruction images* in Chapter 12. What is meant by these two categories will be discussed in those two chapters. Chapter 13 will then start the long-anticipated discussion of radiation therapy—the treatment of cancer (and other disease) using radiation.

But before we proceed with our discussion of projection and reconstruction imaging modalities, let's take a quick glimpse into the future of clinical medical imaging modalities.

10.5 EMERGING TECHNOLOGIES IN MEDICAL IMAGING

Contributed by Lisa G. Whitelock, DMP, Technical Operations Manager, Krueger-Gilbert Health Physics, an Apex Physics Partner

We have thus far discussed some basic ideas associated with medical imaging. The following two chapters will discuss the major imaging modalities used in medical physics today. However new discoveries are always on the horizon. This section will give a brief sampling of recent advances in the medical physics associated with imaging.

Photon counting CT

The first photon counting computed tomography unit was installed at the Mayo Clinic in Rochester, Minnesota in 2014, and human research studies began in August 2015. A second-generation prototype was introduced in 2020 and photon counting CT was approved by the FDA on September 30, 2021.[20]

Photon counting CT uses the direct conversion of x-rays into electrical signals by way of a semiconductor material detector. When x-rays strike the semiconductor material, electron-hole pairs are created and these charges are separated by a strong electric field. Thus it is possible to detect and count each individual x-ray photon as it strikes the detector.[21]

There are several advantages to photon counting CT including elimination of cross-talk between detectors, better geometric dose efficiency, smaller detector pixels, elimination of electronic noise, increased intrinsic spectral sensitivity, and the ability to better detect lower energy photons. These detectors allow the use of lower radiation dose and less iodine contrast while still generating the same if not better diagnostic quality images. Contrast between objects is improved as well as spatial resolution. Physicians are also able to extract multi-energy information to differentiate internal structures and reprocess images without re-scanning the patient.[21]

Dedicated Breast CT (DBCT)

Dedicated breast computed tomography (DBCT) has been in development since 2001, however it is still not as widespread as mammography, which is the gold standard.[22]

DBCT utilizes a cone-beam CT geometry. The patient lies prone, face-down on the exam table with the breast pendulant inside of the imaging area. The x-ray source and the detector rotate around the breast. Imaging can be done with or without contrast dye.[23] Advantages of DBCT include better visualization of malignant lesions, easier integration with other modalities, mitigation of superimposition effects, and there is no need for compression.[22] Future research includes the use of photon counting detectors with these systems.[24]

Solid-State PET/CT

Solid-state detector PET/CT was introduced by Philips at the Radiological Society of North America annual meeting in November 2013.[25]

Solid-state PET/CT uses solid-state silicon photomultiplier detectors (SiPM) instead of the traditional scintillation detectors with multiple photomultiplier tubes. When the photon strikes the detector crystal, the light produced is directly channeled to a silicon pixel and digitized to produce data for the image.[26] The advantages of solid-state PET/CT include a higher count rate detection efficiency, improved time-of-flight resolution, increased image quality, faster scanning, and lower dose.[27]

Fluorescence Image-Guided Surgery

Fluorescence image-guided surgery (FGS) was first introduced in 1948 when fluorescein (a diagnostic contrast agent) was used intravenously to define potential brain tumors during neurosurgery. The first FGS imaging system was approved by the FDA in 2005.[28]

FGS uses a preoperative injection of a photosensitizer contrast agent and then a special imager to illuminate the surgical field and see the tumor. This allows for a better visualization of tumors and an increased likelihood of getting all of the malignant tissue with less damage to healthy tissue.[28]

Theranostics

Theranostics is an emerging healthcare field that merges nuclear medicine and radionuclide therapy. The concept was first postulated in 1900 by Paul Ehrlich as a "magic bullet" that would be a special drug to accurately and precisely kill disease without damaging healthy tissue. In 1936, Dr. Saul Hertz had the idea to examine iodine metabolism using radioactive isotopes of iodine. Animal trials started in 1937 and the first patients were treated for hyperthyroidism using Iodine-131 at Massachusetts General Hospital in 1941.[29]

Iodine-131 and Lutetium-177 are examples of theranostic agents. These agents treat cancer by emitting beta particles and subsequently in their decay, gamma particles are emitted that can be imaged using a nuclear medicine camera. In the 1990s, Indium-111 for treatment of neuroendocrine tumors in humans and Yttrium-90 for treatment of pancreatic neuroendocrine tumors in experimental rats were introduced. These treatments are known as peptide receptor radionuclide therapies or PRRTs.[29]

Theranostic treatments are advantageous because they can be customized to each patient and they allow clinicians to visualize and treat disease with the same agent. Additionally, they target disease while sparing healthy tissue as much as possible.[30]

10.6 QUESTIONS, EXERCISES, & PROBLEMS

10-1. Research and explain in your own words the similarities and differences between *radiology* and *diagnostic medical physics*.

10-2. It was stated in this chapter that Raymond Damadian was the first to point out that cancerous tumors could be detected *in vivo* using NMR. What was not pointed out was that he also received the first patent in the field of MRI for that idea of detecting cancer using NMR, and he produced the first *in vivo* MRI scan through a full human body (the chest). In addition, he developed the first commercial MRI scanner. Nevertheless, the 2003 Nobel Prize in Physiology or Medicine, "for their discoveries concerning magnetic resonance imaging"[31], went to Paul Lauterbur and

Peter Mansfield. Research the work done by these three men and then answer the following questions: Why do you think the Nobel Prize committee did not include Damadian in the 2003 prize for physiology or medicine? Do you think the committee made a mistake not including him? Back up your answers with findings from your research (including references!).

10-3. Discuss the difference between the terms *image quality* and *image clarity*.

10-4. Compare and contrast the units of *absorbed dose* and *equivalent dose*. Are they the same thing, or something quite different? Explain.

10-5. It is stated in this chapter that part of our average annual radiation exposure comes from radioactive sources in our own bodies. Research this further. What are the dominant radioactive sources in our bodies? How do they get there?

10-6. What is the difference between *anatomy* and *physiology*?

10-7. (a) *Research the following*. What is the average dose from a dental x-ray? ...from an x-ray CT scan? ...a PET/CT scan? How do these values compare to the average annual equivalent dose from the non-medical background radiation exposure given in this chapter? (b) NCRP Report No. 160 shows that the average dose from medical procedures in the United States increased by more than a factor of 7 between the early 1980s and 2006. Research and discuss why you think this might be the case. As always, be sure to state your references.

10-8. The last section in this chapter mentions new technologies that have not yet been incorporated into routine imaging procedures used in the clinic. Pick one of the topics mentioned, then research this topic and summarize what you learned. (Don't forget the references!)

10.7 REFERENCES

1. Nobel Prize Outreach AB. Full text of Alfred Nobel's will. https://www.nobelprize.org/alfred-nobel/full-text-of-alfred-nobels-will-2. Accessed July 9, 2019.
2. Nobel Prize Outreach AB. From the First Nobel Prize Award Ceremony, 1901. https://www.nobelprize.org/ceremonies/from-the-first-nobel-prize-award-ceremony-1901. Accessed July 9, 2019.
3. Nobel Prize Outreach AB. All Nobel Prizes in Physics. https://www.nobelprize.org/prizes/lists/all-nobel-prizes-in-physics. Accessed July 29, 2019.
4. Brownell GL. A history of positron imaging. http://websites.umich.edu/ ners580/ners-bioe_481/lectures/pdfs/Brownell1999_historyPET.pdf. Accessed July 18, 2019.
5. Brownell GL, Sweet WH. Localization of brain tumors with positron emitters. *Nucleonics*. 1953; 11: 40-45.
6. Vaughan D, ed. *A vital legacy: Biological and environmental research in the atomic age*. California: Lawrence Berkeley National Lab; 2019.
7. Damadian R. Tumor Detection by Nuclear Magnetic Resonance. *Science*. 1971; 171: 1151-1153.
8. Lauterbur PC. Image Formation by Induced Local Interactions: Examples Employing Nuclear Magnetic Resonance. *Nature*. 1973; 242: 190-191.
9. Godt E. UCLA's Phelps, PET inventor, receives Nuclear Pioneer Award from SNMMI. https://www.healthimaging.com/topics/molecular-imaging/uclas-phelps-pet-inventor-receives-nuclear-pioneer-award-snmmi. Accessed August 6, 2017.
10. U.S. Department of Energy. Molecular Nuclear Medicine Legacy. https://www.lacinybros.com/cmss_files/attachmentlibrary/timeline-1977.pdf. Accessed August 7, 2019.
11. Mansfield P, Maudsley AA. Medical imaging by NMR. *British Journal of Radiology*. 2014; 50(591): 188-194.
12. Mansfield P. Multi-planar image formation using NMR spin echoes. *J. Phys. C: Solid State Phys.* 1977; 10: L55-L58.
13. The Regents of the University of California, Davis campus. EXPLORER Total-body PET Scanner News, Human Images From World's 1st Total-Body Scanner Unveiled. https://explorer.ucdavis.edu/news. Accessed August 6, 2019.

14. Hendee WR, Ritenour ER. *Medical Imaging Physics.* 4th ed. New York: Wiley-Liss; 2002.

15. National Council on Radiation Protection and Measurements (NCRP). *Report No. 160—Ionizing Radiation Exposure of the Populations of the United States.* Bethesda, MD: NCRP; 2009.

16. National Council on Radiation Protection and Measurements (NCRP). *Report No. 115—Risk Estimates for Radiation Protection.* Bethesda, MD: NCRP; 1993.

17. Lin EC. Concise Review for Clinicians: Radiation Risk from Medical Imaging. *Mayo Clinic Proc.* 2010; 85(12): 1142-1146.

18. American Cancer Society. Lifetime Risk of Developing or Dying from Cancer. www.cancer.org/cancer/cancer-basics/lifetime-probability-of-developing-or- dying-from-cancer.html. Accessed August 8, 2019.

19. United States Environmental Protection Agency. Radiation Sources and Doses. https://www.epa.gov/radiation/radiation-sources-and-doses. Accessed August 7, 2019.

20. Grove E. With photon-counting-detector CT, Mayo Clinic at forefront of CT imaging technology. https://newsnetwork.mayoclinic.org/discussion/with-photon-counting-detector-ct-mayo-clinic-at-forefront-of-ct-imaging-technology/. Accessed July 12, 2022.

21. Siemens Healthineers. Understanding the technology behind photon-counting CT. https://www.siemens-healthineers.com/en-us/computed-tomography/technologies-and-innovations/photon-counting-ct. Accessed July 12, 2022.

22. Medical Professionals. Dedicated CT Imaging of the Breast. https://www.medical-professionals.com/en/dedicated-ct-imaging-of-the-breast/. Accessed July 12, 2022.

23. Lindfors KK, Boone JM, Newell MS, D'Orsi CJ. Dedicated breast computed tomography: the optimal cross-sectional imaging solution? *Radiol Clin North Am.* 2010; 48(5): 1043-1054. doi: 10.1016/j.rcl.2010.06.001. PMID: 20868899; PMCID: PMC2972197.

24. Berger N, Marcon M, Saltybaeva N, et al. Dedicated Breast Computed Tomography With a Photon-Counting Detector: Initial Results of Clinical In Vivo Imaging. *Investigative Radiology.* 2019; 54(7):409-418.

25. DAIC. Philips Unveils First Digital Detector PET/CT System at RSNA 2013. https://www.dicardiology.com/product/philips-unveils-first-digital-detector-petct-system-rsna-2013. Accessed July 12, 2022.

26. Zhang J, Maniawski P, Knopp MV. Performance evaluation of the next generation solid-state digital photon counting PET/CT system. https://www.researchgate.net/publication/328770646_Performance _evaluation_of_the_next_generation_solid-state_digital_photon_counting_PETCT_system. Accessed July 12, 2022.

27. Zhang J, Maniawski P, Knopp MV. Performance evaluation of the next generation solid-state digital photon counting PET/CT system. *EJNMMI Res.* 2018; 8(1): 97. https://doi.org/10.1186/s13550-018-0448-7.

28. Nagaya T, Nakamura YA, Choyke PL, Kobayashi H. Fluorescence-Guided Surgery. *Front. Oncol.* 2017; 7. https://doi.org/10.3389/fonc.2017.00314.

29. Gomes Marin JF, Nunes RF, Coutinho AM, et al. Theranostics in Nuclear Medicine: Emerging and Re-emerging Integrated Imaging and Therapies in the Era of Precision Oncology. *RadioGraphics.* 2020; 40(6). https://doi.org/10.1148/rg.2020200021.

30. Miller C, Rousseau J, Ramogida CF, Celler A, Rahmim A, Uribe CF. Implications of physics, chemistry and biology for dosimetry calculations using theranostic pairs. *Theranostics.* 2022; 12(1):232-259. doi: 10.7150/thno.62851. PMID: 34987643; PMCID: PMC8690938.

31. Nobel Media AB. All Nobel Prizes in Physiology or Medicine. https://www.nobelprize.org/prizes/lists/all-nobel-laureates-in-physiology-or-medicine. Accessed August 1, 2019.

Projection Imaging Modalities

CONTENTS

The previous chapter discussed some historical advances in imaging along with some of the general properties of images. In this chapter, we will start our discussion of specific types of imaging modalities. In particular, we will discuss modalities that are formed by means of *projection*. To start off, we will describe what is meant by a projection image.

11.1 THE IDEA OF PROJECTION

We are all well familiar with the idea of shadows—regions of relative darkness formed when the path of light is obstructed by one or more objects, as shown in Fig. (11.1). When we speak of a *projection image* in medical imaging, we are speaking of an image formed by photons—usually x- or gamma-rays—a portion of which has been obscured or attenuated by structures of anatomy.

As we learned in Chapter 8, the attenuation of photons traversing a known material of attenuation coefficient μ is governed by the equation,

$$I(z) = I_0 e^{-\mu z}, \tag{11.1}$$

where I_o is the intensity of radiation incident at the surface of the material, $z = 0$, and $I(z)$ is the intensity remaining after the radiation has passed through a depth z of the material. Let's consider the application of this equation to a more specific scenario.

Consider a beam of photons of incident intensity I passing through the body of a patient. We will schematically represent two structures of anatomy by a sphere and a rectangular box. The photons move down through the patient and are eventually recorded by a photon detector, as shown in Fig. (11.2). We will be interested in three points on the detector, points 1, 2, and 3.

DOI: 10.1201/9781003477457-11

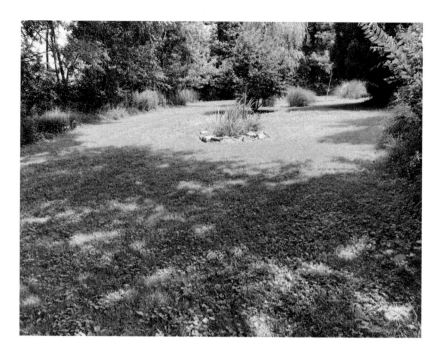

FIGURE 11.1: Shadows formed by the passage of light being blocked by one or more objects.

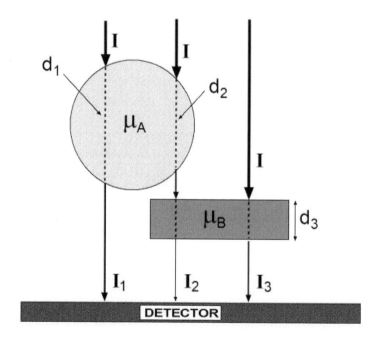

FIGURE 11.2: Incident photons pass through structures in anatomy as they make their way to a photon detector.

Let the absorption coefficients of the spherical and rectangular box structures be denoted μ_A and μ_B, respectively. Any photons reaching the detector without passing through either of these two structures will be detected with the incident intensity I. (For simplicity, we assume that any absorption outside of the structures A and B is negligible.) But photons reaching points 1, 2, and 3 on the detector will have been attenuated by different amounts since they pass through different depths of anatomy, as given by the distances d_1, d_2, and d_3 shown in Fig. (11.2). Indeed, we can see from Eq. (11.1) that the intensities at detector points 1, 2, and 3 will be given by:

$$I_1 = Ie^{-\mu_A d_1} , \tag{11.2}$$

$$I_2 = Ie^{-(\mu_A d_2 + \mu_B d_3)} , \tag{11.3}$$

and

$$I_3 = Ie^{-\mu_B d_3} . \tag{11.4}$$

Assuming that μ_B is significantly larger than μ_A, it would then follow that the shadow of the photons incident on the anatomy in Fig. (11.2) is darkest at point 2 and lightest at point 1. That is, it would then follow that

$$I_2 < I_3 < I_1 , \tag{11.5}$$

as indicated by the width of the intensity arrows shown in the figure. We can thus say that the 2-D image formed by the detector is a shadow image of the anatomy above the detector. This shadow image is called a *projection image* since information about the 3-D anatomy is *projected* onto the 2-D image.

We will discuss different types of projection images in this chapter, starting with the simplest projection image, the radiograph.

11.2   RADIOGRAPHY

The most commonly used imaging technique is *radiography*. A *radiograph*, or is what is commonly known as simply an "x-ray", is a projection image of the patient's anatomy through which the x-rays travel. The x-ray photons that survive the journey through the patient without being absorbed or scattered are then incident on an x-ray sensitive film or screen that is on the other side of the patient.

As discussed in §9.2, x-rays were discovered accidentally on November 8, 1895 by Wilhelm Conrad Röntgen while he was investigating the emissions of rarified gases in cathode ray tubes. After the discovery, Röntgen immediately began investigating the properties of the new mysterious "x-rays". He found that the x-rays produced a glow on a fluorescent screen, so he began placing objects between the source of the x-rays and the screen in order to study the penetrating ability of the new rays. He was amazed to find a projection of the bones in his hand when he placed his hand in front of the screen. On December 22, 1895, Röntgen recorded the image of the hand

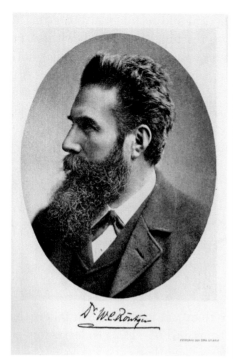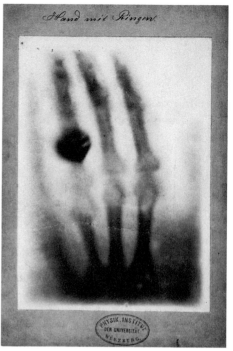

FIGURE 11.3: Left: Wilhelm Conrad Röntgen in 1901. (Public Domain) Right: First x-ray image of human anatomy, taken by Röntgen in 1895. This fuzzy image is of his wife's left hand with her wedding rings. (By Wilhelm Röntgen. - Public Domain.)

of his wife, Anna Bertha Ludwig. This was the first recorded x-ray image of human anatomy and the image that started medical radiography. See Fig. (11.3).[1]

X-Ray Detectors

A modern set-up for a radiograph typically consists of an x-ray source on one side of the patient and a flat detector on the other side. The detector can be either a screen-film detector or a digital detector, although screen-film detectors are rarely used anymore.

A screen-film detector is a flat cassette consisting of two screens on either side of a sheet of film. The screens serve to intensify the radiation that is incident on the film, which is coated on both sides by a light-sensitive emulsion. The screens serve to convert the photon-energy in the form of incident x-rays into visible light, which can then expose the emulsion on the film. After exposure, the film must be removed from the cassette and chemically processed in order to obtain the image. See the left side of Fig. (11.4).[2]

On the other hand, a digital detector—typically called a *flat panel detector*—involves no film and no chemical processing. The digital image can be viewed within seconds after the detector is exposed to the x-rays.

There are various types of flat-panel detectors. Some are constructed with *charge-coupled devices*, or CCDs, while others exploit the properties of *complementary*

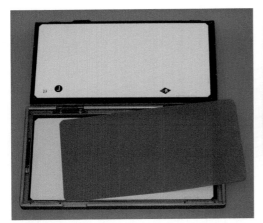 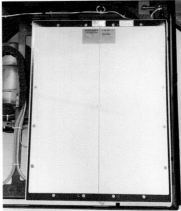

FIGURE 11.4: Left: An open film cassette showing the two screen intensifiers and a sheet of x-ray film. (Open Access) Right: A digital TFT kV x-ray detector. (Courtesy of Joann Prisciandaro and Alexander Moncion.)

metal-oxide semiconductor (CMOS) light-sensitive arrays. Still others use a photostimulable phosphor plate that can release stored energy in a phosphor to form a projection image in a technique called *computed radiography*. However, we will discuss a different type of flat-panel display that is in wide use in clinics today.

A TFT, or *thin-film-transistor*, array detector is made of amorphous silicon and consists of a large number of x-ray sensitive detector elements arranged into a rectangular array, each connected to a transistor and a charge-collection capacitor. The detector element effectively acts like a switch that determines the extent to which a pixel in the desired image is turned ON or OFF, depending on the amount of charge collected by the capacitor. The charge collected by each capacitor is sent to a charge amplifier that produces a voltage that is proportional to the charge collected. This voltage is then used to determine a gray-scale value for the corresponding pixel in the image. This process is represented schematically in Fig. (11.5). The set of all of the gray-scale pixel values are then arranged to form the desired projection image. A TFT flat-panel detector is shown on the right side of Fig. (11.4).

There are two types of TFT detectors: *indirect* conversion detectors and *direct* conversion detectors. Both types of detectors involve producing an electrical signal using the energy of an incident x-ray. The signal is then sent to the TFT element and then to a charge storage capacitor. The amount of charge stored in the capacitor is then used to determine the gray-scale level of the corresponding pixel in the final image. How the two types of detectors differ is in how the electrical signal is produced. We will start by discussing indirect TFT detectors.

In an indirect TFT detector, the x-ray photons that survive the passage through the patient's anatomy first interact with a scintillation layer made of a phosphor that is similar to the intensifying screens found in x-ray film cassettes. The phosphor absorbs the energy of the incident x-ray photon and emits visible-light photons. Since most of the incident x-rays are absorbed toward the front end of the intensifying layer,

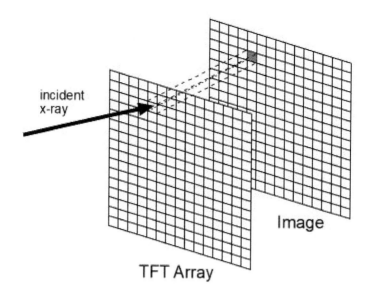

FIGURE 11.5: A schematic representation of a TFT detector array. The energy of an x-ray that is incident on one of the TFT detectors in the array will ultimately determine the shading of a corresponding pixel in the final image.

the emitted photons must effectively traverse the thickness of the scintillation layer in order to make it to the TFT array. This passage through the thickness of the intensifying layer can result in scatter, which degrades the clarity of the image.[3]

As shown in Fig. (11.6), light emerging from the phosphor scintillation layer then interacts with photodiodes that are incorporated into the TFT array.[4] These photodiodes produce the charge (the electrical signal) that is sent to the transistors

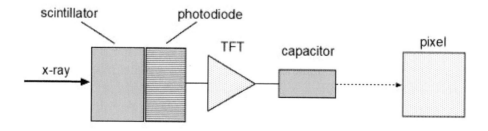

FIGURE 11.6: A schematic diagram showing the basic set-up of an indirect conversion detector. X-rays incident on a scintillation layer undergo interactions within that layer to produce visible-light photons. Those photons then interact with photodiodes that convert the photon energy into an electrical signal. This signal then travels to the thin-film-transistor element (TFT) and to a charge-storage capacitor. The amount of charge stored in the capacitor is then used to determine the gray-scale value of a pixel in the final image.

Direct Conversion

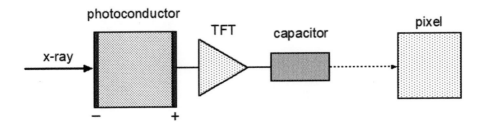

FIGURE 11.7: A schematic diagram showing the basic set-up of a direct conversion detector. X-rays incident on a photoconducting layer undergo interactions within that layer to produce positive and negative charges due to ionization within the material. A voltage maintained between the two surfaces of that layer serve to separate the charges produced in the ionizations, thereby producing an electrical signal. This signal then travels to the thin-film-transistor element (TFT) and to a charge-storage capacitor. The amount of charge stored in the capacitor is then used to determine the gray-scale value of a pixel in the final image.

in the TFT elements and is then collected in the capacitors, thereby determining the gray-scale value for the corresponding pixel in the image.

In contrast to the indirect detector, a direct TFT detector does not need a scintillation layer to produce visible photons from the incident x-ray photons. Instead, the direct detector employs a photoconducting semiconductor layer of amorphous selenium (a-Se) or cadmium telluride (Cd-Te) that is sandwiched between two conducting layers that act as electrodes.[5] This "semiconductor sandwich" is placed immediately before the TFT layer. When an x-ray photon is absorbed in the photoconductor material it produces an ionization pair. A voltage maintained between the two electrodes then readily attracts the positive and negative charges in the ion pair to opposite electrodes. This charge is then collected in the storage capacitor in the TFT detector element. Note that the applied voltage not only keeps the charges in the ion pair from having much lateral motion that would move them to a different pixel detector element, but it also reduces the chance of recombination within the semiconductor material, which would in turn reduce the efficiency of the device.[6]

Digital flat-panel detectors provide for a better image quality and a significant improvement of image storage and sharing over the film cassette. In addition, direct conversion flat-panel detectors typically offer the most efficient conversion of x-ray energy into image information along with the least amount of noise, which can result in a lower dose to the patient for a given image quality. However, the resolution of a TFT flat-panel detector image is limited by the size of the detector elements ("dels"), resulting in a resolution of around $330\,\mu m$ for a typical chest radiograph. This can be contrasted with a resolution of around $170\,\mu m$ for a chest radiograph obtained using a film-screen system.[7,8] Figure 11.8 shows an example of a radiograph obtained with a flat-panel detector.

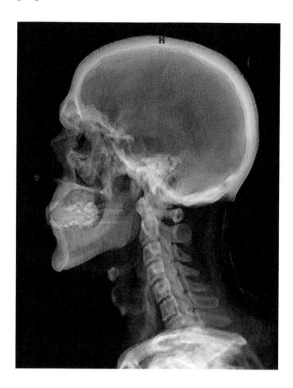

FIGURE 11.8: A digital radiograph produced by a flat-panel detector. It is interesting to note that this is not an image of a person, but rather of a *phantom*—an object made with the shape and basic structure of a person as far as x-ray interactions are concerned. Such an object can be useful to the medical physicist during the treatment-planning process in helping to determine dose distributions to patients. (Courtesy of Joann Prisciandaro.)

11.3 FLUOROSCOPY

Fluoroscopy is a type of medical imaging that results in what is basically a radiographic movie. Fluoroscopic sequences of images can be recorded and stored as part of a patient's record, or they can be used in real time to help a surgeon during a treatment procedure.

A "real-time" movie has at least 30 frames viewed per second since motion seems smooth to the human eye when viewed at this frequency. In fluoroscopy, radiographs are taken in rapid succession and viewed in either real time or from a digital recording. Clearly, in order for fluoroscopy to become feasible, various technological difficulties had to be overcome. We will discuss three of these difficulties.

First, there must be a means of producing rapid "frames" of the x-ray movie. Originally, such images were produced by exposing the patient to a continuous beam of x-rays while "snapshots" having 33 ms acquisition times were taken, one after the other, thereby resulting in a real-time movie. But there were some major problems with this method. Any motion of the anatomy being imaged that occurred during the 33 ms acquisition time resulted in a blurred image. In addition, the continuous exposure to an x-ray beam could result in a relatively large dose to the patient.

These problems were overcome after the 1980s with the advent of a rapidly pulsed x-ray beam. Instead of having patients continuously exposed to an x-ray beam, they were exposed to higher intensity but shorter in duration x-ray pulses. For example, assuming that "frames" of the x-ray movie lasted 33 ms, instead of recording an x-ray image for the full 33 ms, the patient could be exposed to a pulse of duration 3 ms to 10 ms with each pulse starting every 33 ms. This would serve to greatly reduce the blur in the image due to patient movement.[3]

Also, if the motion of the anatomy being recorded is rather slow, the number of frames per second could be reduced—in fluoroscopy the frame rate can vary from 3 fps (frames per second) up to 30 fps. Lower frame rates would result in a lower dose to the patient.

The second difficulty to be overcome was that there must be a detector system that can display or record the image within a very short time interval, and then be ready for the next image. Modern fluoroscopy systems use digital video cameras or digital flat-panel detectors that exploit the electrical properties of fast-response semiconductor devices: *charge coupled device* (CCD) or *complementary metal oxide semiconductor* (CMOS) applications for the cameras, and thin film transistor (TFT) applications for the flat panel detectors.

Lastly, a very rapidly produced image implies a correspondingly very low amount of radiation energy that can be used to produce the image. This results in a very dim image that is difficult to view or record. This problem is overcome with fluoroscopic detectors that can be thousands of times more sensitive than radiographic detectors. These detectors use either an *image intensifier* that exploits the properties of *phosphors* to convert x-ray or electron-beam energy into visible light energy, or TFT detector arrays that exploit charge amplifiers. The increased sensitivity in fluoroscopic detectors does not come without a price, however—these detectors tend to have lower resolution and higher noise than those used in radiography.

Fluoroscopy is used for both diagnostic and therapeutic procedures. Being able to image the beating of the heart or to observe the process of a patient swallowing during a barium swallow study can be invaluable for the physician. In these cases, stand-alone fluoroscopic systems are used. But for cancer treatment with radiation using a linear accelerator (a "linac"), it is useful to be able to do a fluoroscopic study of a patient immediately prior to or even during irradiation. For this reason, some linacs come equipped with fluoroscopic equipment attached to the body of the accelerator to allow for such studies.

Figure (11.9) shows a linac with an arm on either side of its main body, which is called the *gantry*. Each arm can swing from the sides of the gantry in toward the treatment couch where the patient lies for treatment. The arm on the left holds the x-ray source and the arm on the right holds the flat-panel detector. When positioned on either side of the patient, this imaging equipment can produce fluoroscopic imaging to help ensure that the tumor being treated is positioned properly under the gantry

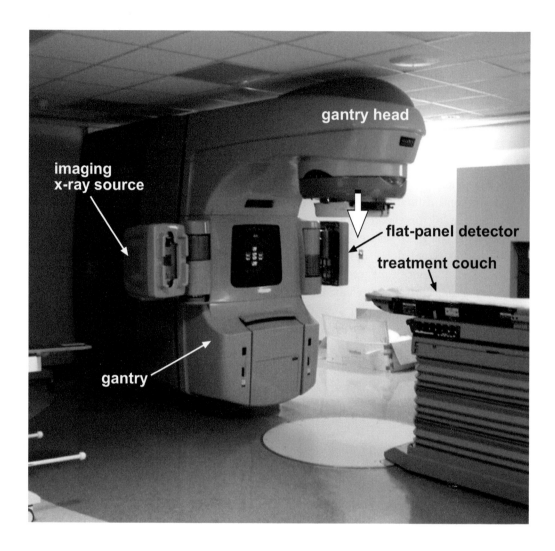

FIGURE 11.9: A linear accelerator (linac) used in radiation therapy cancer treatment. X-rays (represented by the large white arrow in the figure) emerge from the gantry head to treat the patient. The patient is positioned on the treatment couch, which can be moved to the correct position for treatment. The source of the imaging x-rays for radiography or fluoroscopy is on the left side of the gantry, and the flat-panel detector used for detection of the x-rays and production of the image is on the right side. The imaging x-ray source and the flat-panel detector can be swung around from the sides of the linac and positioned on either side of the patient for imaging.

head, from which high-energy x-rays used for treatment emerge, or it can be used to monitor the progress of the treatment fractions.

The ease and utility of fluoroscopic imaging in viewing not only patient anatomy but also patient physiology makes it an invaluable diagnostic as well as therapeutic tool.

11.4   NUCLEAR PLANAR IMAGING

Nuclear medicine is that branch of medical imaging that exploits the properties of radiopharmaceuticals (also called radiotracers) to diagnose and treat disease. These radiotracers can emit high-energy photons—x-rays or gamma rays—or charged particles inside the patient. Since charged particles readily lose their energy and are subsequently absorbed due to the stopping power of the tissue in the body (see Chapter 9), they tend not to emerge from the patient's body, leaving only the high-energy photons to be available for imaging. (Recall that photons tend to have an exponential drop-off in intensity, so some of them will survive the trip through the patient's body. (See Chapter 8.)

The imaging modalities that we have discussed so far in this chapter produce images of *anatomy*—the parts of the patient's body that otherwise would lie unseen beneath the skin. A nuclear medicine image, on the other hand, shows how various parts of the anatomy are *functioning*. As a result, nuclear medicine images give information about the *physiology* of the patient.

This functional imaging is accomplished by using radiopharmaceuticals. A *radiopharmaceutical* consists of a radioactive isotope bound to an organic molecule. The radioisotope is selected based on its half life and on the characteristics of the radiation that it emits—typically gamma- or x-rays. The organic molecule is chosen for the regions of anatomy into which it tends to be selectively absorbed or deposited. The radiopharmaceutical is useful in nuclear medicine when healthy tissue accumulates different amounts of the organic molecule than the corresponding diseased tissue. Given that this is the case, more or less radiation coming from a given region of the anatomy in a nuclear medicine image shows whether that region is functioning properly or not—hence a functional image.

The majority of radiopharmaceuticals in use today for nuclear medicine use an isomer of technetium—Tc-99m—as the radionuclide. The "m" in Tc-99m refers to the fact that the isomer of technetium is *metastable*, having a clinically convenient half-life of 6.02 h. In addition, Tc-99m emits gamma rays as it transitions down to the ground state of Tc-99. These gamma rays will readily emerge from the patient's body and be available for use in producing an image. (See the text around Eq. (7.9) for a discussion of metastable states and isomeric transitions.)

As an example of nuclear medicine, let's consider the case of a patient with thyroid cancer. The thyroid is a gland in the front portion of the base of your neck. Nearly all of the iodine in your body is absorbed by the thyroid, which means that radioactive iodine, I-131, can be used for imaging and treating the thyroid.

I-131 is a radioactive isotope of iodine that undergoes beta decay followed by gamma decay. The emitted electrons can destroy tissue into which the radioactive iodine has been absorbed, while the gamma rays can be used for nuclear medicine imaging. For diagnosis, a very small amount of I-131 is administered to the patient, either in capsule or liquid form. The iodine is quickly absorbed in the bloodstream and subsequently collected in the thyroid.

Figure 11.10 shows a nuclear planar image of a thyroid-cancer patient after having part of her thyroid surgically removed and then undergoing I-131 treatment.[9] The black region in the neck corresponds to gamma emission from the I-131 collected in the remaining portion of the thyroid, while the black regions in the lungs and hip region show that the cancer had spread (*metastasized*). Note how this image shows the regions of the anatomy associated with the thyroid and the metastasized thyroid cancer, but it does not show any clear image of anatomy.

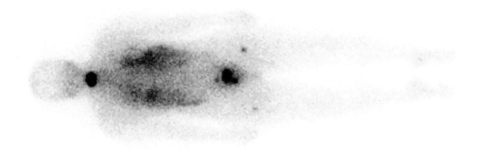

FIGURE 11.10: A nuclear planar image of a thyroid-cancer patient after receiving I-131 treatment. (The head of the patient is to the left and the feet are toward the right.) The black areas show regions of high I-131 concentration. (Image by Lager et al. Available under creative commons license 4.0.)

The Gamma Camera

In nuclear planar imaging, the gamma- or x-rays given off by the radiopharmaceutical are typically recorded by a nuclear scintillation camera, called a *gamma camera* or an *Anger camera* in honor of Hal Anger, who invented the camera in 1956.[10] The scintillation crystal in the camera has a thickness from about 6.4 mm to 12.7 mm,[11] and can have a large area, up to about 60 cm × 40 cm,[3] resulting in a correspondingly large field-of-view.

An issue arises in nuclear planar imaging that does not arise in radiography or fluoroscopy. In radiography and fluoroscopy, the x-ray source is located outside the patient and basically acts like a point source of the radiation. This means that the photons travel in straight lines from the source, through the patient, and onto the detector unless they undergo interactions before they are detected. All of the x-rays entering the patient are, at least initially, headed toward the detector.

This is far from the case for nuclear planar imaging in which the photons emitted by the radiotracers are emitted in random directions. Because these photons are emitted isotropically, this means that the photons arriving at a given point on the detector could have come from any point within the patient containing the radiotracer, resulting in a completely blurred image. What is needed for a useful image is for all of the photons arriving at a given point on the scintillation crystal to have come from a more-or-less fixed direction within the patient—the resulting image will then be a projection image, more like a radiograph.

This is accomplished within the gamma camera by a *collimator* that is positioned on the side of the crystal closest to the patient. The collimator usually consists of a series of thousands of narrow holes drilled in a high-Z material, often lead. Only those photons entering a hole in a direction that is nearly parallel to the hole axis will make it to through to the detector—nearly all other photons will be absorbed by the wall of the hole. The resulting image is, therefore, a 2-D projection of the 3-D distribution of the radiopharmaceuticals within the patient's body.

Figure 11.11 shows a schematic of a typical gamma camera. The bottom of the figure shows a portion of the patient's anatomy. The dark areas A and B represent two regions that have absorbed the radiopharmaceutical. As a result, A and B are both sources of high-energy photons that can be emitted in any direction, as shown by the solid and dashed lines that represent photons emanating from A and B. The

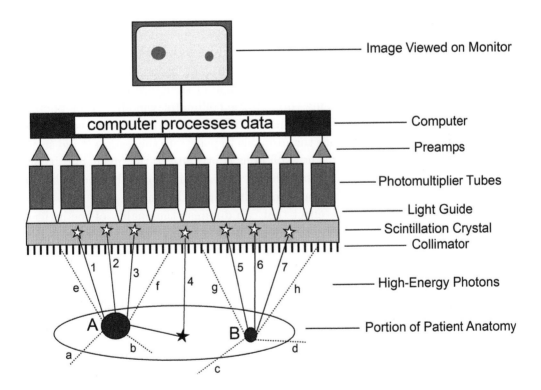

FIGURE 11.11: Schematic of a typical gamma camera. Shaded portions of the patient anatomy have absorbed radiopharmaceuticals and emit gamma rays. Solid lines represent emitted photons that contribute to the final image; dashed lines do not contribute to the image. The black star represents a Compton scattering event and the white stars represent positions where the gamma rays incident in the crystal are absorbed and visible-light photons are emitted. See the text for more information.

majority of the photons leaving A and B will not even head toward the detector, as represented by photons a, b, c, and d in the figure.

Consider photons f and g. These two photons are from very different parts of the patient's anatomy, but they are both headed toward the same region of the detector. If there were no collimator and the photons were actually detected and contributed to the image, then the image would be completely blurred and contain no useful information. For this reason, a collimator is positioned at the bottom of the detector. As mentioned above, the collimator keeps photons trying to get into the detector from different directions from contributing to the same position on the image. In other words, the collimator helps keep the image from getting too blurred to be of clinical use. Careful examination of Fig. (11.11) shows that photons e, f, g, and h are all blocked by the collimator and therefore do not contribute to the image. All of the dashed lines in the figure represent photons that, for one reason or another, never make it into the detector. Indeed, only about 1 in 10000 photons emitted by the source[12] and 1 in 1000 photons incident on the collimator[13] make it through the collimator and into the detector.

The solid lines in Fig. (11.11) represent photons that contribute to the image. These photons are heading in a direction that is close enough to the axis of the holes in the collimator that they are not stopped by the walls of the collimator holes. It can be seen that photons 1, 2, and 3 contribute to the image of structure A in the anatomy, and 5, 6, and 7 contribute to the image of structure B. But very careful inspection of these photons passing through the collimator will show that photon 7 actually hits the wall of the hole that it enters and, therefore, should be absorbed. Photon 7 represents those photons that are able to penetrate the lead wall and survive the trip through the collimator. These photons contribute to the image even though they were heading in a direction that should have been stopped by the collimator. Such photons will therefore contribute to a blurring of the image.

Photon 4 represents another effect that can diminish the quality of the image by contributing to background noise. As photons travel through the body of the patient, they can undergo interactions such as the Compton and photoelectric interactions (see Chapter 8). While the photoelectric interaction results in the absorption of the photon, the Compton interaction results in the photon being scattered, so that it may end up heading in a completely different direction. Photon 4 in the figure was initially moving away from the detector when it was emitted from structure A, but, after being scattered, it ended up moving straight upward and surviving the journey through the collimator. (The black star in the figure represents the scattering event within the patient that changed the direction of photon 4.) It will therefore contribute to the image but provide no useful information about the regions of the patient's anatomy that had absorbed radiotracers.

Once the gamma-ray photons pass through the collimator, they are incident on a scintillation crystal. The purpose of the scintillation crystal is to take the high-energy photons emitted by the radiopharmaceuticals and exchange them for photons in the visible region of the spectrum. The crystal typically used in the gamma camera is NaI(Tl)—sodium iodine doped with thallium.

NaI is a semiconductor that has a relatively large energy gap between the valence and conduction bands—the regions of allowed energy levels for electrons in a semiconductor energy-level diagram. (See Chapter 4 and Fig. 4.3 for a discussion of energy levels and photon emission.) Electrons in the conduction band that make a transition across the gap down to the valence band will emit photons that have too large an energy to be in the visible region of the spectrum. However, when thallium is incorporated into the lattice, energy levels are introduced within the band gap that allow for lower-energy transitions associated with photons in the visible region. NaI(Tl) absorbs gamma rays and emits light in the blue region of the spectrum.[14]

The white stars within the scintillation crystal in Fig. (11.11) denote locations where the incident high-energy photons shown are absorbed and subsequently emit visible-light photons. These photons are then transferred via a light guide to photomultiplier tubes.

Highly efficient *photomultiplier tubes* (PMTs) take the visible light produced in the scintillation crystals and convert that light to bursts of electrons. NaI(Tl) scintillator crystals have the property that, the higher the energy of the incident gamma ray, the more visible-light photons will be generated. As a result, higher gamma-ray energies means greater bursts of electrons from the PMTs. These electron bursts form an electronic signal that is sent to a preamplifier (or *preamp*) that generates a voltage corresponding to the electronic signal. The preamp compares this voltage to a preset threshold voltage. If the voltage of the signal is less than the threshold voltage, then that signal is ignored, thereby removing, for example, contributions from gamma rays that were scattered and have a lower energy than the originally emitted gamma rays from the radiopharmaceuticals. This improvement in the signal-to-noise ratio by the preamp is necessary in order to obtain clinically useful images without too much noise.

The signals from the various PMT-preamp pairs are then sent to a computer where they are analyzed and interpreted to form the final image, which can then be viewed on a monitor or stored for later viewing. Figure 11.12 shows a modern gamma camera.[15]

11.5   ULTRASOUND

A few words are in order before we begin our discussion of ultrasound imaging. First, unlike the other imaging modalities discussed in this book, ultrasound imaging does not use photons traveling through the patient's body to construct the image— instead, it uses *sound waves*. Second, ultrasound is not officially a projection imaging modality. The waves do not travel through the body and emerge on the other side to be detected and form the image. Instead, the ultrasound image is formed as a result of reflections of the sound waves within the body, so it's more of a *reflection* image. Nevertheless, it is still a projection of various reflected waves within the patient, and can thus be considered a type of projection image.

By *sound* waves we mean *pressure* waves—traveling waves of alternating higher and lower pressure regions in the medium through which the sound is propagating. Sound waves traveling through a given medium travel with a speed that depends on

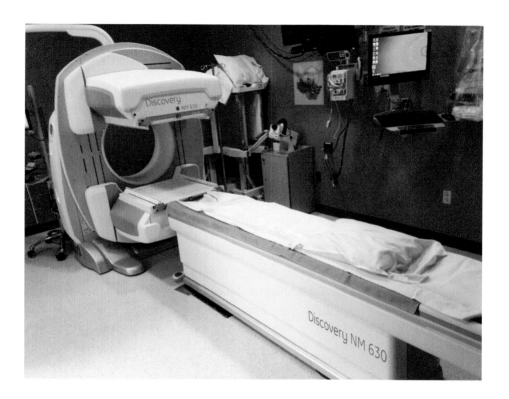

FIGURE 11.12: The Discovery 630 SPECT gamma camera manufactured by GE. (Image by Nightryder84. Available under creative commons license 3.0.)

the physical properties of the medium itself. Sound waves in air are waves that travel with a speed that is dictated by the physical properties of the air: temperature, density, humidity, *etc*. The speed of sound in air at sea level and at $0\,^{o}$C is 330 m/s. In general, the more *stiff* the medium (that is, the more quickly it returns to its equilibrium configuration when displaced), the faster sound travels through that medium. For example, sound travels through soft tissue in the human body at 1540 m/s and through skull bone at 4080 m/s.[3]

On average, humans can hear sound waves with frequencies in the range from about 20 Hz to about 20 kHz. In general, ultrasound waves are high frequency waves above the audible range with frequencies varying roughly from kHz to GHz; ultrasound waves used in diagnostic imaging are typically in the range from 2 MHz to 20 MHz. Ultrasound imaging is also called *sonography*, and the resulting image is called a *sonogram*.

In ultrasound imaging, the ultrasound waves travel through the patient's body in order to image the patient's anatomy. Since waves (light or sound) can be used to image objects as long as the wavelength is smaller than the objects being imaged, it is important to use small wavelength waves—hence, ultrasound frequencies. (Objects about the same size as the wavelength or smaller tend to scatter the waves in all directions, which would tend to produce noise in the image.)

The speed of sound waves in a medium is dictated by the physical characteristics of the medium—its density and an elastic characteristic of the medium called the *bulk modulus of elasticity*. Since sound waves can be both longitudinal and transverse in solids, and since solids, liquids, and gases can all be found inside the human body, ultrasound waves can exist in longitudinal as well as transverse form within the body. But it turns out that only the longitudinal waves are of practical use in the clinic, so we will focus our attention on longitudinal ultrasound waves.

We generally observe objects in our surroundings by means of visible light that reflects off of the surfaces of those objects. The reason light reflects off of objects is that the light is incident on a boundary between two media—the air and a coffee cup, for example—within which the light has different speeds (or, equivalently, different indices of refraction). When we take a picture of the objects in a room, for example, nearly all of the light coming from those objects that is used to form the image is *reflected* light. A photograph is therefore a projection image of the light in the room that was reflected and was subsequently incident on the detector inside the camera.

Likewise, ultrasound images can be formed from high frequency sound waves that are reflected off of boundaries between two media (different tissues) in the patient within which the sound waves have different speeds. More specifically, the *acoustic impedance* of a certain type of tissue depends on the density of that tissue and on its bulk modulus of elasticity. For example, the acoustic impedance values for air, soft tissue, and muscle, in units of $10^{-4} \; kg/(m^2 s)$, are respectively equal to 0.0004, 1.63, and 1.70.

The greater the difference in impedances between two materials on either side of a boundary, the more an incident ultrasonic wave will be reflected at that boundary; if the impedances of the two materials on either side of a boundary are very close, then most of the wave will be transmitted and very little will be reflected. Therefore, if the amplitude of a reflected wave is measured and compared with the amplitude of the wave that was originally sent out, information can be deduced about the medium on the other side of the boundary off of which the sound was reflected.

Figure (11.13) shows the ultrasound equipment used to produce a sonograph.[16] Transducers, shown on the right side of the tray in the picture, will be discussed next.

The Transducer and the Ultrasound Image

How can an image be formed using ultrasound waves? To produce an ultrasound image, an instrument called an *ultrasound transducer* is placed in contact with the patient's skin, as shown in Fig. (11.14).[17] The transducer is a hand-held instrument that serves as both the producer and detector of ultrasound waves.

A key component of the transducer is the *piezoelectric crystal*. This crystal can be used to convert electrical energy (voltage signals) into mechanical energy (vibrations). When placed in contact with the patient, these high-frequency vibrations within the transducer produce ultrasound waves that travel into the patient. After the waves are reflected back by structures in the patient's anatomy, the vibrations of the returning waves are converted by the crystal inside the transducer into voltage signals that are then transferred to the rest of the ultrasound equipment and used to form the image. These conversions in the crystal from electrical signals into mechanical vibrations

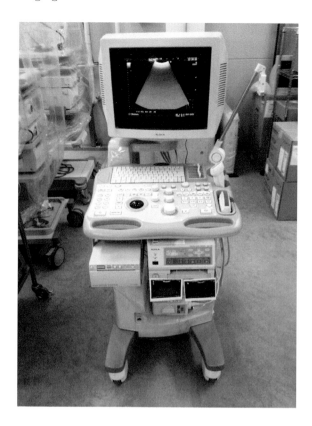

FIGURE 11.13: Ultrasound equipment used to produce a sonograph. (Image by Kitmondo Marketplace. Available under creative commons license 2.0.)

and *vice versa* are accomplished by means of a phenomenon called the *piezoelectric effect*.

The time between the production of the wave pulse produced by the transducer at the surface of the patient and the detection of a wave, or echo, reflected from a boundary between two different materials (for example, an organ or bone embedded in soft tissue) specifies the depth of the boundary into the patient, given the speed of the wave in the intervening tissue. In addition, as mentioned previously, the amplitude of the reflected wave gives us information about the characteristics (impedances) of the two media on either side of the boundary. Information from many such reflected waves can then be used to produce the ultrasound image.

By the *resolution* of an imaging modality we mean the size of the smallest object that can be viewed in the image. The resolution is roughly given by the wavelength of the waves used to produce the image. Given this, one might think that all ultrasound images should be made using waves having the smallest possible wavelength (highest frequency) in order to obtain the best possible resolution in the resulting image. Things are not so straight forward, however. While waves with higher frequencies have a better resolution, they also suffer the greatest attenuation as they traverse the body, so the higher frequency waves will have their amplitudes reduced more, resulting in a lighter image of features that are deeper within the patient's anatomy.

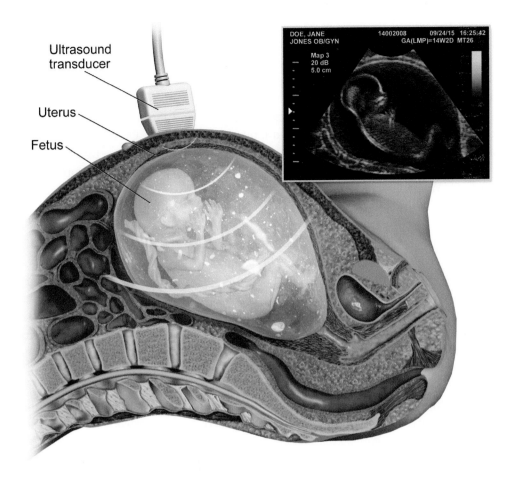

FIGURE 11.14: An ultrasound transducer being used to create a sonograph of a fetus. The insert shows the resulting sonograph. (Image by Bruce Blaus. Available under creative commons license 4.0.)

A good quality image is produced by compromising between high resolution and the depth of features within the patient to be displayed in the image—deeper features will require lower frequencies.

11.6 QUESTIONS, EXERCISES, & PROBLEMS

11-1. In the discussion associated with Fig. (11.2), assume that $\mu_B = 5\,\mu_A$. Also assume that all distances in the figure are to scale. Carefully explain why Eq. (11.5) must then be true. That is, explain why the shadow at the position of the detector is darkest at point 2 and lightest at point 1.

11-2. Compare and contrast direct and indirect conversion TFT detectors. What is being "converted" into what in these detectors?

11-3. Research and explain the imaging process known as *computed radiography*.

11-4. At the end of the section on radiography it is stated that: "In addition, direct conversion flat-panel detectors typically offer the most efficient conversion of x-ray energy into image information along with the least amount of noise, which can result in a lower dose to the patient for a given image quality". Explain why a more efficient conversion of x-ray energy can result in reduced patient dose.

11-5. As mentioned in this chapter, video cameras and flat panel detectors used in fluoroscopy exploit the use of semiconductor devices such as CCDs, CMOS devices, and TFT arrays. Research these devices and explain their basic operation and use.

11-6. It was stated in this chapter that image intensifiers exploit the properties of *phosphors*. What is a phosphor? How can it convert x-ray or electron-beam energy into visible light?

11-7. Linear accelerators (*linacs*) produce x-rays for treatment that have energies on the order of MeVs. It was mentioned in this chapter that arms are sometimes attached to the sides of linacs to add fluoroscopic capabilities. (See Fig. 11.9.) The x-ray source of the fluoroscopy attachment also produces x-rays, but with energies on the order of keVs. Why do medical physicists go through all of this trouble? Why don't they just use the x-ray beam coming out of the linac's gantry to not only treat the patients but also image them? OK—maybe they wouldn't be able to do treatment and imaging at the same time, but they could at least use the MeV x-ray beam to image the patient immediately before and immediately after the treatment with the linac, right? Explain. (Hint: See Chapter 8.)

11-8. Carefully explain why the image obtained using a gamma camera would be completely blurred if it did not have a collimator. Your answer should include a sketch to help clarify your explanation.

11-9. Another factor not discussed in this chapter that affects the quality of an image is *quantum noise*. Research quantum noise and explain how it can contribute negatively to the quality of a medical image. Are all imaging modalities discussed in this chapter significantly affected by quantum noise? Explain.

11-10. As mentioned in the text, NaI(Tl) scintillation crystals are thallium-doped NaI semiconductors. The following questions build off of the discussions on energy-level diagrams in Chapter 4 associated with Fig. 4.3. (Note that the discussions in Chapter 4 are associated with the hydrogen atom. While these questions do not involve hydrogen, the ideas provided in those discussions will be useful here.) You will have to do some research on your own to answer the questions below. (a) Conceptually explain the differences between an insulator, a conductor, and a semiconductor. (b) Draw energy-level diagrams for an insulator, a conductor, and a semiconductor. Your diagrams should show the valence band, the conduction band, and the band gap. (c) Use the energy level diagrams in (b) to explain the differences described in (a). (d) Doped semiconductors are semiconductors into which a small number of impurity atoms have been introduced into the lattice. These impurity atoms introduce energy levels within the band gap of the semiconductor material at the positions of those atoms. Draw a generic energy level diagram for a doped semiconductor, and then explain how the introduction of impurities can allow the semiconductor to emit larger-wavelength photons as electrons make transitions from the conduction band down to the valence band compared to the pure, undoped semiconductor. (e) Explain why this is an important property of a scintillation crystal in a gamma camera.

11-11. Photomultiplier tubes (PMTs) are clearly an important component of the gamma camera. Research how PMTs work and then explain how visible-light photons enter one end of the PMT and a burst of electrons come out the other end. A well-labeled diagram should accompany your explanation. (As always, be sure to list your references.)

11-12. As mentioned in this chapter, clinical ultrasound waves have frequencies in the range from 2 MHz to 20 MHz. Consider ultrasound waves traveling through soft tissue with a speed of 1540 m/s. What are the approximate sizes of the smallest features that can be resolved by waves having the highest and the lowest frequencies of the clinical range of ultrasound frequencies given above?

11-13. As mentioned in this chapter, the speed of sound waves in a medium depends on the bulk modulus of elasticity of the medium and on the density of the medium. (a) Look up and then explain in your own words the definition of the *bulk modulus of elasticity*. (b) Using your answer in part *a*, explain why it makes sense that, if the bulk modulus of medium A is greater than that in medium B, then the speed of waves in medium A should be greater than the speed in medium B if the densities of the two media are the same. (c) Likewise, explain why it makes sense that, if medium A has a larger density than medium B but they have the same value of bulk modulus, then a wave traveling through medium A will move more slowly than a wave moving through medium B.

11-14. It was stated in this chapter that a piezoelectric crystal is used in an ultrasound transducer to produce the ultrasound waves. Research the piezoelectric effect and use the results of your research to explain how piezoelectric crystals in a transducer can be used to produce ultrasound waves.

11-15. Consider the following acoustic impedance values, all given in units of 10^{-4} $kg/(m^2 s)$: air = 0.0004, water = 1.50, soft tissue = 1.63, kidney = 1.62, and muscle = 1.70. Use this information to explain why ultrasound imaging cannot be used to study cancerous tumors in a patient that are within the lungs or on the far side of the lungs from the transducer.

11-16. Consider the following acoustic impedance values, all given in units of 10^{-4} $kg/(m^2 s)$: air = 0.0004, water = 1.50, soft tissue = 1.63, kidney = 1.62, and muscle = 1.70. Use this information to answer the following questions: Two equal amplitude ultrasound waves are sent into a patient. One wave is incident on the kidney, and the another is incident on muscle. Parts of the two waves are reflected and subsequently detected by the transducer. Assume that both waves travel through equal distances of soft tissue before and after the reflections. Which detected wave will have the larger amplitude? Why?

11-17. An acoustic coupling gel is placed on the skin of the patient before the transducer is used to produce the ultrasound waves. The acoustic impedance of the gel is designed to match the impedance of the patient's skin. The purpose of the gel is to eliminate layers of air between the transducer and the patient's skin while the ultrasound waves are being produced and detected. Explain why it is important to eliminate these air layers.

11-18. The average value of the speed of ultrasound waves in human soft tissue is 1540 m/s. The time between the generation of an ultrasound pulse by the transducer and the detection of an echo is measured to be 42.2 μs. What is the distance from the patient's surface at the position of the transducer to the tissue boundary off of which the waves reflected?

11.7 REFERENCES

1. (left) Public Domain. https://commons.wikimedia.org/wiki/File:Wilhelm_Conrad_R%C3%B6ntgen.jpg (Right) Public Domain. https://commons.wikimedia.org/w/index.php?curid=12354709
2. Left Image: EinAnonymerBenutzerVonVielen (https://commons.wikimedia.org/wiki/File:Roentgen-filmkassette_offen.jpg), https://creativecommons.org/licenses/by-sa/4.0/legalcode.
3. Bushberg JT, Siebert JA, Leidholdt EM, Boone JM. *The Essential Physics of Medical Imaging.* 3rd ed. Philadelphia: Lippincott Williams & Wilkins; 2012.
4. Allisy-Roberts P, Williams J. *Farr's Physics for Medical Imaging.* 2nd ed. Edinburgh: Elsevier Limited; 2008.
5. TWI. WHAT IS DIGITAL RADIOGRAPHY AND HOW DOES IT WORK? https://www.twi-global.com/technical-knowledge/faqs/digital-radiography. Accessed July 24, 2021.
6. Seibert JA. Flat-panel detectors: how much better are they? *Pediatr. Radiol.* 2006; 36(Suppl 2): 173-181. doi: 10.1007/s00247-006-0208-0.
7. Nickoloff EL. AAPM/RSNA Physics Tutorial for Residents: Physics of Flat-Panel Fluoroscopy Systems. https://pubs.rsna.org/doi/10.1148/rg.312105185. Accessed August 15, 2022.
8. Huda W, Abrahams RB. X-Ray-Based Medical Imaging and Resolution. *AJR.* 2015; 204: W393-W397.
9. Lager CJ, Koenig RJ, Lieberman RW, Avram AM. Rare Clinical Entity: Metastatic malignant struma ovarii diagnosed during pregnancy—Lessons for management. *Clin Diabetes Endocrinol.* 2018; 4: 13. https://doi.org/10.1186/s40842-018-0064-5. Extracted from Fig. 2g. Open Access, CC license 4.0.
10. Tapscott, E. Nuclear Medicine Pioneer, Hal O. Anger, 1920-2005. *Journal of Nuclear Medicine Technology.* 2005; 33(4): 250-253.
11. Cherry SR, Sorenson JA, Phelps ME. *Physics in Nuclear Medicine.* 4th ed. Philadelphia: Saunders; 2012.
12. Celler A. Nuclear Medicine. In: Lindon J, Tranter G, Koppenaal D, eds. *Encyclopedia of Spectroscopy and Spectrometry.* 2nd ed. Oxford: Elsevier; 2010.
13. Schirrmeister H, Arslandemir C. Diagnosis of skeletal metastases in malignant extraskeletal cancers. In: Heymann D, ed. *Bone Cancer. Progression and Therapeutic Approaches.* New York: Academic Press; 2010.
14. Ahmed SN. *Physics & Engineering of Radiation Detection.* London: Academic Press; 2007.
15. Nightryder84 (https://commons.wikimedia.org/wiki/File:Spectct_cmh_630ge.JPG), "Spectct cmh 630ge", https://creativecommons.org/licenses/by-sa/3.0/legalcode.
16. Kitmondo Marketplace (https://commons.wikimedia.org/wiki/File:ALOKA_SSD-3500SV.jpg), "ALOKA SSD-3500SV", https://creativecommons.org/licenses/by/2.0/legalcode.
17. BruceBlaus (https://commons.wikimedia.org/wiki/File:Fetal_Ultrasound.png), https://creativecommons.org/licenses/by-sa/4.0/legalcode.

Reconstruction Imaging Modalities

CONTENTS

The fundamental ideas behind the imaging modalities discussed in the previous chapter are very straight-forward, even though the details may not be so straight-forward: x-ray photons (or sound waves) work their way through the patient and arrive at a detector. The detector effectively records the numbers and positions of the incident photons (or directions of reflected ultrasound waves) and, with that information, a projection image is formed.

The fundamental ideas behind the formation of images for the modalities discussed in this chapter are not so straight-forward: the challenge is basically to figure out how to construct a 2- or 3-D image of a patient's anatomy or physiology from the information contained in a large number of projection images. The catch is that the image that we'd like to obtain is an image of a planar slice through the patient that is perpendicular to the planes of the projection images from which it is formed. In other words, we wish to obtain an image of anatomy in a plane that is *parallel* to the direction of motion of the incoming radiation, not perpendicular to that direction as is the case for projection images.

We'll start with a discussion of the general ideas of image formation through reconstruction, and then we'll move on to describe CT, MRI, SPECT, and PET imaging. This will then conclude our discussion of imaging modalities.

12.1　THE IDEA OF RECONSTRUCTION

We start by considering a small volume element of the patient's anatomy. Such a volume element is called a *voxel*. For simplicity in our discussion, we will assume that the voxel has a square cross-section of side z and depth Δx, so that the volume of the voxel is $\Delta V = z^2 \Delta x$. We will assume that ΔV is small enough that we may reasonably treat the attenuation coefficient (μ) as constant throughout the volume.

DOI: 10.1201/9781003477457-12

A beam of photons of intensity I_o is incident on the voxel, as shown in Fig. (12.1). We then position a detector on the other side of the voxel to measure the emerging intensity, I. From our previous discussions of the attenuation of radiation by matter, we know that the intensity of radiation emerging from the voxel is given by the equation,

$$I = I_0 e^{-\mu z}. \tag{12.1}$$

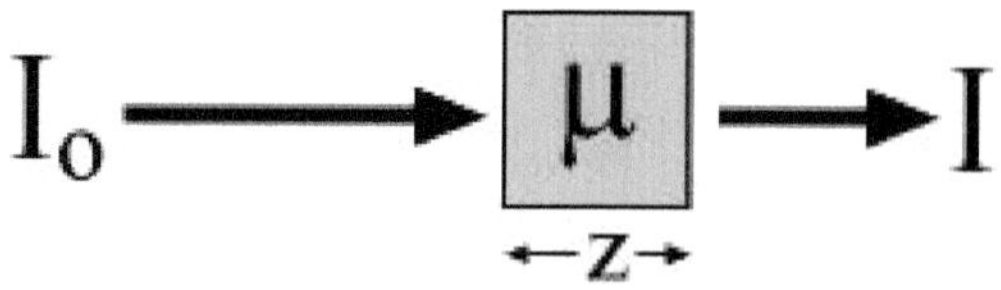

FIGURE 12.1: The attenuation of radiation by a single voxel of patient anatomy. The face of the voxel as shown in this figure has an area z^2. The depth of the voxel (into the page) is Δx.

Since Eq. (12.1) involves one equation with one unknown—μ—we can readily solve this equation for the value of the attenuation coefficient.

Let's now say that, for some silly reason, we wish to form an image of this single voxel of anatomy. In the last chapter our image would simply have been the projection image formed by the intensity of radiation I detected by the detector. That image would have represented the attenuation of radiation traveling through the cross-sectional area $z\Delta x$ as it made its way to the detector. But in this case, we wish to form an image of the voxel as if we were looking at it face-on, as seen in Fig. (12.1)—that is, we wish to form an image of the face of the voxel of area z^2.

Values of the total attenuation coefficient for 100 keV photons incident on human anatomy range from about $1.87 \times 10^{-4} \, cm^{-1}$ for air up to about $0.335 \, cm^{-1}$ for bone.[1] In addition, current computer displays support 256 shades of gray. Grayscale values for pixels vary from 0 to 255, with 0 representing black and 255 representing white. Therefore, we could break up the range of μ values for human anatomy into 255 intervals and assign a grayscale value for each pixel in an image for each value of attenuation coefficient computed from Eq. (12.1). If we were to assign a range of pixels in a monitor to represent the image of the face of our voxel, we could then send the grayscale information to the monitor and have it display the desired image. It wouldn't be much of an image to look at, but it would represent an image having a very different character than the projection images discussed in the previous chapter—it would be our first image of anatomy viewed face-on.

Let's now take a small step in complexity for our image: we'll now consider two adjacent voxels of anatomy. Figure (12.2) shows two voxels, again with incident intensity I_o. Now we use two detectors to measure the intensity of radiation emerging from each of the two voxels, I_1 and I_2. The values of these two intensities are determined by the average values of μ within the two voxels, μ_1 and μ_2, representing the types of anatomy contained within those voxels. The equations that show the functional relations between the measured intensities and the anatomy are given by

$$I_1 = I_0 e^{-\mu_1 z}$$
$$I_2 = I_0 e^{-\mu_2 z} . \qquad (12.2)$$

Equations (12.2) represent a system of two equations with two unknowns, μ_1 and μ_2, which can then be solved for the two unknown values. The two values of attenuation coefficient thus obtained can then be assigned grayscale values, as discussed above, and an image of the two voxels of anatomy can then be formed and displayed on a monitor. Again, the image will not be very interesting, but it nevertheless contains visual information about the anatomy within the two voxels as viewed in a plane that is parallel to the direction of motion of the incident photons.

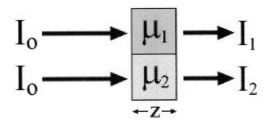

FIGURE 12.2: The attenuation of radiation by two adjacent voxels of patient anatomy.

The two simple sections of anatomy discussed so far have been one dimensional in the sense that the small voxels have been lined up, one after the other, so that the resulting image has also been effectively 1-D. Let's now move on to the somewhat more complicated situation of a two-dimensional array of voxels. The set-up in Fig. (12.3) shows four adjacent voxels arranged in a 2×2 array. There are now four values of μ that need to be determined in order to form the corresponding image of this section of anatomy. That means that we need four independent equations involving the four unknowns. The two detectors (not shown) to the right of voxels 3 and 4 measure the intensities I_{13} and I_{24}, given by

$$I_{13} = I_0 e^{-(\mu_1+\mu_3)z}$$
$$I_{24} = I_0 e^{-(\mu_2+\mu_4)z} , \qquad (12.3)$$

but this forms a set of only two equations. How can we obtained the additional two equations required to solve for the four unknown values of μ?

The idea is very straight-forward: simply rotate the source of the incident radiation and the two detectors about an axis perpendicular to the plane of Fig. (12.3) to give us the set-up shown in Fig. (12.4). This configuration then leads to the two additional equations

$$I_{12} = I_0 e^{-(\mu_1+\mu_2)z}$$
$$I_{34} = I_0 e^{-(\mu_3+\mu_4)z} , \qquad (12.4)$$

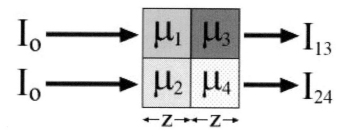

FIGURE 12.3: The attenuation of radiation by four adjacent voxels of patient anatomy.

which give us the information needed to solve for the coefficients μ_1, μ_2, μ_3, and μ_4. These values then allow us to determine the grayscale pixel values for the corresponding 2-D image of patient anatomy.

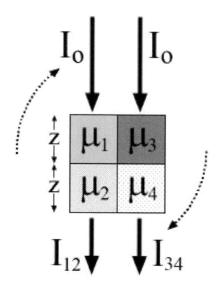

FIGURE 12.4: The source of radiation and the two detectors (not shown) are rotated from the configuration of Fig. (12.3) by 90°, as represented by the dashed arrows. This then generates the two remaining relations needed to solve for the four unknown values of the attenuation coefficient, μ.

It is tempting to think at this point that we have solved the problem of rendering a 2-D image of a cross-section of patient anatomy—after all, we have already seen how to construct a 2-D image of a portion of anatomy in the 2×2 array of voxels shown in Figs. (12.3) and (12.4). A moment's thought will show that we are not quite there, however.

Consider the next step: a 3×3 array of voxels. If we send in an incident beam of radiation to form a projection onto a vertical array of three detectors, similar to the 2×2 case in Fig. (12.3), and then rotate the source-detector system by 90° to get a second projection onto a horizontal array of three detectors, similar to the 2×2 case in Fig. (12.4), then we see that we will only have a system of 6 equations to solve for 9 unknown attenuation coefficients. We clearly need more relations between the unknown and known quantities.

There is a relatively simple solution to this problem, however: we simply rotate the source-detector system by a different angle. For example, Fig. (12.5) shows beams incident on a 3×3 array of voxels at 0°, 45°, and 90°, measured clockwise from the original horizontal direction. Clearly, this will yield sufficient information to allow us to solve for the desired attenuation coefficients. These ideas can then be extrapolated to larger arrays of voxels.

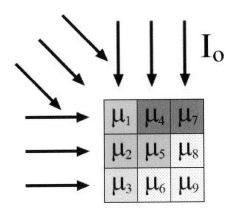

FIGURE 12.5: For larger arrays of anatomy voxels the radiation source and corresponding array of detectors must be rotated about the patient at different angles in order to obtain the information required to solve for the associated voxel attenuation coefficients.

The original scanner for diagnostic radiology that produced a cross section of patient anatomy (the brain), invented by G.N. Hounsfield in 1972, used an 80×80 array of voxels.[2] This scanner obtained projection data for 180 projections with a 1° rotation between each projection. Modern scanners use an array of 512×512 voxels.

Clearly, a significant amount of computer work is required to extract the attenuation coefficient values from the large systems of equations thus generated and to produce the resulting image. While straight-forward in principle, the method of solving for the average μ values for the various voxels becomes unwieldy for large systems of equations. So the problem remains: how can we efficiently reconstruct a cross sectional image of anatomy from the projection data produced in a series of scans?

Hounsfield Units

The discussion in this section has centered on associating a gray-scale value directly with a value for the attenuation coefficient, μ. In practice, this is done indirectly by means of a quantity called the *CT number*. In honor of G. N. Hounsfield, the inventor of the computed tomography (CT) imaging technique that was announced in 1972, the CT number is also referred to as the *Hounsfield unit*, denoted H.

The Hounsfield unit is defined as follows: let μ denote the value of the average attenuation coefficient of the voxel of anatomy in question and let μ_w denote that of water. For 100 keV photons, the attenuation coefficients for water, air, and bone are (to two significant figures): $0.17\,cm^{-1}$, $1.9 \times 10^{-4}\,cm^{-1}$, and $0.34\,cm^{-1}$, respectively.[1] The Hounsfield unit for the given section of anatomy is then defined to be

$$H = 1000\left(\frac{\mu - \mu_w}{\mu_w}\right). \tag{12.5}$$

Using the attenuation coefficient values given above for air and bone, we find that the Hounsfield units for air and bone are equal to -1000 and $+1000$, respectively.

12.2   REFINING THE RECONSTRUCTION PROCESS

The previous section outlined an approach to obtaining the attenuation coefficient as a function of position within a section of human anatomy. An image of that anatomy could then be produced by associating the attenuation coefficient values with gray-scale values for pixels on a monitor. But that approach involved solving a large system of simultaneous equations, which can be computationally intensive and time consuming. As a result, this approach is not used to reconstruct the anatomy in the form of an image. In this section we will discuss some of the approaches that are used for various reconstruction imaging modalities. Our discussion will be very rudimentary, however, as the mathematical complexity associated with a number of these techniques prevents a more complete discussion.

Before discussing reconstruction techniques, we will first mention a few refinements to the data obtained in the production of forward projection.

Geometrical Weighting Factors

Figure (12.5) shows various rays of radiation incident on an array of anatomy voxels in a patient. In the approach discussed in the previous section, the rays incident at different angles were assumed to travel through equal distances of each voxel, but this is clearly not true. As a result, rays emerging from some voxels will need a weighting factor (WF) to correct for the geometry of the ray and voxel.

For example, consider rays incident on the same voxel at different angles, as shown in Fig. (12.6). The left side of the figure shows the assumed configuration with the ray passing through the width z of the voxel. No correction is needed for this ray, and the weighting factor is given the value of *1*. However, the configurations shown in the center and right sections of Fig. (12.6) show rays whose weighting factors are not equal to *1*: if the distance traveled through the voxel is greater than z then we must have that $WF > 1$, and if the distance traveled is less than z, then $WF < 1$. These weighting factors can be determined from the geometry and incorporated into the analysis of the projection data by computer programs used in the production of the image.

Beam Energy Corrections

As discussed in Chapter 8 and shown in Fig. (9.3), photons emerging from the gantry of a clinical linear accelerator (or *linac*) have a broad spectrum of energies. These

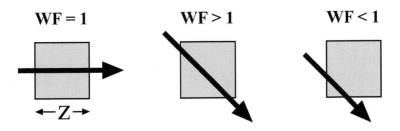

FIGURE 12.6: (*left*) A ray of radiation passing through a distance z of a voxel. (*center*) The ray passes through a distance greater than z, resulting in a weighting factor that is greater than *1*. (*right*) A ray passing through a distance in a voxel that is less than z; the associated weighting factor is therefore less than *1*.

energies extend from very low energies up to a maximum energy that is equal to the energy of the accelerated electrons used to produce the x-ray photons emerging from the linac.

Furthermore, as discussed in §8.14, the average energy of the photons in a linac beam increases as the beam travels through the patient in a process called *beam hardening*. But a higher average photon energy means smaller values of photoelectric and Compton scattering cross sections. See equations (8.58) and (8.59), along with Fig. (8.15). Finally, Eq. (8.54) shows that smaller cross section values result in smaller values of attenuation coefficients.

This all means that, as the ray passes through successive voxels of anatomy, its average energy will increase, resulting in a decrease in the value of the attenuation coefficient for exactly the same tissue. This effect must also be corrected for in computer programs analyzing the projection data before the corresponding image is produced.

Other Corrections

There are other factors that should be addressed in the computer analysis of the projection data. First of all, we assumed in our discussion that the intensity of the incoming beam was uniform—this is generally not the case. While adjustments to the beam are made to make the beam profile as uniform over a given region as possible, the incident intensity will not be constant as the different regions of the beam encounter the region being imaged. This can be addressed by making the beam area very small, as in the case of pencil beams, but this effect needs at least to be considered.

Second, the detectors in general consist of many elements used to detect the emerging intensity of radiation at various positions. But one or more of these detector elements may be malfunctioning or dead, in which case the computer program analyzing the data must interpolate between the readings of adjacent elements to accommodate the missing data.

Next, radiation scatter can compromise the image. This scatter can come from scattering of the radiation as it exits the gantry, or it may come from scattering within the patient. In particular, regions of low signal intensity can be significantly affected by scatter and other sources of image noise. Addressing the sources of scattered radiation and random noise can improve the image quality.

Finally, as shown in Eq. (8.37), the beam intensity has an exponential decrease with depth of tissue traversed. In addition, the beam has a $1/r^2$ decrease with increasing distance r from the source of the radiation. Depending on the distance the radiation must travel through the patient, these corrections could improve the image quality.

We will now discuss various techniques used to generate the information needed to produce an image.

Back Projection

The method of *back projection* was the original technique used for image reconstruction—it is also the most simplistic and, in its original form, is no longer used for the production of images. An improved form of back projection is commonly used, however—this form will be discussed below.

Consider as a very simple example the configuration of nine voxels shown in Fig. (12.7a), representing a small section of patient anatomy. We assume that a uniform beam of radiation is incident on the array from the left, as shown in the figure. We will take this orientation to be the 0° orientation. (Angles will be measured clockwise from this orientation.) To enable us to discuss this technique quantitatively, the incident intensity is taken to be $I_o = 100$, in arbitrary units.

Each voxel that the radiation passes through will absorb some of the radiation. Note that all of the voxels are white with the exception of two of the center-row voxels—the dark shading in these two voxels represents a portion of anatomy that is highly absorbing with a relatively large value of μ. We will take a very simplistic approach in this discussion to allow us to discuss the fundamental ideas involved in backscattering without getting bogged down in mathematical details. To this end, we will assume that each white-colored voxel absorbs 5 units of radiation intensity, while the dark shaded voxels absorb 40 units each. We will further assume that each voxel will absorb the full 5 or 40 units of intensity regardless of whether the ray passes through the full distance z of the voxel or not. That is, we will assume a weighting factor of 1, regardless of the geometry of the voxel and the incident ray of radiation, so that all of the configurations shown in Fig. (12.6) would have $WF = 1$. Computer programs modeling this interaction with radiation would, of course, not make these simplifying assumptions.

Detectors to the right of the array of voxels in Fig. (12.7a) record the intensities of the emerging radiation, I_1, I_2, and I_3. With an incident intensity $I_o = 100$ and the absorptions for the various voxels as discussed in the previous paragraph, it then follows that $I_1 = 85$, $I_2 = 15$, and $I_3 = 85$. These intensities are then assumed to come equally from each of the three voxels through which the emerging ray passed. That is, each of the three voxels in the first row are assumed to contribute $I_1/3 = 28$ units of intensity, rounded to the nearest integer. Likewise, each voxel in the second and third rows are assumed to contribute $I_2/3 = 5$ and $I_3/3 = 28$ intensity units to the emerging ray. The emerging intensities are therefore back-projected onto the

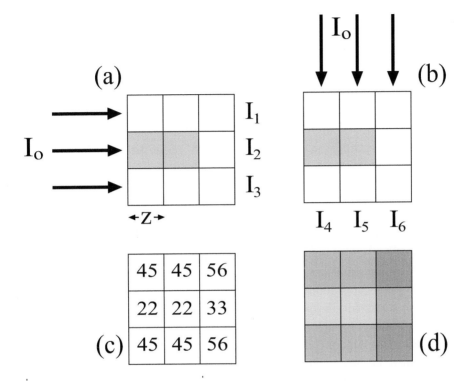

FIGURE 12.7: A small section of anatomy is modeled by a 3 × 3 array of voxels. The dark voxels have a greater attenuation (40 units of intensity) than the white voxels (5 units of intensity). (a) A uniform intensity I_o is incident on the array resulting in detector readings I_1, I_2, and I_3. (b) The intensity source-and-detectors system is rotated clockwise by 90° to allow the measurements of intensities I_4, I_5, and I_6. (c) Assuming an incident intensity of $I_o = 100$ (arbitrary units), distributing the emergent intensities among the voxels in each row in (a) and each column in (b) and summing the results gives us the intensity contributions shown in each voxel. (d) Assigning a grayscale value to each voxel proportional to its intensity contribution shown in (c) results in the simplistic image shown. See the associated discussion in the text for more detail.

voxels traversed by each ray. We could at this point construct our initial image from this information—a zeroth-order image, if you will. We could associate a gray-scale value to each intensity for each voxel and create the image, but this would be a very poor image of the section of anatomy being studied—not much information has been put into it, so not much information can come out.

To get a better-quality image we will rotate the incident radiation and the detectors to an angle of 90°, measured clockwise from the original horizontal orientation, and record the new intensities. This set-up is shown in Fig. (12.7b). With the same incident intensity $I_o = 100$, the new emerging intensities are found to be $I_4 = 50$, $I_5 = 50$, and $I_6 = 85$. Again, these intensities are divided by 3 and back projected into each of the voxels in the corresponding columns. When these intensity numbers are added to the intensity numbers obtained in the set-up of Fig. (12.7a), to total numbers shown in Fig. (12.7c) are obtained.

To produce an image corresponding to the intensity numbers for each voxel as shown in Fig. (12.7c), we can assign a gray-scale value proportional to the intensity values. Thus, higher intensity values correspond to higher gray-scale values. Since higher gray-scale (GS) values correspond to darker shades ($GS = 0$ is white, while $GS = 255$ is black), we see that this procedure should produce an image that is basically the *negative* of the 9-voxel section of anatomy shown in Fig. (12.7a). Note that this mimics typical medical images in that regions of high absorption (such as bone) appear very light in the image while regions of very low absorption (such as air) appear dark. The resulting image is shown in Fig. (12.7d).

This "negative image" in medical imaging was a characteristic of x-ray films in which incident x-rays interacted with grains of silver bromide in the film's emulsion. These interactions resulted in the absorption of x-ray photons and in the deposition of small quantities of metallic silver at that location in the emulsion. This resulted in the formation of a latent image of metallic silver on the film. The final image was then formed by a developing solution that deposited more silver at the positions of x-ray absorption where small quantities of silver had already been deposited; the regions of high silver deposition appeared dark in the image.[3] Hence, regions of high-intensity x-ray emission from the tissue being imaged corresponded to dark regions in the image, resulting in the "negative" characteristic of the image.

While the image shown in Fig. (12.7d) certainly shows some similarities to the original anatomy section shown in Fig. (12.7a), it would certainly not be called a good image of that anatomy. This image displays significant blurring, which is a characteristic of the back projection technique. We can certainly improve the image by adding even more information into it. This can be accomplished by sending radiation in at different angles. But just adding in more information is not good enough—we must make sure that the information that we add in contains *new* information that is not already in the image. For example, sending radiation in at an angle of 180° will simply duplicate the information already added for 0°—it won't make the image any better, it will simply make it darker. To add in more information we will use incident angles of 45° and 135°. These configurations are shown in Figs. (12.8a) and (12.8b).

Invoking the simplifying assumption stated earlier that $WF = 1$ for all geometries of a ray passing through a voxel, independent of the distance traveled through that

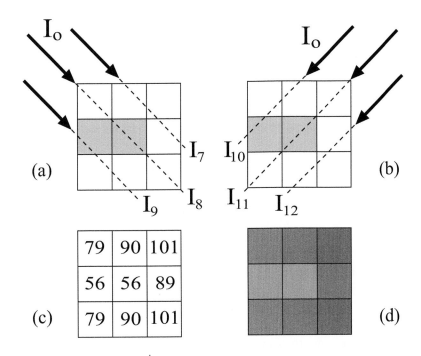

FIGURE 12.8: The source of incident intensity-and-detectors system shown in Fig. (12.7a) is rotated by two more angles to achieve a somewhat higher quality image of the section of anatomy. (a) Rotation angle $= 45°$. (b) Rotation angle $= 135°$. (c) Repeating the process shown in Fig. (12.7) and then adding the intensity-contribution results for each voxel to the values shown in Fig. (12.7c) result in the upgraded values shown in each voxel. (d) The image resulting from the additional information obtained by the new rotation angles. See the text for more details.

voxel, intensity values I_7 through I_{12} can be determined. (For example, $I_7 = 85$ and $I_9 = 50$.) The total intensity values for each voxel resulting from all of the intensity readings I_1 through I_{12} are shown in Fig. (12.8c), and the corresponding image is shown in Fig. (12.8d). It can certainly be seen that this image is sharper than that shown in Fig. (12.7d), but the characteristic blurring is also still apparent.

Filtered Back-Projection
As was mentioned at the beginning of the discussion of back projection, this method is overly simplistic to the extent that the resulting images are not clinically useful. (See the unfiltered image in the second row of Fig. 12.9.) Although it is computationally very simple and therefore very fast, the speed of modern computers renders this advantage moot as more complex algorithms can still be done almost instantaneously. The blurring issue associated with the back projection technique of course results from the projection—or smearing—of the emergent intensities back through the voxels associated with each intensity reading. The blurring in the back projection

technique can be significantly reduced, however, by exploiting an integration method from calculus called *convolution*, resulting in a process called *filtered back-projection*.

In back projection, radiation is first sent at numerous angles from 0° to 180° through the object being imaged, resulting in forward-projected intensity profiles as represented by the attenuation graphs and by the corresponding shaded strips (labeled "forward projection") beneath the figures in the top row of Fig. (12.9).[4,5] If all of the shaded strips from the forward projections are stacked on top of one another, with the 0° strip at the bottom and the 180° strip at the top, the resulting figure is called a *sinogram*. (It's called this since an off-center point in the object will trace out a sine wave in the sinogram.) The sinogram corresponding to the projections for the object shown in the top row of Fig. (12.9) is shown in the center row of the figure. Performing a back-projection procedure using all of the forward projections in the sinogram results in the corresponding image, as shown at right in the center row. The characteristic blurring resulting from back projection is evident in this image.

In filtered back-projection, the sinogram obtained from the forward projections is first filtered using convolution before back-projection is performed. In the convolution process, the forward projections are modified by (*convolved with*) a function called the *kernel* that serves as a kind of mathematical filter. Depending on the form of the kernel, it can serve to smooth out the forward projections or, more typically, to enhance the borders between voxels having sudden changes in transmission values—such as the border between the transmitted intensities I_1 and I_2 in Fig. (12.7a). These enhanced projections then clarify borders in the image when they are used in the back projections. This process involving convolution is what constitutes filtered back-projection. The bottom row of Fig. (12.9) shows the filtered sinogram that results from the convolution of the sinogram in the center row; back projection then results the filtered image shown in the figure. The utility of the filtering process is clear: filtered back-projection yields clinically useful images.

Iterative Methods

An iterative approach to obtaining an image of cross-sectional anatomy tends to be more efficient than filtered back-projection. The images produced using iterative methods can contain less noise using the same forward projected images as filtered back-projection.

The idea behind iterative reconstruction is basically as follows. Start with an initial "guess" image. This initial guess can be a standard guess image, a stored filtered back-projection image, or even an image consisting of a uniform background.[2] Any initial guess can do, although the closer the initial guess is to the final image the fewer iterations will be required to acquire the image with the desired quality. Forward-projection images at various angles through the patient are then obtained and numerically computed forward-projection images are generated by a computer from the initial guess image. The measured and computed images at corresponding angles are then compared and the differences between the images are computed to determine an error matrix, or "error image", if you will. The error image is then back projected by the computer algorithm being used in order to revise, or "correct", the initial guess image. This is the first iteration.

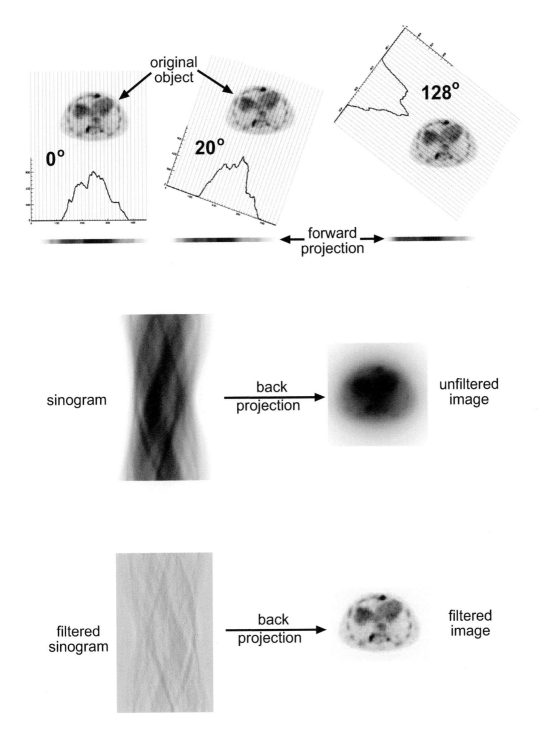

FIGURE 12.9: (Top Row) Forward projections at various angles. (Center Row) The resulting sinogram and the corresponding back-projected image. (Bottom Row) The filtered sinogram and the resulting filtered image. (Images for this figure were captured from animated gifs created by Adam Kesner, with permission.)

The result of the first iteration then replaces the initial guess image, and the process is repeated: forward projection images at various angles are numerically computed and compared with the original projection images of the patient. The iterations are continued until the changes in the guess image from one iteration to the next fall to within pre-specified tolerances. In this way, a set of self-consistent images is produced in that the final cross-sectional image of patient anatomy resulting from the iterative reconstruction algorithm generates forward-projection images that are very close to those obtained for the patient, which, when back projected, would generate the final cross-sectional image of patient anatomy.

Iterative image reconstruction tends to be used with CT, SPECT, and PET imaging modalities—all of the imaging modalities discussed in this chapter other than MRI, which uses Fourier techniques that will be discussed in the section on MRI imaging.

Reconstruction Overview and the Future: Deep Learning

Starting with the first commercially available CT scanners in the early 1970s, filtered back-projection (FBP) was the imaging reconstruction modality of choice. It was fast, reliable, and produced excellent images (high signal-to-noise, good contrast and differentiation between tissue types) as long as the data were low in noise. Unfortunately, lower noise image data meant higher dose to the patients. The era of FBP dominance for CT images lasted for about 30 years until the push for reduced dose to the patients from medical imaging motivated the development of a more efficient algorithm for the production of lower-dose images without compromising image quality.

Iterative reconstruction (IR) started being used in CT image reconstruction around 2008. For a given lower dose to the patient, IR algorithms tended to produce a better quality image than FBP. Model-based IR (MBIR) used full geometric models to produce the forward projections used in the iterations. However, while producing higher-quality images with lower noise, MBIR algorithms were computationally intensive and thus took longer to produce an image. In addition, clinicians were complaining about the apparent texture of the IR images—they sometimes appeared "plastic" or "waxy" compared to FBP images. This texture is associated with the distribution of noise within the image. The noise distribution in IR images could be more correlated, leading to the more artificial look. Nevertheless, IR methods continue to be used with CT, SPECT, and PET imaging.

More recently, a desire has developed for an approach that produces high-quality images with good contrast and low noise while being as fast as IR. In addition, the more "natural" look of the FBP images is preferred over the look of the IR images. The fulfillment of these desires came around 2018 when deep learning approaches started being applied to image reconstruction.

Deep learning (DL) is an approach to computer programming that enables computers to learn by example. It is the technology that allows driverless cars to distinguish between a pedestrian and a lamppost or between a stop light and a street light. DL also enables voice recognition in cell phones and other voice-activated devices. In the world of medicine, computers are being trained with deep learning to recognize cancer at the cellular level.

Deep learning exploits the properties of algorithms that are structured into many layers to form an artificial neural network. DL algorithms basically use information contained in images, text, and sound files to classify input information.[6] In order to do this accurately, DL algorithms require large amounts of data (for example, thousands of images) and a significant amount of computational power.

DL is a subset of machine learning. Whereas machine learning uses pre-constructed filters that are used to guide the learning process, DL algorithms can train themselves given sufficient data. They can also incorporate millions of parameters into the framework of the learning process, whereas MBIR, for example, can only use fewer than a hundred parameters during its image reconstruction process.[7]

The neural network training in deep learning image reconstruction (DLIR) uses high-quality FBP images with natural-looking noise texture so that the resulting image shares the natural look of the FBP images. An additional advantage of DLIR is that it can produce images with higher contrast-to-noise ratios than can be provided by FBP or IR techniques with the same dose to the patient, meaning that DLIR can reduce the patient imaging dose for the same quality of image. Figure (12.10)[8] shows head images produced from the same data using FBP, IR, and DLIR.

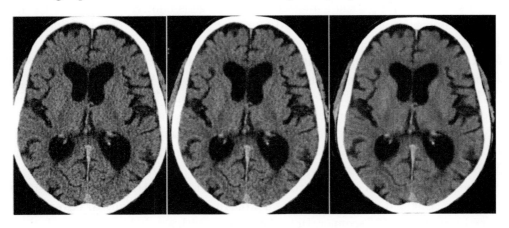

FIGURE 12.10: Three CT images produced from data acquired from a scan at 120 kV and thickness of $2.5\,mm$ with a patient dose of $49.5\,mGy$. Left: Image obtained using FBP. Center: Image obtained using IR. Right: Image obtained using DLIR. Note the reduced noise, improved texture, and increased contrast between grey and white matter (the darker and lighter shades of grey) in the DLIR image. (GE, with permission.)

Data for images is acquired by scanning a slice of anatomy with a pre-specified thickness. The thicker the slice used for the data generation the lower the noise due to scatter, but then the features in the anatomy—in particular, the boundaries between various structures—can be blurred due to the averaging effect inherent in the integration through the thicker slice. It has been shown that thin slice $(1.25\,mm)$ DLIR images produced a noise texture similar to that of a thick slice $(5\,mm)$ FBP image, meaning DLIR can produce high-quality thin-slice images characterized by sharp boundaries between neighboring regions of anatomy.[9] DLIR can also be beneficial in reducing the noise in lower-energy images where scatter tends to increase while improving contrast over corresponding IR images.[7]

Given that technology that is readily available in the clinic seems to lag research and development by some number of years, it may be some time before deep-learning methods are routinely used in most clinical settings. Nevertheless, given that a number of institutions are already regularly using DLIR for many of their clinical protocols, it is clear that we are rapidly moving into the era of deep learning approaches to image reconstruction in the clinic.

This ends our discussion of approaches to image reconstruction. This discussion has, by no means, been comprehensive, but it has covered the general ideas behind the primary approaches to reconstruction. The following sections in this chapter discuss the basic ideas behind the imaging modalities that exploit these reconstruction methods: CT, MRI, SPECT, and PET. The last section in this final chapter on imaging introduces new technology that is emerging in the field of medical imaging.

12.3 COMPUTED TOMOGRAPHY (CT)

Whereas a radiograph is a picture of an x-ray shadow of anatomy, an *x-ray computed tomograph*, or "x-ray CT scan" (often simply called a *CT*), is an image that shows a 2D cross section of a patient's anatomy. This image is numerically constructed from a large number of radiographs formed by many narrow beams of x-rays incident on the patient from different angles. As a result, the CT scan shows significantly more detail than a single radiograph. It also follows that a CT scan will deliver more dose to the patient than a simple radiograph.

The first clinical CT scanner was designed and built by Sir Godfrey Hounsfield, who was a radar operator and electrical engineer at Electric and Musical Instruments (EMI) Central Research laboratories in Hayes, west London. The scanner was first publicly presented at the 1972 meeting of the Radiological Society of North America (RSNA).

The first CT scan of a patient took place in 1971 at the Atkinson Morley Hospital in London, England. The patient was a woman who was thought to have a tumor. Using his prototype CT scanner, Hounsfield, along with a radiologist, James Ambrose, spent about 30 minutes taking the scans. Hounsfield then drove to the EMI Labs with the magnetic tapes containing the scan data and worked for about 2.5 hours processing the data at EMI before the completed image could be captured using a Polaroid camera (see Fig. 12.11).[10,11] The completed image of the patient clearly showed the suspected tumor.

Hounsfield's first CT scan used an 80×80 matrix to produce the image. Today's CTs use a 1024×1024 matrix and can produce an image in seconds—without the drive across town.

CT systems have two major components: the gantry, which contains the x-ray source, detectors, and the patient table, and the computer system that controls the table and scanner and stores and manipulates the acquired data to produce the final CT image. Figure 12.12[12] shows the gantry and the patient table that is used to position the patient within the gantry bore.

Most scanners in clinics today use what is called a "rotate-rotate" geometry in which the x-ray source and the array of x-ray detectors rotate simultaneously as a

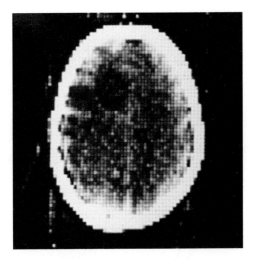

FIGURE 12.11: The first CT image of a patient, taken by Godfrey Hounsfield and James Ambrose at Atkinson Morley's Hospital in England. The image clearly shows a tumor in the frontal lobe of the patient. (Open Access.)

single unit about the patient. This source/x-ray system is connected to a slip ring that allows the system to rotate rapidly about the patient while the scan is taking place. The detectors, which tend to be scintillation detectors (see the discussion of TFT indirect conversion detectors associated with Fig. 11.6), record the forward

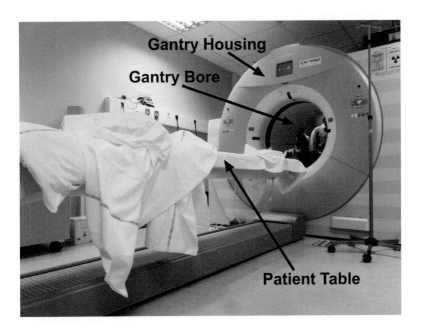

FIGURE 12.12: A typical CT gantry housing and the patient table. The housing contains the x-ray source and detectors that slide along a circular ring as they rotate about the patient to acquire the data for the CT image. (Public Domain.)

projection of x-ray intensities transmitted through the patient. It is these projections that are used to determine the voxel values expressed in the form of Hounsfield Units using either filtered back projection or iterative reconstruction, as discussed in the previous section. Figure 12.13 shows a schematic of a typical CT gantry.

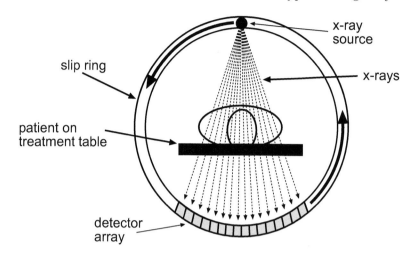

FIGURE 12.13: Schematic of a typical CT gantry showing the x-ray source, the array of x-ray detectors, and the treatment table. The x-ray source and detectors slide along the slip ring in a circular motion of period. The slip-ring design allows the source and detector system to rotate around the patient without tangling cables or compromising connections due to external wires. Current scanners can typically rotate with a period of 0.3 s.

CT scanners can operate in one of three modes: axial, helical, and fluoroscopy.

Axial Mode: the source-detector system within the gantry rotates constantly with a period of about 0.5 s. The x-ray tube is turned off except for a single rotation during which data for a single scan are taken. With the tube turned off, the table is then moved slightly so that the next scan can be made. This process is repeated until the entire anatomical region of interest has been imaged. The x-ray tube is turned off between scans to help reduce dose to the patient. Each scan corresponds to the source-detector system moving along one complete circular path along the slip ring.

Helical Mode: the table moves with a constant speed through the gantry bore as the source-detector system rotates with a constant speed while acquiring data. As a result, the x-ray source (and detectors) traces out a helical path as the data are being taken. This mode of operation tends to result in much quicker scans for the region of interest (often on the order of seconds), although there is a slight compromise in spatial resolution due to the motion of the patient during each rotation of the source-detector system. The quicker scans result in reduced dose to the patient. In addition, discontinuities in images between adjacent portions of anatomy are readily reduced compared to the *point-and-shoot* scans taken in axial mode.

Fluoroscopy Mode: rapidly updated CT images are produced, similar to conventional fluoroscopy (see Chapter 11). This mode of operation is typically used to guide procedures that use a needle or some other instrument. During this mode of operation, the patient table is stationary while the source-detector system continuously rotates while acquiring data needed to update the image.[13]

Dual-Energy CT

That CT could be used in treatment planning in radiation therapy was first proposed in 1983.[14] CT is now routinely used for radiotherapy simulation in which the placement and size of the x-ray beams that will be used during treatment can be determined without having to use the high-energy linear accelerators that are used for the treatment. CT images are invaluable for delineating the treatment volume in the patient.

Not only was CT beneficial for helping to localize tumors, but the attenuation coefficient information obtained in the CT reconstruction process could be used to help treatment planning programs more accurately plan how the incident x-ray energy would be absorbed in regions of inhomogeneous tissue, thereby improving dose calculations.

As discussed in the first section of this chapter, attenuation coefficients of different materials are often specified relative to water in terms of Hounsfield units. Hounsfield units depend not only on the effective atomic number of the material but also on its mass density: high values of atomic number and density typically yield higher Hounsfield units. This can lead to issues in conventional CT images since some materials with a higher mass density can end up having the same Hounsfield unit as a different material that has a higher effective atomic number, thereby rendering the two materials indistinguishable in the CT image.

But while the dependence of the Hounsfield unit for a given material on the effective atomic number depends strongly on the energy of the incident x-ray beam because of the energy dependence of the photoelectric effect (see Chapter 8), the effect of mass density on the Hounsfield-unit value is energy independent.[15] This means that two materials that are indistinguishable at one x-ray energy can be readily distinguished at a different energy. This important idea was pointed out in Hounsfield's seminal 1973 paper[16] in which he described how transverse images of the head could be obtained from x-ray transmission data using values of attenuation coefficients determined from the data that were taken at various angles through the head. He pointed out that these images could be used in the clinic to help expose disease that would otherwise have to be discovered through exploratory surgery. Hounsfield further pointed out that regions of high atomic number could be enhanced so that they could be differentiated in images by using multiple energies of incident x-rays.

Multiple-energy CTs can be produced in different ways. One simple way is to simply produce two consecutive scans at the desired energies. This method causes issues, however, because of the time difference between the acquisition of the two scans—a time during which the patient can move–and because of the dose to the patient being basically doubled.

The time-difference issue was resolved when CT scanners were produced having two separate sets of x-ray source and detector array positioned at different positions about 90° apart on the slip ring in the CT gantry. This allowed for an almost simultaneous acquisition of the two scans at different energies; the scans were offset slightly in time since the lead source-detector system would image a portion of anatomy ahead of the second system by about one quarter of the period of rotation around the slip ring. However, in order to fit both systems into the gantry, one of the tube-detector systems has to be smaller than the other. This means that the smaller system with its smaller field-of-view limits the field-of-view of the larger system since both systems must be imaging the same region of anatomy in order to get a dual-energy CT image.[17]

A third approach is to have a single source-detector system, but the source rapidly switches between two different beam energies. These two energies are then detected by a dual-layer detector whose top layer detects the lower-energy photons while transmitting the high-energy photons, which are then detected by the bottom detector layer.[18]

However it is accomplished, dual-energy CT can provide distinct advantages over conventional single-energy CT.

The first advantage is that the expanded data result in an improvement in dose calculations that rely on the attenuation coefficient information obtained during the scans. Multi-energy scans allow for more precise specification of effective atomic number distribution within the anatomy of interest.

Secondly, iodine is often used as a contrast agent for viewing tumors more clearly in CT images. The presence of iodine in a region of anatomy increases the Hounsfield unit of that region, resulting in greater photon absorption and more contrast with the surrounding tissue. But even with a contrast agent, conventional CT can still result in less-than-desired contrast between the tumor and surrounding healthy tissue. Dual-energy CT has been shown to result in improved contrast-to-noise in the image for certain types of tumors.[18]

An *angiogram* is an image that shows the flow of blood through veins, arteries, and the heart or other organs in the body. In conventional CT images, bones in the patient can obscure the blood flow being studied. The use of dual-energy CT, combined with an iodine contrast agent injected into the blood, allows for the removal of the bone from the image, allowing for the full inspection of the region of interest. This amazing application of dual-energy CT is shown in Fig. (12.14).[15]

Since its introduction into the clinic in the 1970s, CT imaging has become an essential tool not only for diagnosis of disease but also for treatment planning. Indeed, there are over 80 million CT scans performed in the United States alone each year.[19] But CT's reach goes well beyond the medical clinic or doctor's office. CTs have also been used for studying gemstones, fruit flies, nuclear warheads, and rocket assemblies, not to mention the ubiquitous luggage scanners at airports.[20] Indeed, CT imaging has even been used to help produce a sound from the voice of Nesyamun, a 3,000-year-old mummy![21,22] CT imaging has become an integral part of our modern lives.

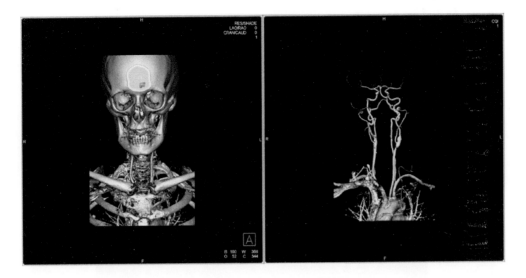

FIGURE 12.14: A 3-D CT angiogram of the head and neck produced using an iodine contrast agent. Such an agent results in Hounsfield unit differences between the iodine and bone that allow for the removal of bone from the image when used with dual-energy CT. Left: The full 3-D CT image. Right: The image with contributions from pixels containing Hounsfield units corresponding to bone removed. (John Wiley and Sons, with permission.)

12.4 MAGNETIC RESONANCE IMAGING (MRI)

Magnetic resonance imaging, or *MRI*, is a very different kind of imaging modality from the others discussed in this and the last chapters, despite the fact that the MRI scanner looks very much like a CT gantry (see Fig. 12.15, for example[23].) In chapters 1 and 2 we discussed the dangers of ionizing radiation—not only can ionizing radiation be used to treat cancer, but it can also cause cancer. There has been an increasing concern over the amount of ionizing radiation received by the public due to medical imaging, a large fraction of which is due to CT imaging. As discussed in Chapter 1, ionizing radiation such as x-rays can cause biological damage due to DNA strand breaks. A huge advantage of MRI is that it does not involve any ionizing radiation. Other than ultrasound imaging, MRI is the only imaging modality discussed in this book that does not exploit the properties of ionizing radiation.

Second, MRI does not involve any kind of "shadow imaging"; there is no back projection to determine the location of the origin of the photons that are detected to help produce the image. Instead, the information for the image is extracted from data of the changing magnetic fields in the tissue being imaged. This is a rather strange means of acquiring an image. With approximately 40 million MRI scans performed in the United States each year, compared to over 80 million CT scans, with the average cost of an MRI scan being about twice as much as a CT scan, it is an imaging modality well worth knowing something about. We start by learning about the magnetic properties of protons.

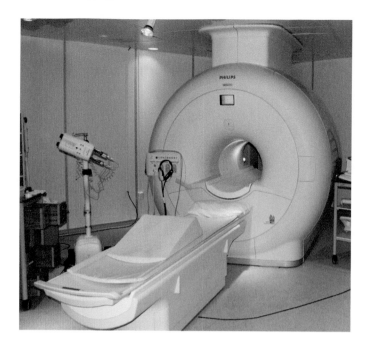

FIGURE 12.15: An MRI scanner by Phillips. Compare this scanner with the CT scanner shown in Fig. (12.12). While the bore in the CT gantry tends to be 65 to 70 cm in diameter, that of an MRI machine is usually between 50 and 60 cm. This, coupled with the fact that the MRI bore is sometimes closed at one end, can lead to a feeling of claustrophobia on the part of the MRI patient. This situation is further exacerbated by the fact that MRI scans can typically take about half-an-hour or more to perform. (Open Access.)

Magnetic Dipoles

In order to understand how MRI works, we first need to understand some fundamental properties of nuclei and their interactions with magnetic fields.

Recall from our discussion in §6.4 that nucleons have a *magnetic spin quantum number*, which is associated with a *magnetic dipole moment*; this means that they act like bar magnets. These tiny magnets produce correspondingly tiny magnetic fields that generally point in the same direction as the magnetic dipole moment vectors. In tissue, these magnetic dipole moments, denoted $\vec{\mu}$, are randomly oriented, so that the associated magnetic fields tend to cancel out, as shown in Fig. (12.16).

However, when the dipoles are immersed in a net external magnetic field, $\vec{B}_{ext}$, the magnetic dipoles experience torques that try to align the magnetic dipole moments with the external field. If we define the positive z-direction to be the direction of the net external magnetic field, so that $\vec{B}_{ext} = B_{ext}\hat{z}$, then the magnetic dipole moments will have a z-component of magnetic dipole moment that is either positive or negative. That is, the dipole moments tend to either align or anti-align with $\vec{B}_{ext}$. Just as we conventionally refer to "up" and "down" as directions relative to an external gravitational field here on Earth, we likewise refer to "up" and "down" for the orientation of a magnetic dipole moment relative to an external magnetic field. We take "up" to mean that the magnetic dipole moment tends to be generally

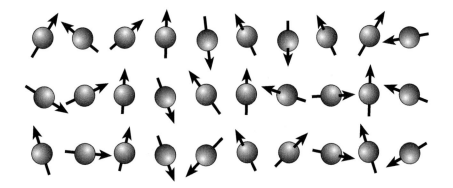

FIGURE 12.16: When there is no net external magnetic field, the hydrogenic magnetic dipoles are randomly oriented in tissue. The arrows shown schematically represent the magnetic dipole moment vectors, $\vec{\mu}$ or, since the magnetic fields produced by the proton dipoles point in the same direction as the dipole moment, the arrows can also be thought of as the magnetic fields generated by the dipoles. The magnetization of a group of such randomly oriented dipoles is zero.

in alignment with $\vec{B}_{ext}$, and we take "down" to mean that it is somewhat anti-aligned. (The alignment is not perfect—we can more precisely think of the z-component of $\vec{\mu}$ being *positive* for *up* and *negative* for *down*.)

For reasons explained below, the magnetic dipole moments that we are interested in are those associated with the protons that make up the nuclei of atomic hydrogen, H-1, so for the remainder of our discussion of MRI, any reference to a magnetic dipole moment will refer to that of the *hydrogenic proton*.

Since protons have a spin quantum number of $s = \frac{1}{2}$, their z-component of spin quantum number can only have two possible values: $m_s = \pm\frac{1}{2}$. It then follows that the z-component of the spin angular momentum of a proton can have the values $S_z = m_s\hbar = \pm\frac{1}{2}\hbar$, where $\hbar$ is the *reduced Planck constant*, $\hbar = h/2\pi$. From quantum mechanics, it turns out that the z-component of the magnetic dipole moment is proportional to the z-component of the proton's spin angular momentum, which means that the z-component of the magnetic dipole moment can only have two possible values. The geometry associated with the external magnetic field, the magnetic dipole moment of the proton, and the z-component of magnetic dipole moment for both up- and down-oriented dipoles is shown in Fig. (12.17).

Since protons in a net external magnetic field experience a torque trying to align them with that external field, it follows that the energy associated with *up* dipoles is lower than that for *down* dipoles—it would take work for us to try to flip a dipole moment and have it point against $\vec{B}_{ext}$. The energy difference between the up and down energy levels is given by

$$\Delta E = 2\mu_z B_{ext}. \tag{12.6}$$

As in our discussion of atomic energy levels, an incident photon that has the energy $E_{photon} = \Delta E$ can be absorbed by the proton, thereby causing it to make a

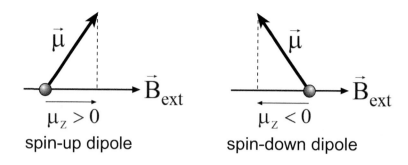

FIGURE 12.17: Since the z-component of spin quantum number for the proton can only have two values, $m_s = \pm 1/2$, the z-component of the proton's magnetic dipole moment can also only have two values, one positive and one negative. Taking the positive z-direction to be the direction of the net external magnetic field, $\vec{B}_{ext}$, the spin-up dipole state is that state with $\mu_z > 0$, and the spin-down state is that state with $\mu_z < 0$.

transition from the lower (up) energy level to the higher (down) energy level. See Fig. (12.18). This, of course, also works the other way: a dipole in the upper-energy state can spontaneously make a transition down to the lower-energy state with the emission of a photon of energy $E_{photon} = \Delta E$.

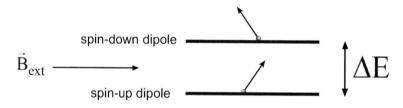

FIGURE 12.18: The energy states associated with spin-up and spin-down dipoles. When a photon of energy $E_{photon} = \Delta E = 2\mu_z B_{ext}$ is absorbed by a lower-energy spin-up dipole, it can undergo a spin flip, ending up in the higher-energy spin-down state. Likewise, when a higher-energy dipole undergoes a spin flip and transitions down to the lower-energy state, it will emit a photon of energy ΔE.

As mentioned previously in our discussion of atomic physics, the energy of a photon is related to its frequency by the equation $E_{photon} = hf$. Combining this with Eq. (12.6) yields the equation for the frequency of photons associated with a spin-flip transition of magnetic dipole moments in a net external magnetic field:

$$f = \frac{2\mu_z}{h} B_{ext}. \tag{12.7}$$

The factor of constants multiplying B_{ext} in Eq. (12.7) is typically denoted $\gamma/2\pi$, so that we can write

$$f = \frac{\gamma}{2\pi} B_{ext}. \tag{12.8}$$

The factor γ is called the *gyromagnetic ratio* for the magnetic dipole. The reason for the presence of the 2π in the denominator of Eq. (12.8) is as follows. Recall that the angular frequency, ω (units: rad/s), is related to the (linear) frequency, f (units: Hz), by $\omega = 2\pi f$. It then follows that Eq. (12.8) can be written in the simpler form

$$\omega = \gamma B_{ext}. \tag{12.9}$$

The frequencies given by Eqs. (12.8) and (12.9) correspond to the classical precessional frequency of the magnetic dipole moment in a net external magnetic field. That is, from the point-of-view of classical physics as shown in Fig. (12.19), the torque exerted on the proton's magnetic dipole moment $\vec{\mu}$ by the net external magnetic field $\vec{B}_{ext}$ would cause the magnetic dipole moment vector to *precess* about the magnetic field direction, just as the spin axis of a spinning top precesses about the direction of the Earth's gravitational field direction.

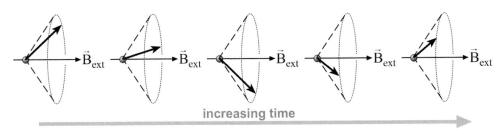

increasing time

FIGURE 12.19: Precession of the magnetic dipole moment vector $\vec{\mu}$ (or the associated dipole magnetic field vector) about the net external magnetic field vector, $\vec{B}_{ext}$. The proper sense of precession is obtained if the initial dipole moment vector on the left is taken to point slightly into the page behind $\vec{B}_{ext}$. Then, as time increases toward the right, $\vec{\mu}$ points further into the page behind $\vec{B}_{ext}$, and then points out of the page in the last two images on the right.

The equation for the precessional frequency was originally derived by Joseph Larmor in 1897. As a result, Eqs. (12.8) and (12.9) are both called the *Larmor equation*, and the values of f and ω are both referred to as the *Larmor frequency*.

Unfortunately, the factor of $\gamma/2\pi$ in Eq. (12.8) is sometimes also referred to as the gyromagnetic ratio, and, even worse, it is sometimes denoted γ, leading to confusion when numerical values are given in various references. With a nod to the reduced Planck constant $\hbar$, we will refer to the factor $\gamma/2\pi$ as the *reduced gyromagnetic ratio*. To be clear, then, it should be noted that the value of the gyromagnetic ratio γ in Eq. (12.9) and the reduced gyromagnetic ratio $\gamma/2\pi$ in Eq. (12.8) for hydrogenic protons are equal to:

$$For\,protons: \quad \gamma = 267.5\,\frac{MHz}{T} \quad and \quad \frac{\gamma}{2\pi} = 42.58\,\frac{MHz}{T}. \tag{12.10}$$

Various nuclei present in the human body have magnetic dipole moments that could be used in MRI, so why do we use the dipole moment of the hydrogenic proton to produce the MRI signal? The reason is really two-fold. First, the hydrogenic proton has the largest value of magnetic dipole moment, μ, thereby making the magnetic effects associated with this dipole moment more prominent and, therefore, easier to detect. Second, the nucleus of the hydrogen atom is by far the most abundant nucleus in the human body—found mostly in water and in fat—again, making the effects stronger by the sheer number of dipoles present in a sample of tissue.

The Magnetization of Tissue

The magnetization vector, $\vec{M}$, is basically the net magnetic field in a material resulting from magnetic dipole moments within that material. (More officially, the magnetization vector is the net magnetic dipole moment per unit volume, which is proportional to the net magnetic field generated by magnetic dipoles in a material.) In tissue without a net external magnetic field, the magnetization is zero due to the random orientation of the dipoles, as shown in Fig. (12.16). But if an external magnetic field is present, we would expect the resulting torque on the dipoles to align all of them with the external field, so they would all be in the lower-energy up state. This turns out not to be the case, however.

Due to random thermal motion of the molecules in the tissue—effectively, the dipole moments bumping into one another via magnetic-field interactions due to the temperature of the tissue—the net external magnetic field tends not to be very successful in trying to align the magnetic dipole moments (and their associated magnetic fields) with the external field. Consider the following: In an external magnetic field of magnitude $B_{ext} = 1.5\,T$, the energy difference between the down and up states is $\Delta E = 4.23 \times 10^{-26}\,J$, as given by Eq. (12.6). In thermodynamic equilibrium at temperature $T = 310\,K$ (the approximate temperature inside a human body), it turns out that, if there are 100,000 magnetic dipole moments in the higher-energy down state, then, on average, there will be 100,001 dipoles in the lower-energy up state—only one extra dipole out of 100,000!

However, since the number of proton magnetic dipoles in a small region of tissue can exceed Avogadro's number (about 10^{23} dipoles), the small excess in up-state dipoles can produce a magnetization that is measurable. For a given magnitude of external magnetic field, this measurable magnetization is the baseline magnetization to which other values of magnetization will be compared. Figure (12.20) shows a greatly exaggerated schematic as far as populations are concerned of the magnetic dipoles in a small sample of tissue in an external magnetic field.

Let's look a bit more closely at the magnetization vector $\vec{M}$ in tissue when an external magnetic field is applied. Figure (12.20) shows a small sample of magnetic dipole moments in tissue with an external magnetic field. The first thing we notice when looking at this figure is probably that some of the dipoles are tending to point up, generally toward the direction of $\vec{B}_{ext}$, and some are pointing down, generally opposite to the direction of the net external field, as previously discussed. Again, letting the direction of $\vec{B}_{ext}$ be the positive-z direction, it then follows that looking at whether the dipoles tend to point up or down is the same as looking at whether the z-components of the magnetic dipole moment vectors—or, equivalently, of the associated magnetic field vectors—are positive or negative. The direction of $\vec{B}_{ext}$ is referred to as the *longitudinal direction*. Since there are more dipoles with positive z-components than negative, we conclude that the z-component, or longitudinal component, of the magnetization vector, $M_z = M_L$, must be positive. We will denote the

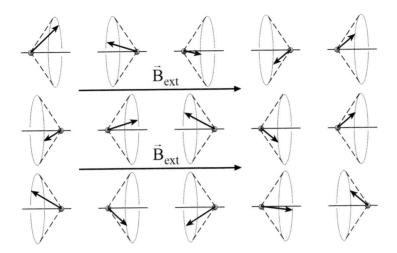

FIGURE 12.20: Schematic representing the magnetic dipoles in a net external magnetic field in thermodynamic equilibrium within the human body. Almost as many dipoles occupy the higher-energy down state as the number occupying the lower-energy up state. Note that the phases of the up and down dipoles are seemingly random—that is, they all seem to point in different directions within their precession cycle—despite the fact that they are all precessing with the same Larmor frequency.

equilibrium value of the longitudinal magnetization resulting from the presence of the net external magnetic field by $M_{L,ext}$.

Let's now consider the direction *perpendicular to* the longitudinal direction. Depending on the orientation of $\vec{\mu}$, this component could point anywhere in the x-y plane; we will refer to this component as the *transverse* component of the magnetization vector, M_T. Note in Fig. (12.20) that the transverse components of the various dipole magnetic fields point in all different directions in the x-y plane. This means that, on average, the transverse components will cancel out, so that $M_T = 0$. Therefore, in thermodynamic equilibrium in a net external magnetic field, the bulk magnetization vector in tissue will point in the same direction as the external field.

Excitation with RF Pulses

We have so far discussed the properties of magnetic dipole moments interacting with a net external magnetic field after reaching equilibrium. We will now see how these magnetic properties are exploited to create an image in MRI.

We've already discussed the fact that a hydrogenic proton in a lower magnetic energy state (spin up) can make a transition to a higher-energy (down) state—that is, the spin magnetic dipole moment of the proton can undergo a "spin flip" from spin up to spin down—if a photon having the proper energy is absorbed. Subsequently, in complete analogy with electrons in atoms, hydrogenic protons in higher magnetic energy levels can spontaneously make a transition down to the lower energy state with the corresponding emission of a photon. Such emitted photons tend to be absorbed in the tissue and serve no purpose in producing the MRI image.

But making magnetic dipole moments undergo a spin-flip when they absorb a photon of the proper energy is not the only effect of the photon absorption. In addition, the dipoles absorbing photons and undergoing spin flips are also set into precessional motions about the external magnetic field that are all *in phase* with one another. Let's see what this means.

Figure (12.20) shows a small section of dipoles in the presence of an external magnetic field, $\vec{B}_{ext}$. As already mentioned, this results in a nearly equal distribution of up- and down-state dipoles. Closer inspection of this figure shows something else— namely, the dipoles are precessing independently of one another. In other words, when one dipole is pointing toward the top of the figure, the others are not necessarily also pointing toward the top. All of the dipoles are precessing with the same Larmor frequency since they are experiencing the same net external magnetic field, but they are not precessing in unison, all pointing in the same direction at the same time. In fact, the direction each dipole is pointing at any instant seems to be random. Such motion is said to be *out-of-phase*. As previously discussed, this means that the equilibrium bulk magnetization vector in the tissue points in the same direction as the external magnetic field: $\vec{M}_{ext} = M_{L,ext}\hat{z}$.

But now let's say that we irradiate the section of tissue with a pulse of photons having energy ΔE equal to the energy separation between the up and down energy states of the dipoles. Since the frequency of these photons, as given by the Larmor equation (12.8), tends to be in the radio region of the electromagnetic spectrum, such photons are said to be radio-frequency photons, or *RF photons*. Not only will dipoles absorbing these photons make the transition from the lower-energy up state to the higher energy down state, but after their transitions they will also be precessing in unison—so-called *in-phase* motion, all pointing in the same direction at the same time, as shown in Fig. (12.21).

Consider once more Fig. (12.20). About half of the dipoles are in the spin-up state, and slightly less are in the spin-down state. When an RF pulse of the appropriate frequency is sent into the tissue, some of the spin-up dipoles will absorb a photon and will undergo a spin flip, ending up in the spin-down state. The dipoles that undergo a spin flip will then precess in phase with one another about the direction of $\vec{B}_{ext}$. But this does not mean that all of the up dipoles will undergo a spin flip—not all of the up dipoles will absorb a photon. The dipoles that did not absorb a photon— both the spin-up dipoles as well as the spin-down dipoles—will continue to precess about the direction of $\vec{B}_{ext}$, but their precessions will be at random phases; they will not be precessing in phase with the dipoles that did absorb a photon and undergo a spin flip. This means that the dipoles precessing in phase after the arrival of the RF pulse may be separated from one another by randomly precessing up and down neighboring dipoles. Since the magnetic fields of neighboring dipoles can interact with one another, it makes sense that the in-phase aspect of the precession of the flipped dipoles may not last long. We will return to this important idea when we discuss relaxation times below.

The excitation of low-energy dipoles into the higher-energy down state and the resulting correlated in-phase motion of the dipoles and their associated magnetic fields have two important consequences. The first is that there is an increased number of

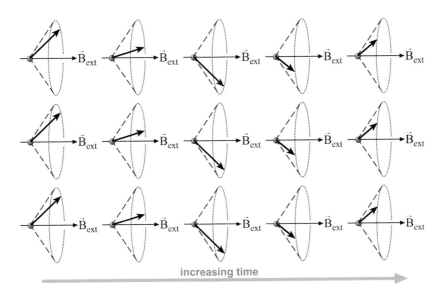

FIGURE 12.21: Three dipoles (top to bottom) precessing in phase with one another as time progresses (toward the right).

dipoles with magnetic fields pointing anti-parallel to $\vec{B}_{ext}$. This means that the value of the longitudinal magnetization will be *decreased*. The resulting value of M_L can be positive, zero, or negative, depending on the strength and duration of the RF pulse and the subsequent number of dipoles making a transition into the higher-energy down state.

The second consequence is that the transverse components of the magnetic fields of the flipped dipoles now *add* as a result of their in-phase precession, instead of canceling each other out as they did when they were in equilibrium before the RF pulse was applied. This means that we end up with a non-zero transverse component of the magnetization vector, M_T. In addition, this component of the magnetization vector must precess with the same Larmor frequency as the dipoles. The non-equilibrium magnetization vector in the tissue after the application of the RF pulse is shown schematically in Fig. (12.22).

In the physics of magnetic fields, Faraday's law states that a closed coil will produce an electric current whenever the magnetic field through the coil changes. This gives us our first real insight into the signal from which an MRI image is formed: a detector coil is placed adjacent to the patient with its axis perpendicular to the direction of $\vec{B}_{ext}$. Then, as M_T sweeps around the direction of $\vec{B}_{ext}$, constantly changing direction as it points toward, then away, then toward the coil, the value of the magnetic field through the detector coil will constantly be changing. From Faraday's law, this then means that the detector coil will produce an alternating current whose frequency is equal to the frequency of precession of M_T—the Larmor frequency, which is in turn determined by the net external magnetic field magnitude, B_{ext}. It is this frequency signal coming from the precessing transverse component of the magnetization vector that is used to produce the image in MRI.

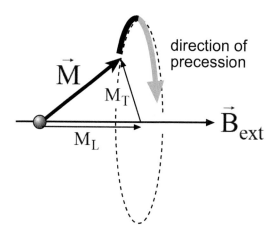

FIGURE 12.22: The magnetization vector, $\vec{M}$ is composed of two components. The longitudinal component, M_L, points in the same direction as the net external magnetic field, $\vec{B}_{ext}$; the transverse component, M_T, points perpendicular to $\vec{B}_{ext}$. Both the full magnetization vector and its transverse component precess at the Larmor frequency about $\vec{B}_{ext}$, moving up, then back into the page and down, as shown.

Relaxation Times

We've now found out what forms the signal in MRI: it's formed by the precessing transverse component of the magnetization vector after an RF pulse has been sent through the portion of anatomy being imaged. But how do we get information for an image from this signal, and how are different structures in the anatomy contrasted with one another?

Let's consider what happens to the dipoles and the associated magnetization vector after the dipoles have been excited into the down state and the M_T signal is obtained.

The first thing that tends to happen is that the magnetic dipoles that are precessing in phase with one another start interacting with the magnetic fields from their neighbors as well as with inhomogeneities in the local magnetic field in the tissue. These interactions effectively give the precessing dipoles little kicks that end up knocking them out of their orderly, synchronized dance. As a result, the transverse components of their magnetic fields start moving out of their in-phase motion, meaning that not all of these transverse components will continue to add up as they did immediately after receiving the RF pulse. It then follows that the value of M_T will decrease from its initial value, which we will denote $M_{T,max}$. As time goes on, more and more of the precessing dipole magnetic fields will depart from the in-phase precession, further decreasing the value of M_T until, eventually, the dipoles will be precessing randomly, out of phase with one another, just as they did when they were in equilibrium before the RF pulse. This means that, as time progresses, the value of M_T will decrease from its initial, maximum value and will gradually approach zero. This decrease in the value of M_T with time is governed by the equation

$$M_T(t) = M_{T,max}e^{-t/T2}.$$ (12.11)

The behavior described by this equation is referred to as *spin-spin relaxation*, and the quantity $T2$ is called the *spin-spin relaxation time constant*. The reason this is called *spin-spin* relaxation is that it results from the interactions of the spin magnetic dipole moments of the in-phase protons with the magnetic fields produced by the spin magnetic dipole moments of neighboring protons in the tissue, which may or may not also be processing in phase.

The second thing that tends to happen after dipoles are excited into the higher-energy down state after the arrival of the RF pulse is that they start to decay back down to the lower-energy up state as they emit a photon, just as excited-state electrons in atoms emit photons as they spontaneously drop down to lower-energy states. As more of the excited-state dipoles undergo a spin flip down to the lower-energy spin-up orientation, their magnetic fields also flip, meaning that fewer and fewer dipole magnetic fields are opposing the external magnetic field. This means that the longitudinal component of the magnetization vector, M_L, will start *increasing*. This increase will continue until, eventually, the longitudinal component will reach the equilibrium value that it had prior to the arrival of the RF pulse, $M_{L,ext}$. This behavior is described by the equation

$$M_L(t) = M_{L,ext}\left(1 - e^{-t/T1}\right). \tag{12.12}$$

This behavior of $M_L(t)$ is known as *spin-lattice relaxation*, since the photons emitted when the dipoles undergo a spin flip to the lower-energy up state interact with and are subsequently absorbed by, the surrounding tissue, which is referred to as the *lattice*. The constant $T1$ in Eq. (12.12) is called the *spin-lattice relaxation time constant*.

The relaxation time constants, $T1$ and $T2$, determine how rapidly the M_L value increases toward $M_{L,ext}$ and how rapidly the M_T value decreases toward zero, respectively. These time constants can depend on the physical characteristics of the tissue being imaged. $T1$ tends to be about 5 to 10 times larger than $T2$,[24] so the shift to out-of-phase precessions by the higher-energy down dipoles happens more quickly than the repopulation of the spin-up state by dipoles that had been excited by the RF pulse. A comparison of these behaviors is shown in Fig. (12.23).

Obtaining the Image: Localization

The first two points listed in our discussion of image clarity in §10.2 were blur and contrast. *Blur* refers to the sharpness of the image, while *contrast* refers to the ability to detect subtle differences in similar, neighboring sections of anatomy in the image. Blur results from not being able to precisely specify the location in the anatomy from which the image information originated.

Image contrast results from information contained in the signal used to form the image that changes as the characteristics of the tissue change. There are, in general, many factors that can affect the signal from which an image is created: mass density, chemical composition, molecular size, constraining forces from boundaries, hydrogenic proton density, magnetic properties of the material, *etc.* In the case of MRI, the "signal" is the change in M_T and M_L values with time. Note that only the changing value of M_T can be directly measured by the detector coil since the magnetic field from M_L does not have a component that passes through the coil

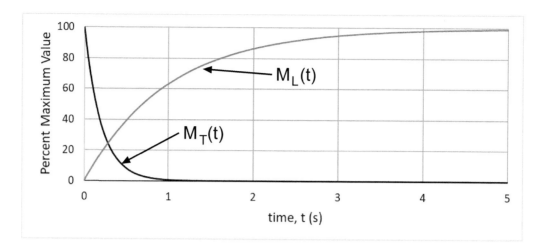

FIGURE 12.23: Transverse and longitudinal magnetization components as a function of time. For this plot, $T1 = 1\,s$ (for the $M_L(t)$ plot) and $T2 = 0.2\,s$ (for the $M_T(t)$ plot). Note that, typically, $T1 = \alpha T2$, where $5 \leq \alpha \leq 10$. For these plots, $\alpha = 5$. For larger values of α, the $M_T(t)$ curve would drop down toward zero even more quickly compared to the build-up of the $M_L(t)$ curve.

along its axis. (Only a changing magnetic field along the axis of the detector coil will produce a current according to Faraday's law.) The changing value of M_L is inferred from information obtained from repeated RF pulses applied to the tissue being imaged.[24]

From the changes in M_T and M_L and the behaviors described by Eqs. (12.11) and (12.12), the relative values of $T1$ and $T2$ can be inferred. In addition, the strength of the magnetization signal reflects the hydrogenic proton density. These quantities are responsible for the contrast in MRI.

The value of the spin-spin time constant, $T2$, depends on the size and mobility of the molecules in the tissue (or fluid within the tissue)—rapidly moving molecules tend to be able to smooth out magnetic field variations within the region of tissue, thereby reducing magnetic field "bumps" between neighboring dipoles and increasing the value of $T2$. On the other hand, the value of the spin-lattice time constant, $T1$, depends on how efficiently energy can be exchanged between the transitioning dipoles and the surrounding tissue. $T1$ values tend to be rather small ($0.1\,s$ to $1\,s$) for soft tissue and relatively large ($1\,s$ to $4\,s$) in fatty tissue.[24]

Different tissues have distinct values of the $T1$ and $T2$ time constants. In addition, diseased tissue—including cancerous tumors—can have different time-constant values from the healthy tissue. The MRI signals (the changing M_T and M_L values) can therefore distinguish these different tissue types. To further improve the contrast, a contrast agent, typically gadolinium (Gd), is often deposited into the tissue being imaged due to its magnetic properties. The presence of the contrast agent lowers the value of the $T1$ time constant, thereby allowing for further contrast.[25]

A very important problem in constructing the image remains—namely, determining the point-of-origin of the signal from within the tissue. In other words, where did the signal come from? This information is obtained by imposing *two* external magnetic fields on the tissue. One magnetic field is constant and points along the length of the patient, say, from the feet toward the head, in the positive-z direction. We will denote this constant magnetic field by $\vec{B}_o = B_o\,\hat{z}$. The second external magnetic field is a gradient magnetic field, denoted $\vec{B}_G$. This gradient field is a function of position, and can typically vary from $1\,mT/m$ up to about $50\,mT/m$ along the length of the patient. Since the direction of $\vec{B}_o$ is taken to be the z-direction, the gradient field is a function of z: $B_G = B_G(z)$. The net external magnetic field is then given by

$$\vec{B}_{ext} = \vec{B}_o + \vec{B}_G\,. \tag{12.13}$$

Since the gradient field is a function of position, it then must follow that the net external field $\vec{B}_{ext}$ is also a function of position. It is the addition of the gradient field—really, three gradient fields, one for each of the three axes x, y, and z—that allows us to locate the origin of the signal within the anatomy being imaged. Let's see how.

Figure (12.24) shows the longitudinal gradient magnetic field as a function of position along the patient. Note that the constant background magnetic field, $\vec{B}_o$, points toward the right in the figure, so that the magnitude of the net external magnetic field, B_{ext}, decreases as z increases. The gradient field is produced by sending an electrical current through a pair of coils that encircle the patient with their axes along the length of the patient. These coils are taken to have a separation of $30\,cm$ for the purposes of this figure and are located at the left and right edges of the graph. The z-component of the gradient field varies from $3\,mT$ at $z = -15\,cm$ to $-3\,mT$ at $z = 15\,cm$ in the graph, with a corresponding gradient of $20\,mT/m$.

To appreciate the significance of the gradient field, consider the vertical line labeled L in the figure. This line is at the position $z = -8\,cm$ at which the z-component of the gradient field has the value $B_{Gz} = 1.6\,mT$. If we take the background field to have a magnitude $B_o = 1.5000\,T$, then the net external field at $z = -8\,cm$ is $B_{ext} = B_o + B_{Gz} = 1.5016\,T$. From Eq. (12.8), we then get that the Larmor frequency for dipole precession at $z = -8\,cm$ is $f_L = 63.938\,MHz$, where the "L" subscript refers to the position of the vertical line labeled L in Fig. (12.24).

Now, looking at the vertical line labeled R in Fig. (12.24), it is at the position $z = -7\,cm$, corresponding to $B_{Gz} = 1.4\,mT$ and, therefore, $B_{ext} = 1.5014\,T$. The Larmor frequency for dipole precession at $z = -7\,cm$ is therefore $f_R = 63.930\,MHz$. This means that the dipoles at $z = -7\,cm$ precess at a slightly lower frequency than those at $z = -8\,cm$. The average of f_L and f_R is $\bar{f} = 63.934\,MHz$, so the range from f_R to f_L can be expressed as $\bar{f} \pm \Delta f = 63.934 \pm 0.004\,MHz$.

Keeping in mind that dipoles will only be excited into the higher-energy down states if they are irradiated with photons having frequencies equal to the Larmor frequencies of the dipoles, we can now appreciate the application of the gradient field: if we irradiate the patient with an RF pulse that consists of photons with frequencies in the range $\bar{f} \pm \Delta f$ computed above, then only dipoles in the 1-cm slice of anatomy between $z = -8\,cm$ and $z = -7\,cm$ will be excited, which means that only transverse

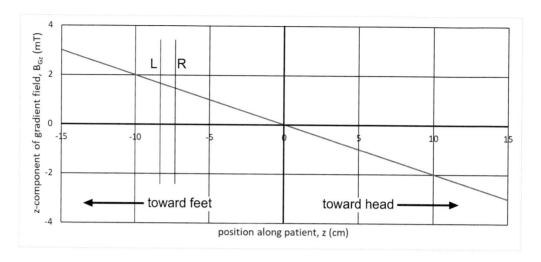

FIGURE 12.24: The longitudinal (z) component of the gradient magnetic field, B_{Gz}, as a function of position z along the length of the patient. The background magnetic field, $\vec{B}_o$, and, therefore, the positive-z direction point toward the right in the figure. The gradient of the magnetic field for this figure was taken to be $20\,mT/m$, and the distance between the two coils producing the gradient field was taken to be 30 cm. The two vertical lines represent the left (L) and right (R) sides, at positions $z = -8\,cm$ and $z = -7\,cm$, respectively, for an image slice of thickness $1\,cm$.

magnetization signals from this slice will be received. By using different values of $\bar{f}$ and Δf we can vary the position of the image slice and its thickness, respectively.

Using transverse gradient fields in analogous but slightly more complicated processes called *frequency encoding* and *phase encoding*, we can likewise localize the signal in the x- and y-directions, transverse to the constant background field $\vec{B}_o$.

As discussed previously, the detected signal is encrypted in the form of frequency data of transverse magnetic field variations. The information needed to produce an image is extracted from the data by means of a numerical process called the *inverse-Fourier transform*, which we will not describe here. Suffice it to say that, by these means, we can associate the signal—meaning the $T1$ and $T2$ values as well as the proton density that comes from the signal strength—with a specific voxel in the patient's anatomy. Associating grayscale values with ranges in the received signals then allows for the production of an image of the cross section of the patient.

There are many examples of images from MRI scans that can be found online, so the image produced by MRI shown below is a very special image. It was produced at the Massachusetts General Hospital in Boston in 2019 using a specially configured MRI scanner.

The scanner was used to produce an image of the brain of a 58-year-old woman who had donated her brain for research. She died of viral pneumonia, so her brain was presumed to be an example of a normal, healthy brain. Using the high background magnetic field $B_o = 7\,T$ and a very long scan time of 100 hours, the researchers were able to obtain the most detailed image of a human brain ever produced. The unusually high resolution of the image, which was able to resolve details smaller than $100\,\mu m$, was possible because the brain was not in a living person, meaning that there was no movement due to breathing or blood flow that would otherwise blur the image. The scan was performed for research, clinical, and educational applications. See Fig. (12.25) for a photograph of the brain along with one of the images obtained from the MRI scan.[26]

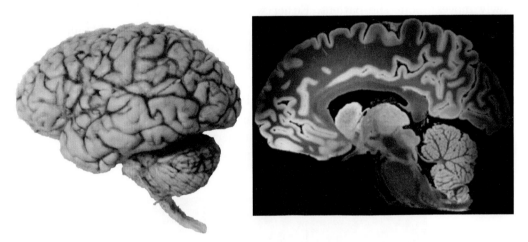

FIGURE 12.25: (Left) Photograph of the brain removed from a 58-year-old woman who had died of viral pneumonia. (Right) One of the images of the brain resulting from a 100-hour-long scan using a specially configured MRI scanner at the Massachusetts General Hospital. The scan used a background magnetic field $B_o = 7\,T$. These are the most detailed images of the human brain ever obtained—a fact that cannot be fully appreciated in this small reproduction of this image. (Open Access.)

12.5 SINGLE PHOTON EMISSION COMPUTED TOMOGRAPHY (SPECT)

We discussed in §11.4 the idea that a nuclear medicine image shows how various parts of the anatomy are functioning. We also discussed the ideas of radiopharmaceuticals and the details of the gamma, or Anger, camera that is used in nuclear medicine imaging. This section on SPECT imaging and the next on PET imaging will build off of the discussions in §11.4, so it would be a very good idea to go back and review that section before continuing on in these last two sections of this chapter.

Single photon emission computed tomography, or SPECT, is a nuclear medicine imaging modality that is closely related to planar imaging. Both modalities use the same radiopharmaceuticals, and both use similar nuclear scintillation cameras. But a planar image is simply a projection of photon emissions from the radioisotopes in the patient's body—it's effectively a photograph of the x- or gamma-rays emanating from the patient's body. A SPECT image, on the other hand, is a compilation of many planar images taken from a series of angular positions around the patient's body.

SPECT produces an image that is computed from data generated by revolving one or more gamma cameras about the patient. The scans tend to cover either 180° or 360° regions about the patient. In the "step-and-shoot" approach, the camera stops, makes a scan, and then moves on to the next angular position before stopping and making another scan. This is repeated until the full angular coverage has been achieved. Some scanners can also do a continuous acquisition of data as the scanner slowly moves about the patient. Either way, the scans produce a series of planar images (see §11.4). These planar images are then used to produce a 3D image of the distribution of the radioisotope throughout the patient's imaged anatomy using either filtered back projection or iterative reconstruction methods, as discussed in §12.2. The physician is thereby provided more detailed information about the distribution of the radioisotope than can be provided by a single 2D planar image.

One of the applications of SPECT imaging is the diagnosis of Parkinson's disease, which is a degenerative disease of the central nervous system. Figure (12.26) shows two SPECT images of the brain: one of a normal brain and one of the brain of a patient suffering from Parkinson's disease.[27]

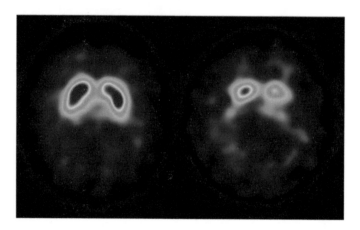

FIGURE 12.26: SPECT brain images of a normal brain (left) and the brain of a patient with Parkinson's disease (right). (Open Access.)

The simultaneous use of multiple detectors allows for multiple planar images to be obtained simultaneously, which can then cut down on the time required for the image. In cardiac imaging, for example, two cameras are positioned at right angles to one another. Each camera is then revolved about the patient for 90°, resulting in scans covering 180°. Typically, these scans are performed as the cameras make 32 stops over their 90° coverage, resulting in 64 planar images covering 180°. Figure (12.27) shows a gamma camera set-up used in cardiac imaging.[28]

Because the photons emitted by the radioisotopes have to traverse the body before they can be detected, attenuation, including scatter, within the patient serves to reduce the resolution of the image, which is typically about $1\,cm$. Resolution can be further hindered by the kinetics of the radiopharmaceutical being used. In addition, SPECT images tend to be noisy as a result of the relatively small number γ-rays

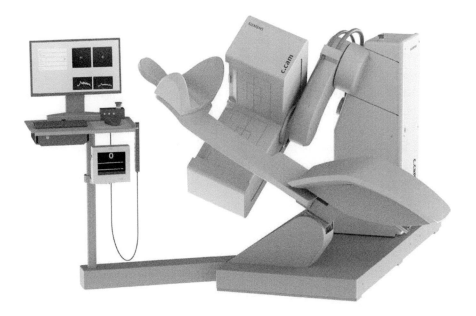

FIGURE 12.27: The c.cam cardiac gamma camera by Siemens is an example of the set-up used in cardiac SPECT imaging. Note the two gamma cameras positioned at right angles to one another about the patient chair. (Courtesy of Siemens Medical Solutions USA, Inc.)

detected, especially as contrasted with the number acquired during CT-data acquisition. This is the reason that SPECT scans are taken over 360°—the duplication of information can help improve the image resolution. But, again, the purpose of using nuclear imaging is not to produce a clear image so much as to provide information about physiological issues. Nevertheless, at times a clear image is desired in addition to functional information. In this case, it is common to combine a CT image with a SPECT image.

12.6 POSITRON EMISSION TOMOGRAPHY (PET)

As with SPECT, in *Positron Emission Tomography*, or PET, high-energy photon emissions are detected by scintillation crystals positioned along a ring at various angular positions around the patient. Unlike SPECT or nuclear planar imaging, however, PET does not involve radioisotopes that undergo gamma decay. Instead, the radioisotopes associated with radiopharaceuticals in PET imaging undergo *positron decay*.

Positron decay is much like beta decay, which was discussed in §7.3. In particular, as was shown in Eq. (7.17), when a nucleus undergoes positron decay, it emits a positron along with a neutrino. The neutrino escapes without any interaction, but the positron is not so lucky. Radioisotopes used in PET imaging tend to emit positrons with maximum energies of around $600\,keV$ up to about 3 MeV.[24] Due to many collisions with tissue atoms, the emitted positrons quickly lose their energy, predominantly resulting in ionization and excitation within the tissue.

The probability of a positron undergoing an annihilation event with a tissue electron increases as the speed of the positron decreases. Eventually, as the positron comes nearly to rest, the inevitable annihilation with an electron takes place. This annihilation can be thought of as an inverse pair-production process (see §8.3) in which a positron and electron combine to produce energy according to Einstein's relativistic energy equation. However, since the electron and positron can be thought of as being nearly at rest at the time of annihilation, and since momentum must be conserved in this process, it follows that not one but *two* photons must be emitted, moving in nearly opposite directions to one another. As explained in Chapter 8, the combined mass-energy of an electron and positron is 1.022 *MeV*, so the energy of each photon emitted in the annihilation process must be 0.511 *MeV*. By the time the positron undergoes annihilation with an electron, it has typically traveled no more than several millimeters from the position where it was released from the radioisotope.[29]

As a result of the two photons being emitted in random but opposite directions, the detector system for PET imaging involves a ring of detectors surrounding the patient. When two detectors on opposite sides of the patient detect 0.511 *MeV* photons at nearly the same time, an annihilation event is recorded. The position of the annihilation must have been somewhere within the patient along the line between the two detectors, called the *line of response*, or (LoR).

Since annihilation events are taking place at random times within the patient, it's important to know when two detected photons are actually a pair of photons emitted in opposite directions during a single annihilation event, or whether they resulted from different annihilation events. As a result, the detectors have a "timing window" of about 5 to 10 *ns*. If two 0.511 *MeV* photons are detected on opposite sides of the patient within the timing window, then a so-called *coincidence event* is declared and an annihilation event is recorded along the associated LoR. While the timing window certainly helps cut down on invalid annihilation events, it certainly cannot eliminate them.

Consider the schematic shown in Fig. (12.28). After being injected with the appropriate radiopharmaceutical and waiting for a given amount of time (up to about an hour) for the radioisotopes to be distributed throughout the patient's system, the patient is positioned inside the gantry within the ring of detectors. Positrons are constantly being emitted by the radioisotopes within the patient's body. They may wander up to a few millimeters away from their point of emission, and then undergo an annihilation event, represented by a white star in the figure. The annihilation event labeled A represents an event in which the two gamma rays are emitted in opposite directions and are subsequently detected at detectors A1 and A2. These two detections take place within the timing window, so an annihilation event is recorded as having taken place somewhere along the LoR between A1 and A2. This is what is referred to as a *true coincidence*.

On the other hand, consider annihilation B in Fig. (12.28). In this case, the two gamma rays are emitted in opposite directions: one is emitted toward the lower-left in the figure is detected at detector B2, while the other is emitted and heads toward detector B1. But before that gamma ray reaches B1, it undergoes a Compton scattering

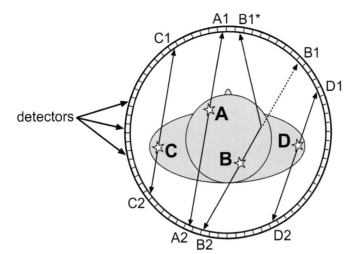

FIGURE 12.28: Schematic of a patient inside a PET gantry. The stars represent annihilation events in which positrons collide with electrons and emit two $511\,keV$ gamma rays moving in opposite directions. A, B, C, and D represent different types of coincidences. See the text for more detail.

event (see Chapter 8) within the patient. As a result, its energy and direction of travel are changed. It is subsequently detected at detector B1*. If the gamma rays detected at B1* and B2 are detected within the timing window, they will be counted as an annihilation event that took place along the LoR drawn from B1* to B2. While this annihilation event did actually occur, the location of the event did not lie along the associated LoR, resulting in a degradation of the resulting image quality. This type of incorrect event recording is called a *scatter coincidence*.

Now let's consider annihilation events C and D in Fig. (12.28). Let's say that these two events occur at nearly the same instant, and that detectors C1, C2, and D1, for example, all detect gamma rays within the timing window—or perhaps all four of the detectors C1, C2, D1, and D2 detect gamma rays within the timing window. When this happens, it is not known how to correlate the detector readings. As a result, these readings are discarded and do not contribute to the image. On the other hand, perhaps only C2 and D1 are detected within the timing window. In this case, an annihilation is incorrectly counted as having taken place along the LoR between C2 and D1, despite the fact that the two photons were not even from the same annihilation event. This is called a *random coincidence*, and contributes to noise in the image.

Once the various annihilation events are recorded, projection images are created from the LoR information. These images are then processed using iterative reconstruction (see §12.2) to produce a 3-D image of the distribution of positron-emitting radionuclides within the body.[30]

The resolution in PET imaging is inherently compromised by three important factors. The first is the discrete size of the detectors within the gantry ring. (See Fig. 12.28.) The second is the distance traveled by the positrons from the point of emission to where they are annihilated—often 2 to 3 mm within tissue. Finally, the conservation of momentum demands that the two photons emitted in the annihilation of the positron with a tissue electron not be emitted in directions exactly 180° apart if the electron-positron system had any net momentum immediately prior to the annihilation event. However, the PET-imaging process assumes that the photons are emitted in exactly opposite directions, resulting in a compromise in the resolution of the image. The net effect of these three factors is a resolution close to 1 cm,[31] resulting in the characteristic blurriness of PET images. See, for example, Fig. (12.31b).

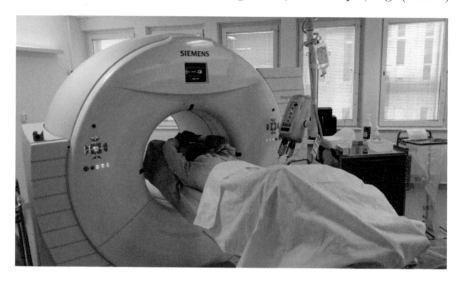

FIGURE 12.29: A patient positioned for imaging in a PET/CT scanner. (Open Access.)

As with SPECT imaging, the relatively small number of annihilation events causes the PET image to show the desired physiological functioning of the body, but sometimes without enough information about where in the anatomy that functioning is taking place. As a result, PET scans are now typically combined with CT scans in order to provide both anatomical and physiological information in the same image. Also, as in SPECT/CT imaging, the absorption-coefficient information from the CT data can be used to help correct the PET data for absorption within the patient as the gamma-ray photons are making their way through the patient and to the detectors. PET/MRI scans are also now available for use in the clinic. An example of a PET/CT system is shown in Fig. (12.29).[32]

From our discussion of the production of PET images from the LoR information, it should be clear that the resolution of the image is not going to be as good as desired—just knowing that the annihilation event took place *somewhere* within the patient along the associated LoR is not helping to localize the information very much. As a result, scintillation crystals that have not only good stopping powers—we need the gamma-rays to be detected within the crystal—but also fast decay times have been developed. A fast decay time means that the time interval between when the two gamma rays were detected in two different crystals can be measured. The time

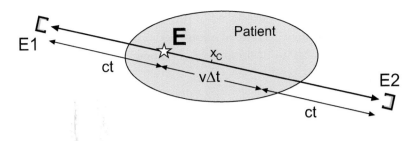

FIGURE 12.30: Schematic showing the spatial significance of the time-of-flight (ToF) for two detected gamma-ray photons after a positron-electron annihilation event, E. Detector E1 detects an annihilation gamma-ray before detector E2. x_C is the position of the center of the LoR between E1 and E2, relative to the position E1.

resolution between the two gamma-ray detections is currently around $500\,ps$. Let's see how this helps improve the resolution of the resulting PET image.

Consider the set-up shown in Fig. (12.30).

An annihilation event occurs at position E, resulting in the emission of two (approximately) oppositely directed 0.511 MeV photons. Let's say that the detector at E1 is the first to detect one of the two annihilation photons. If that photon took a time t to reach E1, then the distance from E to E1 is approximately given by $d = ct$, where c is the speed of light in a vacuum. (We are assuming that the majority of the distance traveled by the photons takes place in air outside the patient, so the speed of the light is c.) Since the second photon detected at E2 is detected after the first photon, it must have traveled a distance $ct + v\Delta t = d + v\Delta t$, where the times t and $t+\Delta t$ are the *times of flight* (ToF) of the two photons, and Δt is the time between the detections of the two photons. Here, we are assuming that the majority of the *extra* distance traveled by the second photon takes place within the patient. The speed of light inside the patient is given by $v = c/n$, where n is the average index of refraction of the tissue through which the light travels. (The index of refraction of water is about 1.33.) Since we don't know the precise time when an annihilation event occurs, we can't measure the ToF t, but we can measure the time interval between the two detections, Δt. Knowing this time interval allows us to localize the annihilation event to a significantly greater extent than in PET systems without ToF capabilities, in which case we only know that the event occurred somewhere along the LoR between detectors E1 and E2.

Letting C represent the center of the LoR between E1 and E2 and letting x_C represent the position of C relative to the detector E1 that detected the first photon, the annihilation event E must have occurred at the position

$$x_E = x_C - \Delta x = x_C - v\Delta t/2. \tag{12.14}$$

This gives the position of the annihilation event to within uncertainties and approximations—for example, not all of the distance d is outside the patient, so the light is traveling with speed v during part of that distance and with speed c for the rest of the distance. Nevertheless, a PET scanner that has ToF capability will certainly have an improved resolution. Current scintillator crystals can measure time intervals between photon detections of down to about $500\,ps,$[30] resulting in an additional uncertainty along the LoR of about $\Delta x = 5.6\,cm$, where we have used the index of refraction of water to approximate the speed of light in the tissue for the calculation.

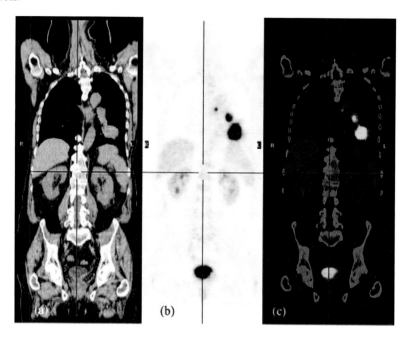

FIGURE 12.31: (a) A conventional CT scan shows the anatomy of a patient, while (b) a conventional PET scan shows the uptake in the positron-emitting radiopharmaceutical (the dark regions). (c) When information from both the CT and the PET scans are combined, the resulting image contains more useful information than both images (a) and (b) separately. (Baños-Capilla et al., with permission.)

An advantage of a PET/CT system is that the reconstruction process for the CT image results in a distribution of attenuation-coefficient values throughout the anatomy being imaged, as discussed earlier in this chapter. This information can then be used to implement attenuation corrections to the PET image. An example of the advantage of a PET/CT scan over a conventional PET scan is shown in Fig. (12.31).[33]

Because of the way PET uses coincidence measurements to detect annihilation events along the LoR, it tends to have a better efficiency and a higher resolution than SPECT, which uses collimators to determine the direction from which a photon entered the detector.[24] PET can be used to detect early signs of cancer by showing areas of abnormal metabolic activity in the way those areas absorb positron-emitting radiopharmaceutials. The most commonly used radiopharmaceutical in PET scans is fluorine-18 fluorodeoxyglucose, or *FDG*. Cancer cells tend to absorb FDG more actively than normal cells, so cancer can show up in PET scans before they might be visible in more conventional scans such as CT and MRI. PET scans can also be used to detect heart disease and brain disorders.

This ends our discussion of medical imaging. The next chapter will start our discussion of cancer treatment, or *clinical medical physics.*

12.7 QUESTIONS, EXERCISES, & PROBLEMS

12-1. Bill Hendee is an accomplished and greatly respected medical physicist with an expertise in medical imaging. Among his many other accomplishments, Dr. Hendee was Acting Dean of the Medical College of Wisconsin, Dean of the University of Wisconsin Graduate School of Biomedical Sciences, President of the Medical College of Wisconsin Research Foundation, President of the American Institute of Medical and Biological Engineering, President and CEO of the Commission on Accreditation of Medical Physics Education Program (CAMPEP), President of the American Association of Physicists in Medicine (AAPM), President of the American Board of Radiology, President of the Society of Nuclear Medicine, and President of the American Institute of Medical and Biological Engineering. He received the William D. Coolidge Gold Medal from the American Association of Physicists in Medicine and the Gold Medal for Distinguished Service to Radiology from the American Roentgen Ray Society.[34] This list barely scratches the surface of Dr. Hendee's accomplishments.

On 23 August 1992, as a part of the series of interviews for the History & Heritage website of the AAPM, Dr. Hendee was interviewed by Dr. Robert Garson.[35] This is a fascinating interview to listen to, not only for anyone interested in the history of medical physics and medical imaging but also for anyone interested in Dr. Hendee's selfless support for those fighting for their civil rights—in particular for reasons of race and sexual orientation—during the tumultuous years of the early 1960s.

As far as medical imaging is concerned, Dr. Hendee describes accepting a position at the University of Colorado Medical Center in 1965. At the time, he was working on radiation therapy using a beam of radiation emitted by a sample of radioactive cobalt-60 (Co-60). Treatment with a Co-60 beam exploits the emission of two high-energy photons—$1.17\,MeV$ and $1.33\,MeV$—as the Co-60 nuclei decay to Ni-60. Despite his background in medical imaging, Dr. Hendee continued working in radiation therapy for several years.

In 1970 and 1971, Bill Hendee became interested in the cross-sectional reconstruction of anatomy using an algorithm for reconstruction by filtered back projection that had recently been developed by Ramachandran and Lakshminarayanan.[36] He was interested in producing grayscale images based on attenuation-coefficient values for use in radiation treatment planning with the Co-60 machine. While he was able to produce images, they were of limited use due to the very poor contrast that characterized them. In 1971 he was at a meeting at which EMI Ltd. first showed images from the prototype unit for CT scans that had been built by Hounsfield and for which he had just received the Nobel prize. The images were exactly like those Hendee was trying to produce, but they were much clearer with significantly better contrast and were therefore much more clinically useful. The EMI images were produced using photons that were about a factor of 10 lower in energy than those that Hendee had used coming from the Co-60 machine. In reflecting on seeing the EMI images, Hendee claimed that he had been "stupid" and that he had "completely missed the point".[35]

What point had Dr. Hendee missed that caused him to claim that he had been "stupid"? Why were the EMI images so much better than those obtained by Dr. Hendee? Explain. (Hint: See Chapter 8.)

12-2. In the brief description of MRI it was stated that the image was obtained from photons emitted by protons in hydrogen atoms making a spin-flip transition from a higher energy spin-down configuration to a lower energy spin-up configuration. The energy difference between these two levels is given approximately by $\Delta E = 2\mu_p B$, where μ_p is the magnetic dipole moment of the proton and B is the magnetic field magnitude at the proton's location. The proton's magnetic dipole moment magnitude is equal to $\mu_p = 1.41 \times 10^{-26} \, JT^{-1}$. (a) Find the approximate value of the frequency of the photon associated with transitions between the two magnetic energy levels of the proton's magnetic dipole moment if the proton is in an external magnetic field of magnitude $1.50 \, T$. (b) What is the wavelength corresponding to this photon frequency? (c) To what part of the electromagnetic spectrum does this wavelength belong? (d) Is this photon radiation in the category of ionizing radiation? Why or why not?

12-3. Describe in your own words the method of iterative image reconstruction.

12-4. In what sense does the method of iterative image reconstruction generate a set of self-consistent images? Explain.

12-5. What is so exaggerated about Fig. (12.20), other than the size of the dipoles in the schematic? (Hint: look at the number of dipoles in the up and down states!) By what approximate factor is this figure exaggerated?

12-6. Figure (12.20) shows a plot of the gradient magnetic field as a function of position. It is stated in the caption to that figure that the slope of the linear behavior shown—the so-called gradient of the gradient field—is $20 \, mT/m$. The slice of anatomy being imaged is 1-cm thick—the distance between the vertical lines L and R in the figure. As discussed in the text, the region of anatomy between these two lines will contain dipoles precessing with a range of Larmor frequencies having an average of $\bar{f}$ and a bandwidth $2\Delta f$. (a) What would the average frequency and bandwidth be if the gradient were changed to $10 \, mT/m$? (b) ...to $40 \, mT/m$?

12-7. In our discussion of the magnetization of tissue in MRI, it was mentioned that, in thermodynamic equilibrium at temperature $310 \, K$ and with an external magnetic field of magnitude $B_{ext} = 1.5 \, T$, there would be an excess of just one extra dipole out of 100,000 in the lower-energy state as compared to the upper-energy state, completely contrary to what we would expect. Let's see if we can verify these numbers. (a) First, verify the value of ΔE given in the text associated with this discussion. (b) In statistical physics, the Boltzmann factor gives the relative number of particles occupying a state of energy E. More specifically, for our two-level system of energies available to the dipoles in an external magnetic field, the ratio of populations N_u/N_ℓ (u = upper; ℓ = lower) is given by

$$\frac{N_u}{N_\ell} = \frac{e^{-E_u/kT}}{e^{-E_\ell/kT}} = e^{-\Delta E/kT}, \tag{12.15}$$

where $\Delta E = E_u - E_\ell$, and $k = 1.38 \times 10^{-23} \, J/K$ is the *Boltzmann constant*. You're going to find that you end up with a tiny number in the exponent of the exponential function. Trying to use a calculator to extract needed information from such calculations can be cumbersome. To help with this, we can use the binomial approximation, which states that, if the magnitude of x is very small compared to 1, that is, if $|x| \ll 1$, then we can write that

$$e^x \cong 1 + x. \tag{12.16}$$

Using Eq. (12.16), compute the ratio of dipole populations in the upper and lower energy states as given in Eq. (12.15) and verify the conclusion drawn in the text concerning 1 extra dipole out of 100,000 in the lower-energy state.

12-8. (a) As mentioned in the text in the discussion on localization in MRI, it was stated that, for a given value of the magnetic field gradient $\Delta B / \Delta z$ (for example, the slope of the line in Fig. (12.24)), the location and thickness of the slice of anatomy being imaged are determined by the average frequency of the RF pulse, $\bar{f}$, and by the bandwidth of the pulse, $2\Delta f$. Explain why this is the case. Assume that the gradient field is zero at the midpoint between the two coils producing that field, as shown in Fig. (12.24). We take the midpoint to be $z = 0$, as in the figure. (b) Let $B_o = 1.5\,T$, and let the field gradient be $\Delta B / \Delta z = 50\,mT/m$. Assuming that the $z = 0$ position is at the midpoint of the coils and that the net magnetic field magnitude B_{ext} is decreasing as z increases, as is the case in Fig. (12.24), find the z-value of the center of the slice of anatomy being imaged along with the thickness of the slice if $\bar{f} \pm \Delta f = 63.724500 \pm 0.005500\,MHz$.

12-9. Information used to form the image in the various imaging modalities tends to come from photons emerging from various regions of anatomy, but the information for an image in MRI is acquired in a very different way. In your own words, briefly summarize what forms the image signal in MRI and how that signal is localized in order to form the image.

12-10. At the end of the MRI section it is stated that the hydrogenic proton density can be determined from the strength of the magnetic signal. Explain why this is the case.

12-11. Figure (12.23) shows the time-dependent behavior of the transverse and longitudinal components of the magnetization vector after the tissue has been irradiated by an RF pulse. These behaviors are governed by Eqs. (12.11) and (12.12). (a) To what percentage of $M_{T,max}$ has the transverse magnetization M_T dropped after a time $t = T2$? Does your answer look reasonable by inspection of Fig. (12.23)? (b) To what percentage of $(M_{L,ext}$ has the longitudinal component of magnetization risen after a time $t = T1$? Does your answer look reasonable by inspection of Fig. (12.23)?

12-12. In Fig. (12.23) we see that the value of $M_T(t)$ decreases with time while the value of $M_L(t)$ increases with time. In terms of what is physically going on with the magnetic dipole moments, carefully explain why these two components of the magnetization vector show this behavior.

12-13. In MRI, explain how the longitudinal component of the magnetization vector can become negative if the RF pulse is left on long enough.

12-14. Clinical MRI scanners can have background magnetic field strengths B_o from $0.2\,T$ up to $7\,T$.[25] What range of Larmor frequencies corresponds to this range of magnetic field strengths?

12-15. (a) Using the numbers given in the associated discussion on back projection in the text, verify the numbers given in Fig. (12.7(c)). (b) Likewise, verify the numbers given in Fig. (12.8(c)).

12-16. (a) Explain in your own words how the time-of-flight measurement, Δt, can be used to localize the annihilation event in PET. (b) Let's say that two detectors, D1 and D2, are $72\,cm$ from one another. They produce a coincidence measurement, so that the corresponding LoR is $72\,cm$ long. What is the most likely position of the annihilation event relative to detector D2, to within given uncertainties and approximations, given that detector D2 detects a gamma-ray photon at a time $\Delta t = 580\,ps$ after D1 detects its photon?

12-17. In our discussion of PET imaging, it was mentioned that a scatter coincidence is when two photons are detected within the timing window, but one of the photons undergoes Compton scattering, so that the direction of the photon can be changed, thereby causing the wrong detector to detect the scattered photon and displacing the LoR from its correct position. But in Chapter 8 we discussed the fact that photons can undergo Compton as well as photoelectric interactions. Why are photoelectric interactions not included in the description of scatter coincidence measurements?

12-18. In the discussion of PET imaging it was stated that there are three major factors compromising the resolution of the PET image: the discrete size of the detectors, the distance traveled by the positrons between emission and annihilation, and the velocities of the emitted photons not being exactly 180° apart. Carefully explain how each of these factors compromises the PET image resolution.

12-19. Explain in your own words and with at least one diagram why electron-positron annihilation results in the emission of *two* photons instead of just one.

12-20. *SPECT is to planar imaging in nuclear medicine as x-ray CT is to radiography.* Explain this statement.

12-21. Radiation dose from medical imaging is discussed at the end of Chapter 10, but in the list of contributions to our annual dose MRI and ultrasound are not listed. Why not? Explain.

12-22. Isotopes of iodine (I-131) and mercury (Hg-203) were often used in nuclear medicine imaging in the 1950s and 1960s.[24] Both of these isotopes decay by beta decay followed by gamma decay, with half-lives of 8.0 days (I-131) and 46.6 days (Hg-203). On the other hand, about 85% of all diagnostic nuclear medicine imaging procedures currently use technetium-99m (Tc-99m).[37] Tc-99m is an isomer of Tc-99 and decays by gamma decay with a half-life of 6.0 hours. As a result, significantly greater activities can be administered to patients undergoing diagnostic nuclear medicine imaging with Tc-99m than those using I-131 or Hg-203, resulting in higher-quality images. Carefully explain the previous sentence.

12-23. *SPECT* stands for Single Photon Emission Computed Tomography. Which imaging modality could be thought of as *TPECT—Two Photon Emission Computed Tomography*? Explain.

12-24. It is stated that the radiation given off by radiopharmaceuticals in nuclear medicine imaging is typically x- or gamma-rays—"typically" meaning not always. What imaging modality is the exception to this? Explain.

12-25. The absorption of photons by tissue is an important consideration in all of the imaging modalities discussed in this brief introduction to imaging except ultrasound imaging and MRI—the signal in ultrasound comes from pressure waves and in MRI the signal comes in the form of time-varying magnetic fields. Photon absorption in radiography and x-ray CT is very different from that in nuclear medicine imaging modalities. Indeed, one could argue that, from the imaging perspective, the absorption of photons by tissue in radiography and x-ray CT is a good thing, while in nuclear medicine imaging it is a bad thing. Explain.

12-26. Explain the difference between anatomical imaging and functional imaging. Then give two imaging modality examples of each, explaining briefly why each modality is an example of anatomical or functional imaging.

12.8 REFERENCES

1. Computed from values for 100 keV photons in Appendices B.2 and D.3 in Attix, H.A., Introduction to Radiological Physics and Radiation Dosimetry, John Wiley & Sons (New York) 1986.
2. Curry, T.S., III, Dowdy, J.E., and Murry, R.C., Jr., Christensen's Physics of Diagnostic Radiology, 4th Ed., Lippincott Williams & Wilkins (Philadelphia) 1990
3. Hendee, W.R. and Ritenour, E.R., Medical Imaging Physics (4th Ed.), John Wiley & Sons (New York) 2002
4. Images for this figure were captured from animated gifs created by Adam Kesner. The gif files were accessed online (15AUG22) on the International Atomic Energy Agency (IAEA) Human Health Campus website at https://humanhealth.iaea.org/HHW/MedicalPhysics/NuclearMedicine/ImageAnalysis/3Dimagereconstruction/index.html
5. Kesner AL, Häggström I. Original Gif Animations to Support the Teaching of Medical Image Reconstruction. *Medical Physics International Journal.* 2019;7(1):9-10. Available online at http://www.mpijournal.org/pdf/2019-01/MPI-2019-01-p009.pdf.
6. Mathworks, Deep Learning. Accessed online on 01/22/2022 at mathworks.com/discovery/deep-learning.html
7. Nett, Brian, Deep Learning CT (from AAPM 2021), from the video series How Radiology Works. 17 August, 2021. Accessed on 15 JAN 22 at https://www.youtube.com/watch?v=WR8TsasTFK4
8. Jiang Hsieh, Eugene Liu, Brian Nett, Jie Tang, Jean-Baptiste Thibault, Sonia Sahney, A new era of image reconstruction: TrueFidelity (Technical white paper on deep learning image reconstruction.) Accessed online 17 MAR 23 at https://www.gehealthcare.com/-/jssmedia/040dd213fa89463287155151-fdb01922.pdf 2019 General Electric Company.
9. Timothy P. Szczykutowicz, Brian Nett, Lusik Cherkezyan, Myron Pozniak, Jie Tang, Meghan G. Lubner, and Jiang Hsieh, Protocol Optimization Considerations for Implementing Deep Learning CT Reconstruction, American Journal of Roentgenology (AJR), June, Vol. 216, No. 6 : pp. 1668-1677.
10. Higgins ES. 50 years ago, the first CT scan let doctors see inside a living skull—thanks to an eccentric engineer at the Beatles' record company. https://theconversation.com/50-years-ago-the-first-ct-scan-let-doctors-see-inside-a-living-skull- thanks-to-an-eccentric-engineer-at-the-beatles-record-company-149907. Accessed December 18, 2021.
11. Taubmann O, Berger M, Bögel M, et al. Computed Tomography. In: Maier A, Steidl S, Christlein V, et al., eds. *Medical Imaging Systems: An Introductory Guide.* Cham (CH): Springer; 2018. Figure 8.2, The first clinical CT scan, acquired October 1971 at Atkinson Morley's Hospital in London. Open Access. Available from: https://www.ncbi.nlm.nih.gov/books/NBK546157/figure/ch8.fig2/. doi: 10.1007/978-3-319-96520-8_8.
12. Romainbehar (https://commons.wikimedia.org/wiki/File:Bron_-_CERMEP_-_Salle_du_scanner_TEP-CT_de_2010,_vue_d'ensemble.jpg), "Bron - CERMEP - Salle du scanner TEP-CT de 2010, vue d'ensemble", https://creativecommons.org/publicdomain/zero/1.0/legalcode.
13. Kalra MK, Rehani MM, Altes, TA, Martinez S, Williams MB. CT Systems (2018). RSNA physics module. https://education.rsna.org/diweb/catalog/launch/package/4/eid/2117643. Accessed January 4, 2022.
14. Dobbs HJ, Parker RP, Hodson NJ, Hobday P, Husband JE. The use of CT in radiotherapy treatment planning. *Radiother Oncol.* 1983; 1(2): 133-41.
15. McCollough CH, Boedeker K, Cody D, et al. Principles and applications of multienergy CT: Report of AAPM Task Group 291. *Medical Physics.* 2020; 47(7):e881-e912

16. Hounsfield GN. Computerized transverse axial scanning (tomography): Part 1. Description of system. *Br J Radiol.* 1973; 46(552): 1016-1022.
17. Patel B. Stanford Healthcare Computed Tomography, Introduction to Dual Energy CT. https://www.youtube.com/watch?v=ntWhwF-p05I. Accessed January 17, 2022.
18. Kruis MF. Improving radiation physics, tumor visualisation, and treatment quantification in radiotherapy with spectral or dual-energy CT. *J Appl Clin Med Phys.* 2022; 23: e13468. https://doi.org/10.1002/acm2.13468.
19. The President and Fellows of Harvard College. Radiation risk from medical imaging. https://www.health.harvard.edu/cancer/radiation-risk-from-medical-imaging. Accessed February 6, 2022.
20. Boone JM, McCollough CH. Computer tomography turns 50. *Physics Today.* 2021; 74(9): 34-40.
21. Howard DM, Schofield J, Fletcher J, et al. Synthesis of a Vocal Sound from the 3,000 year old Mummy, Nesyamun 'True of Voice'. *Sci Rep.* 2020; 10: 45000. Accessed November 27, 2022. https://doi.org/10.1038/s41598-019-56316-y.
22. St. Fleur N. The Mummy Speaks! Hear Sounds From the Voice of an Ancient Egyptian Priest, The New York Times, 23 January, 2020. https://www.nytimes.com/2020/01/23/science/mummy-voice.html. Accessed November 27, 2022.
23. Jan Ainali (https://commons.wikimedia.org/wiki/File:MRI-Philips.JPG), "MRI-Philips", https://creativecommons.org/licenses/by/3.0/legalcode
24. Bushberg JT, Seibert JA, Leidholdt EM Jr, Boone JM. *The Essential Physics of Medical Imaging.* 3rd ed. Philadelphia: Lippincott, Williams & Wilkins; 2012.
25. Jordan D. State of the art in magnetic resonance imaging. *Phys. Today.* 2020; 73(2):34-40.
26. Edlow BL, Mareyam A, Horn A, et al. 7 Tesla MRI of the ex vivo human brain at 100 micron resolution. *Sci Data.* 2019;6(1): 1-10. https://doi.org/10.1038/s41597-019-0254-8.
27. Son SJ, Kim M, Park H. Imaging analysis of Parkinson's disease patients using SPECT and tractography. *Sci Rep.* 2016; Sci Rep 6: Article Number 38070. https://doi.org/10.1038/srep38070.
28. Siemens Medical Solutions USA, Inc. c.cam cardiac camera. https://www.siemens-healthineers.com/en-us/molecular-imaging/spect-and-spect-ct/c-cam. Accessed March 28, 2022.
29. Guy C, ffytche D. *An Introduction to The Principles of Medical Imaging.* London: Imperial College Press; 2000.
30. Gagandeep C, White S, Yester M, et al. PET/PET-CT/Image Quality (2019). RSNA physics module PHYS16-2019. https://education.rsna.org/diweb/catalog/launch/package/4/eid/2645461. Accessed January 4, 2022.
31. Shukla AK, Kumar U. Positron emission tomography: An overview. *J Med Phys.* 2006; 31(1): 13-21. doi: 10.4103/0971-6203.25665. PMID: 21206635; PMCID: PMC3003889.
32. Då.nu (https://commons.wikimedia.org/wiki/File:PET_CT_scanner.JPG), https://creativecommons.org/licenses/by-sa/4.0/legalcode.
33. Baños-Capilla MC, García MA, Bea J, Pla C, Larrea L, López E. PET/CT image registration: Preliminary tests for its application to clinical dosimetry in radiotherapy. *Med. Phys.* 2007; 34: 1911-1917. https://doi.org/10.1118/1.2732031.
34. Hendee WR. Curriculum Vitae, dated March 20, 2013.
35. AAPM. AAPM History Interview with Bill Hendee. AAPM History & Heritage website. https://www.aapm.org/org/history/InterviewVideo.asp?i=61. Accessed January 2, 2022.
36. Ramachandran GN, Lakshminarayanan AV. Three-dimensional reconstruction from radiographs and electron micrographs: application of convolutions instead of fourier transforms. *Proc. Nat. Acad. Sci.* 1971; 68(9): 2236–2240.
37. World Nuclear Association. Radioisotopes in Medicine. https://www.world-nuclear.org/information-library/non-power-nuclear-applications/radioisotopes-research/radioisotopes-in-medicine.aspx. Accessed July 12, 2020.

Overview of Radiation Oncology

CONTENTS

According to a recent report published by the American Association of Physicists in Medicine (AAPM), 77% of medical physicists in the United States and Canada work in radiation oncology. Consequently, radiation oncology is a very important component of the discipline of medical physics, and the remainder of this book will address basic medical physics as applied to radiation oncology.

Radiation oncology involves the use of radiation, primarily ionizing radiation (see Chapter 2), to treat cancer and some benign diseases. Although in the early history of radiation medicine, ionizing radiation was used to treat other conditions, at present, radiation is used almost exclusively to treat malignant disease. The "twenty-five words or less" definition of the role of the medical physicist in radiation oncology is something like "ensuring that the radiation delivered during a radiation treatment is done in such a manner that is safe". In this chapter, and the chapters that follow, we will present some of the fundamental physical principles germane to the treatment of cancer with ionizing radiation and some of the ways these principles are currently applied to make the treatment safe.

In this chapter, in particular, we will first identify why we use radiation to treat cancer. Radiation affects both malignant disease as well as uninvolved tissue, so we will then address why we need to spare uninvolved tissue and how we do it. Finally, we look at the team that is used to treat cancer. Radiation therapy requires a multidisciplinary team, and we will identify who is involved and what they do.

13.1 RATIONALE FOR THE USE OF RADIATION

The goal of radiation therapy is to deliver doses of radiation to a tumor sufficient to kill tumor cells while sparing uninvolved tissue that might be irradiated. To do so, we optimize the treatment of tumor cells using both biology and geometry. By biological optimization, we mean that we take advantage of differences in biological response to radiation between tumor cells and healthy cells. These were discussed in Chapter 2. By geometrical optimization, we mean that we design treatment geometries that irradiate the tumor while keeping radiation doses to uninvolved tissue below specified limits.

Several paths exist toward geometrical optimization. First, we can collimate the radiation beam to restrict the radiation reaching the target volume in order to spare the uninvolved tissue that is lateral to the tumor—that is, in a direction perpendicular to the radiation beam axis. (See Chapter 20 for a more precise definition of *target volume*.) We are likely to use multiple beams directed toward the tumor to help spare normal tissue that is proximal (closer to the radiation source) and distal (more distant to the radiation source) to the tumor. We might also use alternative forms of ionizing radiation such as charged-particle beams instead of photon beams to take advantage of their finite depth of penetration in limiting the extent of the region to be irradiated. Further refinement of the lateral intensity distribution of the beam can be accomplished using the technique of intensity-modulated radiation therapy (IMRT) to further shape the high-dose region.

13.2   NORMAL TISSUE SPARING

As was discussed in Chapter 2, radiation doses to normal tissue can cause damage. This damage can appear in the form of acute effects, which manifest themselves shortly after irradiation, as well as late effects, which may appear many years after the radiation treatment. As a consequence, it is important to spare as much normal tissue as possible to ensure an acceptable quality of life for the patient after treatment. We look at methods for sparing normal tissues both lateral to the tumor as well as proximal and distal to the tumor.

Normal tissue lateral to the tumor is spared by collimation, which limits the lateral extent of the beam by using shielding. Typically, two or three sets of collimators are used. Primary collimators define the largest available field size and consist of a tungsten block with a circular opening. Secondary collimators consist of four blocks, two forming upper jaws and two forming lower jaws. These four blocks define a rectangular field. They may be either symmetric or asymmetric. Figure (13.1) is an illustration of the head of a linear accelerator, indicating the location of the primary and secondary collimators.

Tertiary collimation is usually necessary to further shape the beam to fit the shape of the target volume. This additional collimation was originally achieved by placing rectangular lead blocks on a transparent tray between the treatment machine and the patient. A more precise definition of the radiation field was made possible with the development of a low melting point alloy (Wood's metal, Lipowitz's metal, Cerrobend^{TM}) that could be cast to a specified shape. The low melting point alloy is an alloy of 50% bismuth, 26.7% lead, 13.3% tin, and 10% cadmium by weight. An outline of the treatment field is first cut out in a Styrofoam^{TM} mold. Because the low melting point alloy has a melting point of 158 °F, it can be melted under hot water and poured into the mold. Figure (13.2) illustrates such a cast metal block. The major disadvantage of this approach is the toxicity of the fumes emanating from the molten metal. Consequently, when casting these blocks, one generally works under a hood.

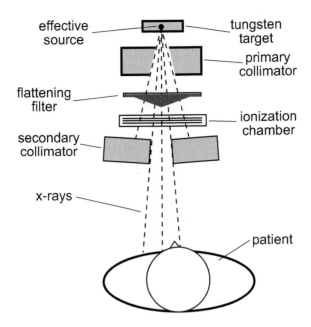

FIGURE 13.1: Schematic diagram of the interior of a linac head (or gantry head) illustrating locations of the primary and secondary collimators. An electron beam (not shown), incident from above, collides with the tungsten target, resulting in x-rays emitted from an effective source point within the target. The x-rays then progress down into the gantry head, as shown. (See Fig. 11.9 for a picture of a linac showing the gantry and the gantry head.)

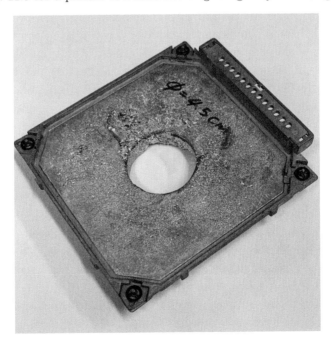

FIGURE 13.2: Example of a cast block of low melting point alloy used in radiation therapy. The hole in the block is formed in the shape of the region of the patient that is to be irradiated. (Photo courtesy of Jay Burmeister.)

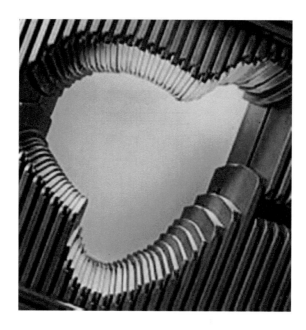

FIGURE 13.3: A multileaf collimator. (Open Source.)

Low melting point alloy blocks have been replaced to a major extent by multileaf collimators (MLC). These have several advantages. They form an integral component of the linear accelerator, so no fabrication is necessary. Moreover, their positions can be controlled through the linear accelerator to achieve customized field shaping, including dynamic field shaping. Figure (13.3)[1] illustrates a multileaf collimator.

Sparing of normal tissue proximal and distal to the tumor can be achieved in one of two ways. If one elects to use indirectly ionizing radiation (e.g., photons or neutrons) sparing can be achieved by the use of multiple beams. As discussed in Chapter 8, uncharged particles exhibit exponential attenuation to first order. Consequently, by aiming multiple beams at the target, it is possible for the target to be irradiated by all the beams while the normal tissue is irradiated by fewer beams and therefore receives a lower dose than the target.

Alternatively, one can use directly ionizing radiation (charged particles) to achieve normal-tissue sparing. In Chapter 9 we saw that charged particles have a finite range that is dependent on the energy of the charged particles. Tissue beyond the range of the charged particles receive very little dose. It should be pointed out, however, that there might be some enhancement of the relative biological effectiveness, or RBE (see Chapter 2), at the end of the range because of the decrease in energy of the charged particles. Uncertainty, therefore, exists as to the magnitude of the RBE dose. Consequently, one typically does not aim the charged particle beam directly at a critical structure lying distal to the target, as the decrease in dose may be offset by an increase in the RBE. Furthermore, although the existence of the Bragg peak results in a low dose proximal to the tumor, the need to spread out the Bragg peak (SOBP) to increase the region of high dose to encompass the tumor also increases

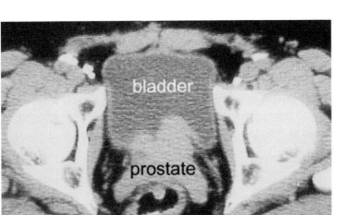

FIGURE 13.4: A CT scan of a transverse plane passing through the prostate, illustrating the prostate "wrapping around" the rectum. (Image from Dr. Robert Miller, with permission.)

the dose proximal to the tumor. (See Chapter 9 for a discussion of the Bragg peak; the SOBP is discussed in Chapter 19.)

The use of collimation and multiple beams to limit the dose outside the target volume results in a high-dose region that is convex. However, in many cases, a target "wraps around" a critical structure resulting in a concave target volume. For example, the prostate often wraps around the rectum (Fig. 13.4).[2] It is now possible to generate a concave region of high dose by modifying the spatial distribution of the intensity of the photon beam by use of dynamic multileaf collimators (Fig. 13.5). This technique

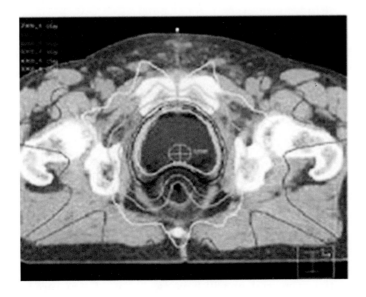

FIGURE 13.5: An IMRT dose distribution illustrating how high-dose region "wraps" around the rectum.

is known as intensity-modulated radiation therapy (IMRT), even though what is being modulated is actually the beam fluence and not the beam intensity. IMRT has become a standard for much radiation treatment using high-energy photon beams.

13.3 THE RADIATION TREATMENT TEAM

One noticeable characteristic of radiation oncology is the fact that it involves a multidisciplinary approach to treatment. In this section, we identify members of the radiation treatment "team", their roles in patient treatment, and the extent and nature of their education and training.

Radiation oncologists oversee the care of the patient undergoing radiation treatment. They assess the patient for the histology and extent of the tumor and for the proximity of critical uninvolved anatomic structures, prescribing a dose and approving a treatment plan that adequately irradiates the tumor while sparing critical structures. During treatment, the radiation oncologist continually monitors the patient, adjusting the treatment, if necessary, to ensure quality care, and treats adverse side effects of the radiation. After treatment, they will regularly monitor the patient to assess the effectiveness of the treatment and mitigate late effects of the radiation. The radiation oncologist is a physician with either an MD or a DO degree. The medical degree is followed by one postgraduate year of general medical training and four years of specialty training as a resident in radiation oncology. Often, the radiation oncologist may receive further specialty training as a fellow. Radiation oncologists can take a certification examination given by the American Board of Radiology that determines if they possess the necessary expertise to practice independently.

As presented earlier in this chapter, the role of the *radiation oncology physicist* (or *medical physicist*) is to ensure that the radiation is delivered to the patient in a manner that is safe. Their role in safety begins when equipment needed in the clinic is originally specified and purchased. The radiation oncology physicist works with the radiation oncologist and administrative personnel to develop a set of equipment specifications to ensure that the machine performance is optimized for the needs of the radiation oncology clinic. Once the equipment is delivered, the physicist performs both acceptance testing to validate the machine performance and safety testing to ensure safe performance of the equipment. The physicist then develops and oversees the ongoing quality assurance program to ensure that the machine continues to perform as specified. (Quality assurance and radiation safety are discussed in Chapter 24.) The physicist also oversees the entry of beam data into the treatment planning system and reviews the treatment plans of each patient. The education of a radiation oncology physicist includes an undergraduate degree in either physics or a physical science or engineering with a strong physics minor, followed by at least two years of graduate education in medical physics leading to a master's degree. Often a graduate student will continue their education and obtain a PhD or ScD degree, especially if they are interested in an academic career. Following the minimum of two years of didactic education, the student will have two years of structured clinical training in the form of a medical physics residency. Some educational institutions have combined the two years of didactic instruction with two years of clinical training into a professional doctorate degree, the DMP. Medical physicists with adequate training and experience can also be certified by the American Board of Radiology.

The radiation oncology physicist is often assisted by a *medical physicist assistant*, especially in a large radiation oncology clinic. The medical physicist assistant performs tasks such as routine quality assurance measurements of treatment machines and dose verification measurements of radiation treatments in support of the practice of the radiation oncology physicist and under the supervision of the physicist. Preparation for a medical physicist assistant is either a bachelor's degree or certification as a radiation therapist, followed by specialty clinical training.

The *dosimetrist* works with the radiation oncologist in developing a treatment plan for the radiation oncology patient. The dosimetrist works on a treatment planning computer, typically taking a CT image data set on which the radiation oncologist has outlined the target volume, calculating the radiation dose distributions for various beam configurations and collaborating with the radiation oncologist and radiation oncology physicist to determine the optimal beam configuration. Dosimetrists either have an undergraduate degree in science or are radiation therapists. They then take a one- or two-year training program in treatment planning. They may obtain certification from the Medical Dosimetry Certification Board.

The *radiation therapist* is the individual who actually sees the patient on a daily basis while delivering the radiation. The radiation therapist sets up the patient in accordance with the treatment plan and follows the treatment plan to deliver the radiation. Often the radiation therapist is the individual who performs the daily checks on the treatment machine prior to treating patients to ensure that the machine is functioning properly. Radiation therapists undergo a two- to four-year training program following high school, either academic-based or hospital-based. They can then be certified by the American Registry of Radiologic Technologists.

Radiation oncology nurses work with the oncologist and the therapist to take care of the patient during treatment. They may evaluate the patient on a regular basis during the course of treatment to assess the patient's response to the treatment, as well as address the concerns of the patients and their family and educate them about the radiation therapy. Radiation oncology nurses are typically registered nurses with additional training in oncology nursing. Mid-level practitioners, such as nurse practitioners or physician's assistants, have had additional training and may take on some of the physician's responsibilities.

Social workers provide counseling to patients and their families, and often arrange for home health care as well as accommodations and transportation arrangements for patients who may live some distance away from the radiation therapy clinic. Social workers typically have a master's degree and pass an appropriate examination.

Larger radiation oncology clinics may have additional personnel such as *service engineers* or *dieticians*. Service engineers maintain the radiation oncology equipment, making repairs as necessary. In smaller clinics, this work is generally handled by the equipment vendor or a third-party service organization. Finally, dieticians work with the patient to ensure that the patient has adequate nutrition while under treatment.

13.4   QUESTIONS, EXERCISES, & PROBLEMS

13-1. Consider a patient lying on a treatment table beneath a radiation source for treatment of prostate cancer. The radiation is incident on the patient from above, as shown in Fig. (13.1). The tumor is located in the prostate well within the patient. Based on the CT image in Fig. (13.4), make a rough sketch of a cross section of the patient showing the incident beam and the tumor. Then label the regions within the patient that are lateral to the tumor, proximal to the tumor, and distal to the tumor.

13.5   REFERENCES

1. Primi11 (https://commons.wikimedia.org/wiki/File:Primer_veclistnega_kolimatorskega_sistema_v_glavi-_linearnega_pospesevalnika.png), https://creativecommons.org/licenses/by-sa/4.0/legalcode.
2. Miller R. Prostate Imaging (CT). https://www.aboutcancer.com/prostate_anatomy_images_ct.htm. Accessed June 10, 2023.

Ethical Considerations

CONTENTS

In this chapter, we address ethical considerations from a clinical point of view. In discussing ethics in this chapter, we briefly move away from the technical aspects of medical physics to address ethics as an important component of the professional practice of medical physics. One reason for the need to address clinical ethics is that instead of aiming a radiation beam at an inanimate target, as we do in many sub-disciplines of physics, in the practice of medical physics, we aim the radiation beam at a human being. Consequently, "It's all about the patient" is a phrase commonly heard in medical physics circles.

This chapter addresses four issues related to professional ethics. We first discuss the definition and implementation of patient privacy. We then describe the component of the Health Insurance Portability and Accountability Act (HIPPA) that regulates the release of a patient's health-related information in the United States. Next, we address codes of ethics, and identify key features of the codes of ethics for various practitioners in radiation oncology, with particular emphasis placed on codes of ethics for medical physicists. Finally, we show how a Code of Ethics evolves to deal with processes and procedures that may not be in place when a Code is published, but bring up new and perhaps unfamiliar ethical issues.

14.1 PATIENT PRIVACY

The guiding rule regarding patient privacy is that patients have a basic right to privacy of their medical records. Procedures must be in place in the clinic to maintain security and confidentiality of patient information. Maintenance of security and confidentiality of information is a major problem in clinical practice because patient information needs to be transferred among healthcare providers. Originally, the records that were used to communicate patient information among providers were written on paper and transmitted either by mailing (internally or externally) or faxing a hard copy of the data. At present, an increasing number of clinical facilities have moved patient information to an Electronic Medical Record (EMR). Whereas the EMR makes information more accessible to providers, it also makes the information more accessible to unauthorized individuals. Consequently, data security has become an issue in clinical practice.

Privacy of patient information is supported by continual training and reminding clinical staff of the need for privacy. Staff must be careful to avoid disclosure of patient information through casual conversation, especially in public regions of the hospital or clinic. Computers accessing patient data must be secured, and media used to transfer data should have the data encoded and protected. Moreover, access to patient information should be limited to those who require the information for patient care.

Further discussion of privacy of patient information will be presented in the following section as this information relates to the Health Insurance Portability and Accountability Act (HIPAA).

Patient privacy extends to research as well. Prior to initiating any research study involving patients or patient information, it is necessary to obtain approval by the institution's Institutional Review Board (IRB). The IRB is typically a committee of peers who review research proposals that involve human subjects or human treatment data and verify that the subjects are treated in a dignified, humane manner. Patient privacy is protected in the case of retrospective treatment plans and data by anonymizing the data and removing patient-specific information from the data to be studied. Special care must be taken with imaging data, in particular, because images often contain headers that contain patient information that should be removed, but such data is not readily displayed. Anonymization operations for such data need to be able to edit the image header and remove patient-identifying information.

14.2   HIPAA RULES

The Health Insurance Portability and Accountability Act (HIPAA), passed by the U.S. Congress in 1996, and signed by President Bill Clinton, is the fundamental law regulating patient privacy in the United States. Title II of HIPAA, in particular, mandates the establishment of national standards for securely processing electronic patient information. Since passing of HIPAA, various rules were established to implement the Act. In particular, the HIPAA Privacy Rule establishes standards for providing protection for individuals' health information for treatment, payment, and other healthcare transactions.

The HIPAA Privacy Rule protects all individually identifiable health information in any form. This information is called Protected Health Information (PHI). More specifically, PHI is any information about the health status, provision of healthcare, or payment for healthcare that is created or collected by a healthcare provider or associate of a provider, and can be linked to a specific individual. This is interpreted rather broadly and includes any part of a patient's medical record or payment history.[1]

Several recommendations have been made to aid in maintenance of PHI. For example, proper disposal of PHI is mandated. In the case of hardcopy records, unused records must be shredded or otherwise destroyed. The analogy related to the EMR would be reformatting of the electronic media in which the data is stored. Another recommendation is the use of two-factor authentication. In two-factor authentication, once a user logs in to a computer system with a user name and password, the system returns to the user a code, generally over a different medium, such as a text message on a mobile telephone. The user must then enter the code in order to access the system. Two-factor authentication prevents an unauthorized user from entering the system even with a compromised user name and password, unless the unauthorized user managed to obtain access to the individual's telephone as well.

14.3 ETHICAL GUIDELINES FOR PRACTITIONERS

One feature common to all practitioners in the health care arena is a code of ethics for their profession. A code of ethics is typically adopted by a professional organization to assist its members in understanding the difference between right and wrong in their specific area of expertise. Codes of ethics are generally cited in the bylaws of a professional organization and are implemented through that organization's Ethics Committee. The Ethics Committee generally has the authority to make specific recommendations regarding ethical issues, and often can take disciplinary action against a member of that organization if the code is violated.

An example of a code of ethics is the code produced by the American College of Radiology (ACR). The ACR is an organization primarily of radiologists and radiation oncologists, but membership also includes medical physicists. The goal of the ACR is promoting and supporting the professional practice of its members. The ACR Code of Ethics can be found in Article XI of its Bylaws. Its Code of Ethics serve as goals of exemplary professional conduct for which members of the ACR are urged to constantly strive. The Code identifies the principal objectives of the professions of its members, supports its members' improving their knowledge and skill in performing appropriate procedures, and also makes reference to moral conduct of its members.

The Code of Conduct of a similar organization, the American Society for Radiation Oncology (ASTRO) includes a commitment to human rights and non-discrimination. It also addresses the business practices of radiation oncology such as relationships with competitors, as well as record keeping and conflicts of interest.

Radiographers and radiation therapy technologists have their own code of ethics, produced by their professional organization, the American Society of Radiologic Technologists (ASRT).

Of most importance to practicing medical physicists, however, is the Code of Ethics of the American Association of Physicists in Medicine (AAPM). The most recent version of the Code of Ethics was released in 2019, and was the work of an AAPM Task Group, which set out to revise a previous version.[2] The Code is divided into three major sections: a set of principles of ethical medical physics practice, guidelines for interpreting the principles, and rules by which a complaint could be adjudicated.

The section on Principles is relatively short, consisting of ten statements that form the basis of ethical behavior on the part of professional medical physicists. The Principles are quoted as follows:

I. Members must hold as paramount the best interests of the patient under all circumstances.

II. Members must strive to provide the best quality patient care and ensure the safety, privacy, and confidentiality of patients and research participants.

III. Members must act with integrity in all aspects of their work.

IV. Members must interact in an open, collegial, and respectful manner amongst themselves and in relation to other professionals, including those in training, and safeguard their confidences and privacy.

V. Members must strive to be impartial in all professional interactions, and must disclose and formally manage any real, potential, or perceived conflicts of interest.

VI. Members must strive to continuously maintain and improve their knowledge and skills while encouraging the professional development of their colleagues and of those under their supervision.

VII. Members must operate within the limits of their knowledge, skills, and available resources in the provision of healthcare. Members must enable practices in which patients are provided the levels of medical physicist expertise and case-specific attention as appropriately supports the modalities of their care.

VIII. Members must adhere to the legal and regulatory requirements that apply to the practice of their profession.

IX. Members must support the ideals of justice and fairness in the provision of healthcare and allocation of limited healthcare resources.

X. Members are professionally responsible and accountable for their practice, attitudes, and actions, including inactions and omissions.

The Principles are relatively general and do not address specific examples, so a rather lengthy set of Guidelines follows. These Guidelines cover behavior in the workplace, such as responsibilities to peers, the profession, the public, and the employer. The Guidelines also include examples of personal behavior, commitment to diversity and inclusivity in the work environment, and general workplace ethics. Another section of the Guidelines addresses responsibilities associated with the clinic, such as responsibilities to patients, caregivers, and other healthcare providers. Yet another section addresses research ethics, including roles of coworkers on the research team, research involving human subjects, research involving animal subjects, publication ethics, and intellectual property. Another section of the Guidelines has to do with education ethics including promotion of a safe environment, respect for students and trainees, confidentiality, and intimate relationships with students and trainees. A final section of the Guidelines addresses business ethics and includes ethics in the employment process, ethics in interactions with vendors, ethics on the part of members who represent vendors, and ethics of self-employed members.

The Code of Ethics is completed with a section on the specific and relatively detailed procedure to be followed when a medical physicist is observed violating a component of the Code.

The fine details of the AAPM Code of Ethics are beyond the scope of this text, and the interested reader should review the original document.

14.4   EVOLUTION OF CODES OF ETHICS

Radiation medicine—and the medical physics associated with it—are evolving disciplines, and the development of new techniques and new procedures may bring about new issues that were unheard of when the original Codes were developed. Consequently, a Code of Ethics must, of necessity, be an evolving document. An example of such new technology is the application of artificial intelligence (AI) in reviewing and interpreting radiological images. In 2019, the question of the ethical use of AI in radiology was addressed by a joint committee of several professional organizations that had connections to radiology, including the ACR and the AAPM.[3] Several topics were brought up including ethics of data, algorithms, and practice, encouraging the various organizations in the radiology community to incorporate issues related to AI into their Codes of Ethics.

14.5   QUESTIONS, EXERCISES, & PROBLEMS

14-1. Identify places in the hospital where one must be extra cautious not to discuss patient information.

14-2. Identify some ways in which patient information can be secured on a computer.

14-3. What patient information can be considered protected health information?

14-4. Present some arguments for and against including an EDI (equity, diversity, inclusion) clause in a Code of Ethics.

14.6   REFERENCES

1. U.S. Department of Health and Human Services. Summary of the HIPAA Privacy Rule. https://www.hhs.gov/hipaa/for-professionals/privacy/laws-regulations/index.html. Accessed October 8, 2019.
2. Skourou C, Sherouse G, Bahar N, et al. Code of ethics for the American Association of Physicists in Medicine(Revised): Report of Task Group 109. *Med. Phys.* 2019; 46(4): e79-e93.
3. Geis JR, Brady AP, Wu CC, et al. Ethics of Artificial Intelligence in Radiology: Summary of the Joint European and North American Multisociety Statement. *J Am Coll of Radiology.* 2019; 16(11): 1516-1521. https://doi.org/10.1016/j.jacr.2019.07.028.

Production of Ionizing Radiation

CONTENTS

Ionizing radiation is the basis for radiation therapy. Consequently, it is important to understand how ionizing radiation is produced. The purpose of this chapter, then, is to describe the production of ionizing radiation that is used for radiation therapy. Three requirements for radiation used in external-beam radiation therapy are that the radiation is sufficiently penetrating to reach the intended target, that the radiation field is relatively uniform over a region of up to 25 cm (although this requirement is often relaxed for x-ray beams), and that the shape of the field can be controlled so that only the tumor receives radiation. The first of these requirements is met by carefully selecting the energy of the radiation beam. The second requirement can be met either by the use of filters designed to flatten the beam or by the use of a scanned beam. The final requirement can be met either by the use of collimators to limit the lateral spread of the beam or by the use of a scanned beam.

Although high-energy x-rays are the most common form of radiation used in external-beam radiation therapy, we will begin our discussion of production of ionizing radiation with electrons. The reason for this is that x-rays are produced from accelerated electrons, so the first component of an x-ray generator is the mechanism for electron production. In addition, we will address the production of heavy charged particles such as protons and carbon ions. The chapter will continue with the production of neutrons and conclude with information regarding the production of radiation from teletherapy sources. A discussion of the production of radiation from brachytherapy sources will be deferred to the chapter on brachytherapy.

15.1 PRODUCTION OF ELECTRON BEAMS

The requirement for producing electron beams used in radiation medicine (diagnosis and therapy) is that the beams be in the energy range of 10 keV to 50 MeV. The lower energies are used for producing x-rays used in diagnostic radiology, while the

DOI: 10.1201/9781003477457-15

higher energies are used either directly for radiation treatment or for producing x-rays used in radiation treatment. Consequently, we need to generate electrons, give them sufficient energy to make them useful, then do something with them, either create a therapeutic electron beam or generate x-rays. The generation of an x-ray beam will be addressed in the next section.

Electrons are initially produced by heating a wire filament until the electrons are "boiled off". The electron source is a thin metal wire with a high melting point. Tungsten meets these specifications in that it can be drawn into thin wires and has a melting point of 3370 °C. The filament is heated by means of an electric current of several amperes. This filament current is sufficient to produce electrons, which can then be accelerated to the desired energy.

Several methods exist for accelerating the electrons. For electrons used to produce x-rays with energies useful for diagnostic imaging, the most common device is the vacuum tube invented by WD Coolidge in 1916. A schematic of a Coolidge tube is shown in Figure (15.1).[1] Electrons are produced at the filament cathode C, and given energy by accelerating them through a potential difference between the cathode and the anode A. They strike a target T, producing x-rays, which are emitted through a window W. The Coolidge tube is practical for production of x-rays with energies up to around 250 keV. At higher energies, the potential difference between the anode and cathode is sufficiently high that safety issues arise. Consequently, alternative means must be used to accelerate electrons to energies useful for radiation therapy. Unlike a Coolidge tube, which accelerates a continuous stream of electrons, most higher-energy electron accelerators produce an electron beam consisting of clumps of electrons.

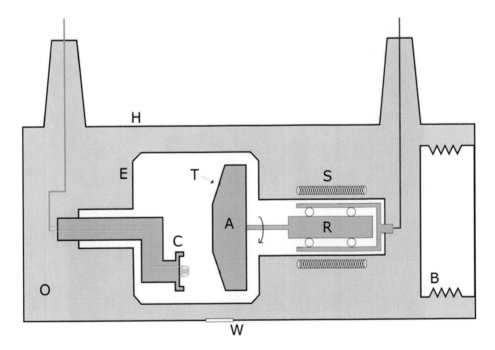

FIGURE 15.1: Schematic of a Coolidge Tube. (Open Source.)

An early device used to accelerate electrons was the betatron, developed in 1935 by Steenbeck and brought into use by Kerst in the 1940s. Electrons are injected into a doughnut-shaped ring in synchrony with a time-varying magnetic field, which accelerates the electrons. Betatrons typically accelerated electrons to energies in the range 2 MeV to 45 MeV, appropriate for radiation therapy. However, because of the relatively low electron fluence, resulting in a low dose rate, the use of betatrons in the clinic has largely been superseded by the use of linear accelerators. The linear accelerator (linac) has become a major source of high-energy electrons and x-rays for clinical applications. Linacs typically produce beams with energies in the range of 6 MeV to 25 MeV. Higher dose rates from a linac have resulted in shorter treatment times than those that were achievable with previous electron accelerators.

A typical linac consists of four parts: a DC power section, a microwave power section, an accelerator, and a treatment head. The DC power section produces pulses of DC power. These pulses are shaped in the pulse-forming network of the modulator and delivered to an electron gun and microwave power section at the proper frequency using a high-voltage switching device (the thyratron). In a manner similar to that by which electrons gain energy from microwaves, the microwave power can be amplified by the deposition of electron kinetic energy of electrons, grouped in "buncher" cavities arrive in "catcher" cavities at the cavities' resonant frequencies. The microwave power section then transmits the amplified microwaves to the accelerator guide. Figure (15.2) is a photograph of a typical linear accelerator used in radiation therapy.

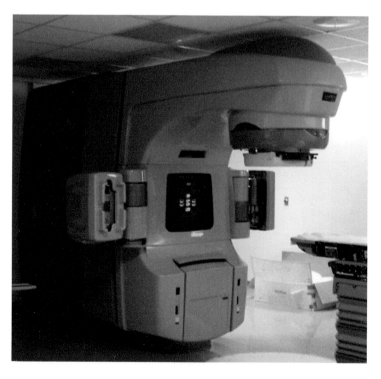

FIGURE 15.2: A typical linear accelerator used in radiation therapy.

The accelerator guide is a cylindrical tube in which electrons, injected by the electron gun, are accelerated by the amplified microwaves. The microwave cavities are configured so that the microwaves phase velocity is matched to the velocity of the electrons traveling through the guide. The accelerated electrons exit the waveguide and enter the treatment head. The treatment head contains the beam shaping, steering, and control components of the linear accelerator. These components are the bending magnet, the scattering foils, dose monitoring chambers, and beam collimation system.

The electrons accelerated in the linac are emitted with a spectrum of energies, so it is necessary to select the energy desired to produce the therapeutic beam. Energy selection is achieved by means of one or more magnets that bend the electron beam and separate the energy components of the electron spectrum.

In the presence of electric and magnetic fields, the force acting on a charge q moving with velocity $\vec{v}$ is given by

$$\vec{F} = q(\vec{E} + \vec{v} \times \vec{B}) \,. \tag{15.1}$$

While the electric field can possibly speed up, slow down, or change the direction of the velocity vector, the magnetic field can at most supply a centripetal force that can try to move the charge along a circular arc. The bending magnet is designed so that the magnetic field is perpendicular to the direction of motion of the electrons. The force magnitude acting on an electron moving through the magnet can then be written as

$$F = evB \,. \tag{15.2}$$

Since the force is perpendicular to the velocity the resulting motion must be circular. Therefore, setting this force equal to the electron mass times the centripetal acceleration,

$$F = m \frac{v^2}{r} \,, \tag{15.3}$$

gives us an expression for the radius of the electron path:

$$r = \frac{mv}{eB} \,. \tag{15.4}$$

Because the radius of the electron's circular path is a function of the electron's energy, by selecting an exit portal corresponding to the desired energy, electrons of that energy are allowed to exit the treatment head.

The electrons exit the bending magnet in a narrow beam. If the linac is to produce an x-ray treatment beam, then the electrons are made incident on a tungsten block immediately after leaving the bending magnet. Collisions between the electrons and the tungsten nuclei will then result in Bremsstrahlung x-ray emission, as discussed in §9.3 and in the next section. However, for treatment with an electron beam, the tungsten block is moved out of the way so the electron beam can continue farther down into the head of the linac.

The narrow electron beam must be broadened in order to generate a therapeutically useful beam. The generation of a beam with uniform fluence is accomplished either by scanning the electron beam using a set of magnets or by passing the beam through scattering foils. In the earlier days of linacs, scanned beam broadening was utilized in some linacs, but presently scattering foils are much more common. The primary foil serves to broaden the narrow incident electron beam by means of electron scattering within the foil; the beam then appears to diverge from a virtual source point as it emerges from the foil. The non-uniform shape of the secondary foil then serves to flatten the profile of the electron beam. The beam then passes through a monitoring chamber, which is a transmission ionization chamber that monitors the dose rate and beam symmetry and is finally collimated to generate a field of a desired shape and size using fixed and moveable collimators, normally made of lead. Figure (15.3) illustrates the interior of the treatment head of an accelerator with a set of dual scattering foils and an electron cone or applicator used for collimation.

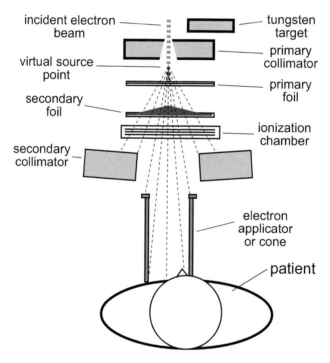

FIGURE 15.3: A schematic of the interior of the head of a linear accelerator showing the primary and secondary scattering foils used to broaden and flatten the electron beam along with an electron applicator or cone used to help collimate the beam near the patient's surface. The tungsten target is moved into the path of the incident electrons if an x-ray beam is desired (see Fig. 13.1).

15.2 PRODUCTION OF X-RAY BEAMS

The basic principle behind the production of x-ray beams for either diagnostic or therapeutic applications is that, when a charged particle decelerates, energy is emitted in the form of electromagnetic radiation. This radiation is called "Bremsstrahlung", or "braking radiation" and is produced in the clinic by having high-energy electrons, produced in one of the methods described in the previous section, striking a metal target. Bremsstrahlung was discussed earlier in §9.3.

The efficiency of Bremsstrahlung production increases as the energy of the incident electron increases. For electrons with energies in the vicinity of 100 keV, the efficiency of Bremsstrahlung production is approximately 0.4%, with most of the rest of the electron energy being converted into heat. Furthermore, the efficiency of Bremsstrahlung production increases with the atomic number Z of the target. Consequently, the target (anode) of the x-ray tube has to be a material with high Z, high melting point, and high specific heat, so that the temperature rise is not significant. Most anodes in x-ray tubes nowadays are made of tungsten embedded in copper. Tungsten has a high atomic number ($Z = 74$) and the highest melting point of all metals (3422 °C). By embedding the target in copper, one takes advantage of the copper to draw excess heat away from the tungsten. Furthermore, anodes in most x-ray tubes are circular in shape, with the tungsten target embedded as a ring in the copper target. The anode then rotates rapidly so that the electron beam strikes each part of the tungsten for only a short period of time. Even so, x-ray tubes typically require external cooling, and care must be used in monitoring the workload of the x-ray tube to prevent breakdown of the target. At higher energies, the production of Bremsstrahlung is much more efficient, and no special cooling mechanism is required.

The x-rays produced in an x-ray tube exhibit a spectrum of energies decreasing linearly from zero energy to the energy of the incident electrons. However, the low-energy component of the x-ray spectrum is not useful from either a diagnostic or therapeutic point of view, because these x-rays are absorbed in superficial tissue, delivering x-ray dose to the superficial tissue, and never reaching either the tumor or an image receptor. Consequently, some means is required to filter out the low-energy component of the x-ray spectrum. Some of the x-rays are filtered by the x-ray tube itself (inherent filtration); more lower-energy x-rays are filtered out by the use of external filters. Figure (15.4) illustrates a typical Bremsstrahlung spectrum, both with and without filtration. The filter of choice is usually aluminum for incident electron energies around 100 keV , whereas copper filtration is often used for higher energies (around 250 keV).

For lower x-ray energies, x-ray production is isotropic, and the useful x-rays are emitted at approximately a 90° angle from the incident electron beam, whereas for higher energies, Bremsstrahlung production is primarily in the forward direction. Because the x-ray beam emanating from a transmission target is highly peaked in the forward direction, a flattening filter is used to selectively absorb the higher-intensity center of the beam. The flattening filter is simply a cone-shaped attenuator (see Fig. 15.5). In recent years, with the advent of intensity-modulated radiation therapy (IMRT), the need for a flat beam is no longer necessary, and flattening filter free (FFF) linear accelerators are becoming more common. These have the advantage of eliminating the lower-energy scattered radiation emanating from x-ray interactions inside the flattening filter.

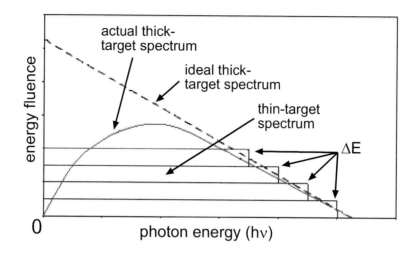

FIGURE 15.4: Filtered and unfiltered Bremsstrahlung spectra.

Next, the x-ray beam needs to be collimated. Collimators were discussed previously in Chapter 13. (See Fig. 13.1.)

Contemporary therapy machines allow a great deal of flexibility of motion in order to be able to precisely and reproducibly irradiate a target from many directions. Recall that this ability is necessary to ensure adequate sparing of uninvolved tissue. The key to this flexibility is the definition of an isocenter. The isocenter is the intersection of the axes of rotation of the gantry, the collimators, and the treatment support unit (the "couch"). In addition to its rotational motion in a plane parallel to the floor of the treatment room as well as three degrees of translational motion, some couches offer an additional two degrees of freedom of rotational motion, in planes perpendicular to the floor of the treatment room.

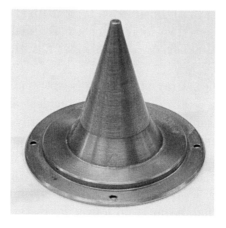

FIGURE 15.5: Example of a flattening filter used in a linear accelerator. (Photo courtesy of Jay Burmeister.)

15.3   PRODUCTION OF HEAVY CHARGED PARTICLES

In this section, we discuss the production of heavy charged-particle beams. In present-day radiation therapy, the overwhelming number of heavy charged-particle beams are proton beams. Consequently, this section will deal primarily with proton-beam production. Much of what is described here, however, is applicable to the production of other heavy charged particles, such as carbon ions.

Although a proton beam can be produced in a linear accelerator using the same principles as was previously discussed in terms of electrons, much more common are accelerators in which the charged particles traverse a circular path while being accelerated. The two major types of circular accelerator are the cyclotron and the synchrotron. The cyclotron produces a proton beam of a single fixed energy; the energy incident on the patient surface is adjusted using a range modulator placed in the machine head to absorb some of the beam energy. The energy of the protons ejected from the synchrotron can be varied, so no range modulator is needed. Instead, spot scanning can be used in which magnetic steering and energy selection is used to move the Bragg peak through the target volume.

As we discussed earlier in Eq. (15.4), charged particles in a magnetic field applied in a direction perpendicular to the plane of motion will move in a curved path with a radius given by

$$r = \frac{mv}{qB},\tag{15.5}$$

where m is the mass of the particle and q is the magnitude of its charge. In a cyclotron, the protons accelerate in two D-shaped electrodes, referred to as "dees", with a high-frequency alternating voltage applied between them. The magnetic field within the dees causes the charged particles to move in a circular arc, while the voltage difference between the two dees results in an electric field that causes the charges to speed up in that region. The result is that the charges will spiral with increasing radius until they leave the accelerating cavity with the desired energy.

Unlike the cyclotron, the synchrotron accelerates protons in spills using a time-dependent magnetic field that is synchronized to the radiofrequency wave that produces the spills. The particles are first accelerated using a linac to several MeV, then injected into the synchrotron and accelerated to the desired energy before being extracted.

Typically, these accelerators have a small duty cycle, that is, the clinical proton beam is directed toward the patient a small fraction of the time the patient is in the treatment room. As a consequence, the beam from a single accelerator can be steered into several treatment rooms, making for more efficient use of the accelerator.

15.4   PRODUCTION OF NEUTRONS

Neutrons, being neutrally-charged particles, cannot be accelerated in an electric or magnetic field. Consequently, neutrons in the therapeutic range of energies must be produced by interactions involving high-energy charged particles. In particular, one of the most common methods of producing neutrons for radiation therapy is by accelerating deuterons or protons in a cyclotron and allowing them to impinge on a beryllium target. In order to produce a neutron beam with sufficient energy to be penetrating, the energy of the incident deuterons or protons must be greater than 50 MeV.

Neutron production from deuteron bombardment of beryllium is a stripping process. Deuterons are accelerated to a high energy and then impinge on a ^{9}Be target. A proton is stripped from the deuteron and added to the Be nucleus producing ^{10}B. The recoil neutron retains some of the incident kinetic energy of the accelerated deuterons. In addition, some gamma rays are produced. The neutron beam consists of recoil neutrons with a spectrum of energies. The spectrum consists of a single peak with a modal value of about 40% of the energy of incident deuterons. Examples of neutron spectra are illustrated in Fig. (15.6).

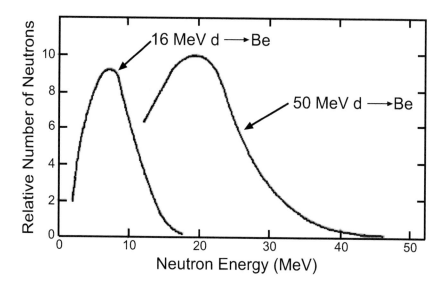

FIGURE 15.6: Neutron spectra produced by 16 MeV and 50 MeV deuterons incident on beryllium.

Neutron production from proton bombardment of beryllium is a knock-out process in which protons are accelerated to a high energy and then impinge on a 9Be target. A neutron is knocked out from the beryllium target to form ^{9}B, producing a neutron beam as well as some gamma rays. In this case, the neutron spectrum is broad, ranging in energy from zero energy to the energy of the incident proton. Figure (15.7) illustrates two neutron spectra resulting from proton bombardment of beryllium. The dashed line is an unfiltered spectrum that was produced from protons accelerated to 43 *MeV*. This spectrum spans a wide range of energies from zero up to the energy of the incident protons. The low-energy neutrons in this spectrum are not penetrating enough for therapy and would cause severe skin reaction. These low-energy neutrons must thus be filtered-out.

A low-Z material such as polyethylene can be used to filter the beam. Polyethylene contains a long chain of hydrocarbons, consequently, there is a large amount of hydrogen to remove the low-energy component. Elastic scatter is the dominant process for lower energy fast neutrons and nuclei with lower mass are more effective on a "per collision" basis for slowing down neutrons. Therefore, a low-Z material like polyethylene, which consists of a long chain of hydrocarbons, would reduce the energy of these neutrons to thermal energies. But, just using polyethylene might just make the problem worse because the beam would have even more low-energy neutrons. However, if the polyethylene were doped with a material like boron, which has a high thermal neutron cross section, it would effectively remove the thermalized neutrons from the beam achieving an overall harder spectrum, as is shown by the solid line in Fig. (15.7). Consequently, it is very likely that boronated polyethylene was used to filter the beam.

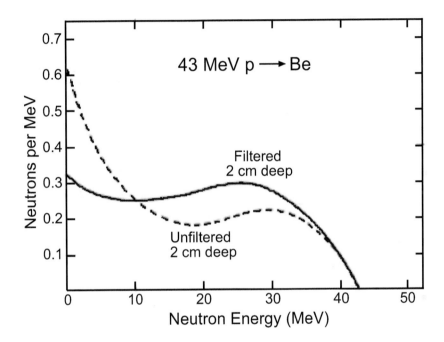

FIGURE 15.7: Neutron spectra from p-Be interactions. Note the reduction in thermal (lower energy) neutrons in the filtered spectrum.

Collimation of neutrons is somewhat more complicated than collimation of x-rays or charged particles. One first uses a hydrogenous material, such as polyethylene, to slow down the neutrons. Material with a high thermal neutron cross section then absorbs the thermal neutrons. Finally, a high atomic number material absorbs the gamma-ray photons produced by neutron activation.

15.5 TELETHERAPY SOURCES

In the early days of radiation therapy, ^{226}Ra was used as a teletherapy source. It has a long half-life (1620 years), so no source replacement is ever required. It is an alpha emitter, decaying to ^{222}Rn, which is also an alpha emitter. Several daughter products in secular equilibrium with ^{226}Ra emit gamma rays yielding a spectrum with maximum energy of around 2 MeV, eventually resulting in stable ^{206}Pb. This energy of gamma rays, although not optimal, provided better penetration than the orthovoltage therapy machines that were available at that time.

^{226}Ra has some serious disadvantages, however. The ^{222}Rn daughter product is a radioactive gas, hence source leakage is a significant issue, especially since the leakage is a radioactive gas. ^{226}Ra also has a relatively low specific activity (1 curie/gram, originally used as the definition of the curie), consequently treatment times using ^{226}Ra were inordinately long. Finally, ^{226}Ra was very expensive, costing in the vicinity of \$50,000/gram in the 1950s.

Fortunately, in the years immediately after World War II, nuclear reactors were developed that allowed the production of ^{60}Co as a radiation therapy source. ^{60}Co decays via beta decay to an excited state of ^{60}Ni, which, in decaying to its ground state, emits two gamma rays, one at 1.17 MeV, the other at 1.33 MeV. Coupled with a high specific activity (1100 curie/gram), the decay of ^{60}Co yields a radiation beam that is significantly more intense that that emitted by ^{226}Ra. Perhaps the only disadvantage of ^{60}Co is its half-life of 5.3 years, which means that the source activity decreases by about 1% each month. Corrections must be made to the output of the machine, and sources must typically be replaced every five years. An advantage of ^{60}Co over a linac is the relative simplicity of the radiation production, thus requiring less resources for continued maintenance than a linac.

15.6 QUESTIONS, EXERCISES, & PROBLEMS

15-1. The basic structure of a linac (linear accelerator) used in the clinic is described in this chapter. Do your own research on the structure of a linac. Then make a schematic diagram of a linac, from the production of pulses of DC power through the bending magnets, labeling the various structures in your sketch. Finally, write a brief description of the function of each labeled structure in your sketch.

15-2. Figure (15.5) shows a flattening filter used in the production of an x-ray treatment beam by a linac. (a) What does the flattening filter flatten? (b) Why is this an important thing to do?

15-3. A linac is used to produce 5 *MeV* electrons. The path of the electrons is bent into a circular arc by a magnetic field of strength 0.7 *tesla* (0.7 *T*) produced by the bending magnets in the head of the gantry. After moving around the circular arc, the electrons are incident on a tungsten target, resulting in the production of x-rays. (a) Why are x-rays produced when the electrons are incident on the tungsten target? (b) What is the radius of the arc of the electron path while the electrons move in the magnetic field of the bending magnets? (*Hint:* Are these electrons relativistic? See Chapter 4.)

15-4. The topic of *filters* was addressed in different contexts in this chapter, notably in the discussion of x-ray Bremsstrahlung spectra and neutron spectra. The purpose of the filtration in each case was to filter out the lower-energy radiation particles. (a) Why is it often desirable to filter out the lower energy particles when treating cancer patients with radiation? (b) What is used to filter out the lower-energy x-rays in a

Bremsstrahlung spectrum? Why is this used? (c) What is used to filter out the lower energy neutrons in a neutron spectrum? Why is this used?

15-5. Figure 15.3 shows a schematic of the interior of the head of a linac (or gantry head) for electron beam treatment, while Fig. (13.1) shows a schematic for an x-ray treatment set-up. How are the gantry-head set-ups similar and how are they different? Explain the reasons for the differences. (Why must the electron beam set-up differ from the x-ray beam set-up?)

15-6. (a) What is meant by "teletherapy"? (b) Compare and contrast the use of ^{226}Ra and ^{60}Co as teletherapy sources. Which, if either, of these sources is used to teletherapy today? Why?

15-7. This problem addresses two radiation-related events that actually occurred. (a) Approximately 50 yr ago, a physicist, instead of measuring the output of a Co-60 source before treating a patient as required, only estimated the decay of the source to save time. The physicist knew the decay constant for Co-60. Unfortunately, he treated the Co-60 source as having a linear decay rather than the correct exponential decay behavior. Assuming that the initial source activity he had recorded 6 months earlier was correct, estimate the error in patient dosage after 6 months. Were patients overdosed or underdosed? (b) Suppose that a linear accelerator were set to deliver a dose of x-rays, but the tungsten target was not in place, meaning that the patient was treated with an electron beam instead of the corresponding x-ray beam. Estimate the error in patient dosage because of the absence of the target. (For more details on these and other radiation-related accidents, refer to https://journals.sagepub.com/doi/pdf/10.1016/S0146-6453(01)00039-2 or search online for "Case Histories of Major Accidental Exposures in Radiotherapy".)

15.7 REFERENCES

1. By wikipedia User:ChumpusRex. This file is licensed under the Creative Commons Attribution-Share Alike 3.0 Unported license. https://commons.wikimedia.org/w/index.php?curid=1433630.

Energy Absorption and Dosimetry

CONTENTS

Perhaps in no branch of medicine other than radiation medicine is accurate measurement as crucial. When prescribing a drug, one often sees dosage expressed as "one or two tablets", indicating an acceptable variation of 100%; in delivering radiation to a tumor, a variation of greater than 5% in dose is not only clinically detectable but can mean the difference between controlling or not controlling a tumor as well as overdosing and causing long-term damage to a critical structure. Because of this tight restriction on dose accuracy, it is important to define terms describing radiation quantity very precisely.

In this chapter, we will define terms related to radiation quantity, both on a microscopic level as well as a macroscopic level. Microscopic quantities describe what is going on at an atomic level while macroscopic quantities are quantities that can be measured. We will also relate the microscopic quantities to corresponding macroscopic quantities. In addition to defining the quantities, we shall also define the units related to these quantities.

It should be noted that some of the discussions in this chapter repeat some of the ideas and definitions presented in Chapter 2. These discussions are fundamental to the topics in clinical medical physics covered in the upcoming chapters, so they bear repeating within the context of this chapter. The notation used in this chapter is that recommended by Report No. 85 of the International Commission on Radiation Units and Measurements.[1]

16.1   RADIOMETRIC QUANTITIES

The first microscopic quantity that we shall define is the *particle number* N. N is simply the number of particles either emitted, transferred, or received. By "particles"

DOI: 10.1201/9781003477457-16

we can mean charged particles, uncharged particles, or photons. The particle number is a dimensionless quantity.

Let us consider a monoenergetic beam of particles. Each of the N particles in a beam carries kinetic energy E. We exclude rest energy for this energy definition. Consequently, R, the *radiant energy* of the beam, is given by $R = NE$. The unit of radiant energy is the joule [J].

A radiation beam consists of moving particles. The quantity that tells us how many particles are moving past a point is the *particle flux* $\dot{N}$. The particle flux is given by $\dot{N} = dN/dt$, where dN is the increment of particle number per unit time dt. The unit for particle flux is the number per unit time $[s^{-1}]$. (Note that we are using the standard dot notation for time derivatives—be very careful of this notation as the dots are easy to miss! Likewise, be careful when you are writing these equations to ensure that the dots are easily visible.)

The beam carries energy. The *energy flux* $\dot{R}$ tells us how much energy is carried by the beam per unit time. The energy flux is given by $\dot{R} = dR/dt$, where dR is the increment of radiant energy per unit time dt. The unit of energy flux is the energy per unit time $[Js^{-1}]$.

Even more useful than the number of particles carried per unit time and the energy transport of these particles are the measures of intensity of the beam, where we look at the number of particles and their energy per unit area. The *particle fluence* Φ is a measure of number of particles per unit area. Specifically, $\Phi = dN/da$, where dN is the number of particles incident on a sphere of cross-sectional area da. The unit of particle fluence is the number per unit area $[m^{-2}]$. In the definition of particle fluence we define the cross-sectional area so that the radiation beam is always *perpendicular* to great circle of area da. We differentiate below the particle fluence from a related quantity, the planar fluence.

As indicated earlier, the particle beam carries energy. The quantity that is a measure of the intensity of the beam as determined by the energy carried by the beam is the *energy fluence* Ψ, given by $\Psi = dR/da$, where dR equals the energy incident on a sphere of cross-sectional area da. The unit of energy fluence is the energy per unit area $[Jm^{-2}]$.

We have defined the energy fluence and energy flux for a monoenergetic beam. However, most radiation beams are polyenergetic with a spectrum of energies. To obtain the energy fluence and the energy flux for a polyenergetic beam, one weights each energy component by the number of particles at each energy.

Combining flux and fluence gives us the *particle fluence rate* $\dot{\Phi}$ given by $\dot{\Phi} = d\Phi/dt$ and the *energy fluence rate* $\dot{\Psi}$ given by $\dot{\Psi} = d\Psi/dt$. The unit for particle fluence rate is the number per unit area per unit time $[m^{-2}s^{-1}]$, whereas the unit for energy is the energy per unit area per unit time $[Jm^{-2}s^{-1}]$.

It should be noted that in disciplines other than radiation physics, the energy fluence has been called the flux and the fluence rate has been called the particle flux density. The International Commission on Radiation Units and Measurements (ICRU), which sets measurement standards in radiation medicine, advises against using those terms.

In defining fluence we look at the number of particles incident on a sphere, but we can also define a quantity, the *planar fluence*, as the number of particles crossing a fixed plane in either direction per unit area of the plane. Figure (16.1) illustrates how planar fluence differs from particle fluence. Consider a case in which we have a beam that is incident on both a sphere of some diameter and a circle of the same diameter. In the left part of the figure, the number of photons crossing the sphere is the same as the number of photons crossing the circle. In the right part of the figure, the beam has been scattered. As a result, a greater number of photons crosses the sphere, whereas the same number of photons crosses the circle. So, even though the planar fluence remains the same, the fluence has increased; consequently the dose delivered to the sphere, which is related to the fluence, will be greater. This exercise demonstrates how the fluence behind an attenuating layer can be greater than the fluence incident on the layer.

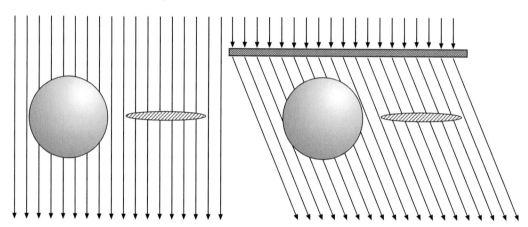

FIGURE 16.1: An illustration of how planar fluence can differ from fluence after a beam is scattered. (Left) A sphere and a circular planar area having the same radius as the sphere are in a radiation field that is uniform and perpendicular to the planar area. The fluence through the sphere is the same as the planar fluence through the circle. (Right) A uniform, planar, non-absorbing scattering medium is now placed above the sphere and circle and perpendicular to the incident radiation, all else being the same. The scattering medium scatters the incident radiation through some fixed angle. The fluence through the sphere is now greater than the planar fluence through the circle, which has remained unchanged.

16.2 DOSIMETRIC QUANTITIES

So far, we have looked solely at microscopic radiometric quantities such as fluence and flux. These quantities are important in order to understand the nature of radiation interactions; however, direct measurement of these quantities can be very difficult. Moreover, we would like to relate them to clinically relevant quantities that we can eventually correlate with cellular and tissue damage.

In order to define a set of dosimetric quantities, we must first recognize the difference between directly ionizing radiation and indirectly ionizing radiation. Ionizing radiation can be divided into these two categories: directly ionizing radiation and indirectly ionizing radiation. Directly ionizing radiation includes all charged particles. These particles interact with electrons through long-range Coulombic charged-particle interactions, and deliver energy to matter directly. Indirectly ionizing radiation include x-rays, gamma rays, and neutrons, all of which are uncharged particles. They will typically interact via a transfer of energy to a single charged particle, and it is the secondary charged particle that delivers much of the energy to the absorbing material. Because both primary and secondary radiation deliver energy to the absorbing material, the macroscopic definition of energy transfer is made considerably more complicated.

Exposure

Some of the earliest attempts at defining dosimetric quantities were based on the unit of measurement. For example, exposure was initially defined to be the number of roentgens, an early unit of measurement of exposure. However, this is not a rigorous way to define a quantity. The definition of a physical quantity must be based on the actual physical phenomenon that is taking place. The first such dosimetric quantity defined in this manner is the exposure.

The formal definition of *exposure* is the absolute value of the total charge of ions of one sign produced in a small mass of air when all electrons liberated by the photons in that mass of air are completely stopped in air, divided by the mass of the air within which the electrons were released. Mathematically speaking, we say that the exposure X is given by

$$X = \frac{dQ}{dm},\tag{16.1}$$

where dQ is the charge produced in a small mass of air and dm is the mass of air.

Let's clarify some of the points made in the definition of exposure. First, the definition speaks of the "absolute value of the total charge of ions of one sign". Because we are dealing with neutral atoms and molecules as targets, the total charge is going to be zero. Consequently, to define exposure we are only going to look at ions of one sign and we are going to look at the total charge of these ions.

Next, we say that the ions are "produced in a small mass of air". Because ionizing events are stochastic (random), we cannot base a definition on a single ionizing event. We need to look at a mass of air that is large enough to have a reasonable number of interactions in order to obtain a mean value, yet small enough so that its location in space can be unambiguously defined.

The final part of the definition of exposure reads "all electrons liberated by photons in air are completely stopped in air". This is perhaps the trickiest part of the definition of exposure. In order to understand this phrase we need to look at what happens when a photon ionizes a target. The photon comes in and interacts with a target atom or molecule and produces an electron. The electron that is produced travels beyond the point of the interaction and causes additional ionizations to take place. So we also have to look a little bit downstream of the initial interaction to follow that electron. We not only have to count the ionization that takes place at the point where the photon interacts, but we also have to somehow count all of the ionizations that take place because of the production of secondary electrons downstream. That causes a lot of issues in how we are going to measure exposure.

We need to look at the initial ionization in a small volume of air, and we need to look at all of the subsequent secondary ionizations produced by that first ionization that take place until that electron gives up all of its energy through ionization processes. Then we divide the number of ionizations by the mass of air because we want an intensive property, that is, one that is independent of the amount of air present. If we have more air, more ionizations will take place. We do not want to say there is more exposure because there is more air so we divide the number of ionizations by the mass of air.

Charged-Particle Equilibrium (CPE)

This definition of exposure causes some limitations. First, exposure is only defined in air. Moreover, it is only defined for photons (x rays and gamma rays). Finally, it is only defined for photons of energies less than approximately 3 MeV. This number appears arbitrary, so some explanation is needed. There is no way to tell the difference between primary and secondary electrons. If we define a volume in which we measure exposure and detect an electron outside this volume, we have no way of knowing whether the electron is a primary or a secondary electron. We can only count the electron in the measurement of exposure if it is a secondary electron produced by an ionization that took place in the defined volume.

In order to get around this issue, we need to introduce the concept of charged-particle equilibrium, *CPE*. CPE exists if the energy deposited by charged particles produced inside a volume is equal to energy deposited by charged particles produced outside the volume and deposited inside the volume. When CPE exists, it is necessary only to measure ionizations inside the volume. CPE exists in most practical measurement situations, but two examples of the violation of CPE occur near radiation sources, where a fluence gradient exists, and near the interface of two different absorbing materials, where there may be a difference in the amount of scatter from one medium to another.

Back to the definition of exposure, for higher-energy photon beams, we would need a volume of dimension around three to four meters for CPE to exist. A room-sized device for measuring radiation quantity would not be practical, nor would it be easy to generate a uniform field of photons of that size. Consequently, once we get beyond an energy of around 3 MeV, it no longer becomes practical to measure exposure, so exposure is not defined beyond that energy.

The ICRU has determined that there be no special unit of exposure. Because exposure is defined to be an amount of charge per unit mass, its units would be $[C\,kg^{-1}]$. An older unit still in use (but not recommended) is the *roentgen* [R], defined such that

$$1\,R = 2.58 \times 10^{-4}\,C\,kg^{-1}. \tag{16.2}$$

The definition of the roentgen was based on an older set of units: the roentgen is equal to $1\,esu$ (an older unit of charge) per cm^3 of air at standard temperature and pressure (STP).

Kerma

The next dosimetric quantity we shall consider is the *kerma*. Kerma, which is actually an acronym for "kinetic energy released in matter", is a quantity that replaced exposure as a dosimetric quantity. Kerma is defined as

$$K = \frac{dE_K}{dm},\tag{16.3}$$

where dE_K is the sum of the initial kinetic energies of all the charged particles liberated by uncharged ionizing particles in material of mass dm.

In order to understand the significance of kerma, it will be necessary to follow the transfer of energy as radiation interacts with matter. A photon interacts with absorbing materials in one of several ways, as discussed in Chapter 8. The photon deposits energy into the target and this energy is used to ionize the target atoms and produce secondary radiation. In determining kerma, we do not look at the secondary radiation and only look at the energy deposited in the initial interaction.

Notice that we are now addressing a local phenomenon. We are not interested in how the secondary electron deposits energy downstream. Nor are we interested in the ionizing events that follow this initial photon interaction. We do not have to track the electron until it deposits all of its kinetic energy in the absorber. We also do not need to be concerned with where the electron is going. All we are interested in is how much kinetic energy the electron has as a result of the immediate interaction with the photon.

Because we are talking about a local phenomenon, we do not need to worry about charged particle equilibrium. We do not have to worry about whether or not we are in air. We could be in any type of material, although there is a specific quantity that we call air kerma, which will be discussed shortly. The concept of kerma has much more generality than the concept of exposure.

The unit of kerma is the unit of energy per unit of mass. The unit of energy is the *joule*, so the unit of kerma is the *joule per kilogram*. Because kerma is important in radiation studies, SI has given kerma its own unit, the *gray* [Gy], defined to be *one joule per kilogram*: $1\,Gy = 1\,J/kg$.

What are the limitations of kerma? There aren't any. Kerma is defined in all absorbing materials; kerma is defined for any kind of *uncharged* ionizing radiation. That might be considered a limitation. We do not talk about kerma for charged radiation, only for uncharged x-rays, gamma rays and neutrons. Kerma is defined at all energies and it can be measured in any way one pleases to measure it. As long the kinetic energy of the electrons that are given off can be measured then one can measure kerma.

A very important quantity related to kerma is *air kerma*. Air kerma is the kerma in a mass of air when radiation interacts with air. This is what we use to quantify, for example, the strength of a radiation source that we use for brachytherapy. The easiest way to measure air kerma is to measure exposure. Multiply the exposure, which is the charge—proportional to the number of electrons—per unit mass of air, by the energy transferred to the medium per ionization, and make the units make sense using conversion factors. It is important, however, to correct for re-radiation, when the secondary electrons can cause production of tertiary photons. We'll deal with that at a later time, although in many cases re-radiation can be ignored, especially when we are dealing with high-energy incident photons.

Example 16.1: Air Kerma and Exposure

Calculate the air kerma that corresponds to an exposure of $1\,R$ (one roentgen).

Solution:

By definition, as given in Eq. (16.2), an exposure of $1\,R$ involves the release of $2.58 \times 10^{-4}\,C$ of charge per kilogram of air. First, we must determine how many ion pairs are produced that corresponds to this amount of charge. Since an ion pair (ip) is a released electron and the resulting positive ion, each of which has a charge magnitude of $e = 1.602 \times 10^{-19}\,C$, we see that the charge magnitude of either sign released per ionization is simply equal to e. This can then be used to convert R to units of ip/kg:

$$1\,R = 2.58 \times 10^{-4}\,\frac{C}{kg}\left(\frac{1}{1.602 \times 10^{-19}\,C/ip}\right) = 1.610 \times 10^{15}\,\frac{ip}{kg}. \tag{16.4}$$

But, recalling from Eq. (2.3) that the average energy deposited in air per ionization is $\overline{W}_{air} = 33.97\,eV/ip$, we see that we can further convert the units of R from ip/kg to eV/kg. We thus get that

$$1\,R = 1.610 \times 10^{15}\,\frac{ip}{kg}\left(33.97\,\frac{eV}{ip}\right) = 5.471 \times 10^{16}\,\frac{eV}{kg}. \tag{16.5}$$

Then, using the definition of an electron-volt $(1\,eV = 1.602 \times 10^{-19}\,J)$, we finally get that

$$1\,R = 5.471 \times 10^{16}\,\frac{eV}{kg}\left(\frac{1.602 \times 10^{-19}\,J}{1\,eV}\right) = 8.76 \times 10^{-3}\,\frac{J}{kg}. \tag{16.6}$$

This is the desired result: an exposure of $1\,R$ is equivalent to $8.76 \times 10^{-3}\,J$ of energy being released in air per kilogram of air. Since $1\,J/kg = 1\,Gy$, and since $1\,cGy = 10^{-2}\,Gy$, we get the final result that

$$1\,R = 2.58 \times 10^{-4}\,\frac{C}{kg} = \boxed{0.876\,cGy}. \tag{16.7}$$

$$\boxed{\textit{End of solution to Example 16.1.}}$$

Absorbed Dose

The final quantity on our list of dosimetric quantities is the *absorbed dose*. Absorbed dose is perhaps the most important quantity in radiation medicine because it defines the amount of radiation a patient receives in the course of a medical procedure. It is really the key quantity when we are looking at the clinical effects of radiation.

Absorbed dose is defined to be

$$D = \frac{d\varepsilon}{dm},$$ (16.8)

where in this case $d\varepsilon$ is the mean energy imparted by the ionizing radiation to the absorbing material of mass dm. The energy here is the energy that is actually transferred from the radiation, whatever the radiation is, to the absorbing material. It does not matter here whether radiation due to primary interactions or radiation due to secondary interactions. This is the major difference between dose and kerma. Kerma deals only with primary interactions, whereas dose deals with all the interactions that take place.

The unit of dose is, again, the unit of energy divided by the unit of mass. That is, the joule per kilogram, or the special SI unit, the gray: $1\,Gy = 1\,J/kg$.

Previously we spoke about limitations of the definition of exposure. Let us examine the limitations of the definition of dose. There are none. Dose is defined in all materials; it is defined for any kind of ionizing radiation and is defined at all energies. So whether we're using x-rays, gamma rays, electrons, protons, negative pions or carbon nuclei, whatever it is, in water, in patients, in air, and whatever energy we want, we can always talk about dose.

Measuring dose is another issue because of the need to account for secondary radiation. We will worry about that later on. Measuring dose can be a little tricky, but at least conceptually, we have a relatively rigorous definition for dose.

16.3   INTERACTION COEFFICIENTS AND ENERGY TRANSFER

In order to quantify the interactions of radiation with matter and examine the transfer of energy from the radiation to the target, we need to introduce some quantities that describe interactions. First, let us define what we mean by an interaction. An *interaction* is an event that changes the energy or direction of the incident radiation or both. We will be covering many such interactions in this text. A *cross section*, σ, is defined to be the probability of such an interaction with a target divided by the fluence of the incident radiation. We can write

$$\sigma = \frac{P}{\Phi},$$ (16.9)

where P is the probability of an interaction with a specified target when the target is bombarded with a specified particle fluence Φ. Thus, if we multiply the cross section times the fluence we will wind up with the probability of an interaction. We will be talking about both probabilities of interactions as well as cross sections of interactions. They are very closely related. Because fluence has the units of reciprocal area, the cross section, now defined as the probability of an interaction per unit fluence, has the units of area. High-energy physicists like to use a special unit for cross section called a *barn* [b]: $1\,b = 10^{-24}\,cm^2$.

Attenuation Coefficients

A very important interaction coefficient is the one called the *linear attenuation coefficient*. When we discuss photon interactions, we often use the linear attenuation coefficient. The linear attenuation coefficient, μ, is equal to the fraction of particles that interact over a specified path distance and is determined by the equation

$$\mu = \frac{dN/N}{dl}, \qquad (16.10)$$

where dN/N is the fraction of particles that are interacting, and dl is the path length. The unit of linear attenuation coefficient is the unit of inverse length, fraction per unit length—inverse meters, for example.

However, the number of interactions that are going to take place is an extrinsic property, that is, the number of interactions is directly related to the number of target particles that are available for interaction—in particular, the particle density. We can generate an intrinsic quantity, independent of the particle density, called the *mass attenuation coefficient*, by dividing the linear attenuation coefficient by the particle density, and expressed as μ/ρ. This quantity is more characteristic of the nature of the material than the linear attenuation coefficient. We will be using both mass attenuation coefficients as well as linear attenuation coefficients to describe attenuation of photon beams. The mass attenuation coefficient is the fraction of particles that interact in a density-weighted path length, $\rho\,dl$. The units of mass attenuation coefficient are the units of length squared divided by mass. In SI units that is m^2/kg. Note that the cross section multiplied by the density-weighted path length has the units of mass, which is the dm in the definition of dose. We are going to be using these interaction coefficients as the tool to connect quantities such as particle fluence, for example—how much radiation there is—to dose, which is how much energy is being deposited. Often, we know the particle fluence and we want to determine the dose. A little bit later down the line we will make that connection.

Stopping Powers

In the world of charged particle interactions, we have a quantity that is analogous to linear attenuation coefficient, called the *stopping power*. Stopping power is the energy loss per unit path length for charged particles and is given by

$$S = \frac{dE}{dl}. \qquad (16.11)$$

The units of stopping power are units of energy divided by units of path length, $[J/m]$ in SI units. We also have a density-independent stopping power called the *mass stopping power*, S/ρ. We probably will be using mass stopping power a lot more than we use stopping power. The units of mass stopping power are units of energy times units of length-squared divided by unit of mass, for example, $J\,m^2/kg$. If we want to know how electrons deposit energy in a medium, we connect the electron fluence with the stopping power to get the energy deposition.

In summary, mass attenuation coefficients and mass stopping powers are analogous quantities. The mass attenuation coefficient is used to describe interactions involving photons, whereas the mass stopping power is used to describe interactions involving charged particles, such as electrons and protons. The mass attenuation coefficient is the fraction of photons interacting per density-weighted path length, while the mass stopping power is the energy loss per density-weighted path length. The mass attenuation coefficient connects photon fluence to dose; the mass stopping power connects charged-particle fluence to dose.

Energy Transfer and Energy Absorption

We will now look at energy transfer probabilities, returning to the linear attenuation coefficient. The linear attenuation coefficient is a measure of the probability of an interaction per unit path length, or another way we described was to say it is the fraction of the photons in a beam attenuated per unit path length. Now we shall look at a photon interaction and follow the energy in such an interaction.

Some of the energy of the incident photon could be transferred to the kinetic energy of a secondary electron. Earlier in this chapter, we defined the energy that is transferred to the kinetic energy of the electron to be the kerma. However, depending on the particular interaction, some energy could be transferred to a scattered photon.

Let us look in particular at the energy that is transferred to electrons. This energy transfer is a stochastic, or random, process—for any particular photon interaction at a given energy we have no idea how much energy is going to be transferred to the electron. What we do know is the *probability* of energy transfer. With the knowledge of the probability of energy transfer for each value of energy transfer, we can determine a mean energy transferred to the electrons. We shall denote this mean energy transfer to kinetic energy of the electrons as $\overline{E}_{tr}$. We can then define a quantity called the *energy transfer coefficient, $\overline{\mu}_{tr}$*, which is the mean fraction of energy transferred to kinetic energy of electrons per unit path length. So, if we start out with a beam which has 10 MeV photons and an average of 5 MeV of energy is transferred to kinetic energy of the electrons per centimeter of path length, the energy transfer coefficient is the fraction of energy transferred, 5 divided by 10, or 0.5, per *cm* of path length. Energy transfer coefficients are also tabulated. If we have energy transfer coefficients and we know the energy of the incident photon, we can determine the energy transferred to the kinetic energy of the secondary electrons per unit path length. This quantity may be important if we are trying to follow the energy. If some energy is being transferred to electrons, we want to determine how much. We can do this using the energy transfer coefficient.

We have shown that kinetic energy is transferred to the electrons. What can happen to this kinetic energy? Some of this kinetic energy can be re-radiated as Bremsstrahlung (see Chapter 9). We know that electrons that are moving can interact downstream with nuclei. These interactions will cause the electrons to deflect and give off Bremsstrahlung. Recall that we addressed this earlier when we discussed the production of x-rays when electrons struck a target. The remainder of the energy, the energy that not re-radiated, is absorbed. The amount of energy that is absorbed is called the *collision kerma*.

So, during a photon interaction, the incident photon energy is transformed into scattered photon energy plus kerma, that is, kinetic energy of electrons. This kerma can then be transformed into Bremsstrahlung, which is re-radiated photons, plus collision kerma. Once we know the collision kerma, we can talk about the *mean energy absorbed*, $\overline{E}_{ab}$, and an *energy absorption coefficient*, $\overline{\mu}_{en}$, which is the mean fraction of incident photon energy absorbed per unit path length. When we talk about radiation dose, we need to look at energy absorbed per unit mass. The *mass energy absorption coefficient*, $\overline{\mu}_{en}/\rho$, is going to be the handle that enables us to connect the incident photon fluence to the radiation dose. So, roughly speaking, fluence multiplied by mass energy absorption coefficient is going to give us radiation dose.

Let us look more closely at the energy transfer coefficient; then we shall look at the energy absorption coefficient. The energy transfer coefficient, which can be defined as the mean fraction of energy transferred to charged particles per unit path length, is the linear attenuation coefficient times the fraction of energy of the incident radiation that is transferred to kinetic energy of charged particles. This fraction of energy is the mean energy transferred divided by the incident photon energy. So we have the equation defining the energy transfer coefficient

$$\overline{\mu}_{tr} = \mu \frac{\overline{E}_{tr}}{h\nu} . \tag{16.12}$$

In this equation, μ is the linear attenuation coefficient, $\overline{E}_{tr}$ is the mean energy transferred to charged particles, and $h\nu$ is the energy of the incident photon. If we want to determine the amount of energy transferred to charged particles, we can rewrite the previous equation as

$$\overline{E}_{tr} = \left(\frac{\overline{\mu}_{tr}}{\mu} \right) h\nu . \tag{16.13}$$

The mean energy transferred to charged particles is then the energy transfer coefficient divided by the linear attenuation coefficient and multiplied by the incident photon energy. Another way of saying this is that the mean energy transferred to charged particles is the fraction of energy transferred to charged particles per unit path length times the energy carried by the beam times the path length.

The next quantity to be determined is the amount of energy actually absorbed by the charged particles. We use the same analysis used previously for energy transfer. The energy absorption coefficient, $\overline{\mu}_{en}$, the mean fraction of energy absorbed per unit path length, is given by the equation

$$\overline{\mu}_{en} = \mu \frac{\overline{E}_{en}}{h\nu} . \tag{16.14}$$

In this equation, analogous to the previous equation, μ is the linear attenuation coefficient, $\overline{E}_{en}$ is the mean energy absorbed by charged particles, and $h\nu$ is the energy of the incident photon. We will give some more precise definitions to energy transferred and energy absorbed later in this chapter. Finally, if we want to determine the amount of energy absorbed by the charged particles, we take the energy absorption coefficient divided by the linear attenuation coefficient and multiply it by the incident photon energy. The mean amount of energy absorbed by charged particles is equal to the fraction of energy absorbed by charged particles per unit path length times the energy carried by the beam times the path length.

The coefficients $\overline{\mu}_{tr}$ and $\overline{\mu}_{en}$ are tabulated, so if we know the incident energy fluence, we can determine how much energy is transferred to the charged particles and how much energy is absorbed by the charged particles. This is really an exercise in accounting. We just have to know where the energy is going and where to place it.

We now know that the energy transferred to electrons is either absorbed or it is re-radiated as Bremsstrahlung. If we let g be the fraction of energy in the charged particles that is lost to Bremsstrahlung, then the energy absorption coefficient is equal to the energy transfer coefficient times $(1 - g)$. At low energies the amount of energy lost to Bremsstrahlung is going to be low, so the energy absorption coefficient will be approximately equal to the energy transfer coefficient. Recall that Bremsstrahlung production is inefficient at low energies. At high energies more Bremsstrahlung is produced, so the energy absorption coefficient will be somewhat less than the energy transfer coefficient.

Let's put some quantities together.

Table (16.1) is a table of attenuation and absorption coefficients for carbon. The first column is photon energy, starting with a very low energy and increasing in powers of 10 through energies we encounter in radiation medicine, from 10 keV to 100 MeV. Notice what happens to the mean energy transfer, which is displayed in the second column. The mean energy transfer starts out for 10 keV photons at 8.65 keV, which is approximately 85% of the energy of the photons. The mean energy transfer then only rises to 14 keV when the photon energy rises to 100 keV, so the fraction of energy transferred goes down to 14%. It then rises to 44% for 1 MeV photons, 73% for 10 MeV photons, and 96% for 100 MeV photons. What this is saying is that, at very low energies and at very high energies, most of the energy of the incident photon gets transferred to kinetic energy of the electrons, but in the range of 100 keV to 1 MeV photons, a much lower fraction of energy gets transferred to electrons, with a larger amount of energy going into scattered photons. So photon scatter is important in intermediate energies.

TABLE 16.1: Attenuation coefficients for carbon. The columns are as follows: (1) energy of incident photon, (2) mean energy transferred, (3) mean energy absorbed, (4) mass attenuation coefficient, (5) mass energy transfer coefficient, and (6) mass energy absorption coefficient

$h\nu$ (MeV)	$\overline{E}_{tr}$ (MeV)	$\overline{E}_{en}$ (MeV)	μ/ρ (m^2/kg)	μ_{tr}/ρ (m^2/kg)	μ_{en}/ρ (m^2/kg)
0.01	0.00865	0.00865	0.2187	0.1891	0.1891
0.1	0.0141	0.0141	0.01512	0.00213	0.00213
1	0.440	0.440	0.00636	0.00280	0.00280
10	7.30	7.04	0.00196	0.00143	0.00138
100	95.62	71.9	0.00145	0.00139	0.00105

Now, let's compare energy absorbed to energy transferred. Keep in mind that the energy not absorbed is re-radiated as Bremsstrahlung. As we would expect, at low energies, all the electron energy is absorbed, and essentially none is re-radiated. At higher energies, such as 10 MeV, and even more so at 100 MeV, a large amount of Bremsstrahlung is produced.

We take the mass attenuation coefficient μ/ρ and weight it by the various fractions of energy transferred and absorbed to obtain the mass energy transfer coefficient and mass energy absorption coefficient.

First, note that at low energies μ/ρ tails off quite quickly with increasing energy, but the curve flattens out at higher energies. During the first power of 10 in energy, we go down by a factor of 20 in μ/ρ, while over the next power of 10, we go down by only a factor of about 2.5, the next power of 10 we go down by a factor of 3, and the last power of 10, we barely go down at all.

Comparing $\overline{\mu}_{tr}/\rho$ to $\overline{\mu}_{en}/\rho$, we see that, at low energies, almost all the kinetic energy is absorbed, but at higher energies some energy is re-radiated.

In the next section, we shall examine more closely the meanings of energy transferred and energy absorbed on a microscopic level.

16.4   MORE ENERGY AND DOSE DEFINITIONS

Before we go more deeply into cavity theory, we need to define more quantities related to energy and energy transfer. A series of diagrams will assist us in these definitions. Figure (16.2) is an example of such a diagram, describing a quantity known as energy transferred. In these diagrams, photons are always shown as squiggly lines while electrons are shown as straight lines. In this diagram, a photon enters a volume V with energy $h\nu_1$. This photon undergoes some sort of interaction. This interaction could be any interaction: a Compton interaction, a pair production interaction, a photoelectric interaction. (See Chapter 8.) In this figure, the interaction happens to be a Compton interaction. A scattered photon is produced with an energy $h\nu_2$. The interaction also

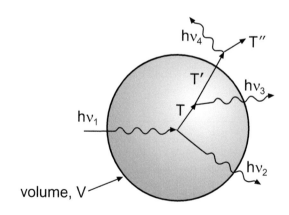

FIGURE 16.2: A diagram of a photon entering a volume, illustrating the interactions that may take place, resulting in energy transfer to the volume V. Lines with squiggles represent photons; straight lines with arrows represent electrons.

sets in motion an electron with kinetic energy T. As this electron traverses its path, it will cause ionizations. But it may also lose energy by production of Bremsstrahlung, losing radiant energy by the production of photons. In Fig. (16.2), we observe that downstream of the initial interaction, the electron emits a photon with energy $h\nu_3$, resulting in an electron energy of T'. The electron exits the volume with this energy T', and undergoes another radiative interaction, emitting a Bremsstrahlung photon of energy $h\nu_4$.

In evaluating the energy quantities defined by these diagrams, we denote the radiant energy of uncharged particles entering the volume as $(R_{in})_u$. The subscript u stands for *uncharged*. Generally the uncharged radiation will be photons. In the example illustrated in Fig. (16.2), the radiant energy of uncharged particles entering volume V is simply the energy of the incident photon $h\nu_1$. The radiant energy of uncharged particles exiting the volume is then defined to be $(R_{out})_u^{nonr}$. Note, however, we exclude the energy that originated from radiative losses of kinetic energy by charged particles while in V. The total radiant energy of uncharged particles exiting V is $h\nu_2 + h\nu_3$. However, we exclude $h\nu_3$ because this photon originated from a radiative process involving a charged particle. So we only include photons that are produced from photon interactions. Finally, ΣQ represents the net energy derived from rest mass in V. If mass is converted to energy, this quantity is positive, whereas if energy is converted to mass, this quantity is negative. In this example, there is no conversion of mass to energy or *vice versa*. On the other hand, if we had a pair production interaction, we would have a conversion of energy into mass, followed by a deposition of energy by the charged particles, followed by a conversion of mass into energy in an annihilation interaction.

We defined a volume V in which the energy transfer takes place. Why did we have to define a volume and how large does this volume need to be? In order to answer this question, we must digress to review the definition of stochastic and nonstochastic quantities. *Stochastic* and *nonstochastic* quantities have to do with random values. Any particular value of a stochastic quantity is determined by a probability distribution. Radiation interactions are random in nature, so quantities that we deal with are often stochastic quantities. We cannot predict whether or not a particular interaction is going to take place; it may take place or it may not. The interaction is a random process. So if we are just looking at a single interaction to determine whether it takes place or not, we really do not know. We may get three interactions in a row or we may wait a long time and get none and then another one comes along; a radiation interaction is a random process.

We have to observe a large number of interactions so that we can get an expectation value. The expectation value of a stochastic quantity is the mean of its measured values as the number of observations approaches infinity. We would like to observe a large number of interactions so we can get the mean value that accurately characterizes the probability distribution, and work with that mean value.

Stochastic quantities vary discontinuously in space and time; it is meaningless to speak of a gradient or rate of change of a stochastic quantity. In dosimetry, we like to deal with nonstochastic quantities, so we can talk about spatial gradients, dose rate gradients, for example, or changes of dose with time. These are all nonstochastic quantities. In the context of ionizing radiation, nonstochastic quantities are related to stochastic quantities by their expectation values.

Radiation dosimetry is nonstochastic dosimetry. Cavity theory will deal with a nonstochastic dosimetric quantity called *absorbed dose*. There is a whole branch of science called microdosimetry that deals with stochastic dosimetry. In order to measure microdosimetric quantities, it is necessary to use specialized devices. Microdosimetry is a fascinating subject, but not one that we generally we deal with in normal everyday life in medical physics.

Returning to our energy definitions, we would like the volume V to be large enough so there are many interactions in it. In that way we can talk meaningfully about the average values due to all the interactions taking place. The size of the volume is completely undefined; we never say how big or small it is, because we really do not know. But we say it has to big enough so that a sufficient number of interactions take place that we can talk about the average values or expectation values, but not so large that the radiation fluence going through the volume would be significantly changed.

We need this volume to make sure we get enough interactions taking place. But the volume needs to be so small so it does not disturb the fluence of these particles in any way. We meet these criteria quite easily, because we are dealing at an atomic level and there are many atoms in a very small space. So these volumes do not need to be very big at all.

We define the *energy transferred* ε_{tr} by the equation

$$\varepsilon_{tr} = (R_{in})_u - (R_{out})_u^{nonr} + \Sigma Q. \qquad (16.15)$$

In this equation $(R_{in})_u$ is the radiant energy of uncharged particle entering V (recall that radiant energy is the particle's energy ignoring the rest mass), $(R_{out})_u^{nonr}$ is the radiant energy of uncharged particles leaving V, except that which originated from radiative losses of kinetic energy by charged particles while in V (*i.e.*, except for the Bremsstrahlung originating in V), and ΣQ is the net energy derived from the conversion of rest mass to energy in V. This means that ε_{tr} must be the energy transferred to charged particles within V.

The radiant energy of uncharged particles (that is, photons) entering the volume in Fig. (16.2) is $h\nu_1$; the radiant energy of uncharged particles exiting the volume is $h\nu_2$; there is no change in rest mass, so the energy transferred is $h\nu_1 - h\nu_2$.

The energy transferred is a stochastic quantity; the nonstochastic quantity, kerma, is the expectation value of the energy transferred to charged particles per unit mass in a volume of interest, divided by the mass of target material in that volume. Kerma is defined for indirectly ionizing radiation only—that is, only for photons and neutrons. For monoenergetic photons, the kerma is related to the energy fluence Ψ by

$$K = \Psi \left(\frac{\mu_{tr}}{\rho} \right), \qquad (16.16)$$

where (μ_{tr}/ρ) is the mass energy transfer coefficient. For polyenergetic photons, we need to integrate the energy-dependent mass energy transfer coefficient over the fluence distribution of the photons.

We have already established that energy can be transferred from non-ionizing radiation to charged particles. The charged particles can deposit energy either via collisional processes or via radiative processes. Because radiative processes carry energy outside our volume of interest, we now want to only consider energy transferred via collisional processes, and not via radiative processes. This requirement introduces a new quantity, the *net energy transferred* ε_{tr}^n, defined to be the radiant energy of the uncharged particles coming into the volume minus the radiant energy of all uncharged particles going out of the volume, including that energy emitted as radiative losses of kinetic energy of charged particles.

The equation that defines the net energy transferred is therefore

$$\varepsilon_{tr}^n = (R_{in})_u - (R_{out})_u^{nonr} - R_u^r + \Sigma Q \,, \tag{16.17}$$

or

$$\varepsilon_{tr}^n = \varepsilon_{tr} - R_u^r \,, \tag{16.18}$$

where R_u^r is the radiant energy emitted as radiative losses by the charged particles that originated in V, regardless of where the radiative loss events occur. Thus ε_{tr}^n does not include energy going into radiative losses, whereas ε_{tr} does.

The net energy transferred in Fig. (16.2) is now the energy transferred, $(h\nu_1 - h\nu_2)$, minus the energy lost due to radiative processes—that is, due to Bremsstrahlung. In the figure, two radiative processes occur after the initial interaction, one giving rise to a Bremsstrahlung photon with energy $h\nu_3$; the second giving rise to another Bremsstrahlung photon with energy $h\nu_4$. Thus, the energy that is lost due to radiative processes is $(h\nu_3 + h\nu_4)$ and the net energy transferred is the energy transferred, $h\nu_1 - h\nu_2 = T$, minus the Bremsstrahlung energy, $(h\nu_3 + h\nu_4)$.

Now that we have defined the net energy transferred, we can use this definition to define the *collision kerma*. The collision kerma is defined by the equation

$$K_c = \frac{d\varepsilon_{tr}^n}{dm} \,. \tag{16.19}$$

It is the expectation value of the net energy transferred to charged particles per unit mass at the point of interest. For monochromatic photon beams, the collision kerma is related to the energy fluence by multiplying it by the mass energy absorption coefficient. For a polyenergetic beam, it is necessary to integrate over the energy fluence distribution.

Absorbed Dose

The next quantity we shall look at is the *energy imparted*, ε, defined to be the energy imparted by ionizing radiation to matter of mass m in a finite volume V. The equation defining the energy imparted is

$$\varepsilon = (R_{in})_u - (R_{out})_u + (R_{in})_c - (R_{out})_c + \Sigma Q \,. \tag{16.20}$$

In this equation, $(R_{out})_u$ is the radiant energy of all uncharged radiation leaving V, while $(R_{in})_c$ and $(R_{out})_c$ are the radiant energies of the charged particles entering and leaving V.

Let's look at each of the terms within the context of Fig. (16.2). First of all, $(R_{in})_u$, the radiant energy of uncharged particles entering the volume, is $h\nu_1$, that is, the energy of the incident photon. Next we look at $(R_{out})_u$, the radiant energy of uncharged particles leaving the volume. We see two photons produced in the volume and leaving the volume, one with energy $h\nu_2$, the other with energy $h\nu_3$. So the radiant energy of uncharged particles leaving the volume is $(h\nu_2 + h\nu_3)$. Because the fourth photon is produced by an interaction that occurred outside the volume, we do not include $h\nu_4$ in the equation. Next, we look at $(R_{in})_c$, the radiant energy of charged particles entering the volume. Since no charged particles are entering the volume, $(R_{in})_c = 0$. Finally, $(R_{out})_c$, the radiant energy of charged particles leaving the volume, is the kinetic energy of the electron leaving the volume, which is T'. Since there is no conversion of mass to energy or vice versa, it follows that $\Sigma Q = 0$. From Eq. (16.20), we finally have that the energy imparted is $(h\nu_1 - h\nu_2 - h\nu_3 - T')$. The energy imparted tells us how much energy stays within the volume of interest.

This leads us to the major dosimetric quantity, the *absorbed dose*. The absorbed dose D at any point P in the volume V is defined by the equation

$$D = \frac{d\varepsilon}{dm} . \tag{16.21}$$

The absorbed dose is the expectation value of the energy imparted to matter per unit mass at a point, a nonstochastic quantity.

So, in summary,

I. The energy transferred looks only at uncharged particles entering a volume of interest and includes energy that goes into radiative losses. The deterministic quantity corresponding to the energy transferred is the kerma.

II. The net energy transferred looks only at uncharged particles entering a volume of interest and does not include energy that goes into radiative losses. The deterministic quantity corresponding to the net energy transferred is the collision kerma.

III. The energy imparted looks at both charged and uncharged particles entering a volume of interest and does not include energy that exits the volume. The deterministic quantity corresponding to the energy imparted is the dose.

Example 16.2: Energy Considerations

A 2.0-*MeV* photon interacts with water via the Compton effect, ejecting a 1.5-*MeV* electron and a 0.5-*MeV* photon. Immediately after its emission, the electron emits a 0.1-*MeV* Bremsstrahlung photon, after which the electron has energy 1.3 *MeV*. Calculate (a) the energy transferred, (b) the net energy transferred, and (c) the energy imparted to a small volume surrounding the location of the Compton interaction.

Solution:
The set-up for this situation is shown in Fig. (16.3). The incident photon has energy $h\nu_1 = 2.0~MeV$. It undergoes a Compton interaction, emitting a photon of energy $h\nu_2 = 0.5~MeV$ and an electron of kinetic energy $T = 1.5~MeV$. We imagine a volume V surrounding the Compton interaction, as shown. We are told that the electron emits a Bremsstrahlung photon *immediately after* its emission, so we take that to mean that the emission takes place within the volume V. A Bremsstrahlung photon of energy $h\nu_B = 0.1~MeV$ is emitted and the electron, now with kinetic energy $T' = 1.3~MeV$, leaves V.

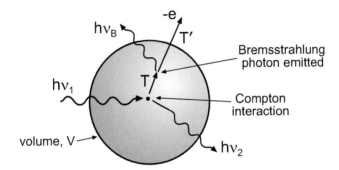

FIGURE 16.3: A schematic of the set-up for Ex.(16.2). An incident photon undergoes a Compton interaction; the emitted electron then immediately undergoes Bremsstrahlung emission.

Applying the definitions given above, we see that the radiant energy carried into the volume V by uncharged particles is $(R_{in})_u = h\nu_1$, while the radiant energy of uncharged particles *not* due to radiative losses (Bremsstrahlung) carried out of V is equal to $(R_{out})_u^{nonr} = h\nu_2$. The radiative losses by charged particles that originated within V are due to the Bremsstrahlung photon that was emitted by the electron after it emerged in the Compton interaction, so $R_u^r = h\nu_B$. (Note that this would not change even if the Bremsstrahlung photon had been emitted by the electron *outside* of V.) This means that the total radiant energy carried by uncharged particles out of the volume V is $(R_{out})_u = h\nu_2 + h\nu_B$. Finally, the radiant energies carried by *charged* particles into and out of V are given by $(R_{in})_c = 0$ and $(R_{out})_c = T'$. Also, since there was no mass converted into energy or *vice versa* in this set-up, $\Sigma Q = 0$. Note that the volume V is small enough that the emitted photons leave V. We are now ready to answer the questions.
(a) The energy transferred is given by Eq. (16.15):

$$\varepsilon_{tr} = (R_{in})_u - (R_{out})_u^{nonr} + \Sigma Q = h\nu_1 - h\nu_2 + 0\,, \qquad (16.22)$$

or,

$$\varepsilon_{tr} = 2.0~MeV - 0.5~MeV = \boxed{1.5~MeV}\,. \qquad (16.23)$$

(b) The net energy transferred is given by Eq. (16.18):

$$\varepsilon_{tr}^n = \varepsilon_{tr} - R_u^r = \varepsilon_{tr} - h\nu_B = 1.5 \ MeV - 0.1 \ MeV = \boxed{1.4 \ MeV}. \qquad (16.24)$$

(c) Finally, the energy imparted is given by Eq. (16.20):

$$\varepsilon = (R_{in})_u - (R_{out})_u + (R_{in})_c - (R_{out})_c + \Sigma Q, \qquad (16.25)$$

or,

$$\varepsilon = 2.0 \ MeV - 0.6 \ MeV + 0 - 1.3 \ MeV + 0 = \boxed{0.1 \ MeV}. \qquad (16.26)$$

$$\boxed{End \ of \ solution \ to \ Example \ 16.2.}$$

Charged-Particle Equilibrium (CPE)

We have one more step to go before we can determine the radiation dose in a cavity. This final step requires recalling the definition of charged-particle equilibrium (CPE): CPE exists if each charged particle of a given type and energy leaving a volume is replaced by an identical particle entering the volume. CPE is a statistical concept, so we always deal with expectation (average) values. When CPE exists, the energy carried out by each of the charged particles is matched by the energy carried in by an identical charged particle. This can be viewed schematically in Fig. (16.4). In this figure, the volume marked with a lower case v is the volume in which we are going to make our measurement. It is a small volume, but now we are going to surround it by a larger volume V. In order to have charged particle equilibrium exist in this small volume v, a larger volume must surround it. So in the figure, the larger volume contains the smaller one. In addition, the boundaries of the large volume V and the small volume v are separated by distance large enough so that any charged particle produced within the outer boundary of V that passes at least partially through v cannot reach the outer boundary of V.

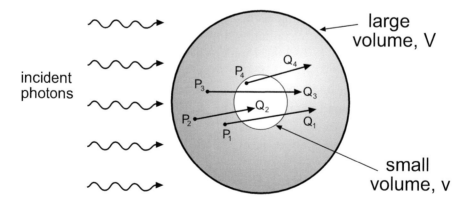

FIGURE 16.4: A schematic illustration of volumes and particle tracks involved in the definition of charged particle equilibrium (CPE).

In Fig. (16.4), we assume that a uniform beam of photons is incident on V. At point P_1 within V an incident photon undergoes an interaction, resulting in the emission of a charge Q_1, which is assumed to have a kinetic energy T. Furthermore, at points P_2, P_3 and P_4, we assume that identical interactions of incident photons result in the emission of identical secondary charged particles Q_2, Q_3 and Q_4, all having the same kinetic energies T.

The charge Q_1 passes completely through v, entering v with energy $3T/4$ and exiting with energy $T/3$. The identical charge Q_2 enters v with energy $T/5$, imparting that energy completely within v. Q_3 also completely passes through v, entering with energy $T/3$ and exiting with energy $T/5$. Finally, charge Q_4 is emitted within v, exiting that volume with energy $3T/4$. Table (16.2) summarizes the energies of the (identical) charged particles entering and exiting the small volume v. Note that one charged particle enters v with energy $3T/4$ and an identical particle leaves with energy $3T/4$. Likewise, one enters with energy $T/5$ and one leaves with $T/5$; another charged particle enters with $T/3$ and an identical particle exits with $T/3$. This is CPE.

TABLE 16.2: Summary of entrance and exit energies for the small volume v of the identical charged particles shown in Fig. (16.4). Note that, for each entrance energy, there is a corresponding equal exit energy for an identical charged particle, and *vice versa*. This is the condition for CPE

Charged Particle	Entrance Energy	Exit Energy
Q_1	$\frac{3}{4}T$	$\frac{1}{3}T$
Q_2	$\frac{1}{5}T$	—
Q_3	$\frac{1}{3}T$	$\frac{1}{5}T$
Q_4	—	$\frac{3}{4}T$

We are always thinking about distances surrounding our point of interest, which is the small volume v. Note that none of the electron paths shown in Fig (16.4) within V and outside of v is greater than the distance between the boundaries of V and v. If a secondary charged particle is emitted on the far side of v from the incident photon field, that particle will not be able to make it to the outer boundary of V.

If we are dealing with neutrons then we are likely to be dealing with other secondary particles, for example, protons. Nevertheless, the concept of CPE is the same.

We are going to identify some conditions such that, if these conditions are satisfied throughout the larger volume, then CPE will exist in the smaller volume. The first condition requires that the medium, both in the large volume and the small volume, be homogenous in both density and composition. We do not want any changes in the medium or in its density, because that affects the attenuation of the primary beam. The second condition is that there exists a uniform field of photons. (Here we will just talk about photons, but it can also be applied to neutrons.) The photons are coming in and interacting in the larger volume V, but we assume that the resulting attenuation of these photons is negligible in traversing this volume. The final condition is that there are no inhomogeneous electric or magnetic fields present. In most cases we do not worry about this, but we don't want anything that is going to disturb the electrons.

If we have CPE, then the radiant energy of charged particles entering our volume of interest is equal to the radiant energy of charged particles exiting the volume. If we now substitute this equality into the expression for energy imparted,

$$\varepsilon = (R_{in})_u - (R_{out})_u + (R_{in})_c - (R_{out})_c + \Sigma Q, \tag{16.27}$$

we get that

$$\varepsilon_{(CPE)} = (R_{in})_u - (R_{out})_u + \Sigma Q. \tag{16.28}$$

We see that under conditions of charged particle equilibrium, the energy imparted is simply the energy of uncharged particles entering the volume minus the energy of uncharged particles exiting the volume plus any changes in mass.

We now recall our energy definitions within the context of Fig. (16.2), but this time under conditions of charged particle equilibrium. First of all, the energy imparted is the radiant energy of the photon entering the volume minus the radiant energy of the photons exiting the volume. The radiant energy of the photon entering the volume is $h\nu_1$, while the radiant energy of the photons exiting the volume is $h\nu_2 + h\nu_3$. The quantity T', the radiant energy of charged particles exiting the volume and ultimately yielding a photon with energy $h\nu_4$, must be compensated for by another T' entering the volume from a photon interaction outside the volume if the volume is, indeed, in CPE.

We next take the expression for energy transferred, that is, the total energy received by charged particles, and insert it into the expression for energy imparted under charged particle equilibrium. From Eq. (16.15),

$$\varepsilon_{tr} = (R_{in})_u - (R_{out})_u^{nonr} + \Sigma Q, \tag{16.29}$$

we get, substituting into Eq. (16.28),

$$\varepsilon_{(CPE)} = \varepsilon_{tr} + (R_{out})_u^{nonr} - (R_{out})_u, \tag{16.30}$$

or, in terms of the set-up in Fig. (16.2),

$$\varepsilon_{(CPE)} = \varepsilon_{tr} + h\nu_2 - (h\nu_2 + h\nu_3) = \varepsilon_{tr} - h\nu_3. \tag{16.31}$$

We find that the energy imparted is equal to the energy transferred plus the radiant energy of photons produced by nonradiative processes exiting the volume minus the radiant energy of all photons exiting the volume. The radiant energy of photons produced by nonradiative processes exiting the volume is $h\nu_2$, and the radiant energy of all photons exiting the volume is $h\nu_2 + h\nu_3$, so the energy imparted under charged particle equilibrium is the energy transferred minus the radiant energy of photons produced by radiative processes exiting the volume, which is $h\nu_3$.

Finally, we observe that the net energy transferred is equal to the energy transferred minus the radiative losses from charged particles originating in the small volume, and, under charged particle equilibrium, we can relate the net energy transferred to the energy imparted. From Eq. (16.18) we have that

$$\varepsilon^n_{tr} = \varepsilon_{tr} - R^r_u, \tag{16.32}$$

so that, from Eq. (16.30),

$$\varepsilon^n_{tr\,(CPE)} = \varepsilon_{(CPE)} - (R_{out})^{nonr}_u - R^r_u + (R_{out})_u. \tag{16.33}$$

Working this out is going to be a bit complicated, and requires some understanding of charged particle equilibrium.

Recall that R^r_u represents the radiative losses from charged particles originating in v and $(R_{out})^{nonr}_u$ is the energy of photons leaving v, except those that are radiative. Under charged particle equilibrium conditions, the following equation holds as long as the volume v is small enough that all radiative-loss photons created in the volume can escape:

$$(R_{out})_{u\,(CPE)} = (R_{out})^{nonr}_u + R^r_u. \tag{16.34}$$

In our small volume, if an electron loses energy by a radiative loss, that radiative loss must be Bremsstrahlung. It is important that the Bremsstrahlung escapes the volume completely. The condition of charged particle equilibrium is needed to ensure that, for every radiative loss contributing to R^r_u outside of v, there is a similar radiative event occurring inside v. The volume must then be small enough that the radiative photon gets out of v to be counted in $(R_{out})_u$. Given that the photon of energy $h\nu_2$ escapes from v, the small-volume condition is satisfied and we are in good shape. This scenario is depicted schematically in Fig. (16.5).

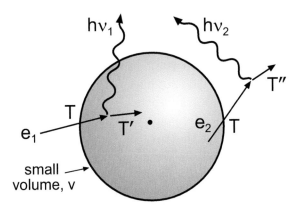

FIGURE 16.5: Tracks of photons and electrons under conditions of charged-particle equilibrium in the small volume v. Each electron emits a Bremsstrahlung photon of equal energy— e_1 emits a photon within v and e_2 emits a photon outside of v.

In the figure, an electron e_1 of energy T enters the volume v and undergoes a radiative loss, emitting a Bremsstrahlung photon of energy $h\nu_1$. Under CPE we may assume that, for each charged particle entering the volume v and undergoing a radiative loss, there is always an identical charged particle with approximately the same energy leaving v and then undergoing a similar radiative loss outside of the volume. Again, we can make that assumption provided we have a large number of events and look at the average values. In Fig. (16.5), we therefore assume that another electron, e_2, emitted within v, exits the volume with kinetic energy T and then emits a Bremsstrahlung photon of energy $h\nu_2 = h\nu_1$.

Considering Eq. (16.34), we first of all see that, for the set-up in Fig. (16.5), the energy carried out of v by all uncharged particles is $(R_{out})_{u\,(CPE)} = h\nu_1$. We also note that there are no photons leaving v that resulted from non-radiative processes, so the corresponding energy of such photons leaving v must be $(R_{out})_u^{nonr} = 0$. Finally, charged particles that were emitted in v and subsequently emitted Bremsstrahlung, no matter whether that Bremsstrahlung was emitted inside or outside of v, contribute to R_u^r. We see in the figure that $R_u^r = h\nu_2$. From Eq. (16.34), we should then have that $h\nu_1 = 0 + h\nu_2$. Under CPE, this equality was already assumed above. We thus have that, under charged particle equilibrium, the radiant energy of photons exiting the volume is equal to the sum of the energy from non-radiative interactions plus the energy from radiative interactions.

Under CPE we can make some important simplifications. The net energy transferred under CPE is the energy imparted in the volume and if we shrink the volumes down, we can take derivatives. The derivative of the net energy transferred per unit mass is equal to the derivative of the energy imparted per unit mass. That is, under conditions of CPE, the absorbed dose is equal to the collision kerma. That is the important equality we want to make at this point.

$$\frac{d\varepsilon_{tr}^n}{dm}\bigg|_{(CPE)} = \frac{d\varepsilon}{dm}. \tag{16.35}$$

When we have CPE at a point in the medium, the absorbed dose is going to be equal to the collision kerma.

Note that the equality of dose and collision kerma is true irrespective of radiative losses. Radiative losses become important at photon energies of about 1 MeV. For energies less than 1 MeV we really do not have to be concerned about radiative losses, but when energies exceed 1 MeV, radiative losses need to be considered, becoming significant at around 4 MeV. So the point where radiative losses in dosimetry come in is right in the range we use for therapy.

The equality of dose and collision kerma under conditions of CPE is important because it relates absorbed dose, a quantity we can measure with a great deal of accuracy, to collision kerma, a quantity we can calculate. This equality, in fact, gives us a way for checking out some of our calculations. If we measure absorbed dose and make the equality with collision kerma, we can see how good our calculations are. This perhaps is the most important result that comes out of it in terms of everyday dosimetry.

Another aspect of the equality is that it allows the ratio of the doses in two media to be calculated. If we have the same photon fluence in each medium, and if CPE holds, then the ratio of the dose in one medium to the dose in another is going to be equal to the ratio of collision kermas, which, in turn, is equal to the ratio of the mass energy absorption coefficients.

$$\frac{D_A}{D_B}\bigg|_{(CPE)} = \frac{(K_c)_A}{(K_c)_B} = \frac{(\bar{\mu}_{en}/\rho)_A}{(\bar{\mu}_{en}/\rho)_B} \equiv \left(\frac{\bar{\mu}_{en}}{\rho}\right)_B^A. \tag{16.36}$$

Often in dosimetry we wish to relate the dose in one medium to the dose in another medium, for example, dose in soft tissue or dose in bone to dose in water. We see here that under conditions of CPE, the ratio of doses is simply equal to the ratio of mass energy absorption coefficients.

Unfortunately, CPE does not exist in many situations in dosimetry. We need to be aware when it breaks down, what to do about it, and how it may affect the theories we deal with.

With high-energy photon beams, CPE can only occur after full buildup has been achieved. That is a reasonable statement. We are looking at the effect of the secondary electrons and how far they penetrate, and it is the secondary electrons that build up in the buildup region. So some kind of equilibrium is necessary before CPE is achieved. The absence of equilibrium in the buildup region for high-energy photons results in one region in which CPE does not exist.

If the attenuation of the photon beam is significant in the distance traveled by the electrons set in motion by the photons, then it is impossible to get CPE. Earlier, we said that a requirement for CPE was there would be no photon attenuation over the range of the secondary electrons. However, a 10-MeV photon beam is attenuated about 7% in the range of its secondary electrons. The 7% is a large number so that CPE cannot exist. For photon energies in the region of about 1 MeV, attenuation is approximately 1%, which is a bit better to get by with, but at 10 MeV the attenuation of the photon beam cannot be neglected. So, for high-energy photons, we do not really have CPE.

Instead, it is necessary to introduce a concept called *transient charged particle equilibrium* (TCPE), which allows us to use the theories and work on the equations. We define TCPE at all points within a region in which the absorbed dose is proportional to the collision kerma. Under CPE we can derive quite rigorously that the dose equals the collision kerma, but when CPE breaks down, if we are fortunate, there is a region in which the dose may not be equal to the collision kerma, but is at least proportional to the collision kerma.

If we look at the standard curve that plots both collision kerma and dose as functions of depth into a medium, as shown in Fig. (16.6), at depths beyond the buildup region, the two curves eventually become parallel. In the region in which the two curves are parallel, we have *transient charged-particle equilibrium* (TCPE). If the energy of the incident beam is low enough, the collision kerma will be approximately equal to the kerma. But this situation does not change much even with radiative losses.

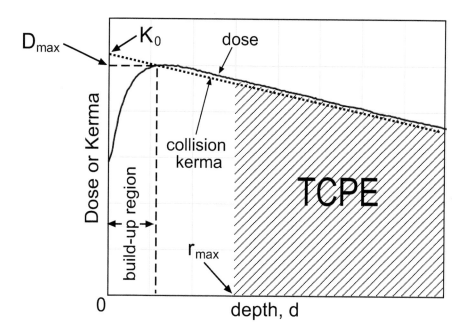

FIGURE 16.6: Plot of collision kerma and dose as a function of depth. The shaded region is the region of transient charged-particle equilibrium (TCPE), where the collision kerma and dose curves are approximately parallel.

In a plot of dose versus depth, the absorbed dose is non-zero at the surface due to backscattered electrons and photons. The depth dose increases as the charged particle fluence builds up and reaches a maximum at the point where the increase is balanced by the decrease due to attenuation of the incident photon beam. The dose maximum, D_{max}, occurs at approximately the point where the dose and kerma curves cross over, and somewhere beyond that is where TCPE exists.

Let's be more specific: at a depth equal to the maximum penetration distance of the secondary charged particles produced at the surface, the dose curve becomes parallel to the kerma curve and hence TCPE exists. Thus, in a typical depth dose curve, the dose starts out not quite zero at the surface but at a relatively low value and increases to a maximum value at some depth. The kerma starts at some value on the surface; there is no build up. Kerma at the surface is denoted K_0. As was pointed out earlier, we have assumed that in this case radiative losses are negligible so the kerma is equal to the collision kerma. The kerma at the surface is K_0 and it attenuates with depth, but with a reasonable approximation it will be exponential with some effective attenuation coefficient.

We continue to go deeper into the target until we reach a depth equal to r_{max}, which is the range of the secondary electrons produced by the incident photons. Beyond that depth we have TCPE and we find that the dose is proportional to the collision kerma. At depths beyond the cross over, the dose curve will always lie above the collision kerma curve. The collision kerma curve will never come out above the dose curve; kerma is always less than the dose.

16.5   CAVITY THEORIES

Let us consider the fluence of charged particles of energy T crossing an interface between two media. In this case the interface is between a medium w and a medium g. We normally talk about w as the wall of an ionization chamber and g as the gas inside the chamber, but it could be the interface between any two materials (Fig. 16.7). (We will discuss ionization chambers in much more detail in the next chapter.)

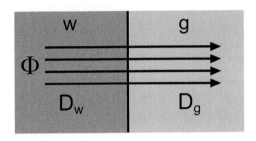

FIGURE 16.7: The interface of two materials, designated as w and g. Φ is the particle fluence (number of particles passing per unit area).

The fluence in w on the left of the interface is the same as the fluence in g on the right of the interface: $\Phi_w = \Phi_g$. Hence we can write that the dose to g equals the fluence times the mass collisional stopping power in g and the dose to w equals the fluence times the mass collisional stopping power in w. We can now write the ratio of the dose in w to the dose in g as the ratio of the mass collisional stopping powers:

$$\frac{D_w}{D_g} = \frac{(S/\rho)_{col,w}}{(S/\rho)_{col,w}} . \tag{16.37}$$

Next, we do a simple thought experiment and place another slab of w on the other side of the slab of g, as shown in Fig. (16.8). We shrink the slab of g so that we have an otherwise homogeneous medium, w, which contains a very thin layer of cavity filled with another medium g.

The cavity g has been made sufficiently thin that we can assume some certain conditions:

I. The thickness of the layer of g is assumed to be so small compared to the range of charged particles crossing it that its presence does not perturb the charged

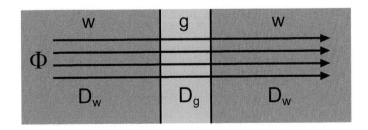

FIGURE 16.8: A thin slab of g embedded in a medium w.

particle field. That is one of the very basic assumptions made in Bragg-Gray theory. That is, when a small cavity or slab of other material is introduced, the presence of this slab does not interfere with the charged particle distribution in either energy or direction.

II. The absorbed dose in the cavity is assumed to be deposited entirely by the charged particles crossing the cavity. This condition is valid for gas-filled cavities in photon beams. That means is we are allowing no interactions to take place within the cavity itself in which energy can be deposited. So all these particles are going to cross the cavity depositing energy in the cavity, and we are not allowing any energy to be deposited by electrons that were set in motion by photon interactions taking place inside the cavity. That is a valid assumption when the cavity is very small and is filled by a material of much lower density than that of the material surrounding it. This condition is valid for gas-filled cavities in photon beams, in which the density of the gas in the cavity is orders of magnitude less than the density of the wall.

The previous relationships were based on fluence from mono-energetic sources. What happens if we have a polyenergetic distribution of charged particles? We define the spectrum-averaged mass collisional stopping power in the cavity medium. That is we are going to average over the energy distribution of secondary electrons. Fortunately, we do not have to do these integrations; someone had done them for us and there are tables of them. But years ago if you wanted your average stopping powers you would have to calculate them yourself and do the integration.

$$\left(\frac{\overline{S}}{\rho}\right)_g = \frac{\int_0^{T_{max}} \Phi(T) \, (S/\rho)_{col,g}(T) \, dT}{\int_0^{T_{max}} \Phi(T) \, dT} = \frac{D_g}{\Phi}. \tag{16.38}$$

If we look at the wall of the chamber, we get the same sort of spectrum-averaged mass collisional stopping power in the wall:

$$\left(\frac{\overline{S}}{\rho}\right)_w = \frac{\int_0^{T_{max}} \Phi(T) \, (S/\rho)_{col,w}(T) \, dT}{\int_0^{T_{max}} \Phi(T) \, dT} = \frac{D_w}{\Phi}. \tag{16.39}$$

Combining these equations, we can relate the dose to the wall as the dose to the gas multiplied by the ratio of spectrum-averaged mass collisional stopping powers. The bars over the S indicate that the average is taken over the energy spectrum of secondary electrons.

$$\frac{D_w}{D_g} = \frac{\left(\overline{S}/\rho\right)_w}{\left(\overline{S}/\rho\right)_g} \equiv \left(\frac{\overline{S}}{\rho}\right)_g^w. \tag{16.40}$$

If the cavity is filled with a gas of mass m in which a charge Q is produced by radiation, ion pairs are going to be created. Recall from Eq. (2.2) that the average energy imparted to a medium per ion pair created is denoted $\overline{W}$. Also recall that the magnitude of charge of either sign created per ion pair is the fundamental charge e.

It then follows that $\overline{W}/e$ is just the energy imparted to the medium per unit charge, so that the dose delivered to the gas is given by:

$$D_g = \frac{Q}{m} \left(\frac{\overline{W}}{e}\right)_g . \tag{16.41}$$

This is the basic equation in the Bragg-Gray cavity. But the equation we obtained is for the dose in the gas; what we really want is the dose in the medium surrounding the gas, w. We are not particularly interested in the dose in the gas, but the dose in the medium is related to the dose in the gas by the ratio of the collision stopping powers, as given by Eq. (16.40):

$$D_w = \frac{Q}{m} \left(\frac{\overline{W}}{e}\right)_g \left(\frac{\overline{S}}{\rho}\right)_g^w . \tag{16.42}$$

These equations make use of the unrestricted collisional stopping powers. The effects of knock-on electrons, that is, secondary electrons produced by the electron-electron interactions, are included in these stopping powers. When we calculate the mean collisional mass stopping power, we integrate over the fluence spectra for primary electrons only.

The dose in the medium equals the measured charge per unit mass in the gas cavity multiplied by $\overline{W}/e$, which is then multiplied by the ratio of collisional mass stopping powers; this is really is the Bragg-Gray relation expressed in the terms of the cavity ionization chamber. If we are only doing Bragg-Gray cavity theory, this is the equation we use. Note that the theory requires charged-particle equilibrium of at least the secondary electrons in the cavity—the knock-on electrons—since this is required in order to use the relationship between dose, fluence, and stopping powers. If there is also charged-particle equilibrium for the primary electron spectrum, certain computational shortcuts are possible.

What has always surprised people is that the Bragg-Gray cavity theory works at all. Because some of the assumptions that we make, such as the neglect of the spectrum of the knock-on electrons, one might think the Bragg-Gray theory would not work. But it works remarkably well. However, it could be improved upon, and the individuals who did the most important work of improving on the Bragg-Gray cavity theory were Spencer and Attix.

In 1955, Spencer and Attix formulated a theory that took these knock-on electrons into account, and developed a very complex procedure for evaluating their theory, assuming CPE held. The Spencer-Attix theory was in much better agreement with the experimental results and this has been the accepted procedure ever since. People always sort of try and modify the Bragg-Gray and Spencer-Attix theories. There are other theories in the literature, which we won't go into. The Spencer-Attix theory has persisted now for a long time and it is the basis for all dosimetry protocols.

The theory still requires the two Bragg-Gray conditions to hold. In fact, Spencer-Attix theory is more stringent because it assumes the entire secondary electron spectrum is not disturbed by the cavity. The basic idea of the Spencer-Attix theory is explicitly to take into account all knock-on electrons above a certain energy threshold, which we will denote by the letter Δ. The theory then considers all other energy losses to be local. It divides the electron spectrum up into two regions. One region is the part of the electron spectrum with energy above the threshold energy Δ, which then gets put back into the primary spectrum, with all electrons with energies below Δ resulting in local energy loss.

Spencer-Attix theory considers the electron fluence to include primary electrons as well as knock-on electrons with energies above Δ, and the integrals for the dose now start at Δ. So rather than integrating over the energy spectrum from zero to a maximum value of energy, now the integrals go from Δ to the maximum energy value. Moreover, rather than using the unrestricted mass collisional stopping powers, Spencer-Attix theory now uses the restricted mass collisional stopping powers. If one sets a value on Δ, the theory gives an energy at which one starts the integrations.

So when the integrations are done, one considers only energy losses creating electrons below energy Δ, because the energy lost to higher energy electrons is explicitly accounted for by the presence of these electrons in the spectrum. Below the value of Δ, one is interested in the energy loss, but above this energy one considers the electrons to be primary electrons.

In analogy with the Bragg-Gray theory, the Spencer-Attix equation is now usually written as:

$$\frac{D_m}{D_g} = \frac{\int_\Delta^{E_{max}} \Phi \left(\frac{L}{\rho}\right)_{\Delta,m} dE + TE_m}{\int_\Delta^{E_{max}} \Phi \left(\frac{L}{\rho}\right)_{\Delta,g} dE + TE_g} = \left(\frac{\overline{L}}{\rho}\right)_g^m, \qquad (16.43)$$

where TE is a term that accounts for track ends. Rather than integrating unrestricted mass collisional stopping power, S/ρ, over energies from zero to the maximum energy value, we now integrate the *restricted* mass collisional stopping power, L/ρ, over energies from Δ to the maximum energy value. The restricted collisional stopping power L is defined the same as in Eq. (16.11) for S, only now dE is the energy loss restricted by the cut-off energy Δ. This ratio is going to be dependent on the value of Δ, but it turns out the specific value of Δ does not really matter too much. Finally, there is a track-end term included to take into account track ends. That is not a big correction; it is for completeness to take into account.

The value of Δ is traditionally taken as the energy of an electron whose range is equal to the mean path length in the cavity. A more physical choice would be based on the mean energy needed for a knock-on electron created in the cavity to escape from it, but Δ is traditionally defined by the first definition. Typical cavities are around 2 or 3 millimeters in diameter, which is the about the size of most ion chambers. An electron with a range of a few millimeters is going to be about 10 keV. Fortunately, in practical situations, the theory is relatively insensitive to the choice of Δ. The value of 10 keV is often used for convenience and the continuous slowing down approximation range of a 10 keV electron is about 2 mm. So that is generally what is used in the calculations.

The track end term, which takes into account the energy deposition by those particles whose energy falls below Δ, represents a significant fraction of the energy deposition. However, this term should be the same in both the medium and the gas since the spectra are assumed to be the same in both cases. The *TE* term can be calculated directly via a Monte Carlo calculation, or estimated by

$$TE = \Phi(\Delta) \left(\frac{S}{\rho}\right)_{\Delta} \Delta, \tag{16.44}$$

where the product of the first two terms (the electron fluence differential in energy and the total mass collision stopping power, both evaluated at the cutoff energy Δ) is roughly equal to the number of stoppers per unit mass.

One advantage of using Spencer-Attix cavity theory is that it does not require charged-particle equilibrium to apply, as long as the cavity does not disturb the electron fluence. So, if the Bragg-Gray cavity conditions exist for a Spencer-Attix cavity, charged-particle equilibrium is not needed because the effect of the secondary knock-on electrons is considered explicitly and the assumption of local energy deposition is accurate on its own without invoking charged-particle equilibrium. Moreover, the Spencer-Attix theory includes an explicit dependence on the cavity size through the choice of Δ.

Table (16.3) depicts the result of calculations of water to air stopping power ratios at a depth of more than halfway into the range of the electrons. The incident electron energies are on the left. The top row indicates the cutoff values in keV of the Spencer-Attix theory, and the column on the right are the Bragg-Gray values. If rather high cutoff values are chosen, the Spencer-Attix values are fairly close to the Bragg-Gray values, but if we go down to very low cutoff energies, we see the difference between Bragg-Gray and Spencer-Attix values is about 2%.

TABLE 16.3: Ratios of water-to-air stopping powers for various values of cutoff energies. The numbers above the double line are the values of the cut-off energy Δ in MeV; the numbers in columns 2 through 5 below the double line are the stopping-power ratios

| Incident | Spencer-Attix Δ (MeV) | | | Bragg- |
Energy (MeV)	0.001	0.01	0.1	Gray
5	1.146	1.131	1.124	1.121
10	1.116	1.102	1.096	1.091
20	1.076	1.064	1.058	1.053

The effect is not large but it is important enough in dosimetry and certainly for standards labs to take this into account. When theory is being compared with very accurate dose measurements using calorimetry or chemical dosimetry, we see that the Spencer-Attix approach is more accurate than the Bragg-Gray.

16.6 DOSIMETRY PROTOCOLS

Essential to the accurate delivery of radiation is the requirement that radiation measurements be consistent from clinic to clinic. In order to achieve consistency, calibration factors, which convert an instrument reading to a dose, are obtained for each measurement device. Calibrations are normally performed using clinical ionization chambers, the design and operation of which will be discussed in the next chapter.

A calibration begins with a measured standard, analogous to standards of length, mass, etc., established in a standardization laboratory. In the United States, the standardization laboratory is the National Institute of Standards and Technology (NIST). In principle, each ionization chamber used for machine calibration in the clinic needs to have a calibration factor traceable to the calibration at NIST. While ideally, a direct comparison of measurements would be made, in practice, a set of Accredited Dosimetry Calibration Laboratories (ADCL) have been established and accredited by the American Association of Physicists in Medicine (AAPM). Round-robin comparisons are regularly made between the ADCLs and NIST. A radiation oncology clinic will typically have an ionization chamber the calibration of which is directly compared to the chamber at an ADCL. Thus, the clinic's chamber calibration is directly traceable to the standard at NIST.

Because clinical measurements of radiation are not absolute measurements of dose, it is necessary to relate a clinical measurement to the measurement that would be made at a standardization laboratory. The basic equation relating a clinical measurement to a dose is

$$D_w^Q = M \, N_{D,w}^Q . \tag{16.45}$$

In this equation, D_w^Q is the absorbed dose to water at point of measurement of ion chamber placed under reference conditions, M is the chamber reading corrected for such factors as pressure, temperature, and humidity, and $N_{D,w}^Q$ is the absorbed dose-to-water calibration factor for beam quality Q. The calibration laboratory provides the clinic with a chamber calibration factor $N_{D,w}^{Co}$, the absorbed dose-to-water calibration factor for a ^{60}Co radiation beam, and the purpose of a dosimetry protocol is to guide the clinic in determining the relationship between the standard laboratory's chamber calibration factor and the appropriate factor to use in the clinic.

These protocols are continually being revised. Older protocols were based on a measurement of exposure of a ^{60}Co gamma-ray beam yielding a calibration factor N_x. One of the earlier protocols was the SCRAD Protocol[2], developed by the AAPM Scientific Committee on Radiation Dosimetry. This protocol was superseded by the AAPM Task Group 21 (TG-21) Protocol[3], which, in turn, was superseded by the AAPM Task Group 51 (TG-51) Protocol[4], which is the dosimetry protocol currently in use in North America.

The TG-51 Protocol is valid for photon beams in the energy range from ^{60}Co gamma rays to 50 MV x-rays, and also for electron beams of energies in the range 4 to 50 MeV. These are the energy ranges most frequently used in radiation oncology. The protocol requires the use of ionization chambers with an absorbed dose-to-water calibration factor $N_{D,w}^{Co}$ traceable to national primary standards (NIST). The quantity D_w^Q, the absorbed dose to water at point of measurement of ion chamber placed under reference conditions, is given by the equation displayed earlier, where $N_{D,w}^Q$, the absorbed dose-to-water calibration factor for beam quality Q, is related to the calibration factor provided by the calibration lab by

$$N_{D,w}^Q = k_Q N_{D,w}^{Co} , \tag{16.46}$$

where k_Q is the quality conversion factor, a chamber-specific value, which converts the calibration factor for a ^{60}Co beam to that for a beam quality Q. Values of k_Q have been tabulated as function of Q for many ionization chambers.

For electron beams, the quality conversion factor is comprised of two factors,

$$k_Q = P_{gr}^Q \, k_{R50} . \tag{16.47}$$

The first factor, P_{gr}^Q , is a gradient correction factor, dependent on the radius of the chamber and ionization gradient at the point of measurement, and must be explicitly measured for each beam by the user. It should be noted that there is actually a gradient correction for photon beams as well, but the gradient correction is the same for all photon beams of the same quality, so P_{gr}^Q is folded into k_Q for photon beams.

In defining the gradient correction, the previous equation separates out the component of k_Q that is independent of P_{gr}^Q, leaving k_{R50}, a quantity that can be written further as the product of two factors, namely

$$k_{R50} = k_{R50}' \, k_{ecal} . \tag{16.48}$$

The second term, k_{ecal}, is fixed for a given chamber model, leaving behind a factor k_{R50}', which is dependent on beam quality. The introduction of this factor may seem arbitrary, but it makes the variation of k_{R50}' among ionization chambers much less than that of k_{R50}. The equation thus defines k_{ecal}, the chamber-specific photon-electron conversion factor that accounts for the variation in calibration factor between that at the cobalt energy and arbitrary energy Q.

The second factor defines k_{R50}', the chamber-specific electron quality conversion factor, which accounts for the variation in calibration factor between Q and the energy defined by R50, the depth where the dose is 50% that of the maximum depth dose.

Let us revisit the corrected dosimeter reading, M, and identify the corrections that must be made to the raw dosimeter reading, M_{raw}. We write

$$M = P_{ion} P_{TP} P_{elec} P_{pol} M_{raw} . \tag{16.49}$$

The following discussions explain the corrections shown in this equation that need to be made to M_{raw}.

The quantity P_{ion} is the correction for ion recombination. The calibration assumes that all ions are collected, but some might recombine. Recombination is function of the dose per pulse. To determine the recombination correction, one makes two measurements, varying the voltage across the ion chamber. The first measurement is at high voltage V_H, giving a reading M_{raw}^H; the other at V_L, approximately $0.5\,V_H$, giving a reading M_{raw}^L. The recombination correction is then given by

$$P_{ion}\,(V_H) = \frac{1 - V_H/V_L}{M_{raw}^H/M_{raw}^L - V_H/V_L} . \tag{16.50}$$

This equation is valid only for pulsed or pulsed-swept beams with $P_{ion} < 1.05$. For higher-order corrections, it is necessary to use published tables.

The next correction, P_{TP}, is a correction for temperature and pressure. This correction is needed because ionization measurements are for a fixed volume of air defined by the ionization chamber, but dose is defined to be energy absorbed per unit mass. The temperature-pressure correction factor, given by

$$P_{TP} = \left(\frac{273.2 + T}{273.2 + T_{st}} \right) \left(\frac{P_{st}}{P} \right), \tag{16.51}$$

corrects for the change in the mass of air within the chamber from the mass at standard temperature, $T_{st} = 22^oC$, and a standard pressure, $P_{st} = 101.33\,kPa$ (1 atmosphere).

The electrometer correction factor P_{elec} is a correction factor for calibration of the electrometer and is included if calibration is performed using a separate chamber/electrometer calibration. Often, calibrations are done for a standard chamber/electrometer pair, so a correction for separate calibration of the electrometer is not needed.

The final factor, P_{pol}, is a correction for chamber polarity. To determine this quantity, one makes two readings changing the polarity of the ionization chamber. Using those two measurements, the chamber polarity correction can be determined by the relation

$$P_{pol} = \left| \frac{(M_{raw}^+ - M_{raw}^-)}{2M_{raw}} \right|. \tag{16.52}$$

(See the corresponding discussion of P_{pol} associated with Eq.22.43.)

One more quantity needs to be defined, and that is the beam quality. The specific definition is not as significant as the need for the definition to be unambiguous, easily measured, and reproducible. The TG-51 protocol calls for a measurement of the percent depth dose at 10 cm depth to be the measure of photon beam quality, and the value of R50, the depth at which the beam dose is 50% of the maximum dose as the measure of electron beam quality.

The procedure for applying the TG-51 protocol to beam calibration is as follows: First, one selects an ionization chamber. The chamber calibration factor $N_{D,w}^{Co}$ is obtained, either directly from an Accredited Dosimetry Calibration Laboratory or by comparison with a dedicated calibrated chamber in the clinic. The beam quality Q is measured in order to determine k_Q, values of which are tabulated for various ionization chambers and the chamber calibration factor is modified for the appropriate beam quality. The machine output M is measured under an appropriate set of reference conditions and corrections are made for temperature, pressure, recombination, and polarity. The calibrated dose output is then found by multiplying the corrected machine output by the chamber calibration factor corrected for beam quality.

A similar procedure is used for electron beam calibration. An ionization chamber is selected, a calibration factor is obtained from the calibration laboratory, the value of k_{ecal} is found from a set of values tabulated for various ionization chambers, beam quality is determined in order to obtain k'_{R50}, machine output is measured under the appropriate set of reference conditions and corrections are made for temperature, pressure, polarity, and recombination, and finally, the gradient correction factor, P_{gr}^{Q}, is obtained. All these quantities are multiplied together to obtain the electron beam calibrated dose output.

One might observe that the protocol is very prescriptive, and this is true. Accuracy and reproducibility are essential in making these measurements. As indicated at the beginning of the chapter, the tolerance level of $\pm 5\%$ in the final dose determination is considered acceptable for clinical use.

A more general protocol that includes calibration of proton beams has been developed by the International Atomic Energy Agency (IAEA)[5]. This protocol, referred to as the TRS-398 Protocol, is similar to the TG-51 protocol in that the dose is determined from a dosimeter reading multiplied by a calibration factor multiplied by a beam-quality factor, but the reference conditions are somewhat different from those described in the TG-51 protocol.[6] In addition the TRS-398 protocol includes proton and heavy ion beams.

16.7 QUESTIONS, EXERCISES, & PROBLEMS

16-1. A boundary region between carbon and aluminum media is traversed by a fluence of 4.10×10^{11} electrons/cm^2 with energy of 12.5 MeV. The ambient temperature is $27\,^{\circ}C$. Ignoring delta rays and scattering, (a) what is the absorbed dose in the carbon adjacent to the boundary, D_C, and (b) what is the dose ratio D_{Al}/D_C, given that the collisional stopping powers of 12.5 MeV electrons in carbon and aluminum are 1.769 $MeV\ cm^2/g$ and 1.658 $MeV\ cm^2/g$, respectively?

16-2. (a) Prove mathematically that the planar fluence through the circle in Fig. (16.1) remains unchanged, but that the fluence through the sphere increases if the incident radiation passes through a scattering, non-absorbing medium, as shown on the right side of the figure. *Hint:* Assume that the incident rays on the left of Fig. (16.1) and at the top of the right-hand figure have a distance d between them, and assume that the rays are scattered through an angle θ. (b) Explain how, when a uniform beam of photons is incident on a scattering, absorbing medium, it is possible for the fluence of the beam beyond the absorbing medium to be greater than that before the medium, while the planar fluence must decrease.

16-3. A 1.50-keV photon interacts with a medium via the photoelectric effect (see §8.1). The binding energy of the ejected electron was $350\,eV$. Immediately after its emission, the electron emits a 0.2-keV Bremsstrahlung photon, after which the electron has energy 0.92 keV. Calculate (a) the energy transferred, (b) the net energy transferred, and (c) the energy imparted to a small volume surrounding the location of the photoelectric effect interaction. Hint: See Ex.(16.2).

16-4. A 3.70-MeV photon interacts with a medium via pair production (see §8.3). The emitted electron and positron each have energy 1.31 MeV. Calculate (a) the energy transferred, (b) the net energy transferred, and (c) the energy imparted to a small volume surrounding the location of the pair-production interaction. Hint: See

Ex.(16.2). Assume that both the electron and positron escape the region of a small volume surrounding the location of the pair-production event.

16-5. A small air-filled cavity has copper walls with thickness equal to the maximum electron range. The cavity volume is $0.100\,cm^3$, the air density is $0.001293\,g/cm^3$, and a given gamma ray exposure generates a charge (either sign) of $7.00 \times 10^{-10}\,C$. (a) What is the average absorbed dose in the cavity air given that the measurement is done in the winter? (b) Apply Bragg-Gray theory to estimate the absorbed dose in the adjacent copper wall assuming a mean energy of $0.45\,MeV$ for the cavity-crossing electrons, given that the collision stopping powers of $0.45\,MeV$ electrons in air and in copper are $1.845\,MeV\,cm^2/g$ and $1.402\,MeV\,cm^2/g$, respectively? (c) Suppose the mean electron energy is in error by 34% and should have been $0.65\,MeV$. Redo part (b). What is the resulting percentage error in D_{Cu}, given that the collision stopping powers of $0.65\,MeV$ electrons in air and Cu are $1.725\,MeV\,cm^2/g$ and $1.312\,MeV\,cm^2/g$, respectively?

16-6. Estimate the linear accelerator beam current necessary to deliver a photon dose rate of $500\,cGy/min$ at a depth of $10\,cm$ in a water phantom. *Hint:* To solve this problem, you will have to make a series of assumptions and approximations. Explicitly identify the assumptions and approximations you are making.

16-7. A ^{60}Co beam of field size $10\,cm \times 10\,cm$ is incident on a water phantom. Estimate the total number of photons hitting the water surface if a dose of $1\,Gy$ is delivered at the depth of maximum dose. Use $(\mu_{en}/\rho)_{water} = 0.0309\,cm^2/g$ at $1\,MeV$ and $0.0282\,cm^2/g$ at $1.5\,MeV$.

16-8. Repeat the calculations in the previous problem for the case of a $10\,MeV$ electron beam. Use $(S_{col}/\rho)_{water} = 2\,MeV\,cm^2/g$.

16.8   REFERENCES

1. The International Commission on Radiation Units and Measurements. *ICRU Report No. 85: Fundamental Quantities and Units for Ionizing Radiation (Revised)*. Gaithersburg, MD: Oxford University Press; 2011.
2. AAPM Scientific Committee on Radiation Dosimetry (SCRAD). Protocol for the dosimetry of x- and gamma-ray beams with maximum energies between 0-6 and 50 MeV. *Phys Med Biol.* 1971; 16:379-396.
3. AAPM Task Group 21. A protocol for the determination of absorbed dose from high-energy photon and electron beams. *Med Phys.* 1983; 10(6):741-771.
4. Almond PR, Biggs PJ, Coursey BM, et al. AAPM's TG-51 protocol for clinical reference dosimetry of high-energy photon and electron beams. *Med Phys.* 1999; 26(9): 1847-1870.
5. IAEA TRS-398. Absorbed Dose Determination in External Beam Radiotherapy: An International Code of Practice for Dosimetry based on Standards of Absorbed Dose to Water, IAEA (2024). https://www-pub.iaea.org/MTCD/publications/PDF/p15048-DOC-010-398-Rev1_web.pdf
6. Huq MS, Andreo P, Song H. Comparison of the IAEA TRS-398 and AAPM TG-51 absorbed dose to water protocols in the dosimetry of high-energy photon and electron beams. *Phys Med Biol.* 2001; 46(11): 2985-3006.

Clinical Dosimetry

CONTENTS

In the previous chapter, we defined many quantities used in radiation measurement. We defined exposure to be the charge released per unit mass, absorbed dose as the energy absorbed per unit mass, and several other quantities that described the transfer of energy from the radiation to the target under various sets of circumstances. In this chapter, we shall address how these radiation quantities are measured.

Dosimetry is the calculation and measurement of absorbed dose. Radiation measurements are of two types: absolute measurements and relative measurements. Absolute measurements are measurements based on the specific definition of the quantity, whereas relative measurements measure a property that changes due to absorption of energy from the radiation. Absolute measurements can be used as measurement standards, whereas relative measurements need to be calibrated, that is, readings on the relative measurement device must be compared to readings on the standard.

In this chapter we shall focus primarily on radiation measurement devices used in clinical applications. In addition, we will investigate two methods of absolute dosimetry. These two methods are included in this chapter because they are presently, or have been previously, used as dosimetric standards.

17.1   THE FREE-AIR IONIZATION CHAMBER

The free-air ionization chamber is a device that directly measures exposure. Recall that exposure is defined to be the charge released per unit mass in air. Figure (17.1) is a schematic of a free-air ionization chamber. The chamber is in a lead-lined box that is isolated from the radiation, because we want to keep stray radiation from entering

DOI: 10.1201/9781003477457-17

the box. Inside the box is a parallel-plate ionization chamber that is filled with air. The top plate is solid, while the bottom plate is divided into two sections. The first section—the center part of the bottom plate—is called the *collecting electrode*. The second section, an annular ring surrounding the collecting electrode, is called the *guard electrode* or the *guard ring*. There is a small gap between the collecting electrode and the guard ring.

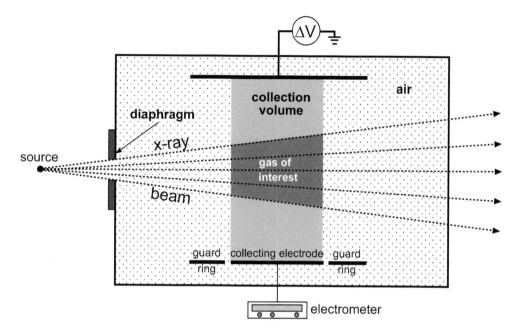

FIGURE 17.1: Schematic of a free-air ionization chamber.

A high voltage is applied from the top plate to the bottom plate. The guard ring serves to define precisely the volume of air from which the charge is collected (the light shaded region in Fig. 17.1). The guard ring ensures that the lines of electric force are as perpendicular to the electrodes as possible. The gap between the collecting electrode and the guard ring must be made very small, but it has to be large enough so that the collecting electrode is insulated from the guard ring. The whole alignment of this is very critical, because a small change in these lines of force (and they can sometimes bow out and sometimes bow in) will change the collection volume. The change in collection volume will change the measurements, which we do not want to happen.

The x-rays enter the ionization chamber through a diaphragm. The diaphragm is extremely carefully machined so that not only is the area of the opening known but also its shape. X-rays enter the chamber and interact with the air, releasing electrons. The electrons then go off and produce additional ionization charges.

An *electrometer* measures the charge that is collected at the collecting electrode. The definition of exposure, Eq. (16.1), says we are interested in all of the ionization charges produced by the electrons that are released within the mass of the *gas of interest*. In this case, the gas of interest is the gas in the volume defined by the electrodes and the diaphragm (the dark shaded region in Fig. 17.1). Note that the gas of interest is a portion of the air within the collection volume.

However, there is a problem in measuring exposure: we must collect all of the charge that is produced as a consequence of electrons released within the gas of interest. It is assumed that all of this charge will remain within the collection volume and will therefore be collected and counted. But, in reality, some electrons released within the gas of interest will leave the collection volume, so the charges produced by these electrons will *not* be collected. On the other hand, some electrons produced within the x-ray beam but outside the gas of interest will enter the collection volume and subsequently produce charges within that volume that *will* be collected.

If the measurement is set up so that an electron produced outside the gas of interest that enters the collection volume and releases charge within that volume is balanced by the charge produced by an electron released within the gas of interest that leaves the collection volume, then a condition called *charged particle equilibrium* (CPE) is achieved. In order to achieve CPE, the distance from the gas of interest to the electrodes must be greater than the range of the secondary electrons produced. (*Secondary electrons* are those electrons released by the primary electrons, which are electrons released by the incident x-rays within the gas of interest.) If we make this distance just greater than the range of the secondary electrons, it provides a good approximation to charged particle equilibrium and primary electrons produced outside the gas of interest will just make it into the collection volume. But they will be compensated for by electrons produced within the gas of interest that barely leave the collection volume. In that way, charged particle equilibrium is achieved.

It is important that *all* of the charge produced by the electrons released within the gas of interest are collected. If the chamber is too small, a secondary electron could reach one of the collecting electrodes directly, depositing some of its energy in the collecting electrode instead of releasing it within the collection volume. So the separation of the plates is determined again by the range of the secondary electrons. Ignoring the fact that the energy of these secondary electrons may be a little lower than that of the primary electrons ejected by the x-ray beam in the forward direction within the gas of interest, we require the separation of the plates to be about twice the range of the secondary electrons. With that condition, an electron produced in the collection volume can deposit all of its energy and stop before it gets to a plate. So the dimensions of the ion chamber are determined by the energy of the x-rays that are being measured, since higher-energy x-rays can release higher-energy electrons. We will soon see how that will create a problem.

The exposure that we measure is then equal to the charge that is collected divided by the mass of the gas interest.

Let's add a slight complication. The definition of the *roentgen* (Eq.16.2), the (old) unit for exposure, is in terms of the mass of air. The use of the term "air" implies dry air. If moisture is present, then the value of energy absorbed per unit charge changes a bit. Exposure is defined for dry air and so corrections may have to be made for humidity.

When we measure ionization, we typically have defined a fixed volume of air, but exposure is defined for a fixed mass of air, so we need to make corrections for temperature and pressure, which change the mass of air in a fixed volume. The normal temperature-pressure correction factor is based on dry air.

We typically do not make humidity corrections on a regular basis when we do calibrations, but the national standardization laboratories certainly do. If there is humid air, it changes the relationship between volume and mass of air. We need to put in a term that takes into account if there is moisture in the air to make sure we can get the mass of the gas accurately.

The collection volume is defined by the entrance aperture and the length of the collecting electrode. The cross-sectional area is defined at a point within the volume of the gas of interest, and not at the entrance aperture. We cannot measure the cross-sectional area inside the volume of interest accurately—there is no easy way of getting to that point inside the chamber. But, if we say the exposure at the entrance of the diaphragm is related to the exposure at a point inside the chamber, the two will be related by the simple inverse-square relationship. The cross-sectional area in the center of the chamber is related to the cross-sectional area of the diaphragm again by the inverse-square relationship, but the relation is now the other way around. This is very convenient because when both these factors are taken into account, the two inverse-square relationships cancel out, giving us a direct relationship between the exposure *at the entrance diaphragm* and the charge collected inside the chamber. We divide the charge collected by the product of the density of air with the cross-sectional area of the *diaphragm* and the length of the collecting electrode to obtain the charge per unit mass of air, which is the exposure at the position of the diaphragm.

In a free-air ionization chamber used for standards work the diaphragm is very carefully machined. The length of the collection volume and the cross-sectional area of the diaphragm are both known very precisely, and the density of the air is determined very precisely as well. The effect of moisture must be taken into account and the charge is measured very precisely. With that information, the exposure in the middle of the entrance diaphragm is determined.

What, then, makes the free-air ionization chamber impractical for clinical use? The problem is that we need to surround the volume of the gas of interest with a sufficient amount of air so that charged particle equilibrium is achieved, and all the charges released by the secondary electrons can be collected. As mentioned earlier, the thickness of the surrounding air needs to be approximately twice the range of the secondary electrons. Table (17.1) gives this range as a function of incident photon energy.

We can infer from this table that, for energies greater than orthovoltage energies (0.1–0.5 MeV), we may have some problems with using a free-air ionization chamber for making radiation measurements. If the plate separation is greater than about a meter, the chamber becomes inordinately large and unwieldly for clinical use. If the chamber is too large, it is not possible to get good straight lines of electrical force to define the collection volume, so the measurement of collection volume becomes inaccurate. Moreover, if the distance between the diaphragm and the collection volume gets very large, significant attenuation of the x-rays in the air in front of the collection volume occurs. And so for energies above about 300 or 400 keV, the size of chambers becomes so large that it is extremely difficult to measure exposure with

TABLE 17.1: Maximum path length of secondary electrons for various photon energies

Photon Energy (MeV)	Maximum Electron Path Length in Air (m)
0.3	0.3
1.0	3.0
3.0	12.2
10.0	40.9

any kind of accuracy, so another approach must be found. That is why we turn to cavity ionization chambers for clinical measurements.

17.2   THIMBLE IONIZATION CHAMBERS

The issue, then, is how to design a chamber that makes ionization measurements and is more mobile than a free-air ionization chamber. To answer that question, we must keep in mind that the free-air ionization chamber has no physical wall to it. The wall, if you like, is an "air wall" surrounding the collection volume that is defined by the diaphragm and the collecting electrode. The rationale for the need of an air wall in the chamber is that the air surrounding the collection volume is used solely to stop electrons that are produced in the collection volume. Consider what would happen if the air wall were "condensed" into "solid air" wall material. A "solid air" wall thick enough to provide electronic equilibrium would permit measurement of exposure with an ionization chamber that would be far more mobile than a free-air ionization chamber. Unfortunately, solid air only exists at extremely low temperatures. However, if we were able to replace the solid air wall with a wall material that interacts with radiation in the same manner as air, we would obtain the same instrument reading as if we had used a solid air-wall chamber. Such a solid material would be called "air-equivalent" and would have radiation parameters, such as the mass energy absorption coefficient, stopping power ratio, stopping power, that are the same as that for air. Although no material is truly air-equivalent, certain materials come very close. Carbon by itself, for example, acts very much like air with respect to these interaction parameters.

It is important to make sure that the walls are equilibrium thickness, but corrections have to be made for attenuation of radiation in the wall. To correct for wall attenuation, ionization measurements must be made for several wall thicknesses. Once this is done, we will have an ionization chamber that has a wall made of air-equivalent material but with caps of different thicknesses. We continue adding to the wall thickness and measuring the ionization. The ionization will initially start to increase, because of increased production of secondary electrons, but then when charged-particle equilibrium is achieved, ionization will begin to decrease because of attenuation. The desired wall thickness will occur where the maximum ionization is reached, just before absorption begins to dominate. However, there is also absorption in the equilibrium thickness of wall, so we plot ionization *vs.* wall thickness and extrapolate the curve back to zero wall thickness to obtain the true ionization value. An ionization chamber designed in this fashion is called a *thimble ionization chamber*. The left side of Fig. (17.2) shows a schematic of such a chamber, while the right side shows three models of thimble chambers.

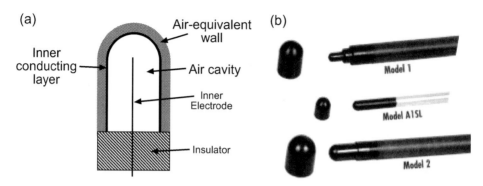

FIGURE 17.2: (a) Schematic of a thimble chamber. The air-equivalent chamber wall allows for electron equilibrium. A high voltage between the inner electrode and the inner conducting layer of the chamber wall allows for the collection of ionization pairs, from which the amount of ionization within the chamber can be determined. (b) Three models of Exradin thimble chambers (Exradin® A1 [REF 92705], Exradin® A1SL [REF 92722], and Exradin® A2 [REF 92718]) manufactured by Standard Imaging® in Middleton, WI, USA. The build-up caps to the left can be attached to the thimble chamber to provide electron equilibrium within the air cavity for different qualities of incident radiation. (Photo courtesy of Standard Imaging.)

The main point to take away from a discussion of a thimble chamber is that the measurement of exposure is no longer an absolute measurement because no solid material is truly air-equivalent. Consequently, a thimble chamber must be calibrated, preferably to an ionization chamber the calibration of which is directly traceable to a national standard. On the other hand, the thimble chamber is much more compact than the free-air ionization chamber and can be used for practical measurements in the clinic.

17.3 THERMOLUMINESCENT DOSIMETRY

Nevertheless, a thimble chamber is a fragile device and much care must be taken in the transportation and handling of the chamber. Moreover, a chamber is still a relatively large device and would not be practical for making in vivo real-time dose measurements while a patient is being treated. The two issues of fragility and size can be overcome by the use of *thermoluminescent dosimeters* (TLDs) for clinical measurements. In order to understand how a TLD works, it is necessary to review a bit of condensed matter physics.

We recall that isolated atoms have electronic energy levels that can be populated with electrons. (See the end of Chapter 4 for a discussion of atomic energy level

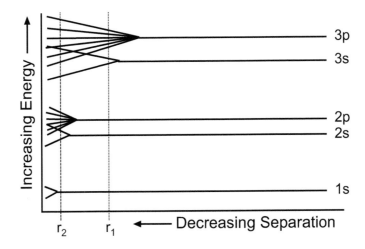

FIGURE 17.3: The splitting of degenerate energy levels as atoms move closer to one another. (Not to scale.)

diagrams.) In the presence of a perturbation such as a nearby atom, the energy levels split, as illustrated in Fig. (17.3). The right-hand side of the figure represents the energy level diagram for an isolated atom, well separated from its neighbors. As the separation between neighboring atoms decreases, the outer electrons of the neighboring atoms start interacting with one another, leading to a splitting of the degenerate higher-energy levels (position r_1). As the separation between atoms decreases even further (position r_2), even the inner electrons start interacting with the electrons in the other atoms, causing a corresponding splitting of their degenerate energy levels, also.

In the limit as the atoms get very close to one another, as in the case of crystalline solids, the energy levels split and overlap so much that they start forming *bands* of energy levels. The filled energy band of highest energy in a solid is the called the *valence band*, analogous to the valence shell of a single atom. The energy band of higher energy that contains unoccupied energy states is the *conduction band*. Electrons in the valence band are bound to the atomic lattice, but electrons with energies sufficiently high to place them in the conduction band can move freely through the entire solid.

Now, suppose that the valence band and the conduction band overlap, meaning that they form a single partially filled energy band. In that case electrons can move freely between bands, and, while in the conduction portion of the band, can travel through the entire material. The material is now capable of conducting electricity and is called a *conductor*. On the other hand, if there is a large energy gap between the valence band and the conduction band, electrons are no longer able to move freely through the material. The material is not able to conduct electricity; this material is an *insulator*. In between these two extremes is a material called a *semiconductor* that has a smaller energy gap than an insulator. Adding impurities to the semiconducting material—a process called *doping*—may introduce energy levels into the energy gap between the valence and conduction bands; it is these impurity energy levels that make TLDs work. Figure (17.4) illustrates energy diagrams for these three types of materials.

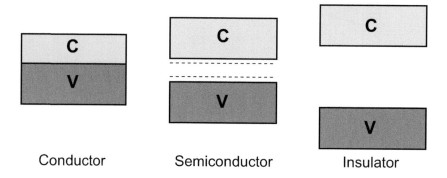

FIGURE 17.4: Conduction (C) and valence (V) bands in a conductor, a semiconductor, and an insulator. The dashed lines within the gap between the valence and conduction bands in a semiconductor show positions of possible impurity energy levels in doped semiconductors.

When a material such as LiF is exposed to radiation, the absorbed energy causes electrons to move from the valence band to the conduction band. The electrons in the conduction band are not stable—they can lose energy by moving into the impurity level within the band gap and are then trapped there. These electrons are in a metastable state, meaning that they can remain in the impurity level for a long period of time. Heating the material gives the electrons sufficient energy to return to the conduction band. They can then drop down to the valence band, recombining with positive charges (holes), and emitting radiation in the form of light. The thermoluminescent (TL) material exhibits a glow peak, in which the wavelength of the light is characteristic of the impurity, and the intensity of light emitted is a function of the TL temperature. The amount of light emitted can then be related to the amount of energy absorbed, that is, the absorbed dose.

LiF doped with Mg and Ti is perhaps the most common material used for TL dosimeters, although other materials exhibit TL behavior. Clinically useful TL dosimeters come in the form of squares, rods, or powder. Consistent handling of the dosimeter material is essential to accurate TL measurements. Prior to irradiation, the TLD is annealed to remove electrons remaining in traps from previous use. Annealing typically involves heating the TL material to a temperature of $400\,^{o}C$ for 1 hour. This annealing resets the trap structure and eliminates electrons from the remaining traps. The TL material is then exposed to radiation. After exposure, it is necessary to anneal the TLD once again, removing unstable, low-temperature traps. Post-irradiation annealing can be done by allowing the material to rest for 24 hr at $80\,^{o}C$, which eliminates the low-temperature traps. Alternatively, one could heat the TL material to $100\,^{o}C$ for 1 hr, emptying the low-temperature traps, but not eliminating the trap structure. The high-temperature traps are much more stable and may remain undisturbed for many years. Cooling can also have a large effect on the TL response. Greatest sensitivity of the TL material occurs if cooling is done on an aluminum plate at room temperature for approximately half an hour.

In order to determine the absorbed dose, the TL material is heated to a temperature of $250-300\,^\circ C$ and the amount of emitted light is measured. The glow curve depends on the readout temperature and the readout time after irradiation. Figure (17.5) illustrates glow curves as a function of time and heating rate. The presence of multiple traps generally makes the glow curves more complicated. Low-temperature glow peaks correspond to the unstable traps that are removed during the post-irradiation annealing.

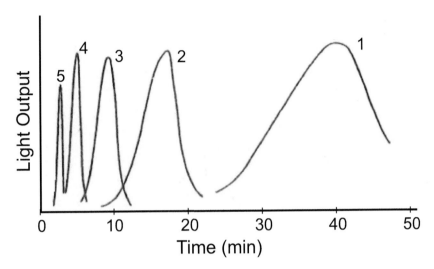

FIGURE 17.5: Glow curves as a function of time and heating rate. 1: 4° per minute; 2: 10° per minute; 3: 20° per minute; 4: 40° per minute; 5: 80° per minute.

The measured TL output is dependent on the batch of TL material and is a function of the temperature of the peak, the heating rate, *etc.* Consequently, a TLD must be calibrated. In the calibration process, TL material from the same batch as the TL used in measurement is exposed to known radiation doses and the amount of emitted light is measured.

The TL response for lithium fluoride doped with magnesium and titanium (LiF:Mg,Ti) is essentially linear up to doses of 5–10 Gy. For greater doses, the TL exhibits supralinear response to around 1 kGy, with damage occurring for doses above 1 kGy. Figure (17.6) illustrates this supralinearity. One can still use a TLD for dosimetry in the supralinear region provided the doses used for calibration are close in value to the estimated dose intended for measurement. For doses beyond 1 kGy, however, because of the potential for damage to the TL material, using a TLD is not advised.

The TL response is also a function of the energy of the radiation. TL over-responds for energies less than that of ^{60}Co radiation, with a maximum over-response in the range of 1.4 to 1.6 at 100 kVp, decreasing at lower energies. A TLD may display an under-response of up to 5% at energies greater than that of ^{60}Co radiation. Consequently, ensuring that the energy at which the TLD is calibrated is identical to the energy of the radiation to be measured is important.

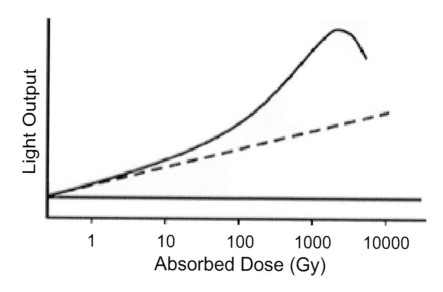

FIGURE 17.6: Supralinear response of a TLD (LiF:Mg,Ti) to radiation.

A TLD has several advantages as a clinical dosimeter. The small size of the TL dosimeter (as small as approximately $1\,mm^3$) makes it very useful for inter-institutional comparisons, as it is easy to transport, for example, using the postal system. Moreover, the small size means that a TLD can be used to measure radiation in regions of rather high field gradients. TLDs exhibit a wide dose range of linearity, and TL dosimeters are reusable as long as proper annealing procedures are followed before and after exposure.

Disadvantages of TLDs include the instabilities in sensitivity of the TL material and its dependence on the handling of the TL material, requiring consistent handling between calibration and measurement. The TL dosimeters are susceptible to surface contamination, but this can be mitigated by keeping the TL material under nitrogen gas during the readout process. Care must be taken to avoid structural damage such as scratches, which affects the light output of the TL material. Consequently, one uses vacuum tweezers for handling TL dosimeters.

Thermoluminescent dosimetry is a precise method for measuring absorbed dose in radiation therapy, with measurement precision of around 2% if appropriate care is taken in the handling of the TL material. Other applications of TLDs for radiation measurements in diagnostic radiology and health physics yield a precision of 5% to 10%.

17.4 FILM DOSIMETRY

The particular property of film that makes it useful for radiographic imaging is that it can detect spatial differences in radiation fluence to high resolution. In this section, we show how the property that film blackening can be related to radiation dose can be applied so that film can be used as a dosimeter.[1] In this section, we begin with the relationship between film optical density and dose.

The *optical density* of a photographic film is an exponential measure of the amount of light that can penetrate the film—a greater optical density means that less light can penetrate. ($OD = 0$ means that all light penetrates; $OD = 1$ means that 10% of the incident light penetrates; etc.) More specifically, the OD is defined to be

$$OD = \log_{10}\left(\frac{I_i}{I_t}\right), \tag{17.1}$$

where I_i and I_t are the incident and transmitted intensities of light.

A Hurter & Driffeld (H&D) curve plots *optical density vs. log(exposure)*. Figure (17.7a) illustrates such an *H&D curve*. A more common representation of this relationship in dosimetry, however, is the *sensitometric curve*, which plots *dose vs. optical density*. An example of a sensitometric curve is illustrated in Fig. (17.7b). The sensitometric curve generally tends to be more linear than the H&D curve, and consequently, interpolates more accurately. The relationship between dose and optical density is a function of many parameters, including dose, dose rate, type of radiation, energy of radiation, depth of measurement, field size, film orientation, and processor conditions. In an optimum film for dosimetry the optical density will be linear with dose as well as dose rate, independent of radiation type and energy, independent of orientation, and independent of processor conditions. Since such independence is generally not achievable, it is important that film be calibrated using radiation of the same type and energy as that being measured. Moreover, it goes without saying that the calibration film come from the same batch as the measurement film, and both types of film be processed under identical conditions.

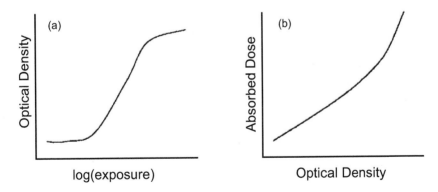

FIGURE 17.7: (a) Example of an H&D curve. (b) Example of a sensitometric curve.

The selection of film type is also important. The useful operating range of the optical density for radiation dosimetry is in the range of 1.0 (10% transmission of radiation) to 3.0 (0.1% transmission). Many types of film are commercially available to enable one to measure dose in various ranges.

Several points should be noted if one wishes to set film up for two-dimensional dosimetry. First, one needs to be very careful in setting up the film embedded in the surrounding phantom. In particular, it is important to minimize air gaps because even small air gaps can cause significant perturbations in film response. As the size of the air gap increases, the magnitude of the air-gap perturbation of the dose distribution also increases. Moreover, misalignment of the film may also cause a perturbation in the receptor response. In order to eliminate these issues, one may vacuum-pack the film. In particular, some modern films used in dosimetry are already vacuum-packed. Film cassettes can ensure reproducible film position as can specially-made phantoms for film dosimetry.

Film dosimetry is especially sensitive to scattered radiation. Because the primary component of film that responds to radiation is the silver halide, a material with an effective atomic number much greater than that of tissue, the sensitivity of film is highly dependent on the energy of the radiation, especially in the region where the photoelectric effect is the primary interaction. The energy of scattered radiation can be very different from that of the primary beam, consequently, the response of the film to the scattered radiation will be different from its response to the primary radiation. Suchowerska et al.[2] used Monte Carlo simulations to demonstrate how the photon spectrum changes with depth as a result of scattered radiation as well as beam hardening, hence, the film sensitivity changes with depth.

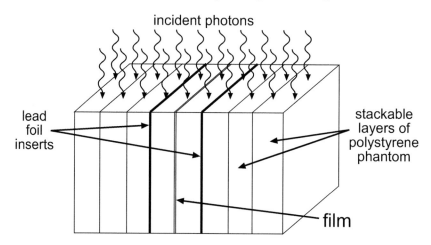

FIGURE 17.8: Film and phantom configuration for depth dose measurement.

Placing a lead filter on either side of the film has been shown by Burch et al.[3] to enable the measurement of dose distributions by reducing scatter. Figure (17.8) shows their set-up: stackable slabs of polystyrene phantom are placed on either side of the film along with two lead foils . Various qualities of radiation can be accommodated by varying the number of slabs to either side of the film.[3,4]

When the effects of scatter are accounted for, film and ion chamber measurements give good agreement for measuring isodose curves[5].

Film dosimetry has the following advantages:

I. Film has excellent spatial resolution with sub-millimeter spatial accuracy.

II. Film enables one to obtain a permanent record of the measurement.

III. Film enables one to obtain a two-dimensional dose distribution with a single exposure.

IV. Film is readily available and relatively inexpensive.

V. Film response is linear at least over a short range of doses, and independent of field size.

Several cautions need to be observed in using film for dosimetry. First, one must keep in mind the strong energy dependence of the sensitivity of film. Film is highly sensitive to low-energy photons due to photoelectric interactions in the high-Z silver ions in the film. Next, careful orientation of the film plane with respect to beam direction is required. The user must be aware of emulsion differences in different batches of film; consequently, in calibrating the film used for dosimetry, it is important to use film for calibration from the same batch as the film used for dosimetry. Moreover, the optical density depends on how the film is processed, including such factors as developer chemistry, temperature, and time. The result of this dependence is that the calibration film must be developed in the same batch as the dosimetry film. Film is highly sensitive to the environment; it can fade due to heat and humidity. As a result, one must be very careful about film storage, both before and after exposure. Furthermore, poor environmental conditions can lead to microbial growth in the gelatin matrix. Finally, film is subject to solarization, a condition observed at very high doses where the optical density of the film decreases with dose.

In summary, radiographic film has been shown as an ideal detector for relative dose measurements, being best suited for planar dose distributions. However, film response is dependent on many extraneous factors including batch, exposure conditions, processing conditions, beam energy, dose, dose rate, *etc.*

Several options have been made available in order to overcome some of these disadvantages of film. For verification imaging, film has been replaced by electronic devices, whereas for obtaining planar dose distributions, some of the aforementioned disadvantages of radiographic film can be overcome by the used of radiochromic film.[6] Radiochromic film is a useful detector over a wide range of doses ($0.01\,Gy - 1000\,Gy$). Radiochromic film consists of a layer of radiosensitive organic microcrystal monomers on a polyester base with a transparent coating. The film color turns blue upon irradiation due to polymerization of the monomer. Analogous to radiographic film, the darkness of radiochromic film increases with increasing dose. However, unlike radiographic film, radiochromic film needs no processing.

Two peaks are observed in the optical absorption spectrum of radiochromic film, a large peak at $633\,nm$, and a lesser peak at $580\,nm$. Optical density can be measured using a He-Ne laser, which generates light at $633\,nm$, and a spectrophotometer or color scanner detector.

Film handling is critical; the ambient temperature must be controlled in a consistent fashion during irradiation, storage, and readout. Film must be handled with care, avoiding dust and fingerprints. Film must be stored in a cool, dry environment to maximize its life. High temperatures (greater than 70^oC) must be avoided, as these temperatures will activate the dye. Film must also be stored in a dark environment because radiochromic film is light-sensitive. After irradiation, at least 24 hours, preferably 48 hours, should pass before readout in order for the film darkness to stabilize.

Similar to that of radiographic film, the response of radiochromic film depends on the film batch, beam quality, readout time, temperature, humidity; consequently, radiochromic film must be calibrated using known amounts of radiation of comparable energy. In addition, the response of radiochromic film depends on the wavelength of light in the scanner. It is also important to calibrate over the linear portion of the calibration curve. Calibration measurements are generally made in a phantom. A water phantom is most desirable, but one should avoid prolonged immersion of film in water. Plastic phantoms can also be used, but it is very important to avoid air gaps between the film and the phantom.

When compared to other types of dosimeters used in clinical applications, radiochromic film is relatively insensitive to radiation. Consequently, it can be used for high-dose dosimetry. Applications include dosimetry of ^{90}Sr ophthalmic applicators, dosimetry in the vicinity of brachytherapy sources where the dose gradient due to inverse-square falloff is large, dosimetry at tissue-metal dental interfaces, dosimetry of small radiation fields used in stereotactic radiosurgery where electronic disequilibrium occurs, and dosimetry in the penumbra of radiotherapy beams where a significant amount of the radiation is low-energy scatter.

17.5   CALORIMETRY

When the energy of ionizing radiation is absorbed by the patient, the energy of the ionizing radiation is converted to heat. If we can measure the amount of heat absorbed by the target material, we can determine the amount of energy absorbed by the target. The absorbed energy is converted to heat, which can be directly measured as temperature. Temperature rise is relatively straightforward to measure using a thermocouple, and can readily be converted to energy absorbed by multiplying the temperature rise by the specific heat of the absorbing material. For example, the specific heat of water it is approximately $4200\,J/kg\,C^o$. Note that because the measurement is a direct measurement of energy absorbed, calorimetry is an absolute measurement of absorbed dose; a calorimeter can be used as a standard. In fact, the present standard for measurement of absorbed dose is established using a calorimeter.

Calorimetry, however, has two major drawbacks that hinder its use in the clinic. The first problem is that of heat loss. One needs a highly insulated volume to minimize heat loss. The second problem is that the temperature rise in water from absorbed dose due to ionizing radiation is very small. Note that the specific heat of water can be written as $4200\,Gy/C^o$. Consequently, a dose measurement of, for example, $1\,Gy$, corresponds to a temperature rise of $0.0002\,C^o$. Because of these two drawbacks, calorimetry is not practical for clinical applications, but is used in standards laboratories.

17.6   CHEMICAL DOSIMETRY

The transfer of energy from radiation to a target can also induce chemical reactions. The conversion of silver halide to metallic silver in radiographic film is an example of such a reaction. Unlike film, several other chemical reactions are less dependent on ambient conditions and can be used as practical dosimeters. As long as a quantitative change in an appropriate material due to a chemical reaction can be accurately measured, the reaction may serve as the basis for a chemical dosimeter.

An example of such a reaction is the oxidation of the Fe^{+2} ion in aqueous solution of $FeSO_4$ in what is known as the *Fricke dosimeter.* In this dosimeter, the amount of Fe^{+3} ion produced is proportional to the amount of energy absorbed. A quantity known as the *G-value* is the proportionality constant, the amount of Fe^{+3} ion produced per unit of absorbed energy. The G-value is slightly dependent on energy and is approximately equal to $1.61\,\mu mol/J$.[7] The ion in solution is colored and absorbs light in the range of $304\,nm$. The technique of Fricke dosimetry involves irradiating an aqueous solution of $FeSO_4$, measuring the extent of attenuation of light through the irradiated solution, converting the extent of attenuation to the number of ferric ions produced, which can then be the related to the amount of energy absorbed. Fricke dosimetry is an absolute measurement, but it is infrequently used in the clinic.

A Fricke dosimeter is prepared by using a solution of 1 mM ferrous ammonium sulfate and $1\,mM$ sodium chloride in $0.4\,M$ sulfuric acid. Sodium chloride is added to reduce sensitivity to organic impurities[8]. After irradiation, readout is accomplished by the use of a spectrophotometer to measure absorption. The ferric ion in solution has two absorption peaks, one at $224\,nm$ and the other at $303\,nm$. Comparing the unattenuated light intensity to the light intensity of the attenuated beam gives us the optical density of the ferric ion solution. Recalling the definition of *OD* given in Eq. (17.1), it can be shown that the optical density (OD) of the ferric ion solution is related to the ion concentration by the relation

$$OD = \log_{10}\left(\frac{I_i}{I_t}\right) = c \cdot L \cdot \epsilon, \qquad (17.2)$$

where c is the ion concentration, L is the length of the absorption vessel, and ϵ is the molar extinction coefficient, a measure of how strongly a chemical species or substance absorbs light at a particular wavelength.

The optical density is measured before and after irradiation. Once the change in optical density has been determined, the (Fricke) dose is calculated using the expression

$$D_F = \frac{\Delta(OD)}{\epsilon \cdot G\left(Fe^{+3}\right) \cdot \rho \cdot L}. \qquad (17.3)$$

All the quantities in the right-hand side of Eq. (17.3) are measurable, so we have an absolute dosimeter. Fricke dose measurements are very reproducible; the precision is typically better than 0.15%. A small energy-dependent response is observed for photons due to the LET of photon radiation, but very little energy dependence is observed for electrons.

Equation (17.3) gives us the dose to the Fricke dosimeter, but we really want to determine the dose in water (because tissue acts very much like water). The dose in water is related to the dose to the dosimeter by

$$D_w = D_F\, f_{w,F}\, P_{wall}\, k_{dd}, \qquad (17.4)$$

where the dose to the dosimeter is multiplied by correction factors, including an f-factor, relating the difference in electron stopping powers, a wall correction factor, and a factor k_{dd} to account for the radial nonuniformity of the beam.

In recent years, Fricke dosimetry has been superseded by other, more convenient clinical dosimetric methods, but several applications of Fricke dosimetry still remain. One of these is absolute dosimetry of low-energy $(4\,MeV - 6\,MeV)$ electrons. The standard for absolute dosimetry is the calorimeter, but, because of the sharp depth dependence of the low-energy electron beam, it is difficult to place a calorimeter at a specified reference depth.

In conclusion, the major advantage of Fricke dosimetry is that it is an absolute measurement of dose. A Fricke dosimeter can be used as a primary dosimeter as long as an accurate G-value is known. The major disadvantage of Fricke dosimetry is its high sensitivity to impurities.[9]

17.7 OPTICALLY-STIMULATED LUMINESCENCE DOSIMETRY

Earlier in this chapter we presented the principles of thermoluminescence. In general, luminescence is the process of emission of light following irradiation. If the interval between irradiation and light emission is less than $10^{-8}\,s$, we refer to the process as *fluorescence*; if the interval is longer, the process is referred to as *luminescence*. Moreover, various forms of luminescence exist. The various forms all have the name "X"-luminescence, where "X" is the method of stimulating the luminescence. If X is heat, that is, heat is used to stimulate the luminescence, we have *thermoluminescence*; if X is light, we have the process known as *optically-stimulated luminescence* (OSL).

OSL has been known for over 50 years. It has been used for many years in luminescence dating. In the 1990s, highly sensitive Al_2O_3:C (Aluminum oxide doped with carbon) was introduced, which led to applications initially in environmental and personnel dosimetry, and, more recently, in radiation therapy.

OSL dosimetry differs from TL dosimetry only in the nature of the detector, and, of course, the material undergoing irradiation. In OSL dosimetry, the stimulation of the exposed detector is done by light, rather than heat. Specific stimulation filters and detection filters are used to focus on specific wavelengths of light emitted in the process of OSL.

Three major methods of OSL stimulation are *continuous-wave OSL* (CW-OSL), *pulsed OSL* (POSL), and *linearly modulated OSL* (LM-OSL). In CW-OSL the stimulation light source is of constant intensity, while the emitted signal of wavelengths different from those of the stimulation light source is recorded. Filtration of the emitted signal is necessary to eliminate detection of the stimulation light. CW-OSL is the most common form of OSL stimulation. In POSL, the stimulation source is pulsed with a duration of hundreds of nanoseconds with a frequency of several thousand Hertz. The detector is blocked during the stimulation, so it is not necessary to filter the emitted light. LM-OSL is similar to CW-OSL except that the intensity of light is ramped and continuously increased. It is not as commonly used as CW-OSL.

Several properties of OSL dosimeters make them quite useful for clinical applications. The ideal OSL dosimeter is small, and does not significantly perturb the radiation field. Measurements using this detector are reproducible. No corrections need to be made for environmental conditions such as temperature, pressure, or humidity. Dose response is linear and independent of dose rate, beam energy. Finally, response is isotropic, independent of orientation of the dosimeter with respect to the radiation field.

Now, let us compare Al_2O_3:C dosimeters with an ideal dosimeter. Early measurements found reproducibility to within one standard deviation of 3.5%,[10] but modified design of detectors can improve reproducibility to within 1.0%. Nevertheless, it is recommended that calibrations of each batch of OSL detectors be done before clinical application. Al_2O_3:C dosimeters are not subject to environmental corrections. Unlike the response of a gas dosimeter, the response of a solid OSL dosimeter is independent of air pressure. Negligible temperature dependence has been observed during irradiation (Fig. 17.9)[11]; some dependence has been observed during readout.[12] Consequently, it is important to keep the readout temperature consistent. One study has shown that dose response is linear from 20 to $400\,cGy$,[13] while another study demonstrated linearity over doses from 1 to $400\,cGy$, but supralinearity at higher doses[14]. No dose rate dependence has been observed from a dose rate of 200 to $600\,cGy/min$.[13] Monte Carlo calculations comparing the response of Al_2O_3:C to that of LiF show an over-response for energies less than that of $250\,kVp$ x-rays, but negligible energy dependence above $6\,MV$ (mean energy around $2\,MeV$)[15], and this has been verified by measurement[16]. The heightened response at lower energies is due to the fact that Al_2O_3 has a greater effective atomic number than LiF. Relatively little work has been done to explore LET dependence, but there is evidence that for higher LET radiation, the sensitivity of the OSL dosimeter decreases.[17] Finally, essentially no directional dependence has been observed.[11]

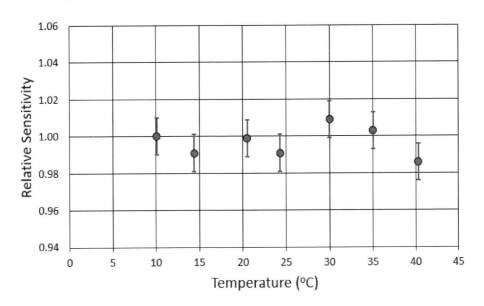

FIGURE 17.9: Temperature dependence of OSL sensitivity.

Fading is another issue that must be addressed. Fading is defined as the loss of signal with time after irradiation. In the case of Al_2O_3:C, fading occurs immediately after irradiation, reaching a steady state in about 5 minutes post-irradiation[17] with a slight decrease in signal after approximately three hours.[11] Consequently, it is important to make measurements consistently at the same time after irradiation. With this caveat, however, recognizing the relative stability of the OSL response, one finds a practical application for OSL dosimetry in remote monitoring of dose and establishing inter-institutional consistency in dosimetry.

Advantages of OSL dosimetry include high sensitivity. An OSL dosimeter can detect a dose as low as $10\,\mu Gy$, making the OSL dosimeter useful for radiation protection monitoring. If there is consistency in the OSL irradiation and readout procedure, OSL dosimeters exhibit high precision. Readout is flexible, fast, non-destructive, and convenient. Because of the small size of the OSL dosimeter, a series of such dosimeters can be used for dose mapping. As was mentioned earlier, after an initial loss of signal, fading is negligible, so dose information can be stored for later readout. There is no need for post-processing such as annealing, which is necessary when one uses TL dosimetry. Finally, OSL dosimeters can be re-used if needed.

Disadvantages of OSL dosimeters include sensitivity to light, requiring storage and handling in light-tight containers. The OSL material is not tissue equivalent, so there is an energy-dependent difference in response between dose to tissue and OSL readout, which may be significant at low beam energies. Finally, only one material has so far exhibited OSL properties and is used for clinical OSL dosimetry.

Clinical applications of OSL dosimetry include dosimetry both in-phantom and in-vivo. Measurements can be made in a phantom to determine percent depth dose and relative output factors[13], showing reasonable agreement with ion chamber measurements. OSL dosimetry can also be used for IMRT quality assurance. In-vivo applications include measurements of external beam entrance dose and exit dose. It is also feasible to perform real-time in-vivo dosimetry by placing a small Al_2O_3:C crystal in a brachytherapy needle and attaching it to a fiber optic system.[18] A final application of OSL dosimetry is its use in remote dosimetry. Dosimeters can be mailed to a number of institutions, irradiated to a specified dose, and returned to a monitoring facility, which can assess the uniformity of dosimetry among the participating institutions. Ensuring uniformity of dosimetry is essential when radiation oncology facilities participate in inter-institutional treatment protocols.

17.8 SCINTILLATION DETECTORS

So far we have looked at two types of radiation detectors that operate by having incident radiation excite electrons in the target medium, followed by a decay of excited-state electrons generating photons; the number of photons is directly proportional to energy deposited in the target. In both TLD and OSLD, the emission of photons that are detected is prompted by the deposition of additional energy, either heat (TLD) or light (OSLD). In principle, scintillation is quite similar to TLD and OSLD, except that the emission of photons is prompt ($10^{-9}\,s - 10^{-7}\,s$) following excitation. These photons are detected using a photodetector, and the light output is correlated to the dose after calibration.

Scintillation materials are of two types: inorganic and organic. The inorganic materials, such as NaI(Tl), CsI(Tl), and CsI(Na), are characterized by high Z and high density. Consequently, these detectors demonstrate an energy dependence significantly different from that of tissue, and care must be taken to calibrate these scintillation dosimeters at the same energy as that of the measurement beam. Organic plastics, such as polyvinyltoluene and polystyrene, are nearly water equivalent, hence the energy dependence of the radiation response is similar to that of tissue. Most of the energy of the incident radiation is transferred to vibrational energy of the phosphor; only about 2.4% of the incident energy is emitted as visible light with wavelength in the range of $450-550\,nm$[19].

Advantages of scintillation detectors are the properties of a linear response to dose, as well as a dose-rate independent response. Moreover, when plastics are used as the dosimetry material, due to the water equivalence of the plastic dosimeter, the response is relatively independent of incident energy; the ratio of dose to dosimeter to dose to water is in the range of 0.97–0.99 over an energy range of $0.2-20\,MeV$.[20] Dose response is also independent of temperature, and scintillation dosimeters exhibit high spatial resolution.

One issue that must be addressed with scintillation detectors is the production of Cerenkov radiation, which occurs when electrons travel through the scintillation medium at a speed exceeding the phase velocity of light in that medium. The Cerenkov radiation appears as a blue light superimposed on the scintillation signal, interfering with it. This component of the emitted light may be significant ($\sim$15%); however, it can be filtered out.[21]

Scintillation dosimetry has several clinical applications including measurement of the output of linear accelerators as part of a routine quality assurance program.[22] Scintillation detectors can also be used to make basic measurements on a radiation beam such as depth dose measurements and generation of isodose distributions.[23] Because of the small size of the scintillation detector, it can be used in making radiation measurements that support radiosurgery.[24] Finally, scintillation detectors can be placed in an array to support quality assurance measurements in intensity modulated radiation therapy (IMRT).[25]

17.9   GEL DOSIMETRY

We have already shown that the absorption of radiation can cause a change in the physical properties of the target material. In the case of the Fricke dosimeter, the physical change is a change in color due to oxidation of the Fe^{+2} ion to the Fe^{+3} ion in aqueous solution. A problem with the Fricke dosimeter, however, is that we are unable to extract spatial information about a dose distribution because of diffusion of the Fe^{+3} ion. If we added a small amount of gelatin ($\sim$5%) to the dosimeter, we would be able to lock the dose distribution in place and be able to extract spatial information about the dose.

Although the Fricke gel dosimeter is feasible, the high atomic number of the Fricke solution negates the tissue equivalence of the dosimeter, consequently, organic polymers, which have a lower average atomic number, are considered much more desirable. Most gel dosimetry is thus effected by the use of the polymer gel dosimeter, whose response to radiation is based on the degree of polymerization of the monomer embedded in the gel matrix.

Gel dosimeters exhibit high three-dimensional spatial resolution. They can be manufactured in anatomical phantoms. They are tissue-equivalent and can measure accumulated dose. Gel dosimeters are primarily used for quality assurance of radiation treatment, verifying that a delivered dose is identical to the planned dose. Disadvantages of gel dosimeters include the need for MR imaging to analyze the extent of polymerization; access to a scanner may not be readily available. In addition, an oxygen-free environment is required to prepare the gel, which happens to be relatively toxic.

The relationship between signal and dose in polymer gel dosimetry is analogous to that of the equation used for Fricke dosimetry. Once a G-value for the polymerization is determined, obtaining the dose is relatively straightforward. A readout is done before irradiation, a readout is done after irradiation, and the difference is taken and converted to dose. Polymer gels often exhibit a threshold dose of a few Gy to evoke a response, but beyond that threshold value, response is linear with dose to about $20\,Gy$. At higher doses, saturation occurs, and there is no increase in signal with dose.

The standard method for reading out gel information is MR imaging, based on changes in the relaxation rate. For Fricke gel dosimeters, the appropriate relaxation rate is $1/T_1$ because the two types of ion relax differently, so one can relate the change in relaxation rate to the amount of Fe^{+3} ion produced. For polymer gel dosimeters, the relaxation rate is $1/T_2$; the polymerization of the gel increases the rigidity of the system, giving rise to a change in relaxation rate. The accuracy of these dosimeters for measuring relative doses is in the range 2–3%, whereas for absolute dose measurements, it is in the range of 3–5%.

CT is another readout methodology for gel dosimetry, in which one can observe the spatial distribution of the relative change of density in the irradiated polymer. An advantage of this system is that radiation oncology facilities have much better access to CT scanners than to MR imagers, whereas, a disadvantage of using CT imaging to determine dose is that the CT signals are somewhat noisy. A system analogous to CT in that it converts attenuation data obtained at various angles to a two-dimensional image is optical CT. In optical CT what is measured are attenuation coefficients of visible light. Changes in optical attenuation coefficients are used to reconstruct a two-dimensional image. For Fricke gels, the two-dimensional image can be correlated to changes in absorption of the incident light beam, whereas for polymer gels, the changes in attenuation are correlated to changes in scatter. These changes in attenuation coefficients have been shown to be linearly proportional to dose in the range of 0–2 Gy.

The first polymer gel used clinically involved the polymerization of N,N'-methylene-bis-acrylamide monomers in aqueous agarose matrix.[26] The acronym for this compound was BANANA, corresponding to the initial letters of the included compounds, "bis", "acrylamide", and "nitrous oxide agarose". BANANA gel did not have the diffusion problem that was present in earlier gels, consequently, it was capable of recording a dose distribution and maintaining the stability of the record. A later refinement of the gel dosimeter had the agarose replaced with gelatin giving rise to the new acronym of BANG.[27]

A major limitation of these gels is that oxygen inhibits the polymerization process. Consequently, these gels must be manufactured in an oxygen-free environment.[28]

Another, more recent, dosimeter is the PRESAGE® dosimeter, manufactured out of a machineable plastic.[29] This dosimeter contains a leuco dye yielding a radiochromic response to radiation. The PRESAGE® dosimeter is a hybrid between the radiochromic dosimeter and the gel dosimeter in that it is radiochromic, but yields a three-dimensional dose response similar to that of a gel dosimeter. The leuco dye is embedded in an optically clear polyurethane matrix, and, upon irradiation, is oxidized to a blue-green color. One then measures the spatial distribution of the optical density of the dosimeter to obtain a three-dimensional map of the dose distribution.

The ability to map a three-dimensional dose distribution is a significant advantage of gel dosimeters. Several disadvantages of these dosimeters include the need to wait at least 12 hours after irradiation of the polymer gel for polymerization to take place. In addition, time must be allotted to readout; if MR imaging is used for readout, one needs at least 30 minutes to 1 hour. Finally, gel dosimeters need to be calibrated using gel from the same batch as was used for measurement.

The primary application of gel dosimetry takes advantage of its ability to depict dose distributions in three dimensions. Consequently it can be used for small-field beam commissioning to obtain dose distributions for small-field radiation beams. One can also use gel dosimeters to commission and verify novel beam configurations and treatment plans in the clinic, and mimic the patient undergoing treatment.

17.10   QUESTIONS, EXERCISES, & PROBLEMS

17-1. In your own words, explain the set-up and operation of a free-air ionization chamber.

17-2. (a) Explain the difference between conductors, insulators, and semiconductors. Energy diagrams should supplement your explanation. (b) Research and explain the purpose of doping, in which impurities are introduced into the crystalline lattice of a semiconductor. What is the difference between p-type and n-type impurities? How do these types of impurities affect the energy diagrams for the semiconductor?

17-3. Explain the operation of a thimble ionization chamber. A well-labeled diagram should accompany your explanation.

17-4. Figure (17.3) shows how degenerate energy levels in atoms are split—that is, the energy levels become no longer degenerate—as the atoms get closer to one another. (a) What is meant by *degenerate* energy levels? (b) The figure shows that the s-energy levels are split into two levels, while the p-energy levels are split into six levels. Explain why. (*Hint:* See Chapter 4.)

17-5. Explain the operation of a TLD—how does it work?

17-6. Explain the basic ideas behind film dosimetry.

17-7. (a) In the section on film dosimetry, it is mentioned that film is especially sensitive to scattered radiation. The reason for this is that scattered radiation will have a lower energy than the incident radiation. When the energy of the scattered photons gets sufficiently low, the photoelectric effect dominates photon interactions and the film will result in a dose measurement that can be significantly greater than the dose in the surrounding phantom material. Use the discussion in this section coupled with information from Chapter 8 to explain this statement. (b) Explain why the insertion of lead foils into the phantom material around the film can reduce the amount of scattered radiation reaching the film, thereby improving the dose measurement. (See Fig. 17.8.)

17.11 REFERENCES

1. Pai S, Das IJ, Dempsey JF, et al. TG-69: Radiographic film for megavoltage beam dosimetry. *Med Phys.* 2007; 34(6): 2228-2255.
2. Suchowerska N, Hoban P, Davison A, Metcalfe P. Perturbation of radiotherapy beams by radiographic film: measurements and Monte Carlo simulations. *Phys Med Biol.* 1999; 44(7): 1755-1765.
3. Burch SE, Kearfott KJ, Trueload JH, Sheils WC, Yeo JI, Wang CKC. A new approach to film dosimetry for high energy photon beams: Lateral scatter filtering. *Med Phys.* 1997; 24(5): 775-783.
4. Yeo IJ, Wang CK, and Burch SE. A filtration method for improving film dosimetry in photon radiation therapy. *Med Phys.* 1997; 24(12): 1943-1953.
5. Williamson J, Khan FM, Sharma SC. Film dosimetry of megavoltage photon beams: A practical method of dosimetry. *Med Phys.* 8(1):94-98.
6. Niroomand-Rad A, Blackwell CR, Coursey BM, et al. Radiochromic film dosimetry: Recommendations of AAPM Radiation Therapy Committee Task Group 55m. *Med Phys.* 1998; 25(11): 2093-2115.
7. International Commission on Radiation Units and Measurements. *ICRU Report 90: Key data for ionizing-radiation dosimetry: Measurement standards and applications.* Bethesda, MD: ICRU; 2016.
8. McEwen M. Primary Standards of Air Kerma for ^{60}CO and X-Rays & Absorbed Dose in Photon and Electron Beams. 2009 AAPM Summer School. https://www.aapm.org/meetings/09SS/documents/15McEwen-PrimaryStandardsfinalforVL.pdf. Accessed March 23, 2020.
9. deAlmeida CE, Ochoa R, Coelho de Lima M, et al. A feasibility study of Fricke dosimetry as an absorbed dose to water standard for ^{192}Ir HDR sources. *PLOS One.* 2014; 9(12): e115155. https://doi.org/10.1371/journal.pone.0115155 (2014).
10. Truscott AJ, Duller GAT, Bøtter-Jensen L, Murray AS, Wintle AG. Reproducibility of optically stimulated luminescence measurements from single grains of Al$_2$O$_3$:C and annealed quartz. *Radiation Measurements.* 2000; 32(5-6):447-451.
11. Data for the graph were taken from Jursinic PA. Characterization of optically stimulated luminescent dosimeters, OSLDs, for clinical dosimetric measurements. *Med Phys.* 2007; 34(12): 4594-4604. https://doi.org/10.1118/1.2804555.
12. Anderson CE, Edmund JM, Damkjaer SMS, Greilich S. Temperature coefficients for in vivo RL and OSL dosimetry using Al$_2$O$_3$:C. *Radiation Measurements.* 2008; 43: 948-953.
13. Viamonte A, daRosa LAR, Buckley L, Cherpak A, Cygler JE. Radiotherapy dosimetry using a commercial OSL system. *Med Phys.* 2008; 35(4): 1261-1266.
14. Schembri V, Heijmen BJM. Optically stimulated luminescence (OSL) of carbon-doped aluminum oxide (Al$_2$O$_3$) for film dosimetry in radiotherapy. *Med Phys.* 34(6):2113-2118.
15. Mobit P, Agyingi E, Sandison G. Comparison of the energy-response factor of LiF and Al$_2$O$_3$ in radiotherapy beams. *Radiat Prot Dosim.* 2006; 119(1-4):497-499.
16. Yukihara EG, McKeever SWS. Optically stimulated luminescence (OSL) in medicine. *Phys Med Biol.* 2008; 53(20): R351-R379.
17. Reft CS. The energy dependence and dose response of a commercial optically stimulated luminescent detector for kilovoltage photon, megavoltage photon, and electron, proton, and carbon beams. *Med Phys.* 2009;36(5):1690-1699.
18. Aznar MC, Anderson CE, Bøtter-Jensen L, et al. Real-time optical-fibre luminescence dosimetry for radiotherapy: physical characteristics and applications in photon beams. Phys Med Biol. 49(9): 1655-1669.

19. Archambault L, Arsenault J, Gingras L, Beddar A S, Roy R, Beaulieu L. Plastic scintillation dosimetry: Optimal selection of scintillating fibers and scintillators. *Med. Phys.* 2005; 32(7 Part 1): 2271-2278.
20. Beddar A S, Mackie T R, Attix F H. Water-equivalent plastic scintillation detectors for high equivalent plastic scintillation detectors for high-energy beam dosimetry: I. Physical characteristics and theoretical considerations. *Phys. Med. Biol.* 37(10): 1883-1900.
21. Archambault L, Beddar S, Gingras L, Roy R, Beaulieu L. Measurement accuracy and Cerenkov removal for high performance, high spatial resolution scintillation dosimetry. *Med. Phys.* 2006; 33(1): 128-135.
22. Beddar AS. A new scintillator detector system for the quality assurance of ^{60}Co and high-energy therapy machines. *Phys Med Biol.* 1994; 39(2): 253-263.
23. Beddar AS, Mackie TR, Attix FH. Water-equivalent plastic scintillation detectors for high equivalent plastic scintillation detectors for high-energy beam dosimetry: II. Properties and measurements. *Phys Med Biol.* 37(10): 1901-1913.
24. Beddar S, Kinsella TJ, Ikhlef A, Sibata CH. Miniature "Scintillator-Fiberoptic-PMT" detector system for the dosimetry of small fields in stereotactic radiosurgery. *IEEE Trans. Nucl. Sci.* 48(3): 924-928.
25. Lacroix F, Archambault L, Gingras L, Beddar AS, Beaulieu L. Clinical prototype of a plastic water-equivalent scintillating fiber dosimeter matrix for IMRT QA applications. *Med Phys.* 2008; 35(8): 3682-3690.
26. Maryanski MJ, Gore JC, Schulz RJ. 3-D radiation dosimetry by MRI: solvent proton relaxation enhancement by radiation-controlled polymerisation and cross-linking in gels. *Proc Intl Soc Mag Reson Med.* New York; 1992.
27. Maryanski MJ, Schulz RJ, Ibbott GS, et al. Magnetic resonance imaging of radiation dose distributions using a polymer-gel dosimeter. *Phys Med Biol.* 1994; 39(9): 1437-1455.
28. Baldock C, Burford RP, Billingham N, et al. Experimental procedure for the manufacture and calibration of polyacrylamide gel (PAG) for magnetic resonance imaging (MRI) radiation dosimetry. *Phys Med Biol.* 1998; 43(3): 695-702.
29. Guo PY, Adamovics JA, Oldham M. Characterization of a new radiochromic three-dimensional dosimeter. *Med Phys.* 2006; 33(5): 1338-1345.

CHAPTER 18

Introduction to External-Beam Treatment Planning

CONTENTS

The process of planning radiation treatments involves computer simulation of the radiation dose distribution to determine a set of beam parameters that will deliver a desired radiation dose distribution. Whereas an ideal dose distribution would deliver a tumoricidal dose to the tumor and no dose to uninvolved tissue outside the tumor, such a dose distribution is, in fact, not possible to achieve. Instead, one must make compromises and, rather than allow the treatment plan to deliver no dose whatsoever outside the treatment volume, we allow some dose to be delivered with the intent, derived from years of clinical experience, that the radiation delivered to uninvolved tissue not lead to serious consequences that adversely affect the patient's quality of life.

In the next three chapters we look at how we plan radiation treatments. We begin this chapter by addressing dose calculations to a single point, from which we are able to calculate the appropriate number of treatment machine monitor units. We then expand the dose calculations to three dimensions, looking at the major types of algorithms used in these calculations. The chapter closes with a brief digression to discuss neutron dose distributions. In the subsequent chapter we present the theory and methodology for calculating charged-particle dose distributions, and in the third chapter we combine our knowledge of dose distributions with our knowledge of clinical consequences of irradiation to present the complete treatment planning and verification process.

DOI: 10.1201/9781003477457-18

18.1 FACTORS AFFECTING POINT DOSE

The most basic form of dose calculation is the determination of dose to a single point within the patient. However, prior to doing so, it is important to understand how patients are set up on a treatment machine.

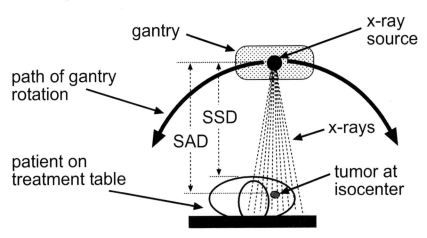

FIGURE 18.1: A schematic showing the x-ray source within the gantry of a linear accelerator (linac) treating a patient with the tumor positioned at the isocenter of the machine. The bold arced arrows show the path of revolution of the gantry. The source-to-surface distance (SSD) and source-to-axis distance (SAD) are also shown.

In the early treatment machines, typically a machine that used ^{60}Co as a source of radiation, the patient was set up with the target at the center of the radiation field at a fixed distance from the radiation source to the patient's surface. This distance is called the source-to-skin distance or source-to-surface distance (*SSD*). Present-day linear accelerators (*linacs*), as well as ^{60}Co teletherapy units, place the source of radiation in a gantry that can revolve around a central axis that is at a fixed distance from the source. (See Fig. 11.9 for a picture of a linac. The circular plate on the floor beneath the gantry can be removed, allowing the gantry to revolve 360° about the patient.) The revolution of the gantry allows the radiation to approach the tumor from different directions through the patient, thereby helping to spare the healthy tissue around the tumor. The *source-to-axis distance* is referred to as the *SAD* and the point that is the intersection of the axis of gantry revolution and the central beam axis is called the *isocenter*. The patient is then set up so a reference point, typically the center of the tumor, is placed at the isocenter. After the patient is treated with one field, the gantry is simply moved to a new position and the patient is treated with additional fields. Figure (18.1) shows a schematic of the gantry and patient set-up.

The dose delivered to points within the photon radiation field consists of dose delivered by interactions involving the primary beam and dose delivered by interactions involving the secondary radiation. The distribution of dose delivered by primary interactions is relatively straightforward to describe based on the exponential attenuation of the primary radiation beam. However, complicating the deposition of dose is the production of secondary radiation—electrons that actually produce most of the ionizations in the radiation target, as well as scattered photons that may deliver dose some distance from the site of the primary interaction.

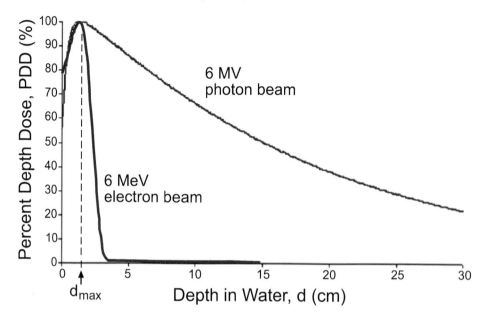

FIGURE 18.2: Percent Depth Dose (PDD) as a function of depth (d) in water for 6 MV x-rays and 6 MeV electrons. Each curve is scaled such that the maximum dose delivered is at 100%. The maximum dose, D_{max}, occurs at the depth denoted d_{max}. The position of d_{max} is shown for the x-ray beam.

At shallow depths, almost all the dose is delivered via primary interactions, as there is no secondary radiation emanating from the air directly above the patient surface. At shallow depths the increase in dose due to scattered radiation is greater than the decrease in dose from the attenuation of the primary beam. Consequently, the dose to the skin surface can be somewhat less than the dose delivered to tissue slightly below the surface. This phenomenon is known as *skin sparing*. As the depth in the patient increases, and the amount of secondary radiation also increases, the dose delivered to the patient increases with depth until an equilibrium is reached between primary and secondary radiation. This depth of maximum dose, d_{max}, increases with the energy of the radiation and can vary from the surface in the case of low-energy $(E < 500\,kV)$ radiation to several centimeters depth for high-energy $(\sim 15\,MV)$ radiation.

The *percent depth dose* (PDD) is defined such that

$$PDD(d) = \left(\frac{D}{D_{max}}\right) \times 100\%,\tag{18.1}$$

where D is the dose delivered at depth d and D_{max} is the maximum dose. Figure (18.2) shows two Percent Depth Dose (PDD) curves, one for x-rays and one for electrons.

At depths beyond d_{max} the effect of exponential attenuation of the primary beam becomes the most dominant factor, and the dose decreases with depth. This decrease in dose is almost, but not quite, exponential, deviating from a simple exponential description because of the contribution of scattered radiation. Rather than explicitly modeling the dose via first physical principles, the quantities used in actually performing point dose calculations are acquired via measurement. They are described in the next section of this chapter.

18.2 DEPTH DOSE QUANTITIES: TAR, TMR, TPR, PDD

Ideally, once a set of beam parameters has been determined and entered into the treatment machine, a phantom with a dosimeter located at a specified point in the phantom would be placed in the radiation beam, the phantom would be irradiated for a specified time, and the dose would be measured. While this task is sometimes done for unusual beam situations, for the most part, beam configurations are relatively straightforward. Consequently, rather than measuring dose every time a new patient needs to be treated, we determine dose to a selected reference point, typically the point where the prescription is specified. We relate the dose to the reference point to the dose to a point at which the output of the machine is calibrated. We then use tabulated data that describes the relationship between the dose to the calibration point and the dose to the reference point.

This section describes in more detail the various central-axis depth dose quantities that we may use to calculate monitor units as further described in the section that follows. The specific quantity that we use and the specific value of that quantity is going to depend on the beam energy, the patient set-up (fixed SSD *vs.* isocentric), the collimator setting, the actual field size, and the depth. In this section we will look at four quantities: the *tissue-air ratio* (TAR), the *tissue-phantom ratio* (TPR), *the tissue-maximum ratio* (TMR), and the *percent depth dose* (PDD).

The first of these quantities, the TAR, is used when a machine calibration is performed in air and the patient is set up isocentrically—that is, the treatment point is placed at the isocenter of the machine. Such a calibration is only done for low-energy beams such as that of a ^{60}Co source undergoing radioactive decay. To make a measurement of the TAR, one measures the machine output in air. Then, without changing any of the machine parameters, one makes a comparable measurement in phantom at the desired depth. The ratio of the two is the TAR. The TAR is thus defined as follows:

$$TAR(E, CS, FS, d) = \frac{O(E, SD, CS, FS, d)}{O(E, SD, CS, FS, air)}. \tag{18.2}$$

In this equation, E is the beam energy, SD is the distance from the source, CS is the collimator setting, FS is the actual field size, d is the depth, and O is the measured output given the beam energy, distance from source, collimator setting, field size, and depth.

Imagine placing an ion chamber in an empty water tank, taking an output measurement, then filling the tank to a desired depth, and repeating the output measurement without moving the ion chamber or the water tank. This is the measurement configuration used to measure the TAR. Figure (18.3) illustrates this measurement configuration.

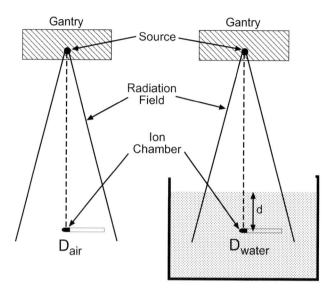

FIGURE 18.3: The configuration used to determine the tissue-air ratio, TAR. (Left) The dose D is measured in air. (Right) The dose D is measured in the same configuration but at a depth d in water. The field size (FS) is the area of the radiation field at the position of the ion chamber and perpendicular to the central beam axis (shown by the dashed lines). The source distance (SD) is the distance from the source to the ion chamber, as shown by the dashed line.

The dependence of the TAR on the various beam parameters is as follows: In general, the TAR decreases with increasing depth due to beam attenuation. The TAR evaluated at the depth of central-axis maximum (d_{max}) is often referred to as the *backscatter factor* (BSF). For shallower depths, depths less than d_{max}, the TAR increases with depth due to the increase deposition of dose from charged particles. Beam energy has an effect on TAR as well. At low energies, the BSF increases with increasing energy due to increased penetration of the photons scattered into the point at central-axis d_{max}. However, at higher energies, the BSF decreases with increasing energy because the scatter, mainly due to Compton interactions, is mainly in the forward direction. The BSF reaches a maximum value in the orthovoltage range of energies, with a beam HVL around $0.4-0.8\,mm$ Cu, where the BSF may be as great as 1.5. (The thickness of copper given is an indication of the penetrating power of the radiation.) This means that about one-third of the dose delivered to central-axis d_{max} for this energy radiation comes from scattered radiation. Next, the TAR increases with increasing field size because of the increased scatter reaching a calculation point, but the effect of field size on TAR is not as great for higher energy beams, again due to the increased fraction of forward-scattered radiation. Finally, the TAR is independent of the distance from the source, because both dose rates incorporated into the definition of TAR are measured at the same distance from the source.

The TAR can be used to calculate the dose rate at distances other than the distance of calibration using the inverse-square relationship to relate the in-air dose rate at one source distance to another. It is important to note that the inverse-square relationship only holds in air, and for relatively small changes in distance from the source. If one is treating a patient at a very large distance from the source, such as when one performs total-body irradiation, then a significant amount of photon interactions with air, along with possible scatter from the walls of the treatment room, mandates a measurement of the machine output at the extended distance from the source. So, for small changes in distance from the source, in order to relate the dose rate in tissue at one distance from the source to another, one calculates the dose rate in air by dividing by the appropriate TAR, uses the inverse-square relationship to relate the in-air dose rates at the two distances from the source, and calculates the dose rate in tissue by multiplying the in-air dose rate by the appropriate TAR.

When calibration measurements are performed in phantom, the TAR is not a useful quantity. In this case, a more common circumstance nowadays, instead of the TAR, one uses a quantity known as the *tissue-phantom ratio* (TPR). The TPR is defined by the following relationship:

$$TPR(E, CS, FS, d, d_{ref}) = \frac{O(E, SD, CS, FS, d)}{O(E, SD, CS, FS, d_{ref})}. \tag{18.3}$$

The TPR differs from the TAR in that the reference measurement is made at some specified reference depth, d_{ref}, within the phantom rather than in air. If the reference depth is the depth of central-axis maximum, d_{max}, then the tissue-phantom ratio is called the *tissue-maximum ratio*, or TMR. Setting the reference depth equal to d_{max} is a common practice in radiation oncology clinics. An issue that one must be aware of is that, for higher energy beams, d_{max} may be a function of field size, so, when performing the reference measurement to obtain TMR values, one must specify whether the reference measurement is performed at a depth for the given field size or at d_{max} for a standard field, typically a $10\,cm \times 10\,cm$ field.

The last of these quantities, the percent depth dose (PDD) is used for fixed SSD setups, and in situations in which a dose is prescribed to a particular isodose line on a treatment plan. The PDD is defined by the relation

$$PDD(E, SSD, CS, FS, d) = \frac{O(E, SSD, CS, FS, d)}{O(E, SSD, CS, FS, d_{max})} \times 100\%. \tag{18.4}$$

(Note that this more precise definition of PDD is equivalent to the definition given earlier in Eq.18.1.) One important point to note is that the percent depth dose is dependent on the source-to-surface distance, SSD. This is because the two measurements are taken at different depths, hence different distances from the source, so the effect of beam divergence has to be accounted for.

In order to derive a relationship between the percent depth dose at one SSD to that at another SSD, it is necessary to derive first a relationship between the percent depth dose and the TAR. To do so, we go from output in tissue (or phantom) to output in air, first at distance from the source $D_{max} \equiv SSD + d_{max}$, then at distance from the source $D \equiv SSD + d$:

$$O(E, D_{max}, CS, FS(D_{max}), d_{max})$$
$$= O(E, D_{max}, CS, FS(D_{max}), d_{max}, air) \times BSF(E, FS(D_{max})), \quad (18.5)$$

and

$$O(E, D, CS, FS(D), d)$$
$$= O(E, D, CS, FS(D), air) \times TAR(E, FS(D), d). \quad (18.6)$$

Now, the in-air dose at distance from the source $D = SSD + d$ is related to the in-air dose at $D_{max} = SSD + d_{max}$ by a beam-divergence factor, giving us

$$O(E, D, CS, FS(D), air)$$
$$= O(E, D_{max}, CS, FS(D_{max}), air) \times \left(\frac{D_{max}}{D} \right)^2. \quad (18.7)$$

Well, that is almost correct. We have neglected the fact that the field size is slightly different at D from what it is at D_{max}, but the effect of the different field sizes is negligible. Combining all these terms, we finally obtain

$$\frac{PDD(E, SSD, CS, FS, d)}{100\%}$$
$$= \frac{O(E, D, CS, FS(D), air) \times TAR(E, FS(D), d)}{O(E, D_{max}, CS, FS(D_{max}), air) \times BSF(E, FS(D_{max}))}, \quad (18.8)$$

or

$$PDD(E, SSD, CS, FS, d) = \frac{TAR(E, FS(D), d)}{BSF(E, FS(D_{max}))} \left(\frac{D_{max}}{D} \right)^2 \times 100\%. \quad (18.9)$$

If we assume that the dependence of the TAR and BSF on field size at two values of the SSD is negligible, then taking the ratio of PDD at one value of the SSD to that at another gives us the relationship

$$\frac{PDD(E, SSD_1, CS, FS_1, d)}{PDD(E, SSD_2, CS, FS_2, d)} = \left[\left(\frac{SSD_1 + d_{max}}{SSD_1 + d} \right) \left(\frac{SSD_2 + d}{SSD_2 + d_{max}} \right) \right]^2. \quad (18.10)$$

Equation (18.10) holds true as long as SSD_1 and SSD_2 are not too different from one another. If they are significantly different, for example, when one goes from a calibration measurement at the machine isocenter to a whole-body treatment at an SSD of perhaps $200\,cm$, then not only are the field sizes different (which may be correctable), but one also has to account for interactions of the x-ray beam with air. Consequently, in such cases, a dose measurement is warranted.

18.3   MONITOR UNIT CALCULATIONS

In this section, we describe a methodology for the calculation of machine settings. Although several protocols for calculating machine settings have been published, these are based on a specific set of machine calibration conditions.[1] Rather than specifying a particular method for calculating machine settings, we attempt to provide here a methodology that allows the physicist to select a particular set of measurement conditions and ensure consistency in the machine setting calculations.

The machine setting M in *monitor units* (MU) is given by the equation

$$M = \frac{D_{ref}}{\dot{D}_{ref}} + EEC \,, \tag{18.11}$$

where D_{ref} is the dose that, if delivered to a specified reference point by a specified reference field, would satisfy the goals of the prescription, $\dot{D}_{ref}$ is the dose rate (cGy/min or cGy/MU) at the reference point (remember that the dot notation stands for the time derivative), and EEC is an end-effect correction (discussed below). Some examples of D_{ref} are as follows: For an isocentric treatment, D_{ref} is typically the prescription dose D_{presc} for the specific field. For a treatment at fixed SSD, D_{ref} is typically the dose delivered at d_{max} for that field. This dose is usually called the *given dose*. D_{ref} is obtained from D_{presc} by the equation

$$D_{ref} = \frac{D_{prescr}}{PDD(d, S, SSD)/100\%} \,, \tag{18.12}$$

in which $PDD(d, S, SSD)$ is the percent depth dose at the depth d of the dose prescription point, field size S defined at the patient surface, and a distance SSD from the radiation source. Here, the percent depth dose has been divided by 100% so it is expressed as a decimal. For isocentric treatments for which the isocenter has been blocked, D_{ref} might be the dose delivered to a point in the unblocked region of the field at the same depth as the isocenter. If the machine setting is to be calculated from output from a treatment planning system, D_{ref} might be the dose delivered to a specified reference point by a specified reference field. For example, if one uses a hard wedge to modify the dose distribution, D_{ref} might be the dose delivered to central-axis d_{max} by the unwedged field with the SSD equal to the source-to-isocenter distance. Another example of D_{ref} might be the dose delivered to central-axis d_{max} by an unwedged, unblocked field with the SSD equal to the source-to-isocenter distance. If one is calculating the dose based on output from a treatment planning system, the specific interpretation of D_{ref} is really dependent on the output representation of the treatment planning system. Finally, EEC is an end-effect correction. It is used when treatments are delivered by a ^{60}Co teletherapy unit; its value is the measured timer correction. The value of EEC for linear accelerators is usually assumed to be zero.

The reference dose rate $\dot{D}_{ref}$ is equal to the calibration dose output multiplied by a set of correction factors that account for the differences in machine output between the calibration condition and the reference condition. The reference dose rate can be written in the form

$$
\begin{aligned}
\dot{D}_{ref} = {} & CDO(d_{cal}, CS_{cal}, SD_{cal}) \cdot OF(CS_{cal}, CS_{ref}) \\
& \times PSF(CS_{ref}, FS_{ref}) \cdot ISF(SD_{cal}, SD_{ref}) \cdot OAF(FS_{ref}, r_{ref}) \\
& \times BMF(FS_{ref}, d_{ref}) \cdot TR(FS_{ref}, d_{ref}).
\end{aligned}
\tag{18.13}
$$

In this equation the factors comprising $\dot{D}_{ref}$ are defined as follows:

$CDO(d_{cal}, CS_{cal}, SD_{cal})$ is the calibration dose output. The calibration dose output is the output of the radiation machine at some specified point under some specified calibration conditions. The calibration dose output is generally expressed either in cGy/MU or in cGy/min. For many linear accelerators $CDO(d_{cal}, CS_{cal}, SD_{cal})$ is set to be 1.0. The calibration dose output is specified either in water at a depth d_{cal}, or in air, for a calibration collimator setting CS_{cal}, and a calibration distance from the source SD_{cal}. If the calibration dose output is specified in water, the calibration depth is usually at d_{max}, although it may be at some other depth, e.g., at 10 cm depth to make the depth consistent with the calibration depth identified in the AAPM TG-51 protocol,[2] which guides treatment machine calibration in the United States. The calibration collimator setting is usually $10\, cm \times 10\, cm$. The calibration distance from the source is either the source-to-isocenter distance SAD, or a distance $SAD + d_{cal}$.

$OF(CS_{cal}, CS_{ref})$ is the output factor. The output factor accounts for the difference between the collimator setting for the reference field CS_{ref} and the calibration collimator setting CS_{cal}. If the calibration dose output is expressed in air, then the output factor is the ratio of doses measured at the same point as that for which the calibration dose output has been specified. The numerator is the in-air dose with a collimator setting CS_{ref}, while the denominator is the in-air dose with a collimator setting CS_{cal}. If the calibration dose output is expressed in water, then the output factor is the ratio of doses measured at depth with the two collimator settings as specified above. The two depths may be different. For example, the depths may be specified to be the values of d_{max} for the two collimator settings. If the values of d_{max} are different for the two collimator settings, then the physicist has the option of selecting either the collimator-setting specific d_{max}, or the d_{max} for the calibration collimator setting. It should be noted, then, that these values of d_{max} must also be the values used in the measurement of TR, the tissue ratio. If the collimator-specific d_{max} is used, then the tissue-ratio becomes the TMR, the tissue-maximum ratio, while if the d_{max} for the calibration collimator setting is used, then the tissue ratio becomes the TPR, the tissue-phantom ratio. Note that the output factor combines factors due to collimator scatter as well as phantom scatter.

$PSF(CS_{ref}, FS_{ref})$ is the peakscatter factor ratio. The peakscatter factor ratio accounts for differences in scattered radiation between the field size determined by the collimator setting and the actual treatment field size. The differences in field size may be due either to the presence of secondary blocking or a reference dose specified at a different distance from the source than that of the calibration dose output. The peakscatter factor ratio is the ratio of either the peakscatter factors or the normalized peakscatter factors at FS_{ref}, the reference field size, and CS_{ref}, the reference collimator setting. The peakscatter factor ratio is used rather than the peakscatter factor because it is a much more slowly varying function of field size. Thus systematic errors in its measurement may not have as deleterious effect on the machine setting calculation as if peakscatter factors alone were used. For high-energy $(E > 10\,MV)$ photons, one can set the PSF equal to 1.0 without significant loss of accuracy. If the conditions under which the dose at the reference position D_{ref} is specified are those that include an unblocked field, then the peakscatter factor ratio is 1.0, because the field size for the unblocked field is the same as the collimator setting. If the output factor is defined at a depth other than at d_{max}, then the peakscatter factor ratio is replaced by a TAR ratio.

$ISF(SD_{cal}, SD_{ref})$ is the beam-divergence ("inverse-square") factor. The beam-divergence factor corrects for the beam intensity from the dose calibration point, at a distance SD_{cal} from the source, to the dose reference point, at a distance SD_{ref} from the source. If the dose calibration point is at the isocenter of the radiation machine and the dose reference point is also at the isocenter, then the beam-divergence factor is 1.0. If the dose calibration point is at the source-to-isocenter distance plus d_{max} and the dose reference point is at the isocenter, then the beam-divergence factor is given by

$$ISF(SD_{cal}, SD_{ref}) = \left(\frac{SAD + d_{max}}{SAD}\right)^2 . \tag{18.14}$$

In general, the beam-divergence factor is given by

$$ISF(SD_{cal}, SD_{ref}) = \left(\frac{SD_{cal}}{SD_{ref}}\right)^2 . \tag{18.15}$$

$OAF(FS_{ref}, r_{ref}, d_{ref})$ is the off-axis factor. The off-axis factor corrects for the fact that the beam intensity is not uniform and a function of field size of the reference field, distance of the reference point from the central axis, and depth of the reference point. The off-axis factor is used when the dose reference point does not lie on the central axis of the radiation beam. Examples include the case when a half-beam block is used or when the field boundary lies close to the central axis so that the isocenter lies in a region of high dose gradient. The off-axis factor can be read from data obtained when the beam is commissioned.

$BMF(FS_{ref}, d_{ref})$ is the beam modification factor. The beam modification factor corrects for the presence of any and all beam modifiers such as trays, wedges, compensating filters, etc. It is important that the beam modifiers be the correct ones for the reference field regardless of the beam modifiers used for the actual treatment field. For example, if the reference field is an unwedged field, then the beam modification factor should not include a wedge factor even if the actual treatment field is wedged. In such a case, the presence of the wedge is reflected in the reference dose, and inclusion of a wedge factor in the beam modification factor would result in the wedge being accounted for twice. Each beam modification factor may or may not be dependent on field size and depth. Whether or not to incorporate these dependencies is a decision to be made by the individual physicist, but the dependencies of the beam modification factors one field size and depth should be determined. For example, the tray factor for $6\,MV$ x-rays from a particular linear accelerator varies by 0.5% from a $5\,cm \times 5\,cm$ field to a $40\,cm \times 40\,cm$ field, and the wedge factor for a 60° wedge varies by 4% from a $4\,cm \times 4\,cm$ field to a $25\,cm \times 25\,cm$ field. Finally,

$TR(FS_{ref}, d_{ref})$ is the tissue ratio. The tissue ratio corrects for the presence of the patient. The various tissue ratios were introduced in the previous section of this chapter. The specific ratio to be used depends on the calibration conditions. If the calibration dose output is specified in air, then the tissue ratio is the TAR evaluated at the field size and depth appropriate to the reference dose. If the calibration dose output is specified in water and the reference depth for the output factor is a field-size independent depth, then the tissue ratio is the TPR evaluated at the field size and depth appropriate to the reference dose and relating to the depth at which the output factor is specified. If the calibration dose output is specified in water and the reference depth for the output factor is d_{max}, which may be field-size dependent, then the tissue ratio is the TMR evaluated at the field size and depth appropriate to the reference dose.

18.4   DOSE-CALCULATION ALGORITHMS

Whereas the previous formalism works for the calculation of doses to individual points, it is not the most practical method nor the most accurate method for obtaining dose distributions that can be used to evaluate the quality of a treatment plan. Perhaps the most accurate method of dose calculation is the Monte Carlo method, which is discussed in greater deal later in this section. Dose-calculation algorithms may tend to be rather time-consuming, so most algorithms currently in use involve some sort of approximations that make the dose calculation more rapid. One such approximation involves the resolution of the rectilinear grid of calculation points. A coarse grid can be used for rapid calculation during the early stages of the development of the treatment plan, switching to a fine grid when the final dose distribution is desired. However, additional speed can be achieved by the selection of the dose-calculation algorithm. It is important for the clinical physicist to understand the dose-calculation algorithm, the approximations made in the calculation, and how they might impact on the final dose distribution.

Perhaps the most commonly used algorithm is the convolution algorithm or one of its variants. In this algorithm, the dose $D(\vec{r})$, at the position $\vec{r}$, is expressed as the convolution of a term related to the primary fluence and a dose kernel:

$$D(\vec{r}) = \int dE \int d^3 r' \, T\left(\vec{r}'; E\right) \, A\left(\vec{r} - \vec{r}'; E\right) . \tag{18.16}$$

In this equation, $A(\vec{r} - \vec{r}'; E)$ is the *dose-spread array*, the relative energy per unit volume deposited at point $\vec{r}$ from a primary photon interaction at point $\vec{r}'$. The dose-spread array is the three-dimensional spatial distribution of energy deposited by electrons and photons spreading from the site of the initial photon interaction. It only needs to be determined once for each energy in a homogeneous, unit-density phantom, and consists of a primary dose-spread array and a scatter dose-spread array. Calculation of the dose-spread array has been done using Monte Carlo calculations, as described later in this section. Values of the dose-spread array are solely a function of the distance of the calculation point from the point of the initial interaction and the energy of the photons at the point of initial interaction. The dose-spread array is sometimes referred to as the "dose kernel". One could think of the dose-spread array as a Green's function, the response of a system to a delta-function input.

The quantity $T(\vec{r}'; E)$ is the *terma* (total energy released per unit mass) at point $\vec{r}'$. The terma is related to the fluence of the primary beam multiplied by the mass attenuation coefficient. In particular

$$T\left(\vec{r}'; E\right) = \frac{\mu}{\rho}\left(\vec{r}'; E\right) \, \Psi\left(\vec{r}'; E\right) . \tag{18.17}$$

The mass attenuation coefficient μ/ρ as a function of $\vec{r}'$ and E depends on the energy E of the beam and can be calculated from the CT value of the voxel located at the point $\vec{r}'$. The primary energy fluence in the patient is written as follows:

$$\Psi\left(\vec{r}'; E\right) = \left(\frac{r_o}{r'}\right)^2 \Phi_o\left(\vec{r}_o; E\right) \, E \, \exp\left[-\int_{\vec{r}_o}^{\vec{r}'} \mu\left(l; E\right) dl\right] . \tag{18.18}$$

In calculating the primary energy fluence, one begins at the patient surface with $\Phi_o(\vec{r}_o; E)$, the in-air fluence on the patient surface. This quantity is obtained during the beam-commissioning procedure and is often performed using an iterative method to fit calculated dose distributions to measured beam data.

In applying the convolution algorithm, one then traces rays through the patient's three-dimensional CT array from the patient's surface to the interaction point $\vec{r}'$. The exponential attenuation of the primary beam is then calculated along the ray. This attenuated primary fluence is then convolved with the dose-spread array to obtain the dose. Finally, this calculation is performed for each energy component of the radiation beam, with the calculation integrated across the energy distribution of the incident beam.

If this sounds like a computationally intensive calculation, it is, especially in the presence of patient heterogeneities. Several simplifications have been proposed to speed up the calculation. If we assume that to first order, the dose-spread array in the inhomogeneous patient is independent of position, we can then take Fourier transforms of terma and dose-spread array and convert the integration into a multiplication. The fast Fourier transform (FFT) algorithm can then be used to speed up the calculation even more.[3] An alternative approach involves first taking energy averages of the terma and dose-spread array and then integrating.[4] In this case, we no longer have a pure convolution; this algorithm is called the *convolution/superposition algorithm*.

Comparing the two algorithms, we find that the FFT-convolution algorithm executes more rapidly than the convolution/superposition algorithm. This is due to two reasons. First, matrix multiplication is faster than calculating a convolution integral. Moreover, rather than calculating the Fourier transform of the dose-spread array for every dose calculation, one could calculate the Fourier transform of the dose-spread array once, then store the Fourier transform rather than the dose-spread array. The FFT-convolution algorithm, however, breaks down for large heterogeneities, because the assumption that the dose-spread array is spatially invariant fails. FFT-convolution algorithm requires a fixed calculation grid of 2^n points in each dimension and computes the dose to the entire grid, whereas the convolution/superposition can compute dose to individual points. Second, the calculation speed of the FFT-convolution algorithm is proportional to the number of energy components in the model photon spectrum, hence this number is kept small, while the calculation speed of the convolution/superposition algorithm is relatively insensitive to the number of energy components because the energy integration is done before the three-dimensional spatial integration.

Some refinements to the convolution/superposition algorithm are necessary, however, for it to be clinically useful. For example, the simple model does not include electron contamination of the primary beam. However, the contribution to dose from electron contamination is small, and virtually nonexistent at depth. Electron contamination can be approximated by a simple empirical function. The effect of modifiers placed in the beam can, to first order, be modeled by attenuating the in-air fluence through the modifier. This model, however, does not include scatter from the beam modifiers. The contribution of scatter can also be modified by the use of an empirical function. A more significant contribution to the in-air fluence is scattered radiation from the head of the linear accelerator, primarily generated from the flattening filter. Head scatter can be modeled by convolving the in-air fluence with a Gaussian smoothing function[5] or by a dual-source model[6].

With the increased speed of computers, so-called "Monte Carlo" calculations have found their way into dose calculations. These calculations received their name from the use of pseudorandom numbers to guide the calculations. Because the numbers are generated according to an algorithm, they are *pseudorandom* numbers rather than strictly random numbers. Monte Carlo calculations are based on following the tracks of individual particles as they exit the therapy machine and traverse through the patient[7,8]. A photon is selected from the phase-space distribution (distribution of positions and momenta) of photons emanating from the therapy machine. The photon then propagates into the patient. Whether or not it interacts with a target in the patient is determined by comparing a pseudorandom number generated by the system with the probability distribution of interactions. The nature of the interaction is then determined by comparing another pseudorandom number with the probability distribution of the types of interactions. The directions and energies of the secondary particles that are generated as a result of the interaction are determined by comparing another pseudorandom number with the probability distribution of energies and directions. These secondary particles are tracked until all the energy has been deposited by the particles or they exit the patient. After many particles have been followed, the energy deposited in each voxel of the patient model is extracted and a dose distribution is generated.

The advantage of using Monte Carlo calculations is clearly the accurate simulation of the interactions the photons undergo depositing energy inside the patient. The disadvantage of these calculations is the intense computational effort required to perform these calculations.

18.5   NEUTRON-BEAM DOSE DISTRIBUTIONS

Because of the relatively limited usage of neutron beams, not as much development has gone into neutron-beam dose calculation methods. However, because neutrons are uncharged particles, as are x-ray photons, the neutron-beam dose distributions are quite similar to those of x-rays.

18.6   QUESTIONS, EXERCISES, & PROBLEMS

18-1. Define the following: (a) SSD; (b) SAD; (c) isocenter. A well-labeled sketch should accompany your definitions.

18-2. Explain how the revolution of the gantry about the patient can result in the sparing of healthy tissue around the tumor.

18-3. Define and explain the phenomenon called *skin sparing*.

18-4. Figure (18.2) shows that the dose deposited by an x-ray beam increases from the surface until it reaches a maximum value, beyond which it decreases. Explain this counterintuitive behavior.

18-5. Figure (18.2) shows that, for comparable energy photon and electron beams, the photon beam deposits dose deep into the patient, while the electron beam deposits its dose very close to the surface. (This is why electron beams are used to treat skin disease instead of photon beams.) Why do electron beams have this rapid drop-off behavior in dose with depth? (*Hint:* See Chapter 9.)

18-6. Figure (18.3) shows the configuration used to determine the TAR. Draw corresponding diagrams for the determination of (a) the TPR; (b) the TMR; (c) the PDD.

18-7. Electron energies as high as 42 *MeV* were once achievable on linear accelerators but are not in widespread use today. Why is this so? (*Hint:* Estimate the impact of range straggling on the depth-dose distribution.)

18-8. Electron arc therapy, in which the electron beam is delivered while the gantry is rotating, was once considered for treatment of chest walls, but is not in widespread use today. Why is this so? (*Hint:* Bremsstrahlung.)

You will have to speak with a clinical medical physicist or visit a radiation oncology clinic to obtain appropriate beam data to do the following problems.

18-9. In most cases, it is necessary to interpolate between values in a table of beam data used in a point dose calculation. One typically uses linear interpolation to perform this procedure. Based on clinical beam data, what is the magnitude of error in a monitor unit calculation when linear interpolation is used?

18-10. Based on clinical beam data, perform a monitor unit calculation for several sets of machine configurations.

18.7 REFERENCES

1. See, for example, Gibbons J, Antolak JA, Followill DS, et al. Monitor unit calculations for external photon and electron beams: Report of the AAPM Therapy Physics Committee Task Group No. 71. Med Phys. 2014; 41(3): 031501 (2014).
2. Almond PR, Biggs PJ, Coursey BM, et al. AAPM's TG-51 protocol for clinical reference dosimetry of high-energy photon and electron beams. *Med Phys.* 26(9):1847-1870.
3. Boyer A, Mok E. A photon dose distribution model employing convolution calculations. *Med Phys.* 1985; 12(2): 169-177.
4. Mackie TR, Scrimger JW, Battista JJ. A convolution method of calculating dose for 15-MV x-rays. *Med Phys.* 1985; 12(2): 188-196.
5. Anesjö A. Analytic modeling of photon scatter from flattening filters in photon therapy beams. *Med Phys.* 1994; 21(8): 1227-1235.
6. Liu HH, Mackie TR, McCullough EC. A dual source photon beam model used in convolution/superposition dose calculations for clinical megavoltage x-ray beams. *Med Phys.* 24(12): 1960-1974.
7. Chetty IJ, Curran B, Cygler JE, et al. Report of the AAPM Task Group No. 105: Issues associated with clinical implementation of Monte Carlo-based photon and electron external beam treatment planning. *Med Phys.* 34(12): 4818-4853.
8. Ma C-M, Chetty IJ, Deng J, et al. Beam modeling and beam model commissioning for Monte Carlo dose calculation-based radiation therapy treatment planning: Report of AAPM Task Group 157. *Med Phys.* 47(1): e1-e18.

CHAPTER 19

Charged-Particle Treatment Planning

CONTENTS

As we learned in Chapter 9, charged-particle interactions with target material differ from photon-beam interactions in that charged particles deposit their energy gradually, transferring a small amount of their energy to the target in each of a large number of interactions. Once the particle has deposited all of its energy, it stops, and, of course, cannot deposit dose beyond that point. Consequently, a charged-particle beam has a finite range. The deposition of dose from a charged-particle beam, to a first approximation, is uniform for depths less than the range of the charged particles, and zero beyond that range. Compare this to the deposition of dose from an uncharged-particle beam (photon beam or neutron beam), for which the dose deposition is approximately exponential.

As a consequence of the depth dependence of a charged-particle beam, one can use a single beam for treating tumors lying at shallow depths, for example, chest walls and shallow lymph nodes. Because of this property, electron beams replaced orthovoltage x-rays for such treatments. (See Fig. 18.2. Note how the dose from the electron beam is confined near the surface, while the photon beam deposits dose well into the patient and beyond, despite the fact that both beams are produced with the same voltage.) In more recent years, photon modalities such as intensity-modulated radiation therapy (IMRT) and volume-modulated arc therapy (VMAT) have partially replaced electron-beam therapy for these applications.

Heavy charged particle (protons and heavy ions) beams have proved promising in the treatment of deeper tumors, with multiple beams targeting the tumor. In many situations, a treatment plan with multiple proton beams, for example, will deliver a more advantageous dose distribution than a multiple-beam x-ray plan. No hard rule exists, however, for predicting in advance whether a proton-beam treatment plan

DOI: 10.1201/9781003477457-19

would be more desirable than an x-ray-beam treatment plan, and sometimes factors other than physical dose distribution enter into the evaluation.

19.1 ELECTRON-BEAM DOSE DISTRIBUTIONS

To a first approximation, the depth dependence of the energy deposition of an electron beam follows what one would expect with a continuous slowing-down approximation. The electron dose would be uniform to a depth equal to the range of the electrons and zero beyond that range. Because electrons in the megavoltage range deposit energy in water at the rate of approximately 2 MeV/cm, a good rule of thumb for approximating the range of the electrons in water, hence in soft tissue, is to take the energy in MeV and divide by 2. That will give you a good estimate as to the range of an electron beam.

Let us be somewhat more precise about our terminology at this time and differentiate between loss of energy and local deposition of energy. The range of a charged-particle beam depends on how the charged particles lose energy. The beam can lose energy either through collisional processes or radiative processes. At low energies almost all energy is lost through collisional processes, whereas at higher energies the fraction of energy lost through radiative processes increases. Range, then, depends on the total stopping power. Dose, however, arises from ionizations. Dose is the energy deposited locally. Consequently, dose is related to the collisional stopping power. That is not much of a difference at lower energies but as we go to really high-energy electrons we have to keep in mind the difference between range and total stopping power versus dose and collisional stopping power.

We also have to be careful when we specify electron energy. Several energy definitions are used clinically. The energy of the electrons emanating from the linear accelerator is not uniform; the energy comes out in a spectrum. We typically define two energies at the surface of the patient. These two energies are $(E_p)_0$, the most probable energy at the patient surface, and $\overline{E_0}$, the mean energy at the patient surface, that is, the modal energy and the mean energy at the patient surface. In addition, we speak of an energy $\overline{E_z}$, the mean energy at depth z. One more quantity related to the energy is the practical range, R_p.[1] Once we understand the factors affecting a central-axis dose distribution, we can introduce a precise definition for the practical range.

The various energy quantities are related to the depth in the patient as follows: The mean energy at the patient surface is related to R_{50}, the depth at which the dose is 50% of the maximum dose, by the relation

$$\overline{E}_0 = 2.33\, R_{50}\,. \tag{19.1}$$

(See Fig. 9.11 for a discussion of R_{50}.) Thus, a measurement of R_{50} will give you the mean energy at the surface.

The most probable energy is related to the practical range as follows:

$$\left(\overline{E}_p\right)_0 = 0.22 + 1.98\, R_p + 0.0025\, R_p^2\,. \tag{19.2}$$

Consequently, to obtain this value, one measures the practical range of the electrons, R_p (discussed below).

Finally, the mean energy at depth is related to the depth and practical range by

$$\overline{E}_z = \overline{E}_0 \left(1 - \frac{z}{R_p} \right) . \tag{19.3}$$

A clinical electron-beam dose distribution is somewhat more complicated than this. Figure (19.1) illustrates this point. At shallow depths, when electrons scatter, the electrons deposit a dose a bit downstream and lateral to the point of initial interaction. We get an enhancement of dose at shallow depth because the electrons are scattering. As a result, the dose at the surface, where all the electrons are coming in straight, will be less than the dose a small distance below the surface where we now have electrons scattering in all directions. This is a very important observation. Because lower-energy electrons are deflected more than higher-energy electrons, given the same incident fluence, the dose below the patient surface will be greater for lower-energy electrons than for higher-energy electrons. Consequently, the surface dose relative to the maximum dose—the *percent skin dose*—will be lower for lower-energy electrons than for higher-energy electrons, typically between 75% and 100% of the maximum electron dose. Note that this is the opposite of the behavior of x-ray beams, for which the percent skin dose is greater for lower-energy x-rays.

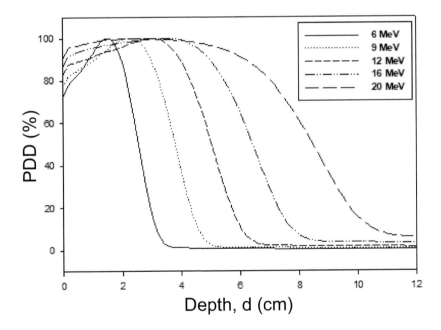

FIGURE 19.1: Central-axis percent depth dose (PDD) curves for various electron beam energies.

At depths beyond the depth of maximum dose, we see the depth-dose distribution taper off, rather than fall quickly to zero. This behavior is primarily due to *range straggling.* Range straggling occurs because the amount of energy transferred from an incident electron to a target electron is not uniform, but rather is statistical. Consequently, the energy distribution of the electron beam spreads out, resulting in a spreading out of the electron range. As the incident energy of the electron beam increases, the slope of the dose fall-off becomes more gradual. The fall-off region begins at approximately the depth of 90% dose. Consequently, when using electrons for radiation treatment, one typically selects an electron energy so that the 90% depth dose encompasses the target volume.

At the end of the fall-off region, beyond the range of the electrons, the dose distribution exhibits a tail due to Bremsstrahlung contamination of the incident beam. The contamination is due to x-rays produced in the head of the linear accelerator. It increases with increasing energy, varies with the design of the accelerator, and can typically be up to around 5% of the maximum dose.

In addition to range straggling and Bremsstrahlung contamination, we must also be familiar with the *practical range* of the electron beam. This topic was discussed in detail in Chapter 9. In particular, see the discussion in §9.11 associated with Fig. (9.11).

19.2   ELECTRON-BEAM TREATMENT PLANNING

Often, when electron beam therapy is used, a single electron beam is used to treat the target. A typical electron-beam dose distribution for a beam incident normally on the skin surface is illustrated in Fig. (19.2). In that case, the field size and energy are selected so that the target volume lies entirely within a specific isodose curve, typically the 90% isodose curve. When selecting a field size, it is important to recognize the

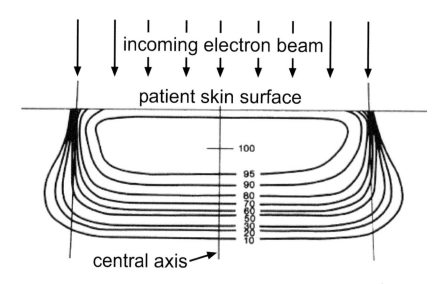

FIGURE 19.2: A typical electron-beam dose distribution. The "100" mark shows the reference position, taken to be maximum (100%) dose. The closed curve labeled "95" encloses the region receiving at least 95% of the maximum dose.

extent of electron penumbra and provide a sufficient margin to enclose the target volume. No hard and fast rule is normally given for the margin between the target volume and the extent of the electron field, but this can be readily determined from the isodose distribution.

The situation becomes somewhat more complicated when the electron beam is not normally incident on the patient surface. The left side of Fig. (19.3) illustrates an isodose distribution for a beam with oblique incidence. In this case, the isodose lines are roughly parallel to the patient skin surface. The depth dose along the central axis is approximately the same as that of a beam incident normally on the patient surface, but some differences occur. The right side of Fig. (19.3) is a graph depicting the change in electron percent depth dose as a function of angle of incidence. Two factors affect the percent depth dose. First, the primary beam fluence changes laterally due to the changes in SSD (Source to Surface Distance) due to the oblique incidence. Then, changes in side scatter will result in an increase in scatter at the depth of maximum dose, denoted d_{max} or R_{100}, resulting in a shift of R_{100} toward the patient surface.

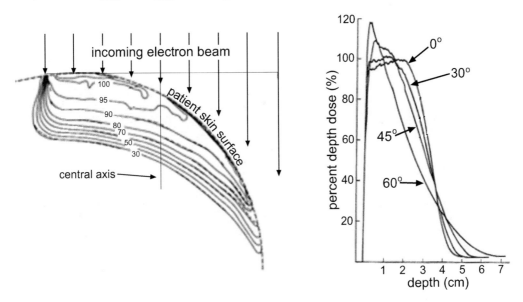

FIGURE 19.3: (Left) Electron-beam isodose distribution for an obliquely incident beam. Note that the angle of incidence and the SSD both vary with position for this set-up. (Right) Central-axis electron depth dose curves for an obliquely incident beam at various angles of incidence. The angle for normal incidence is taken to be 0°. The percentages shown are percents of the maximum dose for the 0° curve.

Often a target is too large to be encompassed by a single electron field. In such a case, multiple matching fields can be used. The difficulty here is in determining the gap between the two fields. Because electron dose spreads with depth due to scattering, *hot spots*—regions of concentrated high dose—and/or *cold spots*–regions of low dose—can result in the region of overlap, depending on the amount of field separation. Figure (19.4) illustrates the dose distributions obtained with two matching 16 *MeV* electron fields with varying gaps. Note the tradeoff between the size of the

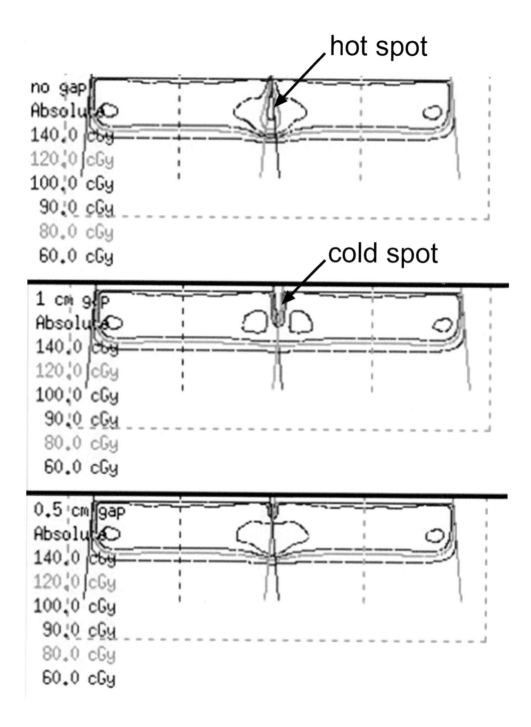

FIGURE 19.4: Isodose curves showing hot and cold spots when two electron fields are matched. Top: no gap. Center: 1-cm gap. Bottom: 0.5-cm gap.

gap and the overdosing or underdosing. With no gap, there is a significant hot spot; with a $1\,cm$ gap the hot spot goes away, but a cold spot appears. The problem is somewhat mitigated with a $0.5\,cm$ gap, but we still see significant dose heterogeneity. To further mitigate this problem, we will often move the junction between the two electron fields several times during the course of treatment, resulting in a smearing out of the hot and cold spots.

Patient heterogeneities characterized by variations in electron densities in tissue have significant effects on the electron beam. Heterogeneities affect the central-axis depth dose, but one can account for them by using a density-weighted depths. A more profound effect is the effect of heterogeneities on electron scatter. Figure (19.5) illustrates this issue. A difference in scatter from the heterogeneity combined with a change in the depth-dose beyond the heterogeneity gives rise to hot (higher dose) and cold (lower dose) spots adjacent to the heterogeneity boundary. In a similar manner, surface irregularities can also give rise to hot and cold spots. Figure (19.6) illustrates the effect of surface irregularities on an electron-beam dose distribution. A serious consequence of the effect of surface irregularities is that they may cause high dose gradients in the vicinity of the depth of maximum dose, d_{max} or R_{100}, making that point unsuitable for dose prescription.

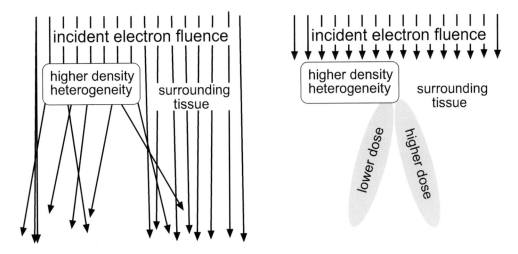

FIGURE 19.5: Effect of a heterogeneity on electron-beam dose distribution. In this case, the density of the heterogeneity is greater than that of the surrounding medium, so the amount of scatter from the heterogeneity is greater than that of the medium. (Left) The scattering of the beam electrons. (Right) The resulting hot and cold spots.

One way in which the effect of heterogeneities on lateral scatter can be modeled is by means of a pencil-beam algorithm.[2] In this model the incident electron beam is approximated by a set of narrow pencil beams. The dose $D(x, y, z)$ at a point (x, y, z) is related to the weight $W(x', y')$ of the pencil beams "convolved" with a Gaussian spread kernel $d(x - x', y - y', z)$

$$D(x, y, z) = \iint W(x', y')\, d(x - x', y - y', z)\, dx'dy'. \tag{19.4}$$

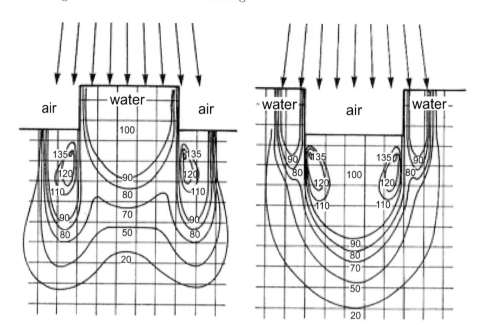

FIGURE 19.6: Effect of surface irregularities on an electron-beam dose distribution. The numbers are the percent of the dose at the position labeled "100".

Note that the word "convolved" in the previous sentence is in quotes, since this equation is not a true convolution; the kernel is not a function of $z - z'$ and the integration is performed over only two dimensions.

The pencil beams are defined at the plane of secondary collimation, that is, the end of the electron applicator and are characterized by a mean angle and an angular spread. We can write the pencil beam kernel as

$$d(x, y, z) = D_\infty(0, 0, z) \frac{\exp\left[-\frac{x^2+y^2}{2\sigma^2(x,y,z)}\right]}{2\pi\sigma^2(x, y, z)}. \tag{19.5}$$

In this equation $D_\infty(0, 0, z)$ is the central-axis dose at depth z for an infinitely broad beam with the same incident fluence at the surface as the pencil beam and $\sigma^2(x, y, z)$ is the mean square lateral displacement of the pencil beam at the position (x, y, z). The quantity $D_\infty(0, 0, z)$ is determined from electron-beam measurements, while $\sigma^2(z)$ consists of two components,

$$\sigma^2(z) = \sigma^2_{\theta_x} (z - L)^2 + \sigma^2_{MCS}. \tag{19.6}$$

The term on the left-hand side of this expression is a measure of the spread of the pencil from the patient surface to a depth z in the patient. $\sigma^2_{\theta_x}$ is the in-air spread of the pencil at the patient surface and L is the distance from the end of the electron collimator to the patient surface. σ^2_{MCS} is a measure of the beam spread due to multiple Coulomb scatter and is obtained from scattering theory to be the second moment of the mass angular scattering power, that is,

$$\sigma^2_{MCS}(z) = \frac{1}{2} \int_{\text{surface}}^{\text{depth, z}} \left[\frac{\theta^2}{\rho l}(z') \right] \rho(z') \, (z - z')^2 \, dz' \, . \qquad (19.7)$$

Two approximations are made in computations involving the pencil-beam equation. First, small angle scatter is assumed, enabling exponential terms to be expressed as the first two terms in a power-series expansion. Second, the effective depth of each point is replaced by the effective depth of the pencil delivering dose to that point. As a consequence, several inaccuracies may result from applications of the model, in particular, modeling the penumbra at large depths, where the small-angle approximation breaks down, calculating the effects of long, thin heterogeneities, where the approximation of point depth by pencil depth breaks down, and in the presence of surface collimation.

Several improvements have been made in the implementation of the pencil-beam algorithm including redefining the pencil-beam parameters at each depth[3] and introducing a polyenergetic electron spectrum[4], but at this point of complexity, calculations using Monte Carlo methods, as described in the previous chapter, incorporate fewer approximations with comparable calculation times.

The final issue in electron-beam treatment planning is how to prescribe an electron dose. That is, if we prescribe a dose to the 90% isodose, we need to know what the 90% refers to, because when we calculate monitor units, we must calculate them to deliver dose to a dose reference point. Typically, the dose reference point is d_{100} for a beam perpendicularly incident on a water phantom at the same SSD as the treatment. This point is well-defined and in a region of low dose gradient. Typically the dose calculation algorithm (pencil-beam or Monte Carlo) will express doses in terms of the reference dose, but this must be verified.

19.3   HEAVY CHARGED-PARTICLE DOSE DISTRIBUTIONS

In Chapter 9, we noted that heavy charged-particle interactions and electron interactions are similar, but several differences between the two types of interactions exist. Perhaps the major difference is that, due to the differences in masses, in the course of an interaction, an incident heavy charged particle transfers very little energy to the target electrons, whereas if the incident particle is an electron, a great deal of energy is transferred. Consequently, the trajectory of an incident heavy charged particle is barely affected by the interaction, but an incident electron can be strongly deflected.

This difference yields several consequences in the dose distribution. First of all, as illustrated in Fig. (19.7), heavy charged-particle dose distributions exhibit a Bragg peak. Because of the inverse relationship between the stopping power of the incident particles and the velocity of the particles, one observes an enhanced deposition of dose near the end of the range of a charged-particle beam, the Bragg peak. (See the discussion on the Bragg peak in §9.7.) If one were to trace the path of a single electron in an electron beam, one would also observe enhanced dose deposition at the end of the trajectory. However, because the electrons are scattered significantly more than the heavy charged particles, the electron trajectories end at a wide range of depths; consequently, the enhanced dose deposition is spread out over a wide range of depths.

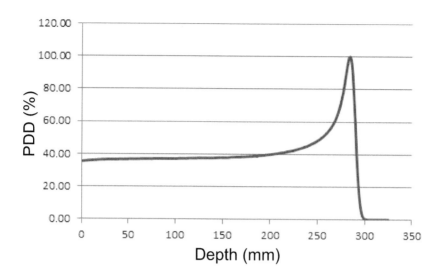

FIGURE 19.7: Central-axis depth dose distribution for a monoenergetic proton beam.

Next, heavy charged particles are only slightly deflected during an interaction, whereas electrons may undergo significant deflection. Consequently, the electron dose distribution displays side-scatter, which is absent in a heavy charged-particle dose distribution. The deflection of the electrons also causes Bremsstrahlung contamination of the beam, whereas heavy charged-particle beams exhibit negligible Bremsstrahlung. Finally, because heavy charged particles have a greater LET than electrons, the RBE is different from 1.0, resulting in a different dose prescription for heavy charged particles from that of photons or electrons. The presently accepted RBE value for protons, for example, is 1.1. Although a constant RBE is easy to incorporate into a dose prescription, such is not the case with heavy charged particles. Because the particles slow down at the end of their range, the LET, and hence the RBE, is increased, and there is great uncertainty as to what value to use. This will have some effect on treatment planning using heavy charged-particle beams, as we shall see in the next section.

19.4 HEAVY CHARGED-PARTICLE TREATMENT PLANNING

As we noted in the previous section, proton beams are characterized by their Bragg peak, followed by almost immediate dose fall-off. In planning for proton radiation therapy, one would select a proton energy so that the target volume fell within the Bragg peak, and would thus receive a significantly greater dose than the uninvolved tissue surrounding the target. However, as we saw in Fig. (19.7), the Bragg peak is very narrow, and would not be sufficiently broad to encompass the target. The solution here is to use a polyenergetic proton beam, weighted so that the Bragg peaks from the various energy components add up to deliver a uniform dose to the target. The *spread-out Bragg peak* (SOBP) is illustrated in Fig. (19.8). The SOBP can be generated using either a range modulator for passively scattered beams, or by multiple energy spots for spot-scanned beams.

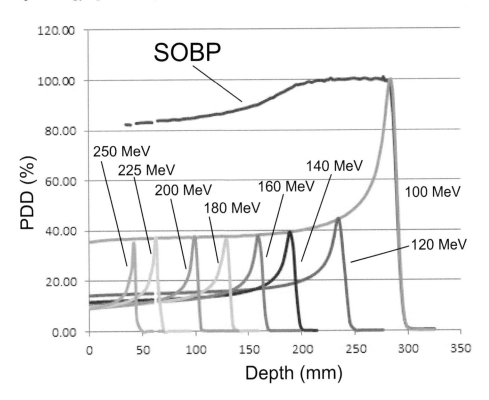

FIGURE 19.8: Combining proton beams of different energies to generate a spread-out Bragg peak (SOBP).

Treatment planning is somewhat different, depending on what method is used to generate the SOBP. When planning with a passively scattered beam, one first selects an energy and field size that encompasses the target, recognizing that the range may be field-size dependent. The field shape is determined using a collimator constructed of brass of approximately $2\,cm$ thickness. Shaping the distal edge of the beam to track the distal edge of the target is achieved using a compensator constructed from tissue-equivalent material such as Lucite or wax. The lateral margins are setup-specific, allowing for both tumor motion and setup uncertainty, whereas the proximal and distal margins are beam-specific. These margins account for uncertainties in the conversion of CT number to stopping power leading to uncertainties in the proton range. As a rule of thumb, the proximal and distal margins are set to be 0.035 times the depth of the proximal/distal edge of target volume plus $3\,mm$. The factor of 0.035 comes from the 3.5% uncertainty in conversion from CT number to stopping power, and the $3\,mm$ comes from uncertainty in the range of the charged particle beam.

Monitor units for proton therapy are calculated as follows: the beam is calibrated to deliver a dose of $1\,cGy/MU$ under a specified calibration condition. For example, a calibration is specified to be a 250-MeV proton beam with a range of $28.5\,cm$ and an SOBP width of $10\,cm$, a $10\,cm \times 10\,cm$ field measured at isocenter, a calibration point depth of $23.5\,cm$ in the center of the SOBP, and a source to calibration point distance of $270\,cm$. Then the number of monitor units, MU, is related to the dose D by the equation

$$MU = \frac{D}{DR}. \qquad (19.8)$$

The dose rate, DR, is given by

$$DR = CDO \cdot ROF \cdot SOBPF \cdot RSF \cdot SOBPOCF \cdot OCR \cdot FSF \cdot ISF \cdot CPSF. \qquad (19.9)$$

The various terms in the expression for dose rate are as follows:

CDO is the calibration dose output under the reference condition, typically taken to be $1\,cGy/MU$.

ROF is the relative output factor that accounts for changes in dose rate due to an energy distribution different from that of the calibration beam. It is a function of beam energy, range modulator, and secondary scatterer.

SOBPF is the SOBP factor accounting for the difference in dose rate for different SOBP widths. In the case of a wide SOBP, the beam passes through a larger number of modulator ramp steps, adding protons with shorter ranges. As the SOBP width increases, the dose rate decreases.

RSF is the range shifter factor that accounts for the difference in dose rate as a function of the thickness of the range shifter. An increase thickness of the range shifter gives a lower dose rate.

SOBPOCF is the off-center SOBP factor, accounting for the change in dose rate if the location of the dose calibration point is away from the center of the SOBP. The $SOBPOCF$ is given by

$$SOBPOCF = PDD \left[\frac{SSD + d_p}{SSD + d_c}\right]^2. \qquad (19.10)$$

In this expression PDD is the percent depth dose along the central-axis of the beam at the depth d_p of the calibration point, and d_c is depth of the center of the SOBP.

OCR is the off-center ratio, which accounts for the fact that the beam is not flat. This quantity is obtained from measured beam profiles.

FSF is the field-size factor, which is the change in dose rate resulting from a change in field size. This term only comes into effect for small fields where the field-size factor is significantly different from 1.0 for field sizes less than $5\,cm \times 5\,cm$.

ISF is the inverse square factor, which corrects the dose rate from the calibration measurement distance to the dose calculation distance.

CPSF is the compensator and patient scatter factor, which accounts for compensator and scatter from patient heterogeneities and is obtained from the treatment planning system.

Planning with spot scanning offers much greater flexibility in beam configurations than planning with a passively scattered beam as a result of the greater number of energies available with a spot-scanned beam. With spot scanning, one can have a treatment with over 100 energies and over 2 million spots. In such a case, treatment planning becomes an optimization problem for spot weights. Spots are first selected to span the target, then the weight of each spot is optimized.

Two methods exists for optimization of spot weights: single-field optimization and multiple-field optimization. In single-field optimization each field is individually optimized to deliver a prescribed uniform dose to the target. This method is generally used when critical structures are not in the beam path. Multiple-field optimization, also referred to as *intensity-modulated proton therapy* (IMPT), is a more complex technique in which all spots from all fields are optimized simultaneously. Using IMPT, one can avoid high doses to critical structures in the beam path. Fields so obtained yield a dose distribution that is more conformal than distributions obtained by single-field optimization, but the quality assurance required to support IMPT is more time-consuming.

Uncertainties in proton treatment planning affect treatment plans in a much different manner than uncertainties in photon treatment planning. The sharp falloff evidenced in proton beams makes proton therapy vulnerable to range uncertainties. As mentioned earlier range uncertainties of approximately 2–3% result from uncertainties in CT number to stopping power conversion. Another source of range uncertainties arises from metal artifacts and heterogeneities in the patient. Internal motion in the presence of heterogeneities, such as encountered in proton therapy of the thorax, complicate matters even more. Finally, one must recognize the impact of uncertainties in the RBE of the proton beam. The RBE is a function of the energy spectrum of the beam, with lower energy protons having a greater biological effect on the target. The distal portion of the SOBP contains a greater number of lower-energy, higher LET protons than the proximal portion of SOBP, hence a greater RBE. The RBE in this fall-off region is not known as precisely as that in major part of SOBP. As a consequence, greater uncertainties impact the effective dose delivered in the fall-off region. Because of range uncertainties and RBE uncertainties, a general rule of thumb in proton treatment planning is not to place a beam so that a critical structure is distal to the target volume along the beam path.

19.5 QUESTIONS, EXERCISES, & PROBLEMS

19-1. Explain in your own words why the PDD curves for electrons as shown in Fig. (19.1) increase as they go from the skin surface ($d = 0$) to depth values of 1 to 2 cm.

19-2. Examination of Fig. (19.1) shows that the PDD curves for lower-energy electrons have a lower percent skin dose at $d = 0$. Explain why this is so.

19-3. The topic of heterogeneities within the patient came up a number of times in the discussion of electron-beam treatment planning. (a) What is meant by a patient *heterogeneity*? What characterizes heterogeneities as far as an incident electron beam is concerned? (b) How do patient heterogeneities affect the dose distribution resulting from an incident electron beam?

19-4. The left side of Fig. (19.3) shows an electron beam incident on a patient whose skin surface curves away from the source of the electron beam. The plot on the right shows percent depth-dose curves for various angles of incidence of the electron beam. (a) Examination of the isodose curves on the left shows that the various curves get closer to each other as we move toward the right past the central axis of the incoming electron beam. Use the plot on the right to explain why. (b) Explain why the depth of maximum dose, R_{100}, decreases as the angle of incidence increases.

19-5. Figure (19.4) shows isodose curves resulting from two electron beams incident on the patient skin surface. Let's dig into these curves a bit more. (a) Why do the isodose curves for a single incident beam as shown in Fig. (19.3) bulge out the way they do on the sides once the electron beam enters the patient? (b) Using the isodose-curve distribution for *one* incoming electron beam shown in Fig. (19.3), sketch two separate but overlapping isodose distributions for *two* incident electron beams that butt against one another with no gap between them as they are incident on the patient skin surface. You need not show numbers associated with the isodose curves, but you should sketch several curves for each incident beam showing the characteristics of the dose distributions. Then make a rough sketch of the total isodose distribution, being sure to show the resulting hot spot. (c) Repeat part (b), but now with a sizeable gap between the two incident beams. You should label the resulting cold spot in your rough sketch showing the total isodose distribution.

19-6. Figure (19.5) shows the formation of hot and cold spots due to electron-beam scattering caused by a heterogeneity that has a higher density than the surrounding tissue. (a) Make sketches corresponding to the left- and right-sides of Fig. (19.5) for the case of a heterogeneity that has a lower density than the surrounding tissue. Be sure to label the hot and cold spots. To help make your point, you may want to exaggerate the scattering in the tissue somewhat more than is done in Fig. (19.5). (b) Explain your thinking behind the sketches you made in part (a).

19-7. Figure (19.6) shows isodose curves resulting from two types of surface irregularities. (a) For each of the two types shown, draw a sketch of the set-up, but instead of sketching the isodose curves, simply draw in and label the hot and cold spots that result from the irregularities. (b) Explain the presence of the hot and cold spots in your sketches for the two types of irregularities.

19-8. The section on Heavy Charged-Particle Dose Distributions has the following statement toward its end: "Because the particles slow down at the end of their range, the LET, and hence the RBE, is increased, and there is great uncertainty as to what value to use". (a) Explain the meanings of LET and RBE. (Don't just write out what the acronyms stand for, but explain what they mean.) (b) Why do the particles in a heavy charged-particle beam slow down as they move through tissue? (c) Explain why the LET and RBE of heavy charged particles in a beam increase as the particles slow down.

19-9. Explain the idea behind a *spread-out Bragg peak* (SOBP). How is it formed? How does it result in a more uniform dose distribution within the treatment volume and therefore a better treatment plan for treating a tumor?

19.6   REFERENCES

1. Khan FM, Doppke KP, Hogstrom KR, et al. Clinical electron-beam dosimetry: Report of AAPM Radiation Therapy Committee Task Group No. 25. *Med Phys.* 1991; 18(1): 73-108.
2. Hogstrom KR, Mills MD, Almond PR. Electron-beam dose calculations. *Phys Med Biol.* 26(3): 445-460.
3. Shiu AS, Hogstrom KR. Pencil-beam redefinition algorithm for electron dose distributions. *Med Phys.* 1991; 18(1): 7-18.
4. Boyd R, Hogstrom KR, Rosen II. Effect of using an initial polyenergetic spectrum with the pencil-beam redefinition algorithm for electron-dose calculations in water. *Med Phys.* 25(11): 2176-2185.

Treatment Planning and Delivery

CONTENTS

Calculating dose distributions, as we have done in the previous two chapters, is just a small, but important, part of the radiation treatment planning process. In this chapter we address the other components of the process. We start with image acquisition and use images in order to construct a computer model of the patient. Next we define our treatment target. In doing so, we will learn about the various factors that enable one to go from a tumor that is visualized on an image to an actual aperture setting on a treatment machine. In the following section we identify various methods of evaluating treatment plans. Next, we look at a method of inverse planning, in which the treatment plans are optimized to deliver the "best" dose distribution. The following section addresses setup uncertainties, how they can be quantified and then mitigated. Then, we address plan verification, ensuring that the radiation is delivered in the same manner as that which had been calculated. The final section of the chapter deals with intensity-modulated radiation therapy, a more sophisticated plan delivery technique that allows for more complex dose distributions.

20.1   IMAGE ACQUISITION FOR TREATMENT PLANNING

A profound shift in image acquisition for radiation treatment planning occurred during the 1980s when the CT scanner became commonplace in radiation therapy clinics. Prior to that time, images for treatment planning were acquired by means of a simulator, an x-ray imaging unit that looked like a skinny linac and simulated the geometries of the treatment beams that were planned to be used with the linear accelerator. The openings through which the x-rays passed in the simulator, called *treatment portals*, were designed on the simulator based on bony anatomy, which was relatively easy to visualize on the kilovoltage simulator image. Most treatments were

DOI: 10.1201/9781003477457-20

delivered using either parallel-opposed fields, three fields at equally-spaced angles, or four fields in a "box" arrangement. The major problem with using a conventional simulator was that, under most conditions, one was unable to visualize the actual tumor because of the relative lack of contrast between a soft-tissue tumor and the surrounding soft-tissue anatomy. (See Fig. 20.3 for an example of a portal image.)

Perhaps no device has had such an impact on radiation treatment planning as the CT scanner. Although the CT scanner was invented in the early 1970s, it was not until 15 to 20 years later that the CT scanner dedicated to radiation treatment planning became an essential component in the radiation oncology clinic. With the CT scanner, one could acquire transverse images of the patient in which the tumor was often plainly visible. (See Chapter 11 for a discussion of CT imaging.) The tumor could be outlined and then, by ray-tracing from a virtual point source, one could determine the relative attenuation of an x-ray beam passing through the patient and obtain a digitally reconstructed radiograph (DRR) with the superimposed projection of the tumor. Finally, the radiation oncologist could visualize directly what he/she intended to treat.

A CT scanner used in radiation therapy imaging differs from one used for diagnostic imaging in that the therapy imaging scanner has a flat couch identical to that on the treatment machine. The patient is placed in the position appropriate for the particular anatomic site to be irradiated, and the location of the isocenter of the treatment machine is identified by external markings. The CT image is acquired and transferred to the treatment planning computer, where the radiation oncologist contours the image of the tumor. Based on this information the treatment planner generates a plan. The process of using a CT scanner to generate simulation images is called "virtual simulation".

For some sites, imaging of internal anatomy may not generate the best images for treatment planning. Additional imaging devices may be used—for example, the PET/CT in which a PET scanner and a CT scanner share the same patient support mechanism. Consequently, a PET scan, which identifies regions of higher metabolic activity (e.g., a tumor) can be superimposed on a CT scan to assist the radiation oncologist in determining a tumor volume. (See Chapter 11 for a discussion of PET scans.)

20.2 TARGET VOLUME DEFINITIONS

As was noted in the previous section, in the early days of radiation therapy, treatment portals were defined by bony anatomy, and dose was calculated to a single point, typically the point at *isocenter*. Treatment planning computers had very limited memory (8 kilobytes in the early computers), and dose distributions were computed in a single transverse plane, the plane containing the isocenter. Dose prescriptions were then presented in the form of a percentage, for example, 180 cGy/fraction to the 95% isodose. (A *fraction* refers to a portion of the prescribed treatment.) But it was not usually clear what "95%" meant. Did it mean 95% of the dose to isocenter, or 95% of the maximum dose, or 95% of the minimum dose in the tumor, or what? This imprecision was not so much of an issue in a single practice, as long as the radiation oncologist was able to correlate clinical responses to whatever he/she defined as "dose", but once clinics collaborated in multi-institutional clinical trials, there had to be some way of precisely defining target volumes and specifying dose prescriptions.

Recognizing the need for precise definition of target volumes within the patient, the International Commission on Radiation Units and Measurements (ICRU) published two reports in order to promote the use of a common set of definitions for specifying and reporting doses in radiation therapy.[1,2] In these two reports, the ICRU identified several volumes that are of relevance in prescribing radiation treatments, and provided guidance for the determination of these volumes.

The first such volume defined by the ICRU is the *Gross Tumor Volume* (GTV). The definition of the GTV is straightforward: it is the extent of the demonstrable tumor. The manner in which the GTV is obtained is not specified; the GTV can be obtained by visual examination, CT, MR, PET, *etc.* Determining the GTV is the responsibility of the radiation oncologist.

The next volume is the *Clinical Target Volume* (CTV). The CTV is a consequence of what some have humorously called the "cockroach principle". This principle is based on the observation that for every cockroach you see, there are many more you do not see. In an analogous manner, for every image pixel that one sees containing tumor, there are many more pixels containing tumor but not observable. The CTV encompasses the GTV and exists due to subclinical disease. The extent of this subclinical disease is determined by the clinical experience of the radiation oncologist, supplemented, in some cases, by pathology studies, e.g., lung studies.[3] Both the GTV and the CTV are based on oncological principles and are much more general than their application to radiation oncology. For example, when a tumor is surgically removed, the surgeon also removes a margin of uninvolved tissue around the tumor. Implicitly, the surgeon recognizes a CTV around the GTV. Consequently, in radiation oncology it is the CTV that must receive the prescribed radiation dose in order to control the tumor.

Tumors may move, for example, due to such activities as respiration or peristalsis. In order to account for this tumor motion, one defines the *Internal Target Volume* (ITV) as the extent of the CTV due to motion. For many years, a population-averaged ITV was determined, to a large extent, by guesswork. However, with the introduction of *four-dimensional CT* (4D CT), in which motion can be explicitly imaged, one can measure an *internal margin* (IM) and determine the ITV directly. This enables us to move from a population-based IM to a personalized IM. The concept of 4D CT will be discussed further in the next chapter.

Finally, we need to acknowledge the fact that the patient is not going to be set up in exactly the same manner for every treatment. Setup uncertainties are a normal part of radiation treatment and will be addressed later in this chapter. Suffice it to say for now that setup uncertainties exist and, in many cases, can be determined. To account for setup uncertainty, one places a setup margin (SM) around the ITV to obtain a *Planning Target Volume* (PTV). The treatment portal is then designed to encompass the PTV.

20.3   TREATMENT PLAN EVALUATION

Once the target volumes have been defined, the treatment planner will typically outline relevant critical structures. Outlining (also referred to as "segmentation") serves two purposes. It allows even soft-tissue structures to be visualized on a *digitally reconstructed radiograph* (DRR), which is not possible in a conventional (film) radiograph. (The DRR is calculated from a CT data set.) It also allows assessment of the radiation dose received by the particular structure, which is important for plan evaluation.

Based on the geometry of the target volume and the critical structures, and also based on the experience and expertise of the treatment planner, a set of beams is identified and treatment portals are drawn to encompass the PTV plus an additional margin to account for the penumbra of the radiation beams. Doses are then calculated and the dose distribution is displayed, superimposed on the images of the patient. Doses are usually displayed by means of isodose curves, in which the treatment planning computer connects points of identical dose. Figure (20.1) illustrates such a dose distribution. Another way in which a dose distribution can be displayed is via isodose surfaces, in which points on a surface of identical dose are superimposed over a three-dimensional image of the patient. However, this display is not as often used as the simple isodose line display.

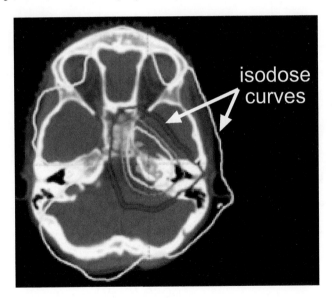

FIGURE 20.1: A distribution of isodose curves for treatment of a brain tumor.

The basic goal of the treatment plan is to ensure that the target volume is adequately covered by the prescription dose and that critical, uninvolved structures are avoided. In recent years, the impact of radiation on normal tissue structures irradiated in treatment has been quantified by the introduction of dose-volume constraints.[4] Dose-volume constraints are typically expressed in the form such as "No more than 20% of the ipsilateral lung may receive more than 20 Gy", and reflect the nature of the organ response to radiation. Organs are typically viewed as either serial structures or parallel structures. Serial structures can have their function destroyed by over-irradiating even a small volume. Thus a dose-volume constraint for a serial structure such as the spinal cord can be expressed in the form "No part of the cord may receive more than 45 Gy". Over-irradiation of even a small portion of the spinal cord may lead to paralysis. On the other hand, a parallel structure such as the lung can receive an excessive radiation dose to part of the structure, destroying it, and still be able to function with the remainder of the structure. The dose-volume constraint quoted earlier is typical of that of the lung. Thus, even though the lung has a relatively low tolerance for radiation, a part of the lung may receive a high dose of radiation and fail to function, but the patient can continue to breathe, and so, if necessary, part of the lung may be irradiated to a high dose of radiation without causing rejection of a treatment plan.

A most effective way to determine how well dose-volume constraints are met is via the *dose-volume histogram* (DVH). The DVH is a plot of the fraction of volume of a region of interest receiving at least a specified dose. Figure (20.2) illustrates such a DVH. From the DVH, it is relatively easy to determine if dose-volume constraints are met, and hence assess the acceptability of a treatment plan.

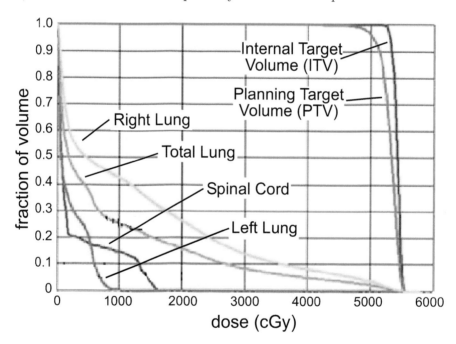

FIGURE 20.2: A dose-volume histogram (DVH).

20.4   INVERSE PLANNING

Conventional treatment planning might well have been called "plan verification". Treatment planning has been a trial and error approach based on the experience and expertise of the treatment planner. A target volume would be defined and critical structures delineated. The planner then used his/her experience to determine a set of beams that are likely to deliver the desired dose distribution, calculated the dose distribution, and evaluated it using one or more of the techniques described in the previous section. If the dose distribution is acceptable, the plan is done; otherwise the planner might vary the beam weights and the beam geometries in an attempt to obtain a more desirable dose distribution. This procedure is continued until the planner has either generated a clinically acceptable dose distribution or run out of time or patience. Moreover, in the case where the patient is planned with *intensity-modulated radiation therapy* (IMRT)—a technique that will be more explicitly described later in the chapter—the plan may have as many as 2000 beamlet weights that have to be optimized.

In the technique called "inverse planning", the planner starts with a desired dose distribution and allows an algorithm to determine a beam configuration that best reproduces that dose distribution. If the dose to a calculation point i is given by D_i, the weight of beam j by W_j, and the dose contribution to point i from beam j is C_{ij}, then the following holds true:

$$D_i = C_{ij} W_j . \tag{20.1}$$

(In the case of IMRT, replace the word "beam" with "beamlet", since the IMRT beam is made up of many small beams.) The total dose to the calculation point is found by summing over all n beam weights:

$$D_i = \sum_{j=1}^{n} C_{ij} W_j . \tag{20.2}$$

Writing this equation in matrix form, we have

$$\mathbf{D} = \mathbf{C} \mathbf{W} , \tag{20.3}$$

where $\mathbf{D}$ is the column matrix of dose values, $\mathbf{W}$ is the column matrix of beams weights, and $\mathbf{C}$ is the $m \times n$ matrix of dose contributions; here, m is the total number of calculation points and n is the total number of beams. Writing the desired dose as $\mathbf{D_0}$ and denoting the associated beam weights that are needed to produce the desired dose by $\mathbf{W_0}$, we can solve for $\mathbf{W_0}$ by operating from the left with the inverse of the dose contribution matrix:

$$\mathbf{W_0} = \mathbf{C}^{-1} \mathbf{D_0} . \tag{20.4}$$

Thus, inverse planning involves inversion of the matrix $\mathbf{C}$. However, in a typical treatment planning problem with IMRT we may have as many as 2000 beamlets depositing dose to 106 calculation points, making the matrix inversion a formidable, if not impossible, task.

Rather than solving the equation and obtaining the exact solution, we want to determine a reasonable dose solution, denoted $\mathbf{D_r}$. We then define an *objective function* $f(\mathbf{D_r}, \mathbf{D_0})$, which is a measure of how close the reasonable solution comes to the desired solution. The goal of inverse planning, then, becomes the minimization of the objective function. For example, if the objective function is written as $f(\mathbf{D_r}, \mathbf{D_0}) = (\mathbf{D_r} - \mathbf{D_0})(\mathbf{D_r} - \mathbf{D_0})^T$, then we have a least squares minimization problem. (By multiplying the column matrix $(\mathbf{D_r} - \mathbf{D_0})$ by its transpose we are adding together the squares of the differences of the reasonable and desired doses.) The variety of choices of objective function and methods for optimizing the objective function provide a wide variety of approaches to the inverse planning problem. Most optimization techniques are iterative, in that one begins with an initial trial solution and the corresponding value of the objective function. Some, or all, of the parameters are modified, and a new objective function is determined. Based on some criteria, either the new solution is accepted, or the old solution is retained, or some combination of the two solutions is used. The process is then repeated until some finalizing criteria are reached, for example, iterations change the value of the objective function by some negligible amount.

A somewhat different approach to optimization is based on the recognition that one may not necessarily want a "best" solution, but rather any solution that meets some well-defined criteria, for example, a solution that meets specified dose and/or dose-volume constraints. Methods for solving this class of problems fall under the category of feasibility-search algorithms, in which one searches for a solution that meets the constraints.

Inverse planning, at the present time, remains somewhat of an art; the quality of a dose distribution obtained by this technique depends to some extent on the ability and experience of the treatment planner; the determination of an optimal inverse planning process remains a topic of current research interest. However, as we shall see in Chapter 25, machine learning may play a significant part in treatment planning.

20.5   SETUP UNCERTAINTIES

Earlier in this chapter, we introduced the existence of setup uncertainties. Setup uncertainties are the unknown differences between the patient's position at treatment-simulation planning or treatment planning as compared to the patient's position at treatment. The fact is that it is not possible to set the patient up in exactly the same position every time, thus these uncertainties occur. Failure to take into account setup uncertainties may result in a geographic miss of the target yielding under-irradiation of the target. Setup uncertainties are different for different time frames: on a daily basis there are differences in patient setup, over longer time frames there may be disease progression or tumor shrinkage. In this section, we will primarily address daily differences in patient setup. These uncertainties result from our inability to set a patient up in exactly the same way each treatment session. Several methods have been used to mitigate these uncertainties including external markings, bony anatomy matching, fiducial markers, and use of reference points. In this section, we also discuss how setup uncertainties may be determined.

Many factors enter into setup uncertainty. Uncertainties may vary from patient to patient. There may be greater uncertainty in the setup of an obese patient compared to the setup uncertainty of a thin patient. Uncertainties may vary for different anatomic sites, being greater in the abdomen than in the head and neck. Uncertainties may also vary for different radiation oncology clinics, for example, in the use of different immobilization devices and simulation techniques. The skill of the radiation therapist may also have an impact on setup uncertainty.

There are two kinds of setup uncertainties: random uncertainties and systematic uncertainties. The understanding of random uncertainties is relatively straightforward; a patient is not going to be set up in exactly the same position every day. The various factors just discussed will play into small variations in the location of the isocenter and the actual position of the patient from treatment to treatment. Systematic uncertainties result from treatment planning based on a single set of images representing one patient setup that may vary slightly from the setups on the treatment machine.

Studies of setup uncertainty have been done using small radio-opaque objects implanted into the patient that can be seen in images. These objects, called *fiducials*, are used to mark reference positions within the patient. In these studies,[5] fiducials were implanted into the tumor or into another region near the target. A planning CT image data set was acquired and a treatment plan was prepared based on the CT data. Daily portal images were acquired of the treatment region. From these portal images, it was possible to determine the mean location of the fiducials as well as the standard deviation of the locations. The standard deviation can then be used as a measure of random uncertainty. The systematic uncertainty can be determined by comparing the location of the fiducials in the planning image to their time-averaged locations in the treatment images. In a similar manner, one may use on-treatment CT images instead of images of fiducials to determine the systematic and random setup uncertainties.[6] Typically, systematic uncertainties are shown to be significantly greater than random uncertainties and also to have a greater impact in determining margins to account for setup uncertainties.

When high precision is desired, systematic uncertainty can be reduced in several ways. A rather straightforward method for reducing systematic uncertainty is tighter immobilization of the patient. When this is not possible, systematic uncertainty can be reduced by acquiring images, either portal images with fiducials or on-treatment CT images for several fractions. After several fractions, one then modifies the patient setup based on either the mean locations of fiducials if portal imaging is used, or the mean position of anatomical landmarks when CT imaging is used. Another method for reducing systematic uncertainty is to acquire several sets of planning CT images in the region around the tumor, determine appropriate target volumes using an average over the planning CT images, and plan based on the mean target volume.

20.6 PLAN VERIFICATION

Once a treatment plan has been developed, the machine parameters have been transferred from the treatment planning computer to the treatment machine, and the patient is ready for treatment, it is important, as part of the quality management process, to verify that the radiation is being delivered as planned. Perhaps the earliest—and most crude—method of plan verification was to acquire radiographic images of the treatment portal, the opening through which the beam passes as it leaves the beam-producing machine. In order to verify the geographic placement of the treatment portal double images were acquired, one of the treatment portal itself, and a second image acquired with an open collimator. Such a portal image is illustrated in Fig. (20.3). With this double image, it was possible to verify the location of the treatment portal relative to the patient's bony anatomy.

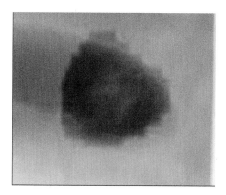

FIGURE 20.3: A portal image of a lung tumor. Note the poor image quality, characteristic of a portal image.

Several problems were evident with this form of portal imaging. The first problem was the use of film as an image receptor—in particular, that film needed to be processed. Although automatic film processors could be used, the development process took up time during which the patient was lying on the treatment couch and could move. This problem, however, was overcome by the use of electronic portal imaging devices (EPIDs). Instead of film, an image receptor was used to produce a digital image of the treatment portal, which could be viewed almost instantaneously after the image was acquired. Moreover, storage of these digital images was more efficient than storage of film images.

The second problem with conventional portal imaging was the poor quality of portal images. Recall that the high contrast of diagnostic radiographic images is due to differences in attenuation of the x-ray beam, primarily due to photoelectric interactions. Recall also that the linear attenuation coefficient for the photoelectric interaction varies as the cube of the atomic number. (See §8.1.) The difference in effective atomic numbers between bone ($Z_{eff} = 13.8$) and soft tissue ($Z_{eff} = 7.4$) is magnified by the Z^3 dependence of the linear attenuation coefficient, thus yielding high contrast between bone and soft tissue. On the other hand the portal image is acquired using high-energy x-rays for which the primary interaction is Compton scatter (see §8.2). Recall that the linear attenuation coefficient for Compton scatter varies roughly as the electron density, which is approximately equal to the mass density. Since the mass density of bone is approximately 1.8 times larger than that of soft tissue, there is less contrast in portal images than that seen in images acquired at lower energies.

Further reducing the contrast in portal images is the scattered radiation resulting from the Compton process. Recall that when Compton scatter occurs, both an electron and a scattered photon are ejected. The electron is absorbed within the patient, whereas the photon could reach the image receptor. It is not possible to determine the source of a photon reaching the image receptor, so it is not possible to ray-trace the scattered photon, determine attenuation along its path, and hence infer structure along the path of the scattered photon. These scattered photons simply add a background of noise to the portal image, further degrading its quality.

Portal image contrast can be improved somewhat by the use of small metallic fiducials implanted in the region of the tumor. These fiducials are much more visible on a portal image and can be used for portal verification. Figure (20.4) illustrates such a portal image with fiducials.

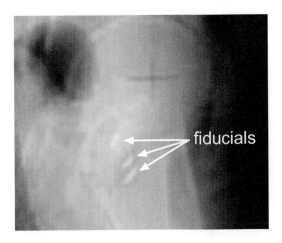

FIGURE 20.4: A portal image taken with several implanted fiducials. The large "+" denotes the center-of-field point.

Once the images are acquired, they are compared to simulation images and possible changes in patient position are made. It is often difficult to determine appropriate shifts based on oblique images, so frequently anteroposterior (AP) and lateral simulation and portal images are acquired rather than images of the treatment portals. Determination of patient shifts are made much simpler and less prone to error from these images.

TABLE 20.1: A comparison of conventional CT to cone-beam CT

	Conventional CT	Cone-beam CT
Beam configuration	Fan beam	Cone beam
Detector	1-dimensional	2-dimensional
Number of slices/rotations	Small number	Many

The use of *cone-beam computed tomography* (CBCT) is another means of plan verification. In CBCT, a two-dimensional image receptor is positioned opposite an x-ray source, the gantry is rotated, and the projections are combined to generate a CT image. Table (20.1) compares CBCT to conventional CT. Figure (20.5) illustrates a CBCT-guided linear accelerator. Note that the x-ray source and image receptor are positioned 90° from the linear accelerator source. The field of view is limited by the size of the image receptor. However, because all the information can be acquired with only a 180° rotation, by partially displacing the image receptor from the central axis of the beam and acquiring data over the full 360° rotation, a much larger field of view can be covered. One study demonstrated a reduction in set-up margins for liver irradiation of a factor of 2 to 3 when fiducial-guided CBCT is used as compared to conventional portal imaging.[7]

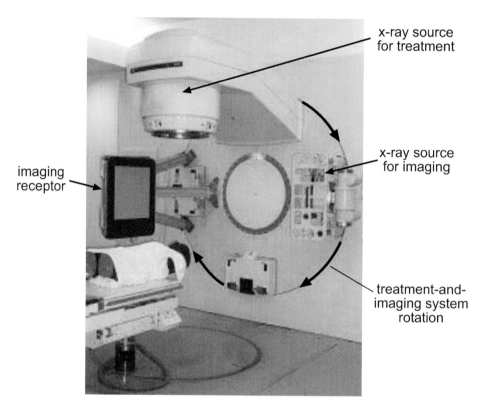

FIGURE 20.5: An x-ray source and receptor forming the CBCT system are oriented 90° from the treatment beam in order to acquire cone-beam CT images. The entire treatment-imaging system rotates together, as shown.

Another method to visualize the patient's anatomy in three dimensions in close temporal proximity to treatment involves the use of a CT scanner that shares the same treatment couch as the linear accelerator. This enables the patient to be scanned on the CT scanner, then treated without having to move the patient. Instead of the treatment couch being moved through the CT scanner as usual, the scanner gantry is placed on wheels and moves on rails during the image acquisition. Using the CT-on-rails allows for millimeter accuracy required for hypofractionated treatments for which high setup accuracy is mandatory. Figure (20.6) illustrates such a CT-on-rails system.

What the CT-on-rails does not do is monitor the movement of the tumor during treatment. To do that requires a real-time image acquisition device that can be

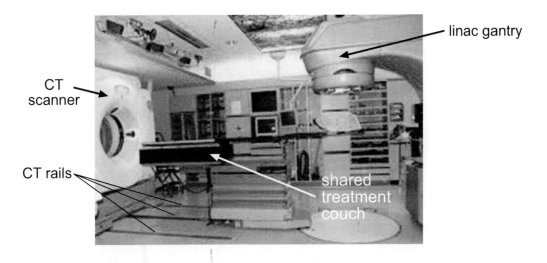

FIGURE 20.6: A CT-on-rails system in which the imaging and treatment equipment use the same treatment couch.

operated while the linear accelerator is delivering radiation. A very promising approach to real-time image acquisition involves the use of magnetic resonance imaging of the patient during treatment.

20.7 INTENSITY MODULATED RADIATION THERAPY

Inverse planning, as described earlier in this chapter, has had only limited success. This limitation is due, in part, to the fact that it is not possible to irradiate a concave target volume using flat beams. See, for example, Fig. (20.7), which illustrates a treatment plan for the irradiation of a tumor in the patient's head. Both regions defined by isodose curves 1 and 2 need to be irradiated to a high dose to control the tumor and tumor spread. Photon beams of uniform spatial intensity are not capable of irradiating the target volume without over-irradiation of the spinal cord. It was found, however, that by modulating the beam fluence, a concave target volume could be irradiated.[8] Intensity-modulated radiation therapy (IMRT) is a technique that uses non-uniform beam intensities to irradiate a target volume of desired shape.

Because it is not obvious how the fluence pattern relates to the dose distribution, IMRT requires a robust inverse planning algorithm. In some respects, IMRT treatment planning remains an art, relying, to some extent, on the skill and experience of the treatment planner. For example, in order to reduce the dose immediately outside the target volume, a planner might introduce a pseudostructure surrounding the target volume. The pseudostructure would then be considered a critical structure and assigned a low tolerance dose to generate an acceptable treatment plan.

Intensity modulation is achieved using a multileaf collimator that is programmed to move during the course of treatment while the radiation beam is on (see Fig. 20.8).[9,10] In some respects, the values of several components of the treatment delivery system need to be known to significantly higher accuracy than the corresponding parameters for static beam delivery. For example, because beam edges have a strong

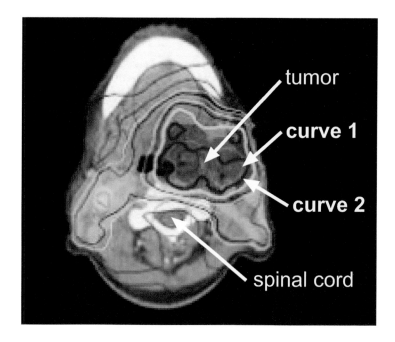

FIGURE 20.7: A treatment plan for irradiation of a tumor in the head.Isodose curves 1 and 2 define regions of high dose designed to control the tumor.

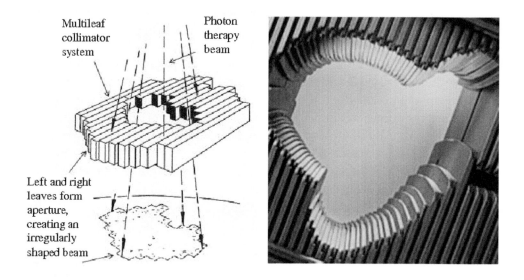

FIGURE 20.8: (Left) Schematic showing the various leaves of the multi-leaf collimator, each of which can move independently of the others. The various leaves can be positioned to generate the desired size and shape of the beam at the position of the tumor, as shown. (Copyright ©2005 Society for Industrial and Applied Mathematics. Reprinted with permission. All rights reserved.) (Right) Photograph of an MLC. (Open Source.)

influence on the dose distribution, it is important to know the location of beam edges to submillimeter precision. Another example of greater accuracy needed for IMRT is the dose per monitor unit output of the linear accelerator, made necessary because of the small numbers of monitor units delivered during each MLC configuration.

Several techniques exist for the delivery of IMRT. Tomotherapy, developed by Mackie and co-workers at the University of Wisconsin[11], was an example of an early use of multileaf collimation to shape dose distributions. The procedure consisted of a 360° rotation of a $6\,MV$ x-ray source around the patient. A photograph of an accelerator used for helical tomotherapy is shown in the left side of Fig. (20.9).[12] It looks somewhat like a CT scanner, but with a megavoltage x-ray source rather than a kilovoltage source rotating around the patient. A binary MLC defines a fan beam approximately 20 cm wide by 1–4 cm thick. The right side of Fig. (20.9)[13] illustrates such a binary MLC. The leaves of the MLC moved in and out during gantry rotation. In an early version of the tomotherapy process, the MLC was attached to the head of a conventional linear accelerator. Radiation was delivered to a transverse slice of the patient during rotation of the gantry. The treatment couch moved longitudinally between the delivery of radiation to each slice. This process was superseded by helical tomotherapy, which combines tomotherapy delivery with MV CT for localization.

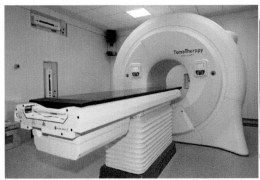 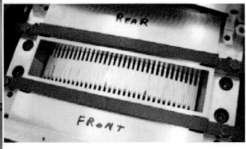

FIGURE 20.9: Left: A helical tomotherapy unit. (Open Source.) Right: A binary MLC (with all leaves closed) used in tomotherapy (Wiley, with permission.).

Another technique for IMRT delivery is "step and shoot". This technique uses a conventional MLC on a linear accelerator, but is based on changing the discrete positions of the MLC during treatment. Step and shoot is a relatively straightforward technique for beam delivery, but its implementation requires a leaf-sequencing algorithm to convert the two-dimensional fluence map obtained from an inverse planning algorithm to a leaf sequence.[14,15]

A third technique for delivery of IMRT is "dynamic MLC". In this technique, the MLC leaves are in motion during the delivery of radiation, with leaf positions changing based on the number of monitor units delivered. In order to achieve dynamic MLC, it is necessary to define a set of control points. At each control point both leaf positions and numbers of monitor units are input. Each MLC leaf is controlled by a separate motor, and the leaf position is indicated by encoders attached to motors.

Consequently, a feedback mechanism verifies the correct leaf positioning, and the beam can be interrupted if the leaf position is outside tolerance levels.

It should be noted that a large number of monitor units is required to deliver the radiation treatment. As a result MLC leakage can be a significant issue, with total MLC leakage exceeding 10% of the prescribed in-field dose.[16]

In a comparison of static MLC IMRT with dynamic MLC IMRT, one finds that static MLC is relatively easy to understand. There is no requirement to control individual leaf speeds resulting in a simpler control system. With dynamic MLC, treatment times are shorter and less of a dosimetric error may occur because the continuous intensity profile is discretized. Also, dynamic MLC has more degrees of freedom. As a result, inverse planning for dynamic MLC will result in a solution equal to or better than that found for static MLC.

Volumetric-modulated arc therapy (VMAT) is an extension of dynamic MLC IMRT in which the gantry is rotated while the MLC leaves are moving.[17] An advantage of VMAT is a significant reduction in treatment times. A typical 5–7 field IMRT treatment typically takes from 5 to 10 minutes for delivery of radiation, whereas a single-arc VMAT treatment takes 1 to 1.5 minutes for treatment delivery. Thus, there is less risk of patient motion with VMAT compared to the other methods of IMRT beam delivery.

20.8   QUESTIONS, EXERCISES, & PROBLEMS

20-1. Define and explain the differences between GTV, CTV, ITV, and PTV.

20-2. Explain the difference between series and parallel organs.

20-3. Explain the general idea behind inverse treatment planning.

20-4. What is the "cockroach principle" and how is it related to the CTV? Explain.

20-5. What is IMRT? What are its advantages over regular radiation therapy?

20-6. Research helical tomotherapy. When was it developed? Explain the ideas behind the operation of the helical tomotherapy unit. What are its advantages?

20-7. This problem addresses two radiation-related events that resulted in patient deaths; these events actually occurred. You will have to make some "reasonable" approximations to answer these questions. (a) Approximately 50 years ago, a physicist, instead of measuring the output of a Co-60 source before treating a patient as required, only estimated the decay of the source to save time. The physicist knew the decay constant for Co-60. Unfortunately, he treated the Co-60 source as having a linear decay rather than the correct exponential decay behavior. Assuming that the initial source activity he had recorded 6 months earlier was correct, estimate the error in patient dosage. Were patients overdosed or underdosed? (b) Suppose that a linear accelerator were set to deliver a dose of x-rays, but the tungsten target was not in place, meaning that the patient was treated with an electron beam instead of the corresponding x-ray beam. Estimate the error in patient dosage because of the absence of the target. (For more details on these and other radiation-related accidents, refer to https://journals.sagepub.com/doi/pdf/10.1016/S0146-6453(01)00039-2 or search online for "Case Histories of Major Accidental Exposures in Radiotherapy".)

20.9   REFERENCES

1. Wambersie A, Landberg T, Akanuma A, et al. *Volume and dose specification for reporting external beam therapy. (The ICRU recommendations).* Bethesda, MD: ICRU; 1997.

2. Landberg T, Chavaudra J, Dobbs J, et al. *Prescribing, recording, and reporting external beam therapy (Supplement to ICRU 50).* Bethesda, MD: ICRU; 1999.

3. Giraud P, Antoine M, Larrouy A, et al. Evaluation of microscopic tumor extension in non-small-cell lung cancer for three-dimensional conformal radiotherapy planning. *Int J Rad Oncol Biol Phys.* 48(4): 1015-1024.

4. Marks LB, Ten Haken RK, Martel MK, eds. Quantitative Analyses of Normal Tissue Effects in the Clinic. *Int J Radiat Oncol Biol Phys.* 76(3 Suppl): S1-S160.

5. Nelson C, Starkschall G, Morice R, Stevens CW, Chang JY. Assessment of lung tumor motion during respiratory gating using implanted fiducials. *Int J Radiat Oncol Biol Phys.* 2007; 67(3): 915-923.

6. Starkschall G, Balter P, Britton K, McAleer MF, Cox JD, Mohan R. Interfractional reproducibility of lung tumor location using various methods of respiratory motion mitigation. *Int J Radiat Oncol Biol Phys.* 79(2):596-601, 2/2011. e-Pub 7/2010.

7. Zhang T, Wang W, Li Y, et al. Inter- and intrafractional setup errors and baseline shifts of fiducial markers in patients with liver tumors receiving free-breathing postoperative radiation analyzed by cone-beam computed tomography. *J Appl Clin Med Phys.* 2015; 15(6): 138-146.

8. Brahme A, Roos JE, Lax I. Solution of an integral equation encountered in radiation therapy. *Phys Med Biol.* 1982; 27(10): 1221-1229.

9. Romeijn HE, Ahuja RK, Dempsey JF, Kumar A. A Column Generation Approach to Radiation Therapy Treatment Planning Using Aperture Modulation. *SIAM Journal on Optimization.* 2005; 15(3): 838–862. https://doi.org/10.1137/040606612.

10. Primi11 (https://commons.wikimedia.org/wiki/File:Primer_veclistnega_kolimatorskega_sistema_v_glavi-_linearnega_pospesevalnika.png), https://creativecommons.org/licenses/by-sa/4.0/legalcode.

11. Mackie TR, Balog J, Ruchala K, et al. Tomotherapy. *Sem. Radiat. Oncol.* 1999; 9(1): 108-117.

12. ASL Reggio Emilia (https://commons.wikimedia.org/wiki/File:Tomotherapy.jpg), "Tomotherapy", https://creativecommons.org/licenses/by-sa/3.0/legalcode.

13. Langen KM, Papanikolaou N, Balog J, et al. (2010), QA for helical tomotherapy: Report of the AAPM Task Group 148. *Med. Phys.* 2010; 37(9): 4817-4853. https://doi.org/10.1118/1.3462971

14. Que W, Kung J, Dai J. Tongue and groove effect in intensity modulated radiotherapy with static multileaf collimator fields. *Phys Med Biol.* 2004; 49(3): 399-405.

15. Kamath S, Sahni S, Palta J, Ranka S, Li J. Optimal leaf sequencing with elimination of tongue-and-groove underdosage. *Phys Med Biol.* 2004; 49(3): N7-N19.

16. Kim JO, Siebers JV, Keall PJ, Arnfield MR, Mohan R. A Monte Carlo study of radiation transport through multileaf collimators. *Med Phys.* 2001; 28(12): 2497-2506.

17. Teoh M, Clark CH, Wood K, Whitaker S, Nisbet A. Volumetric modulated arc therapy: a review of current literature and clinical use in practice. *Brit J Radiol.* 2011; 84(1007): 967-996.

Special Treatment Techniques

CONTENTS

Whereas the previous chapters addressed treatment planning and treatment delivery techniques that could be considered "standard" in radiation oncology, the present chapter will cover some more specialized treatment techniques in radiation therapy. These are techniques that require more than a simple monitor unit calculation or isodose calculation, or even an inverse plan. These techniques are more complex in terms of dose calculation, more sophisticated equipment, specialized quality assurance procedures, and more involvement by physics support. Consequently, not every radiation treatment facility supports these techniques. Four techniques that will be briefly addressed in this chapter are stereotactic radiosurgery, total body irradiation, total skin electron irradiation, and respiratory motion management. It should be noted, however, that as "special techniques" become used more frequently in radiation oncology clinics, they cease to be "special" and could be considered "standard". One could argue convincingly that one or more of the techniques described in this chapter are no longer "special".

21.1 STEREOTACTIC RADIOSURGERY

Stereotactic radiosurgery is a technique that was originally intended for use in neurosurgery. Its basic principle is the use of a single high dose to ablate the tumor, with a stereotactic frame to immobilize the patient and achieve sub-millimeter accuracy in patient positioning. Figure $(21.1)^1$ illustrates such a head frame. When the head frame is typically installed, the patient receives a local anesthetic, and screws are inserted into the patient's skull. The frame is then used for accurate reproduction of patient setup in acquiring planning images as well as in treatment. Images are first acquired with the frame in place. The coordinate system defined by the frame is transferred first to the treatment planning system, and then to the treatment delivery system, where the single, high-dose radiation fraction is delivered.

DOI: 10.1201/9781003477457-21

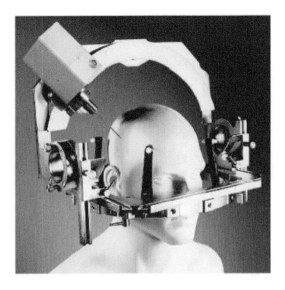

FIGURE 21.1: A head frame used for patient immobilization in stereotactic radiosurgery. (Open Access.)

For the treatment of other regions of the body, a small number of high-dose fractions may be used in what is termed *stereotactic body radiation therapy* (SBRT). As in stereotactic radiosurgery, patient immobilization is paramount. In order to immobilize the patient for SBRT, a vacuum cushion is often used. The vacuum cushion is a large bag filled with small pellets. Figure (21.2) illustrates such a cushion. After the patient has been placed in the bag, air is drawn out of the bag. The creation of a vacuum in the bag causes the bag to harden, thus immobilizing the patient. Alternatively, metallic fiducials can be implanted in the region near the tumor. These are readily imaged prior to planning as well as prior to using the treatment machine.

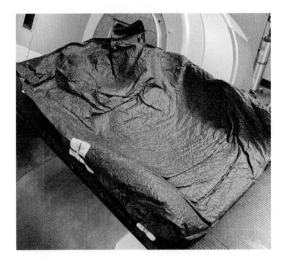

FIGURE 21.2: A vacuum cushion used for patient body immobilization. (Photo courtesy of Jay Burmeister.)

The portal images acquired on the treatment machine are compared against the planning images in order to verify the patient positioning prior to treatment.

Because moving the patient from the CT scanner to the treatment machine prior to the initial treatment setup as well as daily treatment setups introduce uncertainty in the patient positioning, several methods have been devised to minimize these setup uncertainties. The CT-on-rails, as discussed in Chapter 20 and shown in Fig. (20.6), is one such method. The CT on rails is a conventional CT scanner placed in the treatment room. However, unlike a conventional CT scanner in which the patient table moves through the scanner as the image is acquired, the CT-on-rails, as its name implies, places the CT scanner on a track, moving the scanner, rather than the table, during the image acquisition. The same table is then rotated from the CT scanner to the treatment machine, keeping patient motion between the verified setup and the treatment to a minimum.

Images of the patient on the treatment table can also be acquired using cone-beam CT. In this technique, the radiation source is the treatment machine. The gantry is rotated a full 360° around the patient, and projection images are acquired by an image receptor placed opposite the patient. A three-dimensional image can then be reconstructed from these projection images, analogous to those images acquired in a conventional planning CT scan. Anatomic landmarks identified on the cone-beam CT scan can then be compared to the landmarks on the planning scan, and the patient position appropriately adjusted if there is a discrepancy.

One of the devices used for delivery of radiation in stereotactic radiation therapy is the Gamma Knife®, developed by the Swedish neurosurgeon Lars Leksell in the late 1960s for treating cranial tumors as well as other cranial conditions. The Gamma Knife® typically consists of 201 ^{60}Co sources, each of approximately $1\,TBq$ activity, placed in a hemispheric array in a heavily shielded treatment head (see Fig. 21.3[2]). Collimators are used to aim the gamma rays emitted from the sources to a single point. A head frame is attached to the patient's skull and used in the acquisition of images for patient setup as well as patient positioning for treatment in the Gamma Knife®.

Another device for delivering radiation is the Cyberknife® system, which consists of a compact linear accelerator mounted on a robotic arm. Because the source of radiation is in a robotic arm rather than a gantry, there are more degrees of freedom in the position of the radiation source than in the conventional linear accelerator. Figure 21.4[3] illustrates an example of a Cyberknife®. The Cyberknife® is used more for body radiation therapy than for cranial therapy.

21.2   TOTAL BODY IRRADIATION

Total body irradiation is a technique that has been used to kill off leukemia, lymphoma, and myeloma cells as well as to suppress the patient's immune system prior to a stem cell or bone marrow transplant. Doses are typically in the range of $10–12\,Gy$. It should be noted that this dose is greater than the LD-50 of 4.5 Gy. (LD-50—*lethal dose-50*—is the dose delivered to each person in a population that results in the death of 50% of that population.) Destruction of the patient's bone marrow by the

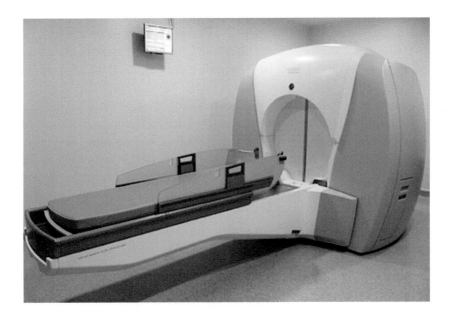

FIGURE 21.3: A Gamma Knife® used for the treatment of cranial tumors. (Open Source.)

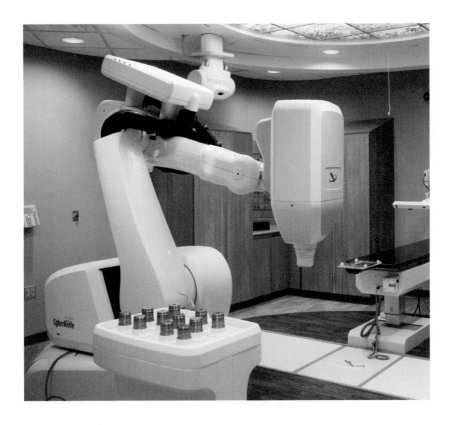

FIGURE 21.4: A Cyberknife®. (Open Source.)

radiation can prove fatal; however, following the total body irradiation with a stem cell or bone marrow transplant prevents death from occurring and allows for restoration of the patient's immune system. It should be noted, however, that total body irradiation has been superseded, to a large extent, by medical intervention—often chemotherapy.

Several issues with total body irradiation are worth noting. First of all, the large field necessary to irradiate the entire patient is achieved by long treatment distances. Because of the long distance between the radiation source and the patient, attenuation in air, in addition to scatter from the walls of the treatment room, results in a breakdown of the inverse square rule for determining radiation intensity. Consequently, measurements of the machine output at the location of the patient are necessary.

Another issue to be considered results from the relatively low tolerance of the lungs to irradiation. The potential for lung damage in the form of pneumonitis at these dose levels is quite real. In order to avoid lung damage, lung shielding is required.

Finally, the long treatment times required by the extended treatment distance may place a heavy workload on a linear accelerator. The delivery of whole body irradiation was a very good application of ^{60}Co irradiation.

21.3   TOTAL SKIN ELECTRON IRRADIATION

Another technique that requires special measurements is *total skin electron irradiation* (TSEI), a technique used to treat mycosis fungoides, a form of cutaneous lymphoma. The treatment goal is a dose of 31–40 Gy to the skin surface in fractions of 1.0–2.0 Gy.[4] In the delivery of radiation, dose inhomogeneity is not to exceed $\pm 10\%$ and photon contamination is not to exceed 0.7 Gy. In order to treat the entire patient an extended SSD of 3–8 m is used, and to protect subcutaneous tissue, low-energy ($\sim 4~MeV$) electrons are used.

In one of the more common treatment methodologies, the patient is treated in a standing position with six electron fields, rotating the patient 60° between fields. If the treatment room is large enough to achieve a 7-m SSD (*source-to-surface distance*), the beam is horizontal, but this is not always the case. In smaller rooms one uses two fields at each patient position, each field angled $\pm 20^o$ from the horizontal.

Because the lowest electron energy available on a linear accelerator is typically 6 MeV, a Plexiglas plate is placed in front of patient. The plate both degrades the energy of the beam and also scatters the electrons to improve the field uniformity at field junctions. Just as in total body irradiation, the SSD is large, so there is significant air and room scatter, resulting in a breakdown of the inverse-square relationship. Consequently, individualized radiation measurements are required.

21.4   RESPIRATORY MOTION MANAGEMENT

Initially, treatment portals for irradiation of lung tumors were determined based on bony anatomy as seen on radiographs. However, dose-volume constraints on the spinal cord and uninvolved lung limited the dose that could be delivered to lung tumors.

When CT imaging was introduced into radiation therapy, treatment portals could be designed based on the extent of tumors. The dose delivered to the tumor could then be increased while maintaining doses to organs at risk keeping the same dose-volume constraints. As we learned in the previous chapter, the expansion of a CTV (clinical target volume) to a PTV (planning target volume) needs to incorporate both internal motion and setup uncertainty. In the case of treating lung tumors, respiratory motion is significant. However, without the ability to measure the tumor motion explicitly, in order to ensure adequate tumor coverage, isotropic margins of 1–2 cm were placed around the CTV.

The use of such a uniform target volume expansion is based on the assumptions that lung tumor motion is identical for all patients, and that the motion is isotropic. CT imaging has shown both assumptions to be incorrect; there is no correlation between tumor motion and size, shape, location, $etc.$[5] By replacing the uniform population-based target margin with a patient-based target margin, that is, by incorporating explicit knowledge of the tumor motion into the treatment plan, we could reduce the margin around the CTV and irradiate less uninvolved lung volume.

The problem with explicitly imaging respiratory motion using CT was that, at the time that the respiratory motion techniques were first being developed (around 2001), the duration of a helical CT scan of the thorax was approximately 10 s. Ten seconds is also the approximate length of a respiratory cycle. Consequently, at first glance, it would not appear possible to capture motion. This problem was solved by taking advantage of the assumption of periodicity of respiratory motion, that is, tumor motion during one respiratory cycle was assumed to be identical to that in all other respiratory cycles. CT information could then be acquired over a series of respiratory cycles at a set of fixed points in each respiratory cycle. A set of three-dimensional CT data acquired at several phases in the respiratory cycle is referred to as a $four\text{-}dimensional\ CT$ (4D CT) data set.

Two approaches have been developed to acquire 4D CT images. In one approach the CT scanner is operated in $cine\ mode$, in which a set of 2D images is acquired at a single table position. The table is then indexed a distance equal to the detector width, and another set of images is acquired. Table indexing and image acquisition is continued until images are acquired of the entire region of interest. A large number (1000-3000) of CT images are thus acquired, each image with a time stamp. By monitoring the respiratory cycle during the acquisition of the CT images, the times of acquisition can then be correlated to the phase of the respiratory cycle. The images are then binned according to the phase of the respiratory cycle to produce the 4D image data set.

A second approach uses helical CT at a very low pitch to acquire projections with a time stamp. These projections are then binned according to phase and then reconstructed to generate the 4D image.

With the need to correlate image acquisition time to the phase of the respiratory cycle, some sort of real-time monitoring of the respiratory cycle is necessary. Several methods have been devised to monitor the respiratory cycle. In one method, a reflective block is placed on the anterior surface of the patient's abdomen. As the patient breathes, the anterior surface of the abdomen moves up and down. The motion of the reflection is monitored and correlated to the elapsed time of image acquisition. Another approach to real-time respiratory monitoring uses an elastic band around the patient's waist. Yet another method monitors the motion of implanted fiducials.

Several methods have been used to account for respiratory motion in the delivery of radiation. In one method, *deep-inspiration breath-hold* (DIBH), the patient is asked to hold their breath upon deep inspiration, with the radiation delivered during the breath-hold. In recent years, DIBH has also been used in radiation treatment of cancer of the left breast to minimize the dose delivered to the heart, which may result in cardiac complications many years after radiation treatment. Another method gates the delivery of radiation to the respiratory cycle, turning the beam on when a specified point is reached in the respiratory cycle, and turning it off when another specified point is reached. Typically, the region of exhalation is used for the gated delivery, because the respiratory motion curve, plotting amplitude of respiration *vs.* elapsed time, is flattest in this region.

It is important to note that whenever either breath-hold or gating is used, the patient must move into the same position at the time of beam delivery. That the patient's position during breath-hold and gating is reproducible was determined by a study in which 4D and breath-hold CT scans were acquired of a set of patients on a weekly basis.[6] The study showed that the location of the tumor relative to that of the vertebral bodies (which do not move under respiration), is consistent over the weekly CT images, certainly within the accuracy of patient set-up.

Alternatively, one could treat the patient under free-breathing. One approach that accounts for respiratory motion is to explicitly delineate an internal target volume (ITV). Recall that the ITV is the CTV along with a margin that accounts for internal motion. Instead of using a population-based margin, one could delineate a CTV on each phase of a 4D-CT image data set, then combine all the CTVs to form an ITV. Delineating GTVs on each phase of a data set, expanding them to generate a set of CTVs, and combining the CTVs may be a rather tedious procedure, so an approximate approach is to determine the envelope of the GTVs, and expand the envelope by an amount equal to the GTV to CTV expansion. One could then determine a PTV and calculate the dose distribution in each phase of the data set. These dose distributions could then be deformed based on the changes in anatomy determined by the 4D-CT imaging, and then combined to form a 4-D data set.

Is it important to explicitly account for respiratory motion in dose calculation? The answer is, "*It depends*". One study compared dose distributions calculated with explicit accounting for respiratory motion with those calculated on the same CT image data set for a single phase, as being representative of approximating respiratory motion.[7] In some cases the DVHs for the data sets that accounted for respiratory motion were significantly different from those cases in which respiratory motion was replaced by a single phase. However, no hard and fast rule could be applied.

A final method for respiratory management is tumor tracking. In this approach, the MLC leaf settings are dynamic, allowing the treatment portal to track the tumor as the patient is breathing. Tracking the tumor can be achieved either by the use of implanted fiducials or by real-time MR imaging.

21.5 QUESTIONS, EXERCISES, & PROBLEMS

21-1. Compare and contrast the Gamma Knife® and the Cyberknife®. Why do you think the Cyberknife® is used more for SBRT than for cranial radiation therapy?

21-2. Compare and contrast *total body irradiation* and *TSEI*.

21-3. In general, all of our anatomy can move around to varying extents as we breath, but no part of the anatomy moves more than the lungs. This can cause major complications when trying to treat a lung tumor with radiation. The last section in this chapter discusses ways in which the motion of a lung tumor can be taken into account when treating a patient. Summarize these approaches to treatment.

21-4. How does stereotactic radiotherapy reduce the setup uncertainty in a radiation treatment?

21-5. If we were to use an SSD of 7 meters to treat a patient with total-body irradiation using a ^{60}Co source, what would be the extent of attenuation of the treatment beam? *Hint:* You will need to look up the mass attenuation coefficient for the appropriate energy gamma rays in air. See Eqs. (8.38) through (8.40) and the associated discussion.

21-6. If we were to use an SSD of 7 meters to treat a patient with total-skin irradiation using a 6 MeV electron beam and place a 1-cm Plexiglas plate in front of the patient, what would be the approximate range of the electrons inside the patient? *Hints:* We can see from Table (9.1) that the mass stopping power for electrons in water (tissue) and solids is $S/\rho \approx 2\ MeV \cdot cm^2/g$ for electron beam energies on the order of 10 MeV; you will need to look up needed densities. See also Eqs. (2.6) and (2.7) and the associated discussion, along with Eq. (9.56) and the first paragraph in §19.1. What happens to the electron beam at an SSD of 7 meters that we neglect at a more typical SSD of 1 meter?

21-7. Besides tumors in the lungs, where else do you think respiratory motion might affect the size of the region being treated?

21.6 REFERENCES

1. Zanotto V, Boscariol P, Gasparetto A, et al. A Master-Slave Haptic System for Neurosurgery. *Applied Bionics and Biomechanics.* 2011; 8: 209-220. https://doi.org/10.3233/ABB-2011-0026. https://creativecommons.org/licenses/by/4.0/.
2. CUF (https://commons.wikimedia.org/wiki/File:Gamma-knife-cuf.jpg), https://creativecommons.org/licenses/by-sa/4.0/legalcode.
3. Communications Manager (https://commons.wikimedia.org/wiki/File:Robotic_CyberKnife_at_St._Marys_Of_Michigan.jpg), "Robotic CyberKnife at St. Marys Of Michigan", https://creativecommons.org/licenses/by/2.0/legalcode.
4. Piotrowski T, Milecki P, Skorska M, Fundowicz D. Total skin electron irradiation techniques: a review. *Postepy Dermatol Alergol.* 2013; 30(1): 50-55.
5. Stevens CW, Munden RF, Forster KM, et al. Respiratory-driven lung tumor motion is independent of tumor size, tumor location, and pulmonary function. *Int J Radiat Oncol Biol Phys.* 2001; 51(1): 62-68.
6. Starkschall G, Balter P, Britton K, McAleer MF, Cox JD, Mohan R. Interfractional reproducibility of lung tumor location using various methods of respiratory motion mitigation. *Int J Radiat Oncol Biol Phys.* 2011; 79(2): 596-601. PMID: 20638189
7. Vinogradskiy YY, Balter P, Followill DS, Alvarez PE, White RA, Starkschall G. Verification of four-dimensional photon dose calculations. *Med Phys.* 2009; 36(8): 3438-3447. PMID: 19746777.

Introduction to Brachytherapy

CONTENTS

Contributed by Alexander Moncion, Ph.D., and Joann Prisciandaro, Ph.D., University of Michigan/Michigan Medicine, Ann Arbor

22.1   A BRIEF HISTORY OF RADIOACTIVITY AND BRACHYTHERAPY

Brachytherapy is a form of radiation therapy that involves the placement of sealed, radioactive sources in or near a lesion. The source is sealed in a capsule or "closely bonded and in a solid form"[1] to contain the radioactive material and give the source rigidity. Additionally, the encapsulation can attenuate short range particles (e.g., alpha or beta particles) that may be emitted during the source decay, if applicable, and/or low energy photons (e.g., characteristic x-rays) that would otherwise increase the dose immediately next to the source rather than contribute to the dose at the desired prescription depth. The term "brachytherapy" was coined in 1931 and is derived from the Greek for "short"—*brachio*—referring to the short distance in which brachytherapy treatments are delivered.[2]

The history of brachytherapy dates to 1896 when Henri Becquerel discovered that uranium salts spontaneously emit radiation. After learning of Wilhelm Röntgen's discovery of x-rays at the 1896 meeting of the French Academy of Sciences, Becquerel, who was already interested in the phenomenon of phosphorescence and uranium, began investigating whether the "phosphorescence" of uranium salts was related to x-rays.[3,4] To test this hypothesis, he placed uranium salts on top of wrapped photographic plates and placed the setup outside so the salts could be exposed to

DOI: 10.1201/9781003477457-22

sunlight. After developing the plates, he observed the outline of the uranium. Becqueral initially believed this effect was due to the salt absorbing the sunlight and then re-emitting the light (i.e., phosphorescence) onto the photographic plates. He was, however, puzzled that the plates would darken whether the salts were exposed to bright sunlight or weak light.[5] After developing the plates from a uranium salt that was not exposed to sunlight (see Fig. 22.1),[6] he soon learned that the penetrating rays originated from the uranium salt itself.

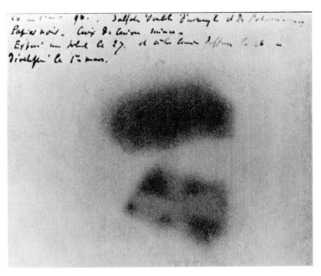

FIGURE 22.1: Photograph of uranium salts that were not exposed to sunlight. This photograph led to the discovery of spontaneous radiation by Henri Becquerel. (Public Domain.)

Fascinated by Becquerel's discovery, Maria Sklodowska-Curie (known more commonly as Marie Curie), a doctoral student at the Sorbonne (a public university in Paris), began working with Becqueral in December 1897. Rather than using photographic plates to quantify the intensity of the uranium rays, Marie Curie employed an ionization chamber, a Curie electrometer[a], and a piezo-electric crystal—a crystal that can generate an electric voltage when put under mechanical stress or in an electric field. (see Fig. 22.2).[7,8] When coupled, an ionization chamber and electrometer can measure electric charges and currents generated within the chamber. Using the piezo-electric crystal as a standard, the emissions from various samples of uranium salts were determined by correcting the electrometer reading for the salts from the reading of the piezo-electric crystal. Marie Curie conducted measurements of uranium in various chemical, physical (e.g., solid, ground), and environmental states (e.g., exposed to heat, light), and found that the emissions were not affected by changing the state of the material.[7,9] Based on these findings, and the fact that the intensity of the emissions from the uranium salts were proportional to the uranium content in the salt, independent of its chemical or physical state, she deduced that the rays

---

[a]A Curie electrometer is a device invented by Pierre Curie and his brother Paul-Jacques, both of whom were physicists who would later become professors at the Sorbonne and the University of Montpellier, respectively.

were the result of an atomic phenomenon in the uranium atom,[5,7] a phenomenon she called "radioactivity".[4,9, 10]

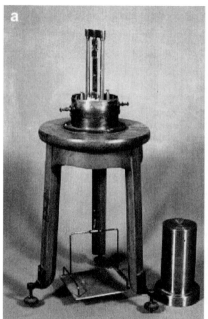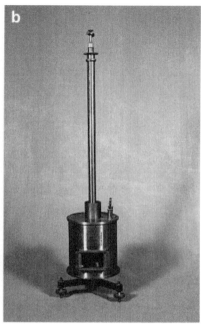

FIGURE 22.2: (a) A piezoelectric quartz device and (b) the Curie electrometer that was invented by Pierre and Paul-Jacques Curie. (Elsevier, with permission.)

Marie Curie also performed measurements on a series of other elements and compounds. She learned that compounds of thorium emitted similar rays, a discovery that was also made by Gerhard Carl Schmidt, a German chemist. With this knowledge, she began conducting studies of ores containing uranium and thorium. Through these studies, she learned that some uranium ores (e.g., pitchblende, chalcolite) were more radioactive than pure uranium, and hypothesized that the ores contained a new element that was more active than uranium.[5,7,9, 11] Collaborating with her husband, Pierre Curie, she chemically separated the more radioactive substances from pitchblende in 1898, leading first to the discovery of polonium, named after Marie's native country of Poland, and then of radium, derived from the Latin word "radius", meaning *ray*. It should be noted that the separation of radium from pitchblende was not trivial. In her initial reports, Marie Curie reported extracting only 6.5 mg of radium from two tons of pitchblende.[12] Due to the short half-life of polonium ($T_{1/2} = 138$ days), she was unable to successfully isolate it.

Shortly after the discovery of radium, its biological effects were investigated. In Germany, Friedrich Giesel, an organic chemist who developed methods to improve the extraction of radium and polonium from pitchblende and later became a commercial supplier of radium,[13] and Otto Walkhoff, a dentist, reported skin burns following self-exposure experiments using radium.[14,15,16] Learning of these effects, Henri Becquerel and Pierre Curie conducted similar experiments, also experiencing radiation burns following prolonged, superficial exposure to radium.[17] The similarity of the effects between x-ray and radium exposures was recognized by Ernest Besnier, a physician and dermatologist at the Hôpital St-Louis, who prompted Pierre Curie to lend a sample of radium to his colleagues, Henri Danlos and Paul Bloch. In 1901, Danlos and Bloch were the first to use radium for the treatment of lupus vulgaris, a cutaneous form of tuberculosis.[14,18] Soon afterwards, radium was used for the treatment of superficial cancers, and with the introduction of radium needles and tubes (see Fig. 22.3), it was used for more deep-seated cancers that could be treated using intracavitary techniques (see §22.3a) such as oral, gynecologic, and anal cancers.

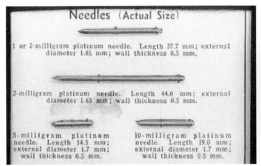
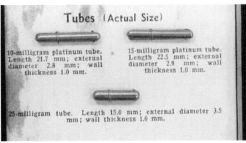

FIGURE 22.3: Samples of radium needles and tubes used for brachytherapy treatments. (ORAU, with permission.)

In 1903, Marie Curie defended her doctoral thesis titled "Recherches sur les substances radioactives" (i.e., "Research on Radioactive Substances"), earning the distinction of being the first woman in France to earn a Ph.D. in physics.[7,19,20] Later that year, Marie[b] and Pierre Curie shared the Nobel Prize in Physics with Henri Becqueral in recognition of "their joint researches on the radiation phenomena discovered by Professor Henri Becquerel".[21]

22.2 COMMONLY USED BRACHYTHERAPY SOURCES—PAST AND PRESENT

As discussed in the previous section, the first radioisotope used for brachytherapy treatments was radium, specifically Ra-226. Radium-226 is a member of a naturally occurring radioactive decay series called the uranium series, which originates with Uranium-238.[22,23] Radium was commercially supplied as a salt, such as radium sulfate ($RaSO_4$), radium chloride ($RaCl_2$), or radium bromide ($RaBr_2$), given the difficulty isolating pure radium and its high chemical reactivity.[24] Radium-226 has a half-life of 1600 years and decays via alpha decay to Radon-222 (Rn-222). Given that Ra-226 has a significantly longer half-life compared with its daughter, Rn-222 ($T_{1/2} = 3.8$ d),

---

[b]Marie Curie was the first woman to be awarded a Nobel prize, and to date, the only female scientist to receive two Nobel prizes. She earned a second Nobel prize in Chemistry in 1911 "in recognition of her services to the advancement of chemistry by the discovery of the elements radium and polonium". (https://www.nobelprize.org/prizes/chemistry/1911/summary/)

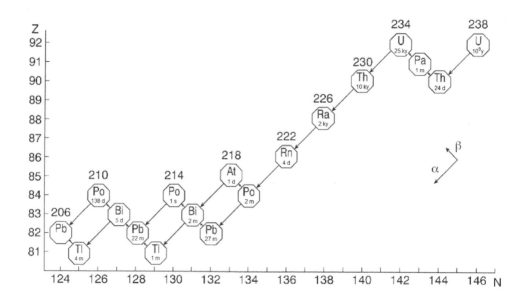

FIGURE 22.4: Decay scheme for the uranium series, of which both Ra-226 and Rn-222 are members. Decay half-lives are given under the chemical symbol. (MDPI, Open Access.)

secular equilibrium (see §7.8) is established between the two isotopes, when contained, within approximately one month. The decay of Ra-226 into Rn-222 is associated with a complex spectrum of alpha, beta, and gamma emissions (see Fig. 22.4).[25] However, given the short range of the emitted alpha and beta particles, these emissions are largely attenuated by at least 0.5 mm of platinum, a common encapsulation thickness that was used for Ra-226 sources. The energy of the gamma rays emitted during the decay of Ra-226 into Rn-222 range from 0.05 to 2.45 MeV, with an average energy of 0.83 MeV. Radium-226 was available in tubes and needles in a range of lengths and activities and was used to treat superficial and deep seeded lesions with intracavitary, interstitial, and surface applications (see §22.3a).

As stated above, Rn-222 is a a decay product of Ra-226. Like Ra-226, Rn-222 was also used for brachytherapy treatments. To isolate Rn-222, a vacuum manifold system known as a radon plant was used (see Fig. 22.5).[24] In this system, radium salts were kept in an aqueous solution. Given that Rn-222 is a radioactive gas, it would build up in and above the solution. When heated, the Rn-222 could then be isolated and encapsulated in a glass or gold capillary tube if it were pinched off and sealed, thereby forming seeds measuring a few millimeters in length.[24]

Following World War II, artificially produced radioisotopes became available for medical use, and eventually came to replace Ra-226 and Rn-222 due to radiation safety concerns associated with these isotopes (e.g., high energy photons, large half-value layers, toxic byproducts, and in the case of Ra-226, long half-life). The selection of radionuclides is based on factors including the types of radiation and energy(ies) emitted, activity and/or specific activity (activity/mass) of the radionuclide, physical half-life, physical form, and radiation safety considerations. Radioisotopes commonly

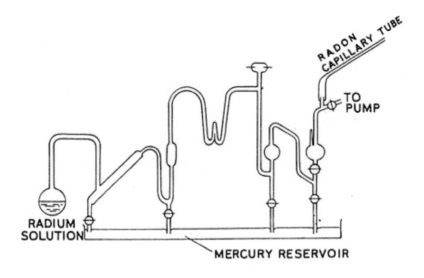

FIGURE 22.5: A schematic of a "radon plant" used to isolate and produce Rn-222 brachytherapy seeds. (Courtesy of the British Institute of Radiology.)

used for brachytherapy are x-ray and gamma-ray emitters, and in the case of very localized therapies, beta emitters. These radionuclides include neutron-rich isotopes produced in nuclear reactors as well as fission byproducts, and accelerator produced radioisotopes.

a. Cesium-137

Cesium-137 is a by-product of nuclear fission and is generated in nuclear reactors. It has a 30-year half-life and undergoes beta decay to an excited state of barium-137 (Ba-137; branching ratio [BR] = 94.7%) followed by the emission of a 0.66 MeV gamma-ray as Ba-137 de-excites to its ground state. Approximately 5.3% of the time, Cs-137 will beta decay directly to the ground state of Ba-137.[26] Cesium-137 is commonly encapsulated in stainless steel, which attenuates beta particles and characteristic x-rays emitted during its decay, yielding a sealed source that is a pure gamma emitter. Based on measured and calculated relative percent dose versus distance in water, the dose distribution of Cs-137 and Ra-226 are nearly identical up to 10 cm from the source (see Fig. 22.6).[27,28] Cesium-137 replaced Ra-226 for *low dose rate* (LDR, see §22.3c) intracavitary, surface and interstitial implants due to the similarities in their dose distribution and the added advantage that Cs-137 has a lower photon energy, and as such, requires less shielding to safely handle this source.

b. Cobalt-60

Cobalt-60 is an artificially produced neutron-rich radioisotope generated in nuclear reactors. It has a half-life of 5.3 years and undergoes beta decay that predominately feeds two excited levels of Ni-60 which de-excite with the release of gamma rays with energies of 1.17 and 1.33 MeV.[105] Cobalt-60 has a similar dose falloff as Ra-226 and Cs-137 (see Fig. 22.6).[28] Given its higher specific activity (i.e., activity per unit mass), smaller sources can be produced with Co-60 than for Cs-137. As such, Co-60

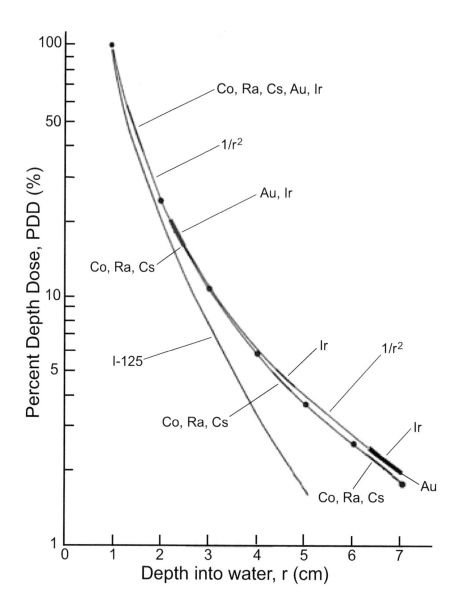

FIGURE 22.6: Percent depth dose (PDD) versus distance (r) into water for point sources of Co-60, Ra-226, Cs-137, Au-198, Ir-192, and I-125. The plot also shows the expected $1/r^2$ behavior of dose due to a point source. Note that the low-energy photon-emitting isotope I-125 falls well below the $1/r^2$ behavior, even at smaller distances.

was often used for LDR interstitial implants. Currently, Co-60 has gained renewed interest as a *high dose rate* (HDR, see §22.3c) source.

c. Iridium-192

Iridium-192 is produced by bombarding Ir-191, a stable iridium isotope, with an intense neutron flux in a nuclear reactor. It has a 73.8 day half-life and undergoes beta decay (BR = 95.2%) to platinum-192 and electron capture (BR = 4.8%) to osmium-192.[105] Iridium-192 has a complex gamma ray spectrum with an average energy of 0.38 MeV.[29] In the past, LDR temporary implants utilizing Ir-192 sources encased in nylon ribbons were used to treat interstitial implants, however, currently, HDR Ir-192 has largely replaced Cs-137 for intracavitary, interstitial, and surface implants.

d. Gold-198

Gold-198 (Au-198) is produced in a nuclear reactor by irradiating Au-197 with thermal neutrons. It has a half-life of 2.7 days and undergoes beta decay with a branching ratio of 99% to an excited state of mercury-198, followed by the emission of a 0.41 MeV gamma ray.[105] Gold-198 seeds or grains were commonly encased in platinum, attenuating beta particles emitted during its decay. For many years, Au-198 was used in place of Rn-222, and given its low energy, it was used for permanent implants, such as prostate seed implants.[29]

e. Iodine-125

Iodine-125 (I-125) is generated through the neutron irradiation of xenon-124 (Xe-124), which produces radioactive Xe-125 and decays via electron capture to I-125. Iodine-125 has a 59.4 year half-life, and decays via electron capture and internal conversion to tellurium-125, with the emission of a 35 keV gamma ray and characteristic x-rays ranging from 27.2 to 31.7 keV.[105,30] It is commonly encapsulated in titanium to absorb low energy electrons and photons.[29] Iodine-125 is chiefly used in permanent LDR implants given its short half-life and rapid dose fall-off, specifically permanent prostate implants.

f. Palladium-103

Palladium-103 (Pd-103) can be produced in a nuclear reactor from Pd-102 and in a particle accelerator by irradiating a rhodium (Rh) target with protons.[31] It decays with a half-life of 17 days via electron capture to Rh-103 with the emission of characteristic x-rays ranging from 20–23 keV and Auger electrons.[105,29,31] Similar to I-125, it is typically encapsulated in titanium and is often used for permanent implants, most commonly permanent prostate implants. With Pd-103's shorter half-life and higher initial dose rate compared to I-125, Pd-103 was initially hypothesized to be better suited for patients with higher grade prostate cancer[32,33] because Pd-103 could deliver dose more quickly, decreasing the number of cancer cells that can repopulate. However, oncologic and morbidity outcomes for patients receiving permanent prostate implants with I-125 and Pd-103 have found that these radioisotopes are equally effective in the treatment of patients with both low and high grade disease.[34,35,36]

g. Cesium-131

Cesium-131 (Cs-131) is generated through the neutron irradiation of barium-130 (Ba-130). When irradiated, Ba-130 captures a neutron producing radioactive Ba-131, which then decays to Cs-131 via electron capture.[37] Cesium-131 has a 9.7 d half-life and decays via electron capture to xenon-131 emitting characteristic x-rays ranging from 4.1 to 34.4 keV.[38] The source material is typically encapsulated in titanium, which attenuates low energy photons (e.g., the 4.1 keV x-ray). The resulting average energy of Cs-131 is 28.5 keV. Cesium-131 is used for permanent implants such as prostate and brain implants.

h. Strontium-90

Strontium-90 (Sr-90) is artificially produced as a fission byproduct in nuclear reactors. It has a 28.9 year half-life and is a pure beta emitter, decaying to yttrium-90 (Y-90) with the emission of beta rays with a maximum energy of 0.5 MeV.[105,31] Yttrium-90 also decays via the emission of beta particles to zirconium-90, a stable isotope, with a half-life of 64 hours. The maximum energy of the beta particles emitted following the decay of Y-90 is 2.28 MeV. It is predominately the betas that are released in the decay of Y-90 that are used in the treatment of superficial lesions, such as malignant and benign ocular conditions (e.g., conjunctival melanoma, pterygium). Additionally, Sr-90 is currently used to treat patients experiencing in-stent restenosis of the coronary arteries following repeat coronary angioplasty and stent placement.

Table (22.1)[105,29,39] provides data for select brachytherapy sources.

22.3   IMPLANT TECHNIQUES AND BRACHYTHERAPY MODALITIES

a. Introduction to Implant Techniques

Brachytherapy treatments may be administered through catheters, needles, or applicators. These devices primarily serve as channels or placeholders for the radioactive source to travel through or reside within. The method of administration depends on the location and size of the cancerous tissue, the physician's intent and expertise, and the available clinical resources. Treatments may be delivered through several techniques including intracavitary, interstitial, intraluminal, intravascular, and surface applications.

One of the most common applications is *intracavitary brachytherapy*, in which an applicator is placed within a body cavity, or a cavity created during a surgical procedure. A common example of intracavitary brachytherapy is when a cylinder is placed in the vaginal canal to treat patients with cervical or endometrial cancer. Interstitial brachytherapy involves the placement of needles and/or radioactive source(s) directly within the tumor or tissue. It is commonly used to treat patients with prostate cancer and advanced gynecological cancers.

Intraluminal brachytherapy is a form of brachytherapy in which radiation is delivered to a lumen or hollow tubular structure. It is used to treat, for example, bronchial and esophageal lesions. Intravascular brachytherapy is a procedure in which a catheter is advanced within a blood vessel, and once positioned, a radioactive source is deployed within the catheter. *Intravascular brachytherapy* may be used to treat patients

TABLE 22.1: Half-life ($T_{1/2}$), energy of emitted photons (E_{photon}), exposure rate constant (Γ), f-factor in muscle (f_{muscle}), and half-value layer ($d_{1/2}$) data for photon-emitting brachytherapy sources that have been or are commonly used. Note that, with the exception of Ra-226, the exposure rate constants listed in this table are for bare (unfiltered) sources

Isotope	$T_{1/2}$	E_{photon} (MeV)	Γ ($R\,cm^2\,h^{-1}\,mCi^{-1}$)	f_{muscle} ($cGy\,R^{-1}$)	$d_{1/2}$ (mm-lead)
Ra-226	1600 y	0.05–2.45 (ave = 0.83)	8.25 (0.5 mm Pt)	0.962	8
Rn-222	3.83 d	0.05–2.45 (ave = 0.83)	10.15	0.962	8
Cs-137	30 y	0.66	3.43	0.962	7.19
Co-60	5.26 y	1.17 and 1.33	12.9	0.965	15.6
Ir-192	73.8 d	0.14–1.06 (ave = 0.38)	4.6	0.964	2.67
Au-198	2.7 d	0.41	2.3	0.965	3.35
I-125	59.4 d	0.027–0.032 (ave = 0.028)	1.75	0.921	0.0211
Pd-103	17 d	0.020–0.023 (ave = 0.021)	1.41	0.921	0.00811
Cs-131	9.7 d	0.029–0.034 (ave = 0.029)	0.679	0.921	0.0262

that experience repeat re-narrowing of a cardiac vessel(s) (restenosis) following the placement of a cardiac stent for patients that have coronary artery disease.

Lastly, *surface brachytherapy* is a technique used to treat superficial lesions such as skin cancers. As its name implies, treatment is delivered using an applicator that is applied to the surface of the afflicted area.

Brachytherapy is a very time and resource intensive procedure. Applicator placement, imaging, and planning typically take place on the same day as the administration of radiotherapy. As such, extreme care is needed to ensure treatments are delivered in accordance with the physician's intent. Commonly used brachytherapy applicators are presented in §22.9.

b. Source Loading Techniques

Brachytherapy sources may be loaded into an applicator, needle, or directly in tissue using a variety of techniques. Hot loading is a technique used when an applicator or needle is pre-loaded with radioactive sources and is then placed into the patient. Although this technique was used almost exclusively in the early days of brachytherapy, except for a few treatment sites (e.g., permanent prostate, temporary eye plaque implants), this technique is not as prevalent today due to radiation exposures received by staff members involved in the procedure. To circumvent this issue, manual afterloading brachytherapy applicators began to emerge in the late 1950s and early 1960s[40] with the introduction of the Henschke applicator and followed shortly by the Fletcher-Suit applicator (see Fig. 22.7).[40,41] These applicators were specifically designed to allow the brachytherapy sources to be introduced after the applicator was placed into the patient either in a procedure or operating room. The patient was then imaged using 2D kV imaging (e.g., C-Arm, fluoroscopic simulator) with dummy sources (non-radioactive "sources" that mimic the size and shape of a source) and a treatment plan was developed based on available brachytherapy sources, or sources that could be ordered and received within a short timeframe, typically within a day. Once available, the sources were then transferred to the patient's room using a lead lined container, known as a "pig". To minimize radiation exposure to staff members involved in the implant, a lead shield was positioned next to the patient, and the radioactive sources were then introduced into the applicator using long handled forceps.

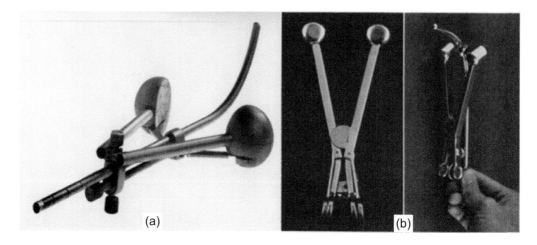

FIGURE 22.7: (a) The Henschke (Elsevier, with permission) and (b) Fletcher-Suit (RSNA, with permission) manual afterloading intracavitary cervical applicators.

Afterloading techniques are credited to Hermann Strebel, who inserted a radium source into a wound after puncturing it with a trocar in 1903, and to Robert Abbe, who inserted a radium source into a hollow tube that was implanted into an abdominal mass in 1909.[42] However, unlike Drs. Henschke and Suit, the intent of the afterloading technique was not for radiation safety purposes,[40] but rather for ease of implantation. In the 1960s, remote afterloading devices were developed.[43] A remote afterloader is a specialized computer driven, mobile device in which the source is housed in a lead lined safe when not in use and extended to pre-programmed positions within an applicator or needle when administering a treatment (see Fig. 22.8). This method further reduces the radiation exposure of healthcare personnel by remotely administering the treatment with the patient in a shielded room, while the staff remotely monitors the patient using cameras and an intercom.

c. Brachytherapy Modalities

There are several different modalities of brachytherapy that are used to treat patients. The modalities are largely distinguished based on the dose rate (low, medium, and

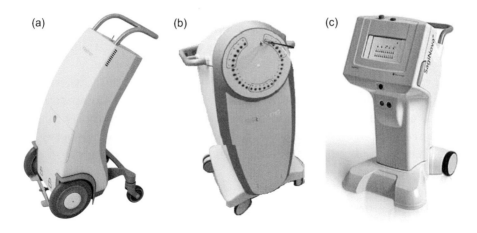

FIGURE 22.8: Examples of commercially available high-dose rate (HDR) brachytherapy afterloaders: (a) Elekta Flexitron (image courtesy of Elekta), (b) Varian Bravos, and (c) BEBIG Medical SagiNova (image courtesy of BEBIG Medical GmbH). Each of these afterloaders utilize an Ir-192 source, with the exception of the SagiNova, which provides the choice between an Ir-192 and a Co-60 source.

high) delivered to the desired prescription point by the source and the source strength utilized for the treatment.[44,45]

Low dose rate (LDR) brachytherapy delivers a dose rate between 0.4 and 2 Gy/h to a point or surface in which the dose is prescribed.[46] LDR brachytherapy was the initial form of brachytherapy used to treat patients and can be used for temporary (treatments on the order of days) or permanent implants.

Medium dose rate (MDR) brachytherapy can deliver a dose rate greater than 2 Gy/h, but less than 12 Gy/h to a point or surface where the dose is prescribed.[45,46] Although less commonly used, MDR treatments are delivered over the course of hours.

High dose rate (HDR) brachytherapy is defined as a modality of brachytherapy in which the prescribed dose rate is at least 12 Gy/h.[45,46] HDR brachytherapy is typically delivered in a matter of minutes, and as such, is strictly used to treat patients with temporary implants.

At many clinics, HDR brachytherapy has replaced treatments that were previously delivered using LDR. The advantage of HDR over LDR brachytherapy include shorter treatment times, the ability to treat patients in an out-patient setting, which in turn can increase patient capacity for this treatment, the ability to optimize the dose distribution by adjusting the time and location of the source within the applicator/needle, and significantly decreased risk of radiation exposure to staff. Although LDR and MDR may be delivered using manual, manual afterloading, or remote afterloading techniques, given the higher dose rate and activity of HDR sources, HDR treatments can only be delivered using remote afterloaders. As such, there are also disadvantages of HDR and/or remote afterloading techniques. This includes the increased complexity of the treatment workflow using a computer driven device, the increased startup and maintenance costs, the need for increased training, and in the event of a device malfunction, a greater risk of radiation exposure.

Although the most common HDR source is Ir-192, in 2003, Eckert & Ziegler BEBIG introduced the first miniaturized HDR Co-60 source.[47] Compared to Ir-192, Co-60 has a considerably longer half-life which allows for significantly longer times between source exchanges, 5 years versus 3 months. This longer period between source exchanges makes Co-60 more fiscally and logistically attractive in low-resource settings, such as developing countries.[48,49,50]

Brachytherapy may also be delivered using *pulse dose rate* (PDR) techniques. PDR combines the best of both LDR and HDR brachytherapy, namely the radiobiological advantages of delivering nearly continuous radiation over the course of treatment as normal tissues repair and maximizing the differential between early and late responding tissues, and the physical advantages of HDR as related to dose optimization and radiation safety.[51] PDR is typically delivered with an MDR source that delivers a series of short exposures (10–30 min) separated by intervals of one or more hours. The resulting dose and treatment time is equivalent to LDR brachytherapy.

In the 1990s a new modality of brachytherapy emerged, electronic brachytherapy.[52] Rather than using a radioactive source, electronic brachytherapy utilizes a miniature x-ray tube to generate low-energy, high dose rate radiation. There are approximately six commercially available systems that are marketed as electronic brachytherapy, operating between 50 and 100 kVp.[53] However, of these, only two can be used to deliver intracavitary, as well as surface therapy, the INTRABEAM® (Carl Zeiss Meditec AG, Jena, Germany) and the Xoft Axxent® (Xoft/iCad, San Jose CA, USA).[54] The INTRABEAM® is a compact x-ray source that was originally designed for stereotactic radiosurgery (see Chapter 21).[52] For the INTRABEAM, electrons are accelerated to a maximum energy of 50 keV and as the beam passes through a drift tube, it is steered and focused on a gold target using a beam deflector, generating x-rays on the inside surface of the probe tip[54,55] (see the top panel of Fig. 22.9). On the other hand, the Xoft system has a similar design as an HDR remote afterloader. It consists of a miniature x-ray tube on a long cable that connects to a control unit. The cable powers the source and carries cooling fluid to prevent the x-ray tube from overheating (see the bottom panel of Fig. 22.9). The average energy of the Xoft x-ray source is between 26 and 35 keV, and the x-ray source can deliver upwards of ten treatments before it needs to be replaced.[55] Compared to HDR brachytherapy, electronic brachytherapy systems have several advantages. Given the low energy emitted from the x-ray source, the dose to neighboring tissues are considerably lower than HDR brachytherapy, the device requires considerably less shielding than an HDR unit, and similar to other x-ray producing devices (e.g., electron linear accelerators, C-arms, CTs), once the device is turned off, radiation is no longer produced.[53,55]

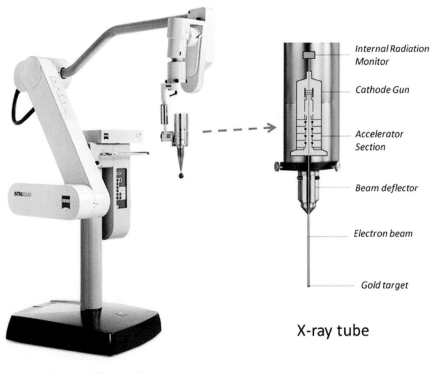

Internal Radiation Monitor

Cathode Gun

Accelerator Section

Beam deflector

Electron beam

Gold target

X-ray tube

Intrabeam Floor Stand

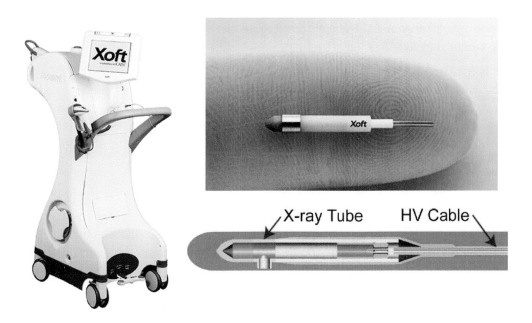

X-ray Tube   HV Cable

FIGURE 22.9: *(Top)* The INTRABEAM® and *(Bottom)* Xoft Axxent® electronic brachytherapy units. (With permission.)

22.4 PROGRESSION OF SOURCE STRENGTH AND BASIC CALCULATION METHODS

a. Milligram Radium (mg-Ra)

Originally, the strength of radium sources was quantified in units of milligrams radium (mg-Ra). Although the source strength was expressed in terms of mass, it was actually measured by comparing its ionization current, that is the emitted radiation, to a radium standard containing a known mass.[22] Based on early measurements, the rate of decay of 1 gram of radium was measured to be 3.7×10^{10} disintegrations per second (this was later updated to 3.61×10^{10} dps), which was defined as 1 curie (Ci), the first unit of activity. Thus, 1 g-Ra = 1 Ci. Since a curie is a large quantity, radium sources were typically expressed in terms of mCi or μCi. In 1975, the becquerel (Bq) was adopted by the International System of Units (SI) as the unit of activity, where 1 Bq = 1 dps. It then follows that[56]

$$1\,\text{mg-Ra} = 1\,\text{mCi} = 3.61 \times 10^7\,\text{Bq}. \tag{22.1}$$

One of the first methods of specifying and prescribing radiation to a patient was to multiply the source strength, in mg-Ra, by the duration of the implant in hours, yielding a quantity in units of *mg-Ra hours*. In an attempt to standardize treatments, several implant systems—Stockholm (1914), Paris (1919), Manchester (1938)—were developed for gynecologic implants.[57] The systems provided details on the number of intracavitary implants, length of the implants, as well loading pattern and relative source strength between the uterine and vaginal applicators. Although these "dose" calculations were simple, they were not meaningful given the absence of details on the source arrangement, the tumor size, and the relative location of the source(s) to the tumor and neighboring structures.

b. Exposure (X)

The earliest attempts to quantify the radiation intensity from gamma and x-ray emitting sources was to measure the ionization produced in air—the exposure, X—at a specified distance from the source, r, assuming the source material was contained within a point in space (the *point source approximation*). The unit of exposure is the roentgen, R, where

$$1\,\text{R} = 2.58 \times 10^{-4}\,\frac{\text{C}}{\text{kg}}. \tag{22.2}$$

The exposure rate is directly proportional to the activity of a photon-emitting source, A, and inversely proportional to the distance squared from the source, where the constant of proportionality is known as the *exposure rate constant*, Γ:

$$\text{Exposure Rate:} \quad \dot{X} = \frac{A\Gamma}{r^2}. \tag{22.3}$$

The exposure rate constant is defined as the exposure rate at a distance of 1 meter from a 1 Ci point source, and depends on the energy and number of photons emitted per decay.[22] In addition, some values of the exposure rate constant include the effects of absorption within the encapsulation material surrounding the active source material. (This is often the case for radium, for example.) A list of exposure rate constants for commonly used brachytherapy sources is provided in Table (22.1).

Example 22.1: Exposure Rate and Exposure

(a) What is the exposure rate from a 20 mg radium source to point P that is located 15 cm away from the source? (b) What is the exposure to point P after 8 hours?

Solution:
(a) We are given the activity, or source strength, in units of mg-Ra: A = 20 mg-Ra. Also, from Eq. (22.1) and Table (22.1), we have that the exposure rate constant for Ra-226 is $\Gamma = 8.25\,\mathrm{R\,cm^2\,h^{-1}\,mCi^{-1}} = 8.25\,\mathrm{R\,cm^2\,h^{-1}\,mg\text{-}Ra^{-1}}$. It then follows from Eq. (22.3) that

$$\dot{X} = \frac{A\Gamma}{r^2} = \frac{(20\,\mathrm{mg\text{-}Ra})\left(8.25\,\frac{\mathrm{R\,cm^2}}{\mathrm{h\cdot mg\text{-}Ra}}\right)}{(15\,\mathrm{cm})^2} = 0.73\,\frac{\mathrm{R}}{\mathrm{h}}. \tag{22.4}$$

It should be noted that the units of Γ for all radioactive sources other than radium are expressed in terms of *activity* in curies (Ci), rather than *mass* in milligrams (mg). Only for radium are the units of Γ usually given as $\mathrm{R\,cm^2\,h^{-1}\,mg\text{-}Ra^{-1}}$.

(b) Since exposure rate is the exposure per unit time, $\dot{X} = X/\Delta t$, it follows that the exposure to point P is

$$X = \dot{X}\,\Delta t = \left(0.73\,\frac{\mathrm{R}}{\mathrm{h}}\right)(8\,\mathrm{h}) = 5.84\,\mathrm{R}. \tag{22.5}$$

End of solution to Example 22.1.

---

c. Milligram Radium Equivalent (mg-Ra Eq)

As new radionuclides began to replace radium, a new term was utilized to specify source strength: milligram radium equivalent (*mg-Ra Eq*). This new term helped to define the source strength of radium substitutes relative to radium. The equivalence was based on an equivalent exposure rate, $\dot{X}$, at the same distance from each source. Therefore, to determine the mg-Ra Eq for a radium substitute, which we will here denote Y, we insist that

$$\dot{X}_{\mathrm{Ra\,Eq}} = \dot{X}_Y, \tag{22.6}$$

from which, using Eq. (22.3), we get that

$$\frac{A_{\mathrm{Ra\,Eq}}\Gamma_{\mathrm{Ra}}}{r^2} = \frac{A_Y\Gamma_Y}{r^2}. \tag{22.7}$$

Solving for $A_{\mathrm{Ra\,Eq}}$ then gives us the *source strength*, or activity, of the equivalent amount of radium-226:

$$A_{\mathrm{Ra\,Eq}} = A_Y\frac{\Gamma_Y}{\Gamma_{\mathrm{Ra}}}. \tag{22.8}$$

Example 22.2: Milligram Radium Equivalent for Co-60

Assume that a 20 mCi Co-60 source is used in place of Ra-226 in the previous example. (a) What is the equivalent mass of radium for the Co-60 source? (b) What is the exposure to point P after 8 hours? (c) Without converting the source strength to mg-Ra Eq, repeat the exposure calculation above using the exposure rate constant for Co-60.

Solution:

(a) From Table (22.1) we get that $\Gamma_{\text{Co-60}} = 12.9\,\text{R cm}^2\,\text{h}^{-1}\,\text{mCi}^{-1}$ and that $\Gamma_{\text{Ra}} = 8.25\,\text{R cm}^2\,\text{h}^{-1}\,\text{mg-Ra}^{-1}$. Note that we have kept the units for $\Gamma_{\text{Co-60}}$ in terms of mCi, as given in the table, and Γ_{Ra} is expressed in terms of $mg\text{-}Ra$, as we did in Ex.(22.1). Let's see why we wrote the units the way we did. From Eq. (22.8), we get that

$$A_{\text{Ra Eq}} = A_{\text{Co-60}}\frac{\Gamma_{\text{Co-60}}}{\Gamma_{\text{Ra}}} = (20\,\text{mCi})\left(\frac{12.9\,\frac{\text{R cm}^2}{\text{h·mCi}}}{8.25\,\frac{\text{R cm}^2}{\text{h·mg-Ra}}}\right) = 31.3\,\text{mg-Ra Eq}. \quad (22.9)$$

First of all, note how the units canceled to give us the desired units of *mg-Ra*—this is why we wrote the units for exposure rate constants the way we did. Second, note that we expressed the final units of *mg-Ra* as *mg-Ra Eq*, denoting the activity of the Co-60 source in terms of the equivalent amount of radium.

(b) From Eq. (22.3),

$$\dot{X}_{\text{Ra Eq}} = \frac{A_{\text{Ra Eq}}\Gamma_{\text{Ra}}}{r^2} = \frac{(31.3\,\text{mg-Ra})\left(8.25\,\frac{\text{R cm}^2}{\text{h·mg-Ra}}\right)}{(15\,\text{cm}^2)} = 1.15\,\frac{\text{R}}{\text{h}}, \quad (22.10)$$

so that,

$$X_{\text{Ra Eq}} = \dot{X}_{\text{Ra Eq}}\,\Delta t = \left(1.15\,\frac{\text{R}}{\text{h}}\right)(8\,\text{h}) = 9.18\,\text{R}. \quad (22.11)$$

(c) Likewise, using the values for Co-60 instead of Ra-226, we get that

$$\dot{X}_{\text{Co}} = \frac{A_{\text{Co}}\Gamma_{\text{Co}}}{r^2} = \frac{(20\,\text{mCi})\left(12.9\,\frac{\text{R cm}^2}{\text{h·mCi}}\right)}{(15\,\text{cm}^2)} = 1.15\,\frac{\text{R}}{\text{h}}, \quad (22.12)$$

so that, as before,

$$X_{\text{Co}} = \dot{X}_{\text{Co}}\,\Delta t = \left(1.15\,\frac{\text{R}}{\text{h}}\right)(8\,\text{h}) = 9.18\,\text{R}. \quad (22.13)$$

Of course, the approaches in parts (b) and (c) must yield the same result since both ways are describing the exposure due to the same source, as given by the condition in Eq. (22.6).

End of solution to Example 22.2.

It is important to remember that, if the source strength is converted to mg-Ra Eq, the remaining parameters used in the calculations should be for Ra-226. For instance, in Example 22.2, the exposure rate constant for Ra-226 should be used in the calculation if the source strength is expressed in mg-Ra Eq.

d. Absorbed Dose Under conditions of charged particle equilibrium (*CPE*—the number of particles entering a volume is equal to the number leaving the volume), absorbed dose can be calculated from exposure, where the dose in a given medium is equal to the collision part of kerma (see Chapter 16). Dose in air under CPE can be determined using (see Eqs. 16.1 and 16.41)

$$D_{air} = \left(K^{col}\right)_{air} = X\left(\frac{\overline{W}}{e}\right)_{air}, \tag{22.14}$$

where $\overline{W}$ is the mean energy to produce an ion pair in dry air (33.97 eV/ion pair) and e is the fundamental electronic charge ($e = 1.602 \times 10^{-19}$ C). Since 1 eV = 1.602×10^{-19} J, it follows that $\overline{W}/e = 33.97$ J/C.[29] Recalling from Eq. (22.2) that 1 R = $2.58 \times 10{-}4$ C/kg, we can write that [*required units for algebraic quantities in the following equations are given in square brackets*]

$$D_{air}\left[\frac{J}{kg}\right] = X[R]\left(33.97\,\frac{J}{C}\right)\left(2.58 \times 10^{-4}\,\frac{C}{R \cdot kg}\right), \tag{22.15}$$

or,

$$D_{air}\left[\frac{J}{kg}\right] = X[R]\left(8.76 \times 10^{-3}\,\frac{J}{R \cdot kg}\right). \tag{22.16}$$

Further, since 1 rad = 10^{-2} J/kg (= 1 cGy), we finally get that

$$D_{air}[rad] = X[R]\left(8.76 \times 10^{-3}\,\frac{J}{R \cdot kg}\right)\left(\frac{1\,rad}{10^{-2}\,J/kg}\right), \tag{22.17}$$

or,

$$D_{air}[rad] = X[R]\left(0.876\,\frac{rad}{R}\right). \tag{22.18}$$

Therefore, exposure (or exposure rate) can be converted to dose (or dose rate) in air by applying a conversion factor of 0.876 rad/R. This conversion factor is known as the *Roentgen-to-rad*, or simply the *f-factor*:

$$f = 0.876\,\frac{rad}{R}. \tag{22.19}$$

It then follows that the dose in air can be written as

$$D_{air}[rad] = X[R] \cdot f. \tag{22.20}$$

| Example 22.3: Dose to Air |

Considering the 20 mCi Co-60 source from Example 22.2, calculate the total dose delivered to air.

Solution:

From Eq. (22.20), we see that we need the exposure in *roentgen*. From Ex. 22.2b or c, we have that X = 9.18 R. It then follows from Eqs. (22.20) and (22.19) that

$$D_{air} [rad] = X[R] \cdot f = (9.18\,R) \left(0.876\, \frac{rad}{R} \right) = 8.04\,rad = 8.04\,cGy. \qquad (22.21)$$

| *End of solution to Example 22.3.* |

To calculate the dose or dose rate in a medium other than air, the f-factor for the medium, f_{med}, should utilized. This factor includes a correction to the in-air f-factor that accounts for the differences in the mean mass energy absorption coefficients between air and the medium:

$$f_{med} = f \cdot \left(\frac{(\bar{\mu}_{en}/\rho)_{med}}{(\bar{\mu}_{en}/\rho)_{air}} \right). \qquad (22.22)$$

It then follows that the dose to the medium at a distance r from the source can be written as:

$$D_{med} = X \cdot f_{med} = \dot{X}\,\Delta t \cdot f_{med}, \qquad (22.23)$$

or,

$$D_{med} = \frac{A\Gamma}{r^2}\,\Delta t \cdot f_{med}, \qquad (22.24)$$

where use has been made of Eq. (22.3).

A list of f-factors for muscle for commonly used brachytherapy sources is provided in Table (22.1).

To improve the point source approximation calculation, the following more complex expression can be utilized that accounts for additional perturbations of the photons emitted from the source as they interact with the medium they are traversing:

$$D_{med}(r) = X \cdot f_{med} \cdot T(r) \cdot \bar{\varphi}_{an}(r). \qquad (22.25)$$

Here, $T(r)$ accounts for radial attenuation and scatter in the medium, and $\bar{\varphi}_{an}(r)$ is a constant that corrects for the radial anisotropy (non isotropic, asymmetric) of the dose distribution given that the source is not a point, but rather the source material extends over a finite length. This factor accounts for self absorption of the emitted photons within the source material and differences in attenuation and scatter within the source encapsulation (see Fig. 22.10)[28].

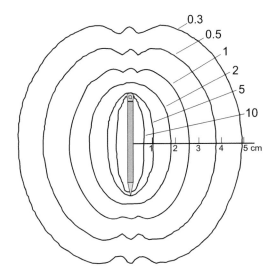

FIGURE 22.10: Isodose distribution in units of rad/h (cGy/h) around a 1 mg radium needle.

For the higher-energy gamma emitters, the dominant factor influencing the dose close to the source is the distance from the source in the form of the $1/r^2$ point-source behavior of intensity with distance. This is due to the fact that the effects due to attenuation and scatter tend to compensate one another closer to the source. With increasing distance, however, tissue attenuation begins to dominate and the percent dose curve will fall below the $1/r^2$ behavior, as illustrated in Fig. (22.6).[28] For low-energy photon emitters (e.g., I-125), tissue attenuation dominates, and the percent depth dose curve is well below the inverse-square curve.

e. Historical Implant Systems

In the early days of brachytherapy, before the advent of electronic calculators and computers, calculations involving multiple sources were time consuming and prone to error. To mitigate this situation, implant systems were developed, each providing detailed rules regarding the distribution of source material to generate reproducible implant arrangements, graphs or tables to look up the dose, and dose specification criteria. Three variations of these early dosimetry systems are the Manchester (Patterson-Parker) system, the Quimby system, and the Paris system.

The Manchester system was developed at the Holt Radum Institute in Manchester, England in the 1930s by Ralston Paterson and Herbert Parker. The objective of this system was to achieve a dose homogeneity of ±10% within the implanted volume with the exception of localized hot spots around the sources. To accomplish this, the activity of the radium sources was distributed in a non-uniform manner. Planar implant tables could be used to look up mg-h Ra per 1000 R based on the treatment area and distance from the implant plane. Similarly, volume implant tables were generated to determine the mg-h Ra per 1000 R based on the implanted volume.

The Quimby system was developed at New York Memorial Hospital in the 1930s by Edith Quimby. The Quimby system used a uniform distribution of sources with uniform source strength, which produced a non-uniform dose distribution that was hotter in the center versus the periphery of the implant. The tables developed for planar implants provided data on mg-Ra hr to produce 1000 R in the center of the treatment plane, effectively yielding the maximum dose in the plane of the implant. Additionally, tables for volume implants were available, where the minimum dose within the implant could be determined.

The Paris system was designed for Ir-192 wire sources and was developed in the 1960s. Using this system, uniform activity sources were ideally implanted straight and parallel to one another and were equidistant.[58] Similar to the Quimby system, a non-uniform dose distribution was produced using this technique, with a higher dose in the center of the implant relative the periphery of the implant.

These systems were typically used to develop a plan prior to a patient implant to determine the number of sources required, their source strength, and the geometric distribution of the sources.[59] Although these implant systems helped to standardize the procedure, it was often difficult to implant the sources based on pre-planned positions and, as such, the actual dose delivered to patients differed from that calculated based on the plan.

f. The Sievert Integral and the Line Source Approximation

Up until this point, we have reviewed basic exposure and dose calculation methods using a point source approximation. However, in reality, radioactive material within a brachytherapy source is distributed along the length of the source. To calculate the exposure rate around a line source, a more robust equation using the Sievert integral is utilized. We will now derive this equation; the set-up for the derivation is shown in Fig. (22.11).

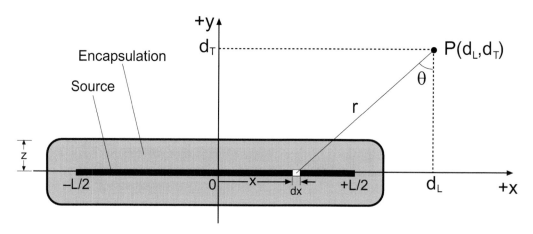

FIGURE 22.11: Set-up for the derivation of the Sievert integral, which is used to determine exposure and dose.

The radioactive brachytherapy source of length L is encapsulated within a material of thickness z. We wish to find the dose D within a medium at some point P outside the source.

We take the x-axis to be along the length of the source and the y-axis to be perpendicular to the source length. The origin of coordinates is taken to be at the center of the source. The point P is at the position $x = d_L$ and $y = d_T$. Here, d_L is called the *longitudinal distance*—in other words, the *distance along* the length of the source. Likewise, d_T is called the *transverse distance* and is a measure of the *distance away* from the length of the source. Note that these distances are measured from the center of the source, which is at the origin.

There are some points we must consider as we work toward finding the dose within the medium.

1. The source is not a point source.

Our starting point in finding the dose at P is Eq. (22.3), which gives the exposure rate in air at some distance r from a point source of radiation. Use of Eq. (22.23) will then allow us to compute the dose within some medium having an f-factor f_{med}. The problem with these equations is that they assume that the source can be treated as a point source, which violates our assumption of a source of length L.[c] However, if we break the source length up into many tiny (differential) pieces of length dx, we will be justified in treating each tiny piece as a point source, and can then use Eqs.(22.3) and (22.23).

Figure (22.11) shows a differential segment of length dx located at the position x from the origin (the center of the source length). This differential segment is at an angular position θ, measured from the vertical, as viewed from the point P. If the source of length L has a total activity A, then the activity per unit length of the source must be A/L. It then follows that the tiny segment of source dx must have a corresponding tiny activity dA, given by $dA = (A/L)\, dx$. Likewise, from Eq. (22.3), the tiny activity dA must result in a tiny exposure rate at point P (in air), $d\dot{X}$, given by

$$d\dot{X} = \frac{dA \cdot \Gamma}{r^2} = \frac{A}{L}\frac{\Gamma}{r^2}\, dx. \qquad (22.26)$$

2. Some of the radiation is absorbed within the encapsulation material.

Since the radiation must pass through the encapsulation material before entering the treatment medium, some of the radiation from the point source of length dx will be absorbed within that encapsulation material. For some active source materials such as Ra-226, the tabulated value of the exposure rate constant Γ already includes these encapsulation-absorption effects. (See Table 22.1.) For most active-source materials, however, this is not the case, so we must incorporate these attenuation effects into our formalism.

If the attenuation coefficient of the encapsulation material is denoted μ, then the radiation from the point source will be attenuated by an amount $e^{-\mu d}$, where d is the distance the radiation must travel through the encapsulation material. (See Eq. 8.37 and Fig. 8.9.)

---

[c]It is a good approximation to use a point-source equation for the dose at P if the distance r from the center of the source is very large compared to the source length L, typically three times the length of the source. However, we are not making that approximation here.

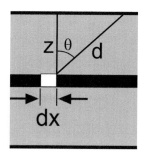

FIGURE 22.12: Magnified view of the distance d of the encapsulation material traversed by the radiation leaving the portion of the source within the length dx and heading toward the point P.

Figure (22.12) shows a portion of Fig. (22.11) around the point source dx. Since the thickness of the encapsulation material is z, it follows that the distance the radiation from dx must travel through the encapsulation material is $d = z\,sec\theta$. Taking the absorption within the encapsulation material explicitly into account, we can then rewrite Eq. (22.26) in the form

$$d\dot{X} = \frac{A}{L}\frac{\Gamma}{r^2}\,e^{-\mu z\,sec\theta}\,dx\,. \qquad (22.27)$$

But this is just the exposure rate at point P due to a tiny piece of the entire source of length L—we want the exposure rate at P due to the *entire* source. This means that we must add up, or integrate, the contributions from all of the point sources of length dx, starting at $x = -L/2$ and going up to $x = +L/2$. Thus,

$$\dot{X} = \int d\dot{X} = \frac{A\Gamma}{L}\int_{-L/2}^{+L/2}\frac{1}{r^2}\,e^{-\mu z\,sec\theta}\,dx\,, \qquad (22.28)$$

where A, Γ, and L were pulled out of the integral since they do not change as the position of the point source dx changes.

3. The variables x and θ are not independent.
The problem with the integral in Eq. (22.28) is that, as x increases, θ decreases—these two variables are related to one another. This means that we must write the integral in terms of x only or in terms of θ only—we can't have a mixture of the two. From Fig. (22.11), we can see that

$$d_L - x = d_T\,tan\theta\,, \qquad (22.29)$$

from which we get that, taking differentials of both sides,

$$dx = -d_T\,sec^2\theta\,d\theta\,. \qquad (22.30)$$

We can also see from Fig. (22.11) that r and θ are related by

$$r = d_T\,sec\theta\,. \qquad (22.31)$$

We choose to write the integral in Eq. (22.28) in terms of the angular variable θ. Substituting Eqs.(22.30) and (22.31), and using the minus sign to switch the limits, finally gives us that

$$\dot{X} = \frac{A\Gamma}{L \, d_T} \int_{\theta_1}^{\theta_2} e^{-\mu z \sec\theta} \, d\theta , \qquad (22.32)$$

where the limits on the integral are given by

$$\theta_1 = \tan^{-1}\left(\frac{d_L - L/2}{d_T}\right) \quad \text{and} \quad \theta_2 = \tan^{-1}\left(\frac{d_L + L/2}{d_T}\right). \qquad (22.33)$$

4. The dose is computed from the exposure rate.
We can now use Eq. (22.32) in Eq. (22.23) to find the dose at the point P within the medium for a dwell time Δt:

$$D = \dot{X}\,\Delta t \cdot f_{med} = \frac{A\Gamma}{L \, d_T}\,\Delta t \cdot f_{med} \int_{\theta_1}^{\theta_2} e^{-\mu z \sec\theta} \, d\theta . \qquad (22.34)$$

The integral in Eqs. (22.32) and (22.34) is called the *Sievert integral*. This integral cannot be solved analytically, but it can be approximated numerically. As computerized brachytherapy treatment planning software packages began to emerge in the 1950s and 1960s, they were used to perform these numerical approximations. However, even with computerized planning software, look-up tables still remain useful to perform quick calculations for secondary dose calculation checks and for teaching purposes.

In 1969, Shalek and Stoval[60] published tables of computed dose rates for Ra-226 based on calculations using the Sievert interval, and in 1978 Krishnaswamy[61] published similar tables for Cs-137 (see Tables 22.2[60] and 22.3[61], respectively). Using these tables, dose and dose rates to a point near a source can be determined based on the longitudinal distance d_L from the center of a linear source *along* its length, and the perpendicular, or transverse, distance d_T *away* from the source axis, as shown in Fig. 22.13. (Note that these distances are the same as were used in the set-up for the Sievert integral, as given in Fig. 22.11.) These tables are known as *along and away* tables and are commonly compiled for radioactive source models used for brachytherapy treatments. It should be noted that along and away tables are specific to a given radioisotope, active source length, and thickness of the encapsulation material.

> **Example 22.4: Sample Along and Away Calculation**

Determine the dose to a point in air that is 4 cm along and 2 cm away from a 10 mg-Ra Eq Cs-137 source that is left in place for 5 hours.
Solution:
Since we have a Cs-137 source, we will use along and away Table (22.3) for a linear Cs-137 source. Given the "along" (longitudinal) distance $d_L = 4$ cm and the "away" (transverse) distance $d_T = 2$ cm, we get that the dose in air per mg-Ra·h is equal to

$$\frac{D_{air}}{A_{Ra\,Eq} \cdot \Delta t} = \frac{0.38\,cGy}{\text{mg-Ra}} . \qquad (22.35)$$

TABLE 22.2: Dose (cGy) per mg-Ra·h delivered in air at various distances from a Radium-226 linear source. The source has an active length of 1.5 cm and is filtered by 0.5 mm platinum. d_L = distance along (*longitudinal distance*); d_T = distance away (*transverse distance*). See Fig. (22.13)

d_L (cm)	Transverse Distance, d_T (cm)										
	0.25	0.5	1	1.5	2	2.5	3	3.5	4	4.5	5
0.25	50.67	20.26	6.67	3.20	1.85	1.20	0.83	0.61	0.47	0.37	0.30
0.5	43.75	16.95	5.89	2.96	1.76	1.15	0.81	0.60	0.46	0.36	0.29
1	11.94	8.18	4.10	2.38	1.52	1.04	0.75	0.57	0.44	0.35	0.28
1.5	3.34	3.38	2.52	1.74	1.23	0.89	0.67	0.52	0.41	0.33	0.27
2	1.48	1.70	1.55	1.24	0.96	0.74	0.58	0.46	0.37	0.30	0.25
2.5	0.81	1.00	1.01	0.89	0.74	0.60	0.49	0.4	0.33	0.28	0.23
3	0.50	0.64	0.69	0.65	0.57	0.49	0.41	0.35	0.29	0.25	0.21
3.5	—	0.44	0.5	0.48	0.45	0.40	0.34	0.3	0.26	0.22	0.19
4	—	0.31	0.37	0.37	0.35	0.32	0.29	0.26	0.23	0.20	0.17
4.5	—	0.23	0.28	0.29	0.28	0.26	0.24	0.22	0.20	0.18	0.16
5	—	0.18	0.22	0.23	0.23	0.22	0.21	0.19	0.17	0.16	0.14

TABLE 22.3: Dose (cGy) per mg-Ra Eq·h delivered in air at at various distances from a Cs-137 linear source. The source has an active length of 1.5 cm and is filtered by 0.5 mm stainless steel. d_L = distance along (*longitudinal distance*); d_T = distance away (*transverse distance*). See Fig. (22.13)

d_L (cm)	Transverse Distance, d_T (cm)									
	0.5	1	1.5	2	2.5	3	3.5	4	4.5	5
0	20.27	6.67	3.20	1.85	1.19	0.83	0.61	0.47	0.37	0.30
0.5	17.25	5.93	2.97	1.76	1.15	0.81	0.60	0.46	0.36	0.29
1	8.79	4.20	2.40	1.53	1.05	0.75	0.57	0.44	0.35	0.28
1.5	3.83	2.64	1.78	1.24	0.90	0.67	0.52	0.41	0.33	0.27
2	2.03	1.67	1.29	0.98	0.75	0.58	0.46	0.37	0.31	0.25
2.5	1.25	1.12	0.94	0.76	0.62	0.50	0.41	0.34	0.28	0.24
3	0.84	0.79	0.70	0.60	0.50	0.42	0.35	0.30	0.25	0.22
3.5	0.60	0.58	0.53	0.47	0.41	0.35	0.31	0.26	0.23	0.20
4	0.45	0.44	0.42	0.38	0.34	0.30	0.26	0.23	0.20	0.18
4.5	0.35	0.35	0.33	0.31	0.28	0.25	0.23	0.20	0.18	0.16
5	0.27	0.28	0.27	0.25	0.24	0.22	0.20	0.18	0.16	0.14

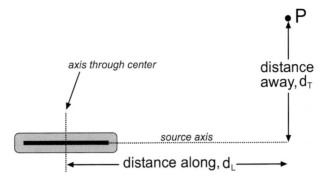

FIGURE 22.13: Schematic of the along and away geometry from a radioactive source to the measurement point, P. The *distance along* is the longitudinal distance measured from the center of the source, d_L; the distance away is the *transverse distance* measured from the source axis, d_T.

We are given that the source activity is $A_{Ra\,Eq} = 10$ mg-Ra Eq and the dwell time is $\Delta t = 5$ h. The dose in air at the specified point is then

$$D_{air}(4,2) = \left(\frac{0.38\,cGy}{\text{mg-Ra}}\right) A_{Ra\,Eq} \cdot \Delta t = \left(\frac{0.38\,cGy}{\text{mg-Ra}}\right) (10\,\text{mg-Ra}) (5\,h)\,, \qquad (22.36)$$

or,

$$D_{air}(4,2) = 19\,\text{cGy}\,. \qquad (22.37)$$

$$\boxed{\textit{End of solution to Example 22.4.}}$$

g. Air Kerma Strength (S_k)

The current recommended measure of source strength is *air kerma strength*, denoted S_k. The term *kerma* is defined as the *kinetic energy released in matter*. Air kerma is a special case of kerma where the measurements are performed in air (see Eq. 22.14). In 1985, the International Commission on Radiation Units and Measurements (ICRU) recommended the use of the air kerma rate as a means of characterizing photon-emitting brachytherapy sources.[46] The air kerma rate, $\dot{K}(\ell)$, is defined as the kerma rate to air at a reference distance of $\ell = 1$ m, where ℓ is measured from the center of the source along the perpendicular bisector of the source length. In 1987, the American Association of Physicists in Medicine (AAPM) introduced the concept of air kerma strength as a method of characterizing photon-emitting sources.[62] Air kerma strength is the product of the air kerma rate and the square of the measurement distance, ℓ:

$$S_k = \dot{K}(\ell) \cdot \ell^2\,. \qquad (22.38)$$

The units of air kerma strength are typically μGy·m^2/h or cGy·cm^2/h. This combination of units for air kerma strength is simply denoted U:

$$1\,U = 1\,\frac{cGy \cdot cm^2}{h} = 1\,\frac{\mu Gy \cdot m^2}{h}\,. \tag{22.39}$$

Air kerma strength measurements must be performed with a source-to-detector distance large enough that the source can be treated as a point source and the detector can be treated as a point detector.[62] Since low-energy photons (e.g., characteristic x-rays) are attenuated in the encapsulation material surrounding the source, only photons above a cutoff energy δ should be considered for air kerma strength measurements:[63]

$$S_k = \dot{K}_\delta(\ell) \cdot \ell^2\,. \tag{22.40}$$

The air kerma strength has several advantages over previous expressions of source strength: (1) knowledge of the air kerma strength of a sources allows for quick approximation of dose at clinically relevant distances, (2) it is independent of dummy variables (e.g., exposure rate constant), and (3) air kerma strength measurements are independent of source encapsulation thicknesses. Overall, air kerma strength measurements are less prone to error than earlier measures of source strength. With the introduction of air kerma strength, the AAPM improved dose calculations at the individual patient level and reduced dosimetric errors introduced by factors used in prior calculation methods. This was partially achieved through recommendations on source traceability and calibration certificates expressed in air kerma strength supplied by source vendors for each source shipped with uncertainty tolerances.[62]

22.5 SOURCE CALIBRATION

The Nuclear Regulatory Commission (NRC), a federal agency that regulates the medical use of radioactive materials[64] (see §22.9.b), requires that brachytherapy sources be assayed using dosimetry equipment that has a calibration that is directly traceable to the National Institutes of Standards and Technology (NIST).[62] This is also recommended by the American Association of Physicists in Medicine (AAPM),[63,65] a professional society dedicated, in part, to providing evidence-based clinical practice guidelines. The initial characterization of a brachytherapy source can be performed on-site at the radioactive source manufacturing facility, NIST, or an accredited dosimetry calibration laboratory (ADCL). The activity for these sources are commonly provided in units of air-kerma strength (U). Although not required by the NRC, the AAPM further recommends that all institutions providing brachytherapy services perform an independent air-kerma strength verification measurement of the source using NIST traceable dosimetry equipment even in scenarios where the manufacturer provides the activity.[66] A more detailed explanation of general dosimetry methods is provided in §16.6.

The most common equipment used to perform an independent assay include a well-type ionization chamber, an electrometer, a thermometer, and a barometer. Well-type ionization chambers can used in brachytherapy assays because of their reproducible, near 4π geometry, and high charge-collecting capabilities. There are two types of well chambers: open and sealed. The gas in the cavities of open well-type chambers have the same temperature and pressure as the room in which the chamber is located. Sealed chambers, however, are pressurized and have a combination of gases that are separated from the atmosphere of the room in which the measurements will be performed. Sealed chambers are unaffected by temperature and pressure variations.

Electrometers are devices capable of applying a high voltage to the well ionization chamber (usually around 300 V), and they quantify the ions created and collected by the electrodes of the chamber. The ADCLs provide a calibration factor for the chamber (N_{cal}, units of Gy·m^2 h^{-1} A^{-1}) along with an electrometer calibration factor (E_{cal}, unitless). Temperature and pressure readings are also acquired to correct for the impact the environmental conditions may have on the mass of air in an open chamber relative to the standard temperature and pressure ($T_{st} = 22.0\,^{o}C$ and $P_{st} = 101.33$ kPa, respectively) at time of the ADCL/NIST calibration measurements. (These corrections are unnecessary if a sealed chamber is used.) This correction is accomplished as follows:[67]

$$P_{TP} = \left(\frac{273.2 + T}{273.2 + T_{st}} \right) \left(\frac{P_{st}}{P} \right), \tag{22.41}$$

where T (in ^{o}C) and P (in kPa) are the measured temperature and pressure, respectively, and P_{TP} is the correction factor.

Another correction factor to consider when determining the source strength is the ion recombination factor, P_{ion}. This factor corrects for charge collection inefficiencies due to the recombination of ion pairs before they are collected at the electrodes of the ion chamber and is defined as[67]

$$P_{ion}(V_H) = \frac{1.0 - (V_H/V_L)^2}{(M_{raw}^H/M_{raw}^L) - (V_H/V_L)^2}. \tag{22.42}$$

This equation provides a method of estimating the ion recombination in a continuous beam of radiation, where V_H is the normal operating voltage (usually 300 V) and M^H is the reading acquired with bias V_H applied to the chamber. V_L is the reduced bias voltage, which is typically reduced by at least a factor of 2 from V_H, and M^L is the reading acquired when V_L is applied to the chamber.

The final correction factor applied is P_{pol}, which accounts for the collection inefficiencies from polarity effects introduced by differences between the electric field within the ion chamber for a positive charge versus negative charge bias. This correction factor can be computed as follows:

$$P_{pol} = \left| \frac{M_{raw}^+ - M_{raw}^-}{2M_{raw}} \right|, \tag{22.43}$$

where M_{raw}^+ and M_{raw}^- are the raw chamber readings when the chamber has a positive bias and a negative bias, respectively, and M_{raw} (either M_{raw}^+ or M_{raw}^-) is the same bias voltage as that used during the chamber calibration at the ADCL or NIST. The volume of air within a well-type chamber is large compared to the dimensions of the source, so it is important to find the optimal position to place the source for measurements within the chamber in order to maximize the reading. This can be accomplished by taking a series of measurements at different positions along the central axis of the chamber and finding the position that results in the highest charge reading.

Putting all of this together, the air-kerma strength can now be determined using the following equation:

$$S_k = M \cdot N_{cal} \cdot E_{cal} \cdot P_{TP} \cdot P_{ion} \cdot P_{pol}, \tag{22.44}$$

where M is the raw chamber reading. The measured air-kerma strength should be within ±3% of the value provided by the brachytherapy source vendor.

22.6 CURRENT DOSE CALCULATION METHODS

a. Task Group No. 43 (TG-43)

In 1995, the AAPM released Task Group Report No. 43 (TG-43), which aimed to update the dose calculation formalism by moving away from table-based dosimetry techniques that did not account for differences in source encapsulation or the internal construction of the source, and to include factors that account for source-to-source differences that are mostly determined from measurements.[68,69] The coordinate system for TG-43 is shown in Fig. (22.14).[69] The generalized 2D formalism used to calculate dose rate (units: cGy h^{-1}), $\dot{D}(r,\theta)$, to a point in space, P(r,θ), is given by:

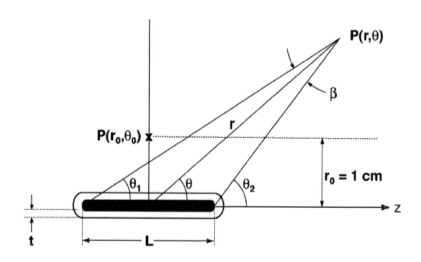

FIGURE 22.14: Coordinate system for the TG-43 formalism. (Open Access.)

$$\dot{D}(r,\theta) = S_k \Lambda \frac{G_x(r,\theta)}{G_x(r_o,\theta_o)} g(r) F(r,\theta), \tag{22.45}$$

where S_k is the air-kerma strength (units: U), Λ is the dose rate constant (units: cGy h^{-1}U^{-1}), $G_x(r,\theta)$ is the geometry function (where $x = P$ or L, depending on whether the source is considered a *point* source or a *line* source; units: cm^{-2}), g(r) is the radial dose function (unitless), and F(r,θ) is the anisotropy function (unitless).

The dose rate constant, Λ, accounts for the effects of the source geometry, the spatial distribution of the source, the source encapsulation, self filtration, and scattering in the medium around the source.[68]

The geometry function, G(r,θ), accounts for the dose falloff with distance relative to a reference point, P(r$_o$,θ_o), located at a radial distance of 1 cm from the center of the source measured along the bisector of the source (r$_o$ = 1 cm and θ_o = $\pi/2$) and is dependent on the distribution of the source activity.[68] For a point source, dose falls off as $1/r^2$, whereas for a line source, dose falls off by approximately $1/r$:

$$\text{Point Source:} \qquad G_P(r,\theta) = G_P(r) = \frac{1}{r^2} \qquad (22.46)$$

$$\text{Line Source } (\theta \neq 0): \qquad G_L(r,\theta) = \frac{\beta}{L\,r\sin\theta} \qquad (22.47)$$

where, as shown in Fig. (22.14), β is the angle (in radians) subtended by the source as viewed from the measurement point, P(r,θ), and L is the active source length. If the point P lies along the source axis ($\theta = 0$), then the line-source result takes on the form:

$$\text{Line Source } (\theta = 0): \qquad G_L(r,0) = \frac{1}{r^2 - L^2/4}. \qquad (22.48)$$

The radial dose function, g(r) in Eq. (22.45), accounts for attenuation and scatter along the axis perpendicular to the source:

$$g(r) = \frac{\dot{D}(r,\theta_o)}{\dot{D}(r_o,\theta_o)} \cdot \frac{G_x(r_o,\theta_o)}{G_x(r,\theta_o)}. \qquad (22.49)$$

Lastly, the anisotropy function, F(r,θ), accounts for the angular and radial dependence of attenuation and scatter in the encapsulation and in the medium:

$$F(r,\theta) = \frac{\dot{D}(r,\theta)}{\dot{D}(r,\theta_o)} \cdot \frac{G_x(r,\theta_o)}{G_x(r,\theta)}. \qquad (22.50)$$

b. Model-Based Dose Calculation Algorithms

TG-43 is the current standard for brachytherapy dose calculations. However, there are limitations to the TG-43 formalism: mainly, a lack of tissue heterogeneity correction (the TG-43 formulism assumes a water medium), it does not account for inter-seed attenuation, and it assumes full scatter conditions, ignoring patient boundaries. These limitations can introduce variations in the dose calculation.

Model-based dose calculation algorithms (MBDCAs) have been introduced into commercial brachytherapy treatment planning software, and can overcome these limitations by using patient imaging data with more advanced dose calculation methods: 1D ray tracing, collapsed cone convolution/superposition, grid based Boltzmann-equation solvers, and Monte Carlo calculations.[70] It is important to note that the accuracy of dose reporting from modern dose calculation techniques is dependent on high quality, volumetric imaging data (i.e., the imaging data that encompasses the target and organs-at-risk (OAR) of interest and is devoid of major artifacts) and accurate tissue delineation on the imaging data (i.e., the target and OARs are properly identified and contoured).

The transition from TG-43 to MBDCAs should be done with great care. The differences in dose calculation results for identical plans when using TG-43 *vs.* MBDCAs should be evaluated, as dose prescriptions may need updating. The implementation can be done in several ways, some of which may include dual calculations on phantoms, retrospective comparisons using data from previously treated patients, and prospective parallel calculations. These studies can be performed to evaluate the differences in the resulting dose calculations.

c. Point vs. Volume-Based Planning

Traditional brachytherapy treatments are based on prescribing dose to a reference point relative to the brachytherapy applicator. This practice is known as *point-based treatment planning*. The main advantages of point-based treatment planning are that it allows for a consistent prescription point that is comparable from patient-to-patient, planning is relatively quick and easy, and the treatment plan is not overly sensitive to small changes in applicator position.

For gynecological patients treated postoperatively (i.e., following a hysterectomy) to the vaginal cuff (upper portion of the vagina that has been sewn and closed off following the removal of the cervix) with a vaginal brachytherapy cylinder, two prescription points are commonly used: the surface of the applicator (i.e., depth of 0 cm) and a distance of 0.5 cm from the surface of the cylinder.[71]

Similarly, up until the early the 2000s, patients treated for cervical cancer with an intact uterus were almost exclusively treated with a point-based treatment plan. The reference point utilized was originally defined in the 1930s by a team in Manchester, England and became known as the Manchester System. According to this implant system, dose was prescribed to a reference point labeled point A, located "2 cm lateral to the central canal of the uterus and 2 cm from the mucous membrane of the lateral fornix in the axis of the uterus". (see Fig. 22.15).[72,73] Although the goal of the system was to treat the "cervix, uterus, vaginal vault, parametria, including, if possible, the obturator node", dose was limited by the tolerance of the neighboring normal tissues.[72] Tod and Meredith were particularly concerned with the dose received by the blood vessels, and defined a reference point, point A, which was intended to correspond to the location where the uterine artery crossed the uterer. A second point, point B, was also defined to represent the obturator node, 3 cm lateral to Point A, at the same level,[74] as shown in Fig. (22.15).

The definition of these points has gone through a series of modifications based on the landmark used to define the vaginal fornices, which resulted in variations in the identification of these points between individual institutions. To standardize the definition of point A, the American Brachytherapy Society published updates with illustrations based on the brachytherapy applicator selected for the treatment[75,76] (see Fig. 22.16).[76]

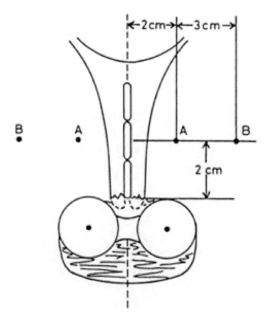

FIGURE 22.15: Diagram showing the locations of point A and point B relative to the ovoid surface and tandem/central uterine canal. (Open Access.)

As computed tomography and magnetic resonance imaging have become more widely available, volume-based treatment planning in brachytherapy has become more commonly utilized in clinics and hospitals in industrialized countries. Volumetric images provide better visualization of the tumor and neighboring anatomy, which allow treatment plans to be developed that conform to the target while minimizing dose to the normal tissues. Volume-based plans are typically prescribed to the *clinical target volume* (CTV); since the applicator or needles are directly implanted in the tumor, a margin for setup uncertainties is unnecessary, resulting in the CTV being the same as the *planning target volume* (PTV). For prostate brachytherapy, the CTV consists of the prostate plus a 1–5 mm margin, typically excluding an extension into the bladder and rectum.[77,78,79] Organs at risk are also contoured and prioritized within the optimization algorithm to ensure dose is minimized to these structures while delivering at least 90% of the prescription dose to at least 90% of the CTV (D90 ≥ 90%).

Beginning in the early 2000s, a transition from point to volume-based cervical treatment planning was initiated, largely based on guidance documents[80,81,82,83] developed by the Groupe Européen de Curiethérapie and the European Society for Radiotherapy & Oncology (GEC-ESTRO) and a European trial on MRI-guided brachytherapy in locally advanced cervical cancer, called the EMBRACE protocol.[80-84] This transition was possible due to the increased availability of MRI, which provides superior soft tissue resolution compared to CT and the clear distinction of target from normal tissues, which allows for improved organ-at-risk sparing and the potential of dose escalation to targets. The first published guidance

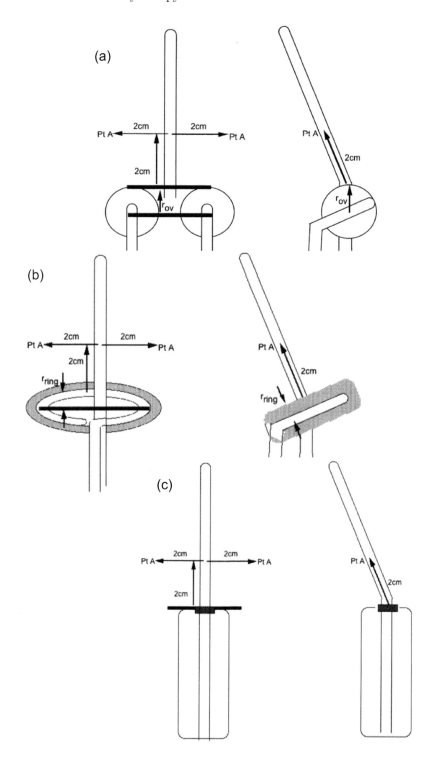

FIGURE 22.16: Schematics illustrating the location of point A for (a) a tandem and ovoid applicator with reference to the superior surface of the ovoid caps, (b) a tandem and ring applicator relative to the superior ring surface, and (c) a tandem and cylinder applicator based on the apex of the cylinder. (Elsevier, with permission.)

document from GEC-ESTRO was aimed at establishing a common language and means of delineating target volumes, which improves data transfer and comprehension between clinics and improves retrospective data analysis.[81] In this publication, three CTV structures were defined (see Fig. 22.17)[81]:

- *High risk CTV (HR CTV):* The volume that contains the initial macroscopic disease plus any residual disease at time of brachytherapy, including the whole cervix and the any presumed extracervical tumor extension;

- *Intermediate risk CTV (IR CTV):* The volume that contains the initial macroscopic disease plus residual microscopic disease at time of brachytherapy (i.e., HR CTV plus a margin ranging from 5 to 15 mm depending on tumor size, location, growth/regression, and treatment technique); and

- *Low risk CTV (LR CTV):* The volume that contains the initial macroscopic disease plus any potential microscopic tumor spread.

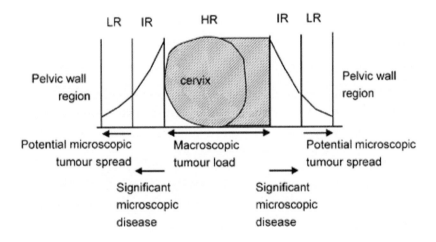

FIGURE 22.17: Schematic of clinical target volumes (CTVs) based on tumor spread. (Elsevier, with permission.)

It should be noted that, although dose is commonly prescribed to the HR CTV or IR CTV (with the intent of covering a minimum of 90% of the target volume with 90% of the prescription dose), the LR CTV is not specifically targeted with brachytherapy—rather, it is treated with surgery and/or external beam radiotherapy.

The GEC-ESTRO working group also published guidance documents on volumetric parameters that are used to easily report the delivered dose to the target and OARs,[80] guidance on how to characterize brachytherapy applicators on MR images so that they are represented accurately in the treatment planning system,[82] and MRI imaging specifications that are relevant to adequately image gynecological patients.[83] Additional international[85] and national[86] recommendations on transitioning to volumetric-based planning have since been published given this method of planning is more advanced, requires an increased level of staff training, utilizes advanced imaging technologies (i.e., CT and/or MRI), and requires a more robust quality assurance program.

d. Biologically Effective Dose (BED) Calculation

Many brachytherapy treatments are adjuvant and are commonly administered after an initial treatment using another treatment modality. An example would be locally advanced cervical cancer, which is often initially treated with chemotherapy and an external beam dose of 45–50 Gy delivered in 1.8–2 Gy fractions. The treatment is then followed by a localized brachytherapy. Given the differences in the dose and fractionation scheme between the external beam and brachytherapy, their doses cannot be simply summed. This complexity is introduced, among other things, by the response of cells to different amounts of radiation and by the type of cell irradiated. Instead of using physical dose, a biologically effective dose (BED) that considers the cell's response to radiation can be calculated. There are several commonly used BED equations utilized for brachytherapy treatments. If the brachytherapy implant is temporary and delivered in a fractionated manner (e.g., HDR brachytherapy), the BED can be calculated as follows:

$$\text{BED} = \text{nd}\left(1 + \frac{\text{d}}{\text{D}_{\alpha\beta}}\right), \tag{22.51}$$

where n is the number of fractions for a given treatment plan, d is the dose per fraction, and $D_{\alpha\beta} = \alpha/\beta$ is the crossover dose at which the rate of cell death caused by a single particle of radiation and cell death from two particles of radiation are equal.[77,87] (See the discussion of the crossover dose, $D_{\alpha\beta}$, at the end of §2.9, as well as the discussions of fractionation found in §3.5 and §3.7.)

If the implant is permanent (e.g., a permanent LDR prostate implant), the BED can be determined based on the following equation, assuming a single isotope is used for the implant:

$$\text{BED} = \text{D}(\text{T}_{\text{eff}})\text{RE}\left(\text{T}_{\text{eff}}\right) - \ln 2\,\frac{\text{T}_{\text{eff}}}{\alpha \text{T}_{\text{p}}}, \tag{22.52}$$

where

$$\text{RE}\left(\text{T}_{\text{eff}}\right) = 1 + \left(\frac{\beta}{\alpha}\right)\frac{\dot{\text{D}}_o}{\mu - \lambda}\frac{1}{1 - e^{-\lambda \text{T}_{\text{eff}}}}\left(1 - e^{-2\lambda \text{T}_{\text{eff}}} - \frac{2\lambda}{\mu + \lambda}\left(1 - e^{-(\mu + \lambda)\text{T}_{\text{eff}}}\right)\right) \tag{22.53}$$

and

$$\text{T}_{\text{eff}} = 1.44\,\text{T}_{1/2}\,\alpha \text{D}(\text{T}_{\text{eff}})\left(\frac{\text{T}_p}{\text{T}_{1/2}}\right). \tag{22.54}$$

In these equations, $\text{D}(\text{T}_{\text{eff}})$ is the total dose delivered over the time period T_{eff}, $\dot{\text{D}}_o$ is the initial dose rate, μ is the repair rate constant, λ is the decay constant, and T_{p} is the doubling time for tumor cells.[77,87] Thus, for two different fractionation schemes to achieve the same effect, the same BED should be delivered. The BED is useful in allowing healthcare providers to compare treatments across different treatment modalities, and to generate a composite dose across radiotherapy modalities.

22.7   IMAGING

In general, acquisition of high-quality medical images within radiation oncology is an extremely important step in the care of patients. Images provide valuable information on the intended target or focus of treatment and allows the physician to weigh the risks between irradiating healthy tissue and delivering the intended treatment to the target(s). In the case of brachytherapy, in addition to visualizing the target and neighboring healthy tissues, it is also essential to visualize and identify the brachytherapy applicator(s) and needles within the treatment planning software to accurately calculate dose.

An important step leading to this assessment is the accurate reconstruction/digitization of the brachytherapy applicator. This is a crucial step in brachytherapy treatment planning since the placement of the radioactive source, and hence the dose distribution, is highly dependent on an accurate representation of the applicator structure relative to the patient's anatomy. During the brachytherapy treatment workflow, imaging may be acquired prior to the applicator implant to guide the applicator placement and/or soon after to assess the placement of the applicator implant relative to target and critical normal structures to plan the treatment accordingly. The use of medical imaging in brachytherapy depends on many factors, including but not limited to the treatment site, the available technological resources, and the expertise of the care team. Although there are many imaging modalities that are available, in this section we will focus on four common imaging modalities commonly used during brachytherapy workflows and their clinical applications: two dimensional kilovoltage imaging, ultrasound, computed tomography, and magnetic resonance imaging; see Fig. (22.18). (See Chapters 10–12 for a more complete discussion of imaging modalities.)

a. Kilovoltage (kV) Two-Dimensional (2D) Imaging
Two-dimensional kV imaging was the standard imaging modality used in brachytherapy for many years. Two-dimensional images provide sharp subject contrast between objects with significantly different attenuations, allowing for the visualization, for instance, of bony anatomy and the brachytherapy applicator. However, it was not very useful for differentiating between different soft tissues, and thus it was not optimal for treatment planning techniques that required more precise differentiation between malignant and healthy tissue. When 2D imaging is used, treatment planning techniques aim to deliver a desired dose to a fixed distance from the applicator that can easily be discerned on kV images.

b. Ultrasound (US)
Ultrasound imaging allows for real-time visualization of the patient's anatomy without the need to expose the patient and personnel to ionizing radiation. In certain situations, this allows the treatment team to determine where the applicator is with

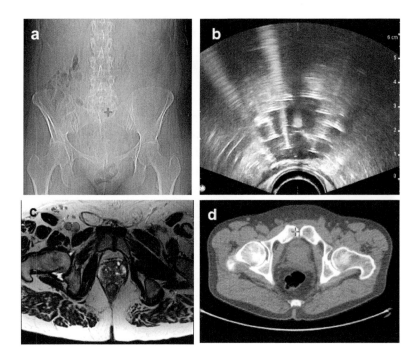

FIGURE 22.18: Sample images of (a) 2D kV radiograph of a pelvis, (b) ultrasound and (c) magnetic resonance imaging, and (d) computed tomography at the level of the prostate. There are advantages and disadvantages to each of these imaging modalities and it is up to the treatment team to assess which available modality provides the most appropriate imaging for the patient's treatment.

respect to the disease site and organs-at-risk of interest, prior to securing the applicator in place. An additional benefit of ultrasound is that transducers, the devices that transmit and receive the ultrasound waves used for image formation, are manufactured in many shapes and sizes. This gives the treatment team greater flexibility in choosing the transducer that best fits the treatment application. An example of this would be in HDR (High Dose Rate) prostate brachytherapy, in which a transrectal transducer is used due to the proximity to the prostate and OARs (*organs at risk*—e.g., rectum, bladder). A downside of ultrasound imaging is the relatively poor image quality. However, an ultrasound expert should be able to mitigate some of these deficiencies by optimizing the image acquisition parameters and being familiar with the ultrasound image representation of the anatomy of interest. Ultrasound images are often 2D, but with the addition of proper hardware and software, a 3D image can be created to utilize in treatment planning.

c. Computed Tomography (CT)

Computed tomography is a very common imaging modality and is the backbone of modern radiotherapy treatment planning. Many improvements to CT technology have been made over decades, resulting in a well-rounded modality that strikes a good balance between acquisition speed and image quality. However, the use of CT may not be adequate for all brachytherapy cases, as the soft tissue contrast resolution may not be sufficient in certain regions of the patient's anatomy to discern between different tissue types. Nonetheless, CTs can provide 3D images in which target and OARs can be delineated/contoured for plan optimization and dosimetric assessments. Computed tomography images would also be beneficial to institutions that use model-based dose calculation algorithms since electron density information can be used for tissue characterization.

d. Magnetic Resonance Imaging (MRI)

Magnetic resonance imaging units use very strong magnetic fields and radiofrequencies to excite and map the precession of protons within the hydrogen atoms of water molecules found within the body. It is an advanced imaging modality that produces three-dimensional images with superior soft tissue contrast compared with the other imaging modalities discussed above. This helps physicians and treatment planners to distinguish between targets and OARs. In addition to better soft tissue contrast, MR images are acquired without the need to expose patients to ionizing radiation. However, image acquisition on an MR unit takes much longer than on a CT—on the order of an hour versus minutes. Additionally, brachytherapy applicators can be very difficult to identify on MR images as they often appear black. Since MRI machines do not use ionizing radiation, no information on electron density is available, which is needed for many modern dose calculation algorithms. If heterogeneity-corrected dose calculations are needed, tissues can be assigned bulk densities,[88] MR images can be converted to synthetic CT,[89,90,91] or a CT can be acquired in a multi-modality approach.

The use of MR in brachytherapy poses a challenge since patients have applicator implants that are constructed from a variety of materials. Commercial brachytherapy are labeled as MR-safe, MR-conditional, or MR-unsafe.[92,93] MR safe applicators pose no known hazard in MRI environments. MR-conditional applicators are safe for use in an MR under specific conditions, but if those conditions are changed the device may no longer be safe for use. MR-unsafe devices should not be used near an MR machine.

There are many MR acquisition sequences that can be used to acquire an image. T2-weighted (T2W) 2D MRI images are recommended for target delineation and T1W scans may be helpful for applicator reconstruction. (See Fig. 22.19).[94,95] A combination of these sequences is often used to highlight certain tissue features or to improve visualization of the applicator during treatment planning.

22.8   CLINICAL APPLICATIONS AND APPLICATORS

Brachytherapy applicators come in many styles to accommodate the intended treatment site. Even within a particular style of applicator, various sizes may be available to account for differences in patient's body habitus. In this section we will focus on the four common brachytherapy treatment sites and the applicators that are commonly used to treat these sites. Note, however, that a modern brachytherapy service may provide treatments for more body sites than the ones presented in this section.

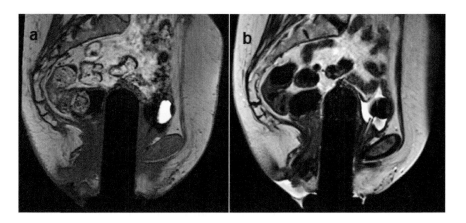

FIGURE 22.19: (a) T1-weighted and (b) T2-weighted MR images of a brachytherapy patient. A cylinder applicator is being used to deliver dose to the vaginal mucosa. These two MR sequences can be used to highlight different tissue contrast that can be advantageous for target and organ-at-risk contouring during planning.

a. Female Reproductive Organs

Gynecologic (GYN) cancers pertain to malignancies involving a woman's reproductive organs. To accommodate these structures, intracavitary and interstitial applicators are typically utilized. The most common GYN cancers treated with brachytherapy are endometrial and cervical cancer. Endometrial cancer affects the tissue of the endometrium, the lining of the uterus.[96] Surgery is the primary treatment for patients with endometrial cancer. For patients in which surgery is not an option, definitive radiotherapy (i.e., external beam and/or brachytherapy), with or without chemotherapy, may be utilized. For patients that have received a hysterectomy, vaginal cuff brachytherapy serves as an adjuvant post-operative treatment for endometrial cancer. Treatment usually starts 4–6 weeks after the surgery. A cylindrical applicator is inserted in the vagina and is secured in place to ensure accurate dose delivery (Fig. 22.20a). For patients with an intact uterus, a cylinder and tandem or an applicator with multiple intrauterine applicators may be used (Fig. 22.20b) to deliver dose to the uterine lining. Interstitial brachytherapy needles (Fig. 22.20c) may be used to deliver dose directly in or near the tumor for cases where the cancer has spread to the pelvic side walls and is inaccessible with an intracavitary applicator alone.

Similar to endometrial cancer, cervical cancer can be treated with surgery followed by radiation or by definitive radiotherapy. Brachytherapy may be used as an adjuvant therapy following external beam radiotherapy or as a stand-alone definitive treatment for early stage disease.[97] Patients receiving brachytherapy for cervical cancer are typically treated with tandem & ovoids (Fig. 22.21a) or ring & tandem (Fig. 22.21b) applicator set. Interstitial needles may also be used if the tumor is bulky. The number of needles implanted is dependent on the size and shape of the target.

b. Breast

Breast conserving surgery (i.e., *lumpectomy*) is the standard of care for patients with early-stage breast cancer.[98] This is commonly combined with radiotherapy.

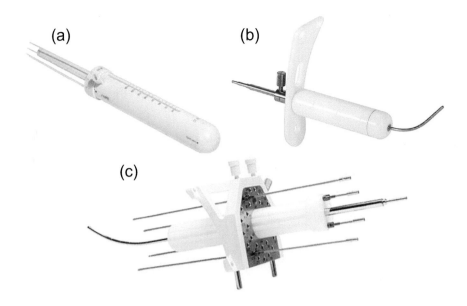

FIGURE 22.20: Three brachytherapy applicators that can be used for the treatment of endometrial cancer: (a) a vaginal cylinder (image courtesy of Elekta), (b) a cylinder and tandem (image courtesy of BEBIG Medical), and (c) a cylinder, tandem, and needle applicator (image courtesy of BEBIG Medical).

Traditionally, patients have been treated with adjuvant whole breast external beam radiation. However, partial breast irradiation has emerged based on studies that have shown breast tumors recur at or near the lumpectomy bed.[99] Further, this technique has the added advantage of limiting the volume of normal tissue irradiated and, given the small volume treated, allows for an accelerated course of treatment.

Partial breast radiation can be delivered using external beam or brachytherapy. Focusing on brachytherapy, interstitial brachytherapy was the first brachytherapy technique used to deliver partial breast irradiation. This is achieved by implanting interstitial catheters in and near the lumpectomy bed. Originally, this procedure was typically performed at the time of surgery, but currently, the procedure is often

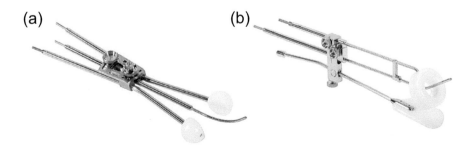

FIGURE 22.21: (a) Henschke tandem & ovoid and (b) ring & tandem applicators used for the treatment of cervical cancer. (Images courtesy of BEBIG Medical.)

delayed 1–2 weeks following the lumpectomy to allow for pathologic results to be available to help guide the implant of the catheters.[99] The catheters are typically spaced 1–1.5 cm apart and if multiple implant planes are needed, they are spaced by approximately 1.5–2.0 cm.[99] Like GYN brachytherapy, the number of catheters implanted depends on the size and shape of the target (see Fig. 22.22a).[100]

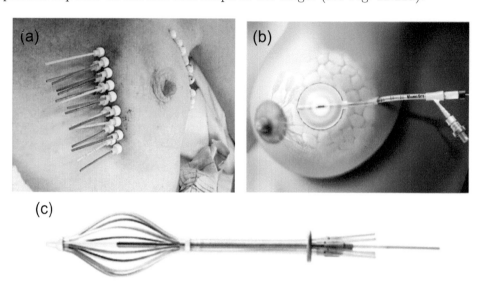

FIGURE 22.22: (a) An example breast brachytherapy implant showing the placement of the catheters. Breast brachytherapy can also be administered with (b) a balloon-style applicator such as the MammoSite, or an applicator that provides the benefits of both intracavitary and interstitial brachytherapy, such as (c) the SAVI applicator. (All images are from Elsevier, with permission.)

Given the complexity of interstitial implants, intracavitary balloon applicators have emerged as an alternative for partial breast brachytherapy.[99,101] The first balloon style brachytherapy applicator was the MammoSite applicator (Hologic Inc., Bedford, MA). The applicator was originally designed as an inflatable spherical balloon with a single *lumen*—the channel through which the source is transported—and a single position in which the source can reside (i.e., at the center of the balloon). The applicator is now available with spherical and elliptical shaped balloons, and with multiple lumens (a central lumen and three peripheral lumens),[99] which allows the applicator to better conform to the lumpectomy bed and allows the treatment planner an enhanced ability to sculp the dose distribution. The uninflated balloon applicator can be placed into the lumpectomy bed either at the time of the lumpectomy procedure or postoperatively. Once implanted, the balloon is typically filled with saline and contrast (see Fig. 22.22b).[102]

To take advantage of the benefits of both intracavitary and interstitial brachytherapy, the Strut-Adjusted Volume Implant (SAVI) (Merit Medical, Jordan, UT) hybrid applicator was introduced. The SAVI consists of a central lumen and 6–10 peripheral lumens,[99] and is available in multiple sizes (in length and diameter). Like the

MammoSite, it can be implanted at the time of lumpectomy or postoperatively with the lumens collapsed, after which the applicator is expanded to conform to the shape of the lumpectomy cavity (see Fig. 22.22c).[99]

c. Prostate

Prostate brachytherapy is delivered through an interstitial application via the perineum. This route allows relatively easy access to the prostate and is often combined with transrectal ultrasound imaging for real-time assessment of needle placement and treatment planning.

i. LDR Prostate

LDR (Low Dose Rate) brachytherapy involves permanently implanting radioactive seeds (e.g., I-125, Pd-103, Cs-131) in the prostate to deliver radiation over an extended period (Fig. 22.23). There are several implant techniques that have been used for LDR prostate brachytherapy: uniform loading, peripheral loading, and modified peripheral loading (Fig. 22.24), although the later two are the most common techniques currently used. Uniform loading involves implanting the seeds equidistant, about 1 cm apart center-to-center, peripheral loading involves placing the seeds along the periphery of the prostate gland, and modified peripheral loading is similar to perpherial loading, with the removal of seeds in the central portion of the gland to reduce the dose to the urethra. Seeds can be placed using pre-loaded needles, seeds in sture, or a loose seeds using a grid and an applicator such as the Mick® applicator (Fig. 22.25). An interstitial grid template is used to assist with spacing the placement of seeds within the prostate. Seed placement can be confirmed with a mobile x-ray unit capable of 2D radiographs and/or transrectal ultrasound.

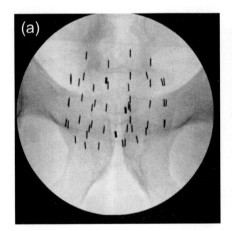 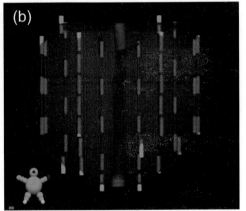

FIGURE 22.23: (a) A pelvic radiograph following an LDR prostate implant. The radioactive seeds can be clearly seen in the image; an image like this could be used for relative seed placement verification. (b) A 3D representation of a prostate (red contour) with LDR seeds (green dashed lines). This is a representation of the patient's anatomy (prostate and urethra—the solid green tube) and seeds based on the contours drawn by the treatment planning team.

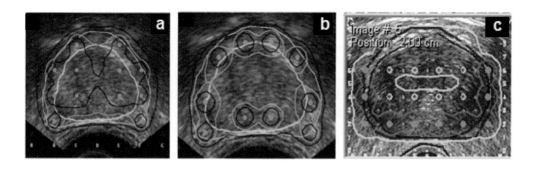

FIGURE 22.24: An example of (a) uniform seed loading, (b) modified peripheral seed loading, and (c) peripheral seed loading.

ii. HDR Prostate

HDR (High Dose Rate) prostate brachytherapy, similar to LDR, involves the placement of interstitial needles using an interstitial grid template (Fig. 22.26). The template is mounted on a device known as a stepper, which allows for fine positioning of the grid. The needles are implanted under US (ultrasound) guidance into the tissue using the interstitial grid template, which also serves to index the needle placement, and the transrectal probe that is coupled to the stepper to help reconstruct the position of the implanted needles on the ultrasound image. A computerized treatment planning system is used to optimize the position and dwell times of the source using US or CT images to deliver the desired dose to the prostate while sparing the organs-at-risk (e.g., rectum, bladder, and urethra). Unlike LDR, once an optimal treatment plan is generated, the needles are connected to a remote HDR afterloader (see Fig. 22.8), and treatment is delivered, and at the completion of treatment the source is retracted and the needles are removed.

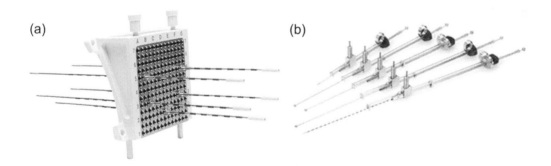

FIGURE 22.25: (a) A prostate grid template with needles used for needle guidance and seed indexing, and (b) Mick® TP and TPV applicators used for LDR seed placement. (Images courtesy of BEBIG Medical GmbH.)

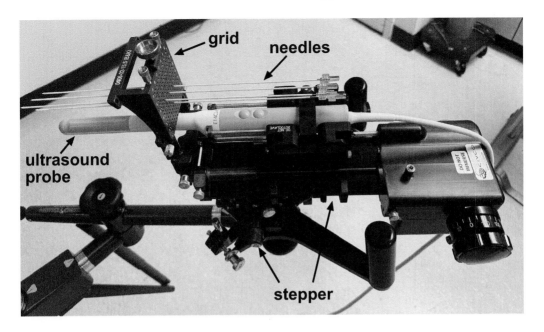

FIGURE 22.26: A stepper holding a transrectal US (ultrasound) probe along with an interstitial grid template with needles used in prostate brachytherapy.

d. Skin

Two common treatment techniques for skin cancer are surgery and radiotherapy. Brachytherapy is an option for patients that are poor surgical candidates or that have a risk of wound complications with surgery. The use of brachytherapy for skin lesions involves bringing an HDR source near the skin lesion. This can either be accomplished using flap-style applicators that cover the affected area (Fig. 22.27a) or conical applicators such as the Valencia™ applicator (Fig. 22.27b) that irradiates an area within a fixed geometry.

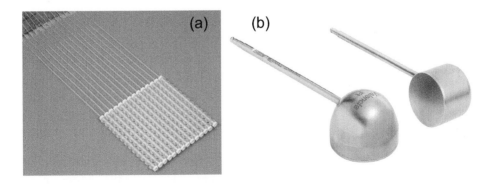

FIGURE 22.27: (a) A flap-style brachytherapy applicator and (b) the Valencia™ applicator, a superficial applicator. (Images courtesy of Elekta.)

22.9 RADIATION SAFETY, REGULATIONS, AND QUALITY ASSURANCE

a. Radiation Safety Advisory Agencies

Radiation protection is managed through the interactions of regulatory and scientific advisory bodies, as well as users of radioactive materials and equipment.[103] The first scientific advisory bodies were created shortly after x-rays and radium sources were introduced into medical clinics and scientific laboratories. As early as 1898, the Roentgen Society convened a committee to investigate "the alleged injurious effects of Roentgen rays", such as erythema (i.e., skin burns) and dermatitis, that were reported by scientists, physicians, and technologist using x-rays.[104] These advisory bodies exist at national and international levels and their recommendations often form the foundation of radiation safety legislation developed by regulatory bodies. A list of several key national and international regulatory and scientific advisory bodies are provided below.

i. International Atomic Energy Agency (IAEA)

The IAEA was created in 1957 as an international autonomous organization within the United Nations intended to promote peaceful, safe, and secure use of nuclear technology.[105] The mission of the IAEA is to:[106]

- Assist its Member States to plan and use nuclear science and technology for peaceful purposes;
- Develop nuclear safety standards and promote safety in the application of nuclear energy; and
- Verify that Member States comply with the IAEA commitment to use nuclear technology for peaceful purposes.

ii. International Commission on Radiological Protection (ICRP)

During the Second International Congress of Radiology in 1928, the International Committee on X-ray and Radium Protection (ICXRP) was formed to respond to concerns and develop standards for the safe use of x-rays and radium[103] in medicine. The ICXRP was restructured and renamed the ICRP in 1950 to account for uses of radiation outside of medicine. The ICRP provides recommendations and guidance on protection of radiation through quarterly publications in the Annals of the ICRP.

iii. International Commission on Radiation Units and Measurements (ICRU)

The International X-Ray Unit Committee was established during the First International Congress of Radiology (ICR) in London in 1925.[107]

The Committee was formed with the intent of proposing units of radiation dosage for use in therapeutic application in medicine, and they adopted the roentgen as the first international unit of x-ray intensity in 1928. In 1950, the Committee expanded its role and was renamed a Commission during the Fifth International Congress of Radiology. The mission of the ICRU is to develop and promote "internationally accepted recommendations on radiation related quantities and units, terminology, measurement procedures, and reference data for the safe and efficient application of ionizing radiation to medical diagnosis and therapy, radiation science and technology, and radiation protection of individuals and populations".[108]

iv. National Council on Radiation Protection & Measurements (NCRP)

In 1929, the American Roentgen Ray Society, the Radiological Society of North America, and the Radium Society agreed to consolidate their efforts and establish a national advisory body, the Advisory Committee on X-ray and Radium Protection (ACXRP). The ACXRP operated as an informal association of scientists to make information and recommendations available on radiation protection and measurements,[109] effectively playing a comparable role to the ICRP but on a national level. In 1934, both the ICXRP and ACXRP published recommendations on an occupational whole body tolerance dose, which was based on a limit of 1/100 of skin erythema dose per month.[103] Following World War II, the role of radiation safety extended beyond medical clinics and scientific laboratories, affecting a larger segment of the population.[110] Given these changes, the ACXRP recognized that it could no longer function in an informal manner and recommended that its charter by expanded. In 1946, the ACXRP was reorganized and renamed the National Committee on Radiological Protection.[103,111] The Committee was reorganized once more in 1964 and is now known as the National Council on Radiation Protection and Measurements.[112]

The mission of the NCRP is to "formulate and widely disseminate information, guidance and recommendations on radiation protection and measurements" and to cooperate with other organizations concerned with radiation protection and measurements.[112]

v. United Nations Scientific Committee on the Effects of Atomic Radiation (UNSCEAR)

The UNSCEAR was established in 1955 to access and study the effects of radiation exposure. They originally investigated the effects of radiation on the Japanese survivors of the atomic bombs in 1945, as well as on other groups that were accidentally exposed to large doses of radiation or received chronic exposures of many years.[104] Today, UNSCEAR's mission has not significantly departed from its initial charge—it serves as an international body that reports on the radiation exposure of people worldwide and based on scientific data, it will access and report on the effects radiation exposure.[113]

vi. Conference of Radiation Control Program Directors (CRCPD)

In 1959, Congress revised the Atomic Energy Act to authorize the Atomic Energy Commission (AEC, now the Nuclear Regulatory Commission, NRC), to enter into agreements with individual states to assume regulatory responsibility for certain types of artificially produced radioactive material, and assume the responsibility of health and safety.[114,115] This amendment was in response to concerns voiced by states regarding the civilian use of nuclear energy authorized by the 1954 Atomic Energy Act, and the adequacy of federal protections against radiation hazards.[114] States participating in the Agreement State Program are permitted to develop rules and regulations governing reactor and accelerator produced radioactive materials, although their regulations were required to be at least commensurate with the AEC (now NRC). As the Agreement State Program was rolled out in the 1960s, participating states began to independently develop their own radiation control programs and regulations. As state radiation control directors began holding regional meetings, they noted inconsistencies and conflicts between their programs.[115] As a result, in 1968, the Conference of Radiation Control Program Directors (CRCPD) was established. The CRCPD consists of radiation professional in local and state government who work in partnership to provide a forum to exchange ideas and communicate with the federal government on issues related to radiation protection.[116]

b. Regulatory Agencies

Shortly after the end of World War II, congressional and military leaders began to debate about who should control atomic energy within the United States, the military or the civilian government. In 1946, the Atomic Energy Act (AEA) was signed into legislation.[111] The 1946 law transferred the control of the nation's atomic energy program (i.e., management, development, use, and control for military and civilian applications) to a newly formed civilian agency, the Atomic Energy Commission (AEC).[111,117] However, the law did not permit private or commercial application of atomic energy.[110]

By the 1950s, federal officials began to reconsider the limitations imposed by the 1946 AEA given the advancements made by other countries in commercial development and use of atomic power. In 1954, the AEA was amended to allow for the development of commercial nuclear power for entities that are licenced and subject to the rules and regulations of the AEC. Under this revised law, the AEC was responsible for the development and production of nuclear weapons, promoting and regulating civilian uses of nuclear material, and establishing rules and regulations to protect the public against the hazards of radiation.[110]

During the 1960s, the AEC's credibility as a guardian of public health and atomic weapons program began to be questioned. Critics charged that the AEC's regulations were insufficiently rigorous in areas such as "radiation protection standards, reactor safety, plant siting, and environmental protection".[118] In 1974, the AEC was abolished by the Energy Reorganization Act, and was replaced by two new agencies, the Energy Research and Development Administration (ERDA) and the Nuclear Regulatory Commission (NRC). The ERDA was charged with managing energy research and development, nuclear weapons, and naval reactors programs, and was later combined with the Federal Energy Administration in 1977 to form the U.S. Department of Energy. The NRC was given the responsibility of overseeing reactor safety and security, administering reactor licensing and renewal, licensing radioactive materials, radionuclide safety, and managing the storage, security, recycling, and disposal of spent fuel.[103]

To date, the NRC is an independent, federal agency tasked with protecting public health and safety and the environment through the regulation of source material (uranium and thorium), special nuclear material (enriched uranium and plutonium), and byproduct material (i.e., accelerator or reactor produced radioactive material).[119]

Portions of the NRC's regulatory authority can be relinquished to an individual state if the state enters into an agreement with the NRC, such as the authority to license and inspect byproduct, source, or special nuclear material used or possessed within the state limits. To become an Agreement State (see part *iv* on the CRCPD in §22.9a), the state must demonstrate that their regulatory program is compatible with the NRC's and that the program can adequately protect public health and safety.[103] In 1962, Kentucky became the first Agreement State, and as of February 2023, 39 states have entered into this Agreement with the federal government.[120]

States, Agreement or Non-Agreement, are responsible for regulating the use of x-ray producing devices such as linear accelerators, CT scanners, and fluoroscopy units. Additionally, individual states are responsible for the regulation of electronic brachytherapy.[100]

c. Regulations

The codification/arrangement of general and permanent rules and regulations of the executive departments and agencies of the U.S. federal government is known as the Code of Federal Regulations (CFR).[121] The CFR is divided into 50 titles representing broad areas subject to federal regulation. Title 10 of the CFR has rules and regulations pertaining to energy, including atomic energy. Several parts within this title are of particular relevance for the medical use of sealed radioactive material, specifically brachytherapy sources.

i. Title 10 of the Code of Federal Regulation Part 20 (10 CFR 20)

Title 10 of the Code of Federal Regulations Part 20 (10 CFR 20), "Standards for Protection Against Radiation", is focused on legislation to protect radiation workers from ionizing radiation and establishing regulations on the receipt, possession, use, transfer, and disposal of radioactive material.[122] Key components of this part details the agency's requirements on:

- Radiation safety programs;
- Dose limits for radiation workers and members of the public;
- Surveys and occupational monitoring;
- Storage and control of licensed material;
- Posting and labeling;
- Receiving and opening packages with radioactive material;
- Waste disposal; and
- Records, reports, and violations.

ii. Title 10 of the Code of Federal Regulation Part 35 (10 CFR 35)

Title 10 of the Code of Federal Regulations Part 35 (10 CFR 35), "Medical Use of Byproduct Material", codifies rules and regulations on the medical use of byproduct material for diagnosis and therapy for the safe use of these materials for radiation workers, patients, human research subjects, and the general public.[62] This part of the Code of Federal Regulations highlights:

- General administrative requirements such as required content within written directives (i.e., prescriptions), training of authorized personnel (i.e., radiation safety officers, authorized medical physicists, authorized nuclear pharmacists, authorized user physicians), and recentness of training;
- General technical requirements including possession, use, and calibration of measurement instruments; possession requirements for sealed sources; and labeling of vials and syringes for unsealed sources;
- Unsealed byproduct materials used for therapy and diagnosis (discussed in Chapter 23);
- Manual brachytherapy (sealed) sources materials;
- Photon-emitting remote afterloader units, teletherapy units, and gamma radiosurgery units; and
- Records, reports, and violations.

For the medical use of byproduct material, the NRC provides definitions of a *medical event*, an event in which radiation is improperly administered (with the exception of events that resulted from the intervention of a patient). The NRC provides definitions of a medical event based on whether the administration is a permanent brachytherapy implant.

Administration of permanent brachytherapy implant[123]
For permanent implant brachytherapy, a medical event is defined as an implant that resulted in:

o The total administered source strength differing by greater or equal to 20 percent of the documented total source strength in the post-implant section of the written directive; or

o The total administered source strength outside of the treatment site exceeding 20 percent of the documented total source strength in the post-implantation section of the written directive; or

o An administration involving:

 - The wrong radioisotope;
 - The wrong patient or human research subject;
 - Sealed source(s) implanted into a location discontiguous from the treatment site; or
 - A leaking sealed source resulting in a dose greater than 0.5 Sv to an organ or tissue.

Administration of unsealed source or temporary brachytherapy implant[123]

For all other administrations of byproduct materials, a medical event is defined as an administration that resulted in:

o A dose that differs from the prescribed dose by greater than 0.05 Sv effective dose equivalent, 0.5 Sv to a tissue or organ, or 0.5 Sv shallow dose equivalent to the skin; and

o The total administered dose differing by greater or equal to 20% from the prescribed dose; or

o The fractionated administered dose from a single treatment fraction differing from the prescribed dose by greater or equal to 50%; or

o An administration involving:

 - The wrong radioactive drug or radioisotope;
 - The incorrect route of administration ;
 - The wrong patient or human research subject;
 - The incorrect mode of treatment; or
 - A leaking sealed source.

Following the discovery of a medical event, licensees are required to contact the NRC Operations Center by the next calendar day, and submit a written report detailing the event within 15 days of the discovery of the event.

22.10 QUESTIONS, EXERCISES, & PROBLEMS

22-1. A radionuclide has a half-life of 74 days. If the activity after 370 days is 10 mCi, what was the initial activity of the source? [*Answer:* 320 mCi]

22-2. The purpose of this problem is to get a better understanding of the temperature-pressure correction factor, P_{TP}. The standard temperature and pressure (STP) for the P_{TP} correction factor are $T_{st} = 22\,^{\circ}\text{C}$ and $P_{st} = 101.3$ kPa. Unless stated otherwise, all parameter values are held constant at STP values. Be sure to explain the reasoning behind all of your answers below. (a) What happens to the value of the correction factor P_{TP} as the pressure P increases to a value $P > P_{st}$? (b) Thinking about the mass of air contained within a given ionization chamber, how does the mass inside the chamber at pressure P compare to that inside the same chamber in STP? (c) For a given beam of incident radiation, how would the ionization-charge reading of the chamber at pressure $P > P_{st}$ compare to the reading at STP? (d) If the chamber reading at pressure $P > P_{st}$ were used to predict the dose produced inside a patient by the same incident beam, would this predicted dose be greater than or less than the actual value of dose delivered to the patient? Would this then result in the patient being overdosed for a given radiation prescription, or underdosed? (Neither of these situations is good.) (e) To help avoid this error, the chamber reading is multiplied by the correction factor P$_{TP}$. In light of this, does your answer in part (a) make sense?

22-3. The purpose of this problem is to get a better understanding of the temperature-pressure correction factor, P$_{TP}$. The standard temperature and pressure (STP) for the P$_{TP}$ correction factor are $T_{st} = 22\,^\circ\mathrm{C}$ and $P_{st} = 101.3$ kPa. Unless stated otherwise, all parameter values are held constant at STP values. Be sure to explain the reasoning behind all of your answers below. (a) What happens to the value of the correction factor P$_{TP}$ as the temperature T increases to a value $T > T_{st}$? (b) Thinking about the mass of air contained within a given ionization chamber, how does the mass inside the chamber at temperature $T > T_{st}$ compare to that inside the same chamber in STP? (c) For a given beam of incident radiation, how would the ionization-charge reading of the chamber at temperature $T > T_{st}$ compare to the reading at STP? (d) If the chamber reading at temperature $T > T_{st}$ were used to predict the dose produced inside a patient by the same incident beam, would this predicted dose be greater than or less than the actual value of dose delivered to the patient? Would this then result in the patient being overdosed for a given radiation prescription, or underdosed? (Neither of these situations is good.) (e) To help avoid this error, the chamber reading is multiplied by the correction factor P$_{TP}$. In light of this, does your answer in part (a) make sense?

22-4. Consider an implant involving three 10 mg-Ra Eq Cs-137 sources. Each of the sources has a physical length of 2 cm; the length of the active source material within each of the sources is 1.5 cm. The three sources are arranged in the implant so that they abut one another end-to-end in a straight line. Using the *along and away* tables, calculate the total dose in air to a point located 1.5 cm from the center point of the implant as measured along the perpendicular to the length of the sources. *Hint:* Start with a good sketch of the set-up, then determine d_L and d_T for the dose point relative to the center of each source. [*Answer:* 25.3 Gy]

22-5. The typical strength for a new HDR Ir-192 source is 10 Ci. (a) What is the exposure rate from an unshielded source at 0.5 m? (b) What is the exposure rate at a point that is 0.5 m from the source during treatment assuming that the patient's body effectively acts like two half-value layers of attenuator? For simplicity, consider a mono-energetic source model. *Hint:* See the discussion of half-value layer in §8.13. [*Answers:* (a) 18.4 R/h (b) 4.60 R/h]

22-6. *Background:* As mentioned in this chapter, a *remote afterloader* is used to treat patients using high dose rate (HDR) brachytherapy. The afterloader contains a highly active radioactive source that is attached to the end of a flexible wire. The wire and source are typically stored within a lead-lined storage container in the afterloader. For the HDR procedure, small catheters are surgically implanted into the patient next to and within the tumor. During treatment, the radioactive source is placed within the catheter. The remote afterloader is then programmed to automatically move the source through the catheter, stopping it at various positions for specified dwell times in order to deliver the prescribed dose to the tumor. When finished, the afterloader pulls the source back into the storage container.

Problem: An Ir-192 HDR treatment prescription using a GammaMed HDR Ir-192 model Plus source is written with the intent to deliver a dose to a depth of 0.5 cm into the vaginal tissue using a 3 cm diameter vaginal cylinder. (This means that the dose is to be delivered 0.5 cm beyond the outer wall of the cylinder.) Five dwell positions (x,y) are used in the treatment plan: (0,0), (1,0), (2,0), (3.0), and (4,0), where y = 0 corresponds to the cylinder's central axis and the x-value specifies the position of the center of the source along that axis. (All coordinates are expressed in centimeters.) The dwell time for each position is 44 seconds. The prescription point P to which the dose is to be delivered resides along the perpendicular to the central cylinder axis that passes through the central dwell position. Assume that the source strength is $S_k = 40700$ U, which corresponds to an activity of 10 Ci. (Tables needed for this problem can be found at the end of these homework problems.) (a) Draw a schematic diagram showing the vaginal cylinder, the dwell positions, and the prescription point, P. (b) Calculate the (x,y) coordinates of the prescription point, P. (c) Using the along and away Table (22.4), calculate the total dose delivered to the point P by this treatment. *Hint:* Watch the units of the numbers in the along and away table. (d) Perform a TG-43 calculation using Tables (22.5) and (22.6) to compute the dose delivered to the treatment point P. How does this calculation compare with the along and away calculation performed in part (c)? What is the percent difference between the two values? *Hints:* See the discussion after Eq. (22.45). Assume that the

TABLE 22.4: Dose rate per source strength (cGy h^{-1} U^{-1}) delivered in air at at various distances from a GammaMed HDR Ir-192 model Plus source. d_L = distance along (*longitudinal distance*); d_T = distance away (*transverse distance*). See Fig. (22.13)

| d_L (cm) | Transverse Distance, d_T (cm) | | | | | | |
	0.5	1	1.5	2	3	4	5
0	4.32	1.117	0.501	0.283	0.1259	0.0707	0.0451
0.5	2.21	0.892	0.449	0.266	0.1225	0.0696	0.0446
1	0.820	0.545	0.343	0.225	0.1130	0.0664	0.0432
1.5	0.384	0.326	0.243	0.1776	0.0998	0.0617	0.0412
2	0.215	0.205	0.1711	0.1367	0.0857	0.0560	0.0385
3	0.0935	0.0970	0.0913	0.0816	0.0607	0.0442	0.0325
4	0.0521	0.0548	0.0543	0.0513	0.0428	0.0339	0.0266
5	0.0337	0.0352	0.0354	0.0344	0.0307	0.0259	0.0214
6	0.0235	0.0243	0.0246	0.0243	0.0226	0.0200	0.01720
7	0.01719	0.01771	0.01798	0.01795	0.01711	0.0156	0.01386

TABLE 22.5: TG-43 g(r) values (no units) for a GammaMed HDR Ir-192 model Plus source. (Dose-Rate Constant: $\Lambda = 1.117\,\mathrm{cGy\,h^{-1}\,U^{-1}}$)

r (cm)	g(r)
0.25	0.997
0.50	0.996
1.00	1.000
1.50	1.003
2.00	1.006
3.00	1.006
4.00	1.004
5.00	0.999
6.00	0.993
8.00	0.968
10.00	0.935

source can be treated as a point source. You will need to do linear interpolations for some values from the tables. You should get a small value for the percent difference. [*Answers:* (c) 500.64 cGy (d) 496.35 cGy]

22-7. A treatment plan for a temporary low dose rate (LDR) Ir-192 brachytherapy implant was generated using five seeds having an activity of 0.79 mCi/seed. (See Table 22.1 for values of the exposure-rate constant, Γ.) The f-factor for the medium of interest is $f_{med} = 0.971$ cGy/R. (a) Assume that the total activity of the five seeds is concentrated 2 cm from the prescription point. Calculate the total dose delivered

TABLE 22.6: TG-43 F(r,θ) values (no units) for a GammaMed HDR Ir-192 model Plus source. (Dose-Rate Constant: $\Lambda = 1.117\,\mathrm{cGy\,h^{-1}\,U^{-1}}$)

θ (°)	Distance from Active Source Center, r (cm)									
	1.00	1.25	1.50	1.75	2.00	2.50	3.00	3.50	4.00	5.00
0	0.608	0.615	0.634	0.625	0.629	0.648	0.654	0.660	0.683	0.702
10	0.738	0.741	0.740	0.748	0.752	0.755	0.765	0.772	0.778	0.799
20	0.852	0.853	0.852	0.858	0.858	0.862	0.865	0.870	0.869	0.878
30	0.912	0.913	0.912	0.918	0.918	0.918	0.921	0.923	0.923	0.927
40	0.948	0.949	0.946	0.950	0.951	0.950	0.953	0.955	0.954	0.958
50	0.971	0.972	0.971	0.972	0.973	0.973	0.974	0.975	0.974	0.977
60	0.985	0.987	0.985	0.987	0.988	0.989	0.989	0.988	0.988	0.989
70	0.995	0.996	0.993	0.996	0.996	0.996	0.996	0.996	0.996	0.996
80	0.999	1.000	0.998	1.000	1.000	1.000	1.000	1.000	1.000	0.999
90	1	1	1	1	1	1	1	1	1	1
100	0.999	0.998	0.998	0.998	0.998	0.999	0.999	0.999	0.999	1.000
110	0.995	0.995	0.993	0.995	0.994	0.995	0.995	0.995	0.995	0.995
120	0.985	0.986	0.984	0.987	0.987	0.987	0.987	0.988	0.989	0.988

to prescription point following a 72-hour implant. Ignore the effects of decay, tissue attenuation, and anisotropy. (b) After the implant, it was discovered that the Ir-192 sources that had been ordered and subsequently implanted had a source strength of 0.79 mg-RaEq/seed instead of the prescribed 0.79 mCi/seed. What was the actual dose delivered to the patient? (c) According to the Nuclear Regulatory Commission, would this administration be considered a medical event? Explain. [*Answers:* (a) 317.58 cGy (b) 569.56 cGy]

22.11 REFERENCES

1. International Atomic Energy Agency, Radiation Protection and Safety of Radiation Sources: International Basic Safety Standards. Vienna: International Atomic Energy Agency; 2014.
2. Forssell, G. La lutte social contre le cancer. *Journal de Radiologie.* 1931; 15: 621-634.
3. Dutreix J, Dutreix A. Henri Becquerel (1852-1908). *Medical Physics.* 1995; 22(11): 1869-1875.
4. Chodos A, Ouellette J, Tretkoff E. This Month in Physics History: March 1, 1896: Henri Becquerel discovers radioactivity. APS News, 2008; 17(3).
5. Friedlander G, Kennedy JW. *Introduction to Radiochemistry.* 5th ed. New York: John Wiley & Sons; 1954.
6. Augustin M, Maiani C, Reynard G, Rouillier E, Martin A. The Curie Method - The discovery of uranium rays. https://lamethodecurie.fr/en/article12.html. Accessed May 2, 2023.
7. Chavaudra J. Pierre and Marie Curie-Sklodowska. *Medical Physics.* 1995; 22(11): 1877-1887.
8. Molinié P, Boudia S. Mastering picocoulombs in the 1890s: The Curies' quartz-electrometer instrumentation, and how it shaped early radioactivity history. *Journal of Electrostatics.* 2009; 67: 524-530. With permission from Elsevier.
9. Chodos A, Ouellette J. This Month in Physics History: December 1898: The Curies Discover Radium. *APS News.* 2004; 13(11).
10. Blaufox MD. Becquerel and the discovery of radioactivity: Early concepts. *Seminars in Nuclear Medicine.* 1996; 26(3): 145-154.
11. Mould RF. The discovery of radium in 1898 by Maria Sklodowska-Curie (1867-1934) and Pierre Curie (1859-1906) with commentary on their life and times. *The British Journal of Radiology.* 1998; 71(852): 1229-1254.
12. Mould RF. *A Century of X-rays and Radioactivity in Medicine.* Bristol and Philadelphia: Institute of Physics Publishing; 1993.
13. Soddy F. Researches Relating to Radium. *Nature.* 1904; 69(1787): 297-299.
14. Mould RF. Priority for radium therapy of benign conditions and cancer. *Curr Oncol.* 2007; 14(3): 118-122.
15. Giesel F. Über radioactive stoffe. *Berichte der deutschen chemischen Gesellschaft.* 1900; 33(3): 3569-3571.
16. Walkhoff F. Unsichtbare, photographisch wirksame Strahlen. *Photographische Rundschau.* 1900; 14: 189-191.
17. Becquerel H, Curie P. Action physiologique des rayons du radium. *Compt. Rend. Acad. Sci.* 1901; 132: 1289-1291.
18. Danlos H, Bloch P. Note sur le traitement du lupus érythémateux par des applications du radium. *Ann Dermatol Syphilog.* 1901; 2: 986-988.
19. Mould RF. Marie and Pierre Curie and radium: History, mystery, and discovery. *Medical Physics.* 1999; 26(9): 1766-1772.
20. NobelPrize.org. Marie Curie—Biographical. https://www.nobelprize.org/prizes/physics/1903/marie-curie/biographical. Accessed March 12, 2022.
21. NobelPrize.org. All Nobel Prizes in Physics. https://www.nobelprize.org/prizes/lists/all-nobel-prizes-in-physics. Accessed August 28, 2022.
22. Johns HE, Cunningham JR. *The Physics of Radiology.* 4th ed. Springfield, IL: Charles C. Thomas; 1983.
23. Friedlander G, Kennedy JW, Macias ES, Miller JM. *Nuclear and Radiochemistry.* 3rd ed. New York: John Wiley & Sons; 1981.
24. Selman J. *The Basic Physics of Radiotherapy.* 2nd ed. Springfield, IL: Charles C. Thomas; 1976.
25. Katz SA. The Chemistry and Toxicology of Depleted Uranium. *Toxics.* 2014; 2(1): 50-78. https://doi.org/10.3390/toxics2010050.
26. International Atomic Energy Agency. Live Chart of Nuclides. https://nds.iaea.org/relnsd/vcharthtml/VChartHTML.html. Accessed April 18, 2023.

27. Meisberger LL, Keller RJ, Shalek RJ. The effective attenuation in water of the gamma rays of gold 198, iridium 192, cesium 137, radium 226, and cobalt 60. *Radiology*. 1968; 90(5): 953-957.

28. Adapted from Khan FM. *The Physics of Radiation Therapy*. 3rd ed. Philadelphia, PA: Lippincott Williams & Wilkins; 2003.

29. Khan FM. *The Physics of Radiation Therapy*. 3rd ed. Philadelphia, PA: Lippincott Williams & Wilkins; 2003.

30. Pouliot J, Beaulieu L. Modern Principles of Brachytherapy Physics: From 2-D to 3-D to Dynamic Planning and Delivery. In: Hoppe RT, Phillips TL, Roach M, eds. *Leibel and Phillips Textbook of Radiation Oncology*. 3rd ed. W.B. Saunders: Philadelphia; 2010.

31. Nath R. Chapter 3: Sources and Delivery Systems I: Radionuclides. In: Thomadsen B, Rivard MJ, Butler WM, eds. *Brachytherapy Physics*. College Park, MD: American Association of Physicists in Medicine; 2005.

32. Porrazzo MS, Hilaris BS, Moorthy CR, et al. Permanent interstitial implantation using palladium-103: The New York Medical College preliminary experience. *International Journal of Radiation Oncology*Biology*Physics*. 1992; 23(5): 1033-1036.

33. Ling CC, Li WX, Anderson LL. The relative biological effectiveness of I-125 and Pd-103. *International Journal of Radiation Oncology*Biology*Physics*. 1995; 32(2): 373-378.

34. Cha CM, Potters L, Ashley R, et al. Isotope selection for patients undergoing prostate brachytherapy. *International Journal of Radiation Oncology*Biology*Physics*. 1999; 45(2):391-395. doi: 10.1016/s0360-3016(99)00187-x.

35. Peschel RE, Colberg JW, Chen Z, et al. Iodine 125 Versus Palladium 103 Implants for Prostate Cancer: Clinical Outcomes and Complications. *The Cancer Journal*. 2004; 10(3): 170-174.

36. Stone NN, Skouteris VM, Rosenstein BS, Stock RG. I-125 or Pd-103 for brachytherapy boost in men with high-risk prostate cancer: A comparison of survival and morbidity outcomes. *Brachytherapy*. 2020; 19(5): 567-573.

37. Meikrantz, D.H., Snyder, J.R., Methods for producing cesium-131. US Patent Application; 2009.

38. Chen Z, Bongiorni P, Nath R. Dose rate constant of a Cesium-131 interstitial brachytherapy seed measured by thermoluminescent dosimetry and gamma-ray spectrometry. *Medical Physics*. 2005; 32(11): 3279-3285.

39. Smith DS, Stabin MG. Exposure rate constants and lead shielding values for over 1,100 radionuclides. *Health Phys*. 2012; 102(3): 271-291.

40. Aronowitz JN. Afterloading: The Technique That Rescued Brachytherapy. *International Journal of Radiation Oncology*Biology*Physics*. 2015; 92(3): 479-487.

41. Suit HD, Moore EB, Fletcher GH, Worsnop R. Modification of Fletcher Ovoid System for Afterloading, Using Standard-Sized Radium Tubes (Milligram and Microgram). *Radiology*. 1963; 81(1): 126-131.

42. Aronowitz JN. Robert Abbe: Early American brachytherapist. *Brachytherapy*. 2012; 11(6): 421-428.

43. Holt J. AAPM Report No. 41: Remote afterloading technology. *Medical Physics*. 1993; 20: 1761.

44. International Commission on Radiation Units and Measurements. *Dose and volume specifications for reporting intracavitary therapy in gynecology, in ICRU Report No. 38*. Bethesda, Maryland: ICRU; 1985.

45. Nuclear Regulatory Commission. *Medical use of byproduct material*. NRC Regulations Title 10, Code of Federal Regulations; 2018. https://www.nrc.gov/reading-rm/doc-collections/cfr/part035/index.html.

46. Rath GK, Sharma DN, Julka PK. ICRU report 38: has the radiation oncology community accepted it? International Commission on Radiation Units & Measurements. *Clin Oncol. (R Coll Radiol)*. 2002; 14(5): 430-431.

47. Bebig Medical. Co-60 in HDR Brachytherapy. https://www.bebigmedical.com/static/upload/file/20230403/1680501496664618.pdf. Accessed April 21, 2023.

48. Strohmaier S, Zwierzchowski G. Comparison of (60)Co and (192)Ir sources in HDR brachytherapy. *J Contemp Brachytherapy*. 2011; 3(4): 199-208.

49. Andrassy M, Niatsetsky Y, Perez-Calatayud J. Co-60 versus Ir-192 in HDR brachytherapy: Scientific and technological comparison. *Rev Fis Med*. 2012; 13(2): 125-130.

50. Shukla AK, Jangid PK, Rajpurohit VS, et al. Dosimetric comparison of (60)Co and (192)Ir high dose rate source used in brachytherapy treatment of cervical cancer. *J Cancer Res Ther*. 2019; 15(6): 1212-1215.

51. Yavaş G. Dose Rate Definition in Brachytherapy. *Turkish Journal of Oncology*. 1999; 34: 44-55.

52. Dinsmore M, Harte KJ, Sliski AP, et al. A new miniature x-ray source for interstitial radiosurgery: Device description. *Medical Physics*. 1996; 23(1): 45-52.

53. Ramachandran P. New era of electronic brachytherapy. *World Journal of Radiology*. 2017; 9(4): 148-154.

54. Thomadsen BR, Biggs PJ, Cardarelli GA, et al. Electronic intracavitary brachytherapy quality management based on risk analysis: The report of AAPM TG 182. *Medical Physics*. 2020; 47(4): e65-e91.

55. Eaton DJ. Electronic brachytherapy—current status and future directions. *Br J Radiol*. 2015; 88(1049): 20150002.

56. National Institutes of Standards and Technology. Taylor BN, ed. *The International System of Units (SI)*. Gaithersburg, Maryland: NIST; 1991.

57. Anjali VR. Evolution of Brachytherapy. In: Mallick S, Rath GK, Benson R, eds. *Practical Radiation Oncology*. Singapore: Springer Singapore; 2020.

58. Pierquin B, Dutreix A, Paine CH, Chassagne D, Marinello G, Ash D. The Paris System in Interstitial Radiation Therapy. *Acta Radiologica: Oncology, Radiation, Physics, Biology*. 1978; 17(1): 33-48.

59. Aronowitz JN, Rivard MJ. The evolution of computerized treatment planning for brachytherapy: American contributions. *J Contemp Brachytherapy*. 2014; 6(2): 185-190.

60. Shalek RJ, Stovall M. Dosimetry in Implant Therapy. In: Attix FH, Tochilin E, eds. *Sources, Fields, Measurements, and Applications*. 2nd ed. Academic Press; 1969.

61. Krishnaswamy V. Dose Distribution Around an 125I Seed Source in Tissue. *Radiology*. 1978; 126(2): 489-491.

62. Nuclear Regulatory Commission. Title 10 of the Code of Federal Regulations, §35, Medical use of byproduct material. https://www.nrc.gov/reading-rm/doc-collections/cfr/part035/index.html. Accessed August 29, 2022.

63. Kutcher GJ, Coia L, Gillin M, et al. Comprehensive QA for radiation oncology: Report of AAPM Radiation Therapy Committee Task Group 40. *Med. Phys.* 1994; 21(4): 581-618.

64. Nuclear Regulatory Commission. About NRC. https://www.nrc.gov/about-nrc.html. Accessed March 15, 2023.

65. Nath R, Anderson LL, Meli JA, Olch AJ, Stitt JA, Williamson JF. Code of practice for brachytherapy physics: report of the AAPM Radiation Therapy Committee Task Group No. 56. *Med Phys*. 1997; 24(10): 1557-1598.

66. Butler WM, Bice WS Jr, DeWerd LA, et al. Third-party brachytherapy source calibrations and physicist responsibilities: Report of the AAPM Low Energy Brachytherapy Source Calibration Working Group. *Medical Physics*. 2008; 35(9): 3860-3865.

67. Almond PR, Biggs PJ, Coursey BM, et al. AAPM's TG-51 protocol for clinical reference dosimetry of high-energy photon and electron beams. *Medical Physics*. 1999; 26(9): 1847-1870.

68. Nath R, Anderson LL, Luxton G, Weaver KA, Williamson JF, Meigooni AS. Dosimetry of interstitial brachytherapy sources: recommendations of the AAPM Radiation Therapy Committee Task Group No. 43. American Association of Physicists in Medicine. *Med Phys*. 1995; 22(2): 209-234.

69. Rivard MJ, Coursey BM, DeWerd LA, et al. Update of AAPM Task Group No. 43 Report: A revised AAPM protocol for brachytherapy dose calculations. *Med Phys*. 2004; 31(3): 633-674. https://doi.org/10.1118/1.1646040

70. Beaulieu L, Tedgren AC, Carrier JF, et al. Report of the Task Group 186 on model-based dose calculation methods in brachytherapy beyond the TG-43 formalism: current status and recommendations for clinical implementation. *Med Phys*. 2012; 39(10): 6208-6236.

71. Small W Jr, Beriwal S, Demanes DJ, et al. American Brachytherapy Society consensus guidelines for adjuvant vaginal cuff brachytherapy after hysterectomy. *Brachytherapy*. 2012; 11(1): 58-67.

72. Tod MC, Meredith WJ. A Dosage System for Use in the Treatment of Cancer of the Uterine Cervix. *The British Journal of Radiology*. 1938; 11(132): 809-824.

73. Figure available under Creative Commons License 2.5 (https://creativecommons.org/licenses/by-sa/2.5/). See the license for the Disclaimer of Warranties and Limitation of Liability. Figure accessed at http://rtnotes.wikidot.com/gyn-cervix-brachy and modified slightly.

74. Tod M, Meredith WJ. Treatment of Cancer of the Cervix Uteri—A Revised "Manchester Method". *The British Journal of Radiology*. 1953; 26(305): 252-257.

75. Anderson J, Huang Y, Kim Y. Dosimetric impact of point A definition on high-dose-rate brachytherapy for cervical cancer: evaluations on conventional point A and MRI-guided, conformal plans. *J Contemp Brachytherapy*. 2012; 4(4): 241-246.

76. Viswanathan AN, Thomadsen B. American Brachytherapy Society consensus guidelines for locally advanced carcinoma of the cervix. Part I: General principles. *Brachytherapy*. 2012; 11: 33-46.

77. Nath R, Bice WS, Butler WM, et al. AAPM Recommendations on dose prescription and reporting methods for permanent interstitial brachytherapy for prostate cancer: Report of AAPM Task Group 137. *Medical Physics*. 2009; 36: 5310-5322.

78. Yamada Y, Rogers L, Demanes DJ, et al. American Brachytherapy Society consensus guidelines for high-dose-rate prostate brachytherapy. *Brachytherapy*. 2012; 11(1): 20-32.

79. King MT, Keyes M, Frank SJ, et al. Low dose rate brachytherapy for primary treatment of localized prostate cancer: A systemic review and executive summary of an evidence-based consensus statement. *Brachytherapy*. 2021; 20(6): 1114-1129.

80. Potter R, Haie-Meder C, Van Limbergen E, et al. Recommendations from gynaecological (GYN) GEC ESTRO working group (II): concepts and terms in 3D image-based treatment planning in cervix cancer brachytherapy-3D dose volume parameters and aspects of 3D image-based anatomy, radiation physics, radiobiology. *Radiother Oncol*. 2006; 78(1): 67-77.

81. Haie-Meder C, Potter R, Van Limbergen E, et al. Recommendations from Gynaecological (GYN) GEC-ESTRO Working Group (I): concepts and terms in 3D image based 3D treatment planning in cervix cancer brachytherapy with emphasis on MRI assessment of GTV and CTV. *Radiother Oncol*. 2005; 74(3): 235-245.

82. Hellebust TP, Kirisits C, Berger D, et al. Recommendations from Gynaecological (GYN) GEC-ESTRO Working Group: considerations and pitfalls in commissioning and applicator reconstruction in 3D image-based treatment planning of cervix cancer brachytherapy. *Radiother Oncol.* 2010; 96(2): 153-160.

83. Dimopoulos JC, Petrow P, Tanderup K, et al. Recommendations from Gynaecological (GYN) GEC-ESTRO Working Group (IV): Basic principles and parameters for MR imaging within the frame of image based adaptive cervix cancer brachytherapy. *Radiother Oncol.* 2012; 103(1): 113-122.

84. GEC-ESTRO. A European study on MRI-guided brachytherapy in locally advanced cervical cancer (EMBRACE). https://www.embracestudy.dk/. Accessed November 11, 2022.

85. Swamidas J, Mahantshetty U. ICRU report 89: prescribing, recording, and reporting brachytherapy for cancer of the cervix. *Journal of Medical Physics.* 2017; 42(suppl. 1): 48.

86. Prisciandaro J, Zoberi J, Cohen GA, et al. AAPM task group report 303 endorsed by the ABS: MRI implementation in HDR brachytherapy—Considerations from simulation to treatment. *Medical Physics.* 2022; 49(8): e983-e1023.

87. Nath R, Bice WS, Butler WM, et al. Erratum: AAPM recommendations on dose prescription and reporting methods for permanent interstitial brachytherapy for prostate cancer: Report of Task Group 137 [Med. Phys. 36, 5310-5322, 2009]. *Med Phys.* 2019; 46(6): 2780.

88. Lambert J, Greer PB, Menk F, et al. MRI-guided prostate radiation therapy planning: Investigation of dosimetric accuracy of MRI-based dose planning. *Radiother Oncol.* 2011; 98(3): 330-334.

89. Johansson A, Karlsson M, Nyholm T. CT substitute derived from MRI sequences with ultrashort echo time. *Med Phys.* 2011; 38(5): 2708-2714.

90. Korhonen J, Kapanen M, Keyriläinen J, Seppälä T, Tenhunen M. A dual model HU conversion from MRI intensity values within and outside of bone segment for MRI-based radiotherapy treatment planning of prostate cancer. *Med Phys.* 2014; 41(1): 011704.

91. Edmund JM, Kjer HM, Leemput KV, Hansen RH, Andersen JAL, Andreasen D. A voxel-based investigation for MRI-only radiotherapy of the brain using ultra short echo times. *Phys Med Biol.* 2014; 59(23): 7501-7519.

92. Kanal E, Barkovich AJ, Bell C, et al. ACR guidance document on MR safe practices: 2013. *J Magn Reson Imaging.* 2013; 37(3): 501-530.

93. Glide-Hurst C, Paulson E, McGee K, et al. Task group 284 report: magnetic resonance imaging simulation in radiotherapy: considerations for clinical implementation, optimization, and quality assurance. *Medical Physics.* 2021; 48(7): e636-e670.

94. Dimopoulos JC, Petrow P, Tanderup K, et al. Recommendations from Gynaecological (GYN) GEC-ESTRO Working Group (IV): Basic principles and parameters for MR imaging within the frame of image based adaptive cervix cancer brachytherapy. *Radiother Oncol.* 2012; 103(1): 113-122.

95. Prisciandaro J, Zoberi JE, Cohen G, et al. AAPM task group report 303 endorsed by the ABS: MRI implementation in HDR brachytherapy—Considerations from simulation to treatment. *Medical Physics.* 2022; 49(8): e983-e1023.

96. Schwarz JK, Beriwal S, Esthappan J, et al. Consensus statement for brachytherapy for the treatment of medically inoperable endometrial cancer. *Brachytherapy.* 2015; 14(5): 587-599.

97. Viswanathan AN, Thomadsen B. American Brachytherapy Society consensus guidelines for locally advanced carcinoma of the cervix. Part I: General principles. *Brachytherapy.* 2012; 11: 33-46.

98. Shah C, Vicini F, Shaitelman SF, et al. The American Brachytherapy Society consensus statement for accelerated partial-breast irradiation. *Brachytherapy.* 2018; 17(1): 154-170.

99. Hepel JT, Wazer DE. A comparison of brachytherapy techniques for partial breast irradiation. *Brachytherapy.* 2012; 11(3): 163-175.

100. Vicini FA, Arthur DW. Breast brachytherapy: North American Experience. *Semin Radiat Oncol.* 2005; 15(2): 108-115.

101. Shah C, Martinez A, Kolar M, Vicini F. Modern Approaches for Breast Brachytherapy. *Seminars in Radiation Oncology.* 2020; 30(1): 61-67.

102. Kacprowska A, Jassem J. Partial breast irradiation techniques in early breast cancer. *Reports of Practical Oncology & Radiotherapy.* 2011; 16(6): 213-220.

103. Stabin MG. *Radiation Protection and Dosimetry.* New York, NY: Springer; 2007.

104. Martin C. The Development of Radiation Protection. In: Martin CJ, Sutton DG, eds. *Practical Radiation Protection in Healthcare.* Oxford University Press; 2014.

105. International Atomic Energy Agency. The "Atoms for Peace" Agency. https://www.iaea.org/about/about-iaea. Accessed March 15, 2023.

106. International Atomic Energy Agency. The IAEA Mission Statement. https://www.iaea.org/about/mission. Accessed March 15, 2023.

107. Tailor L. History of the International Commission on Radiological Units and Measurements (ICRU). *Health Phys.* 1958; 1(3): 306-314.

108. International Committee for Radiological Units. About ICRU. https://www.icru.org/about-icru/. Accessed April 25, 2023.

109. National Council on Radiation Protection and Measurements. Mission. https://ncrponline.org/about/mission/. Accessed March 15, 2023.

110. Walker JS, Wellock TR. A short history of nuclear regulation, 1946-2009 (NUREG/BR-0174, Revision 2). U.S. Nuclear Regulatory Commission; 2010.

111. Jones CG. A review of the history of U.S. radiation protection regulations, recommendations, and standards. *Health Phys.* 2005; 88(2): 105-124.

112. National Council on Radiation Protection and Measurements. https://ncrponline.org/. Accessed April 25, 2023.

113. United Nations Scientific Committee on the Effects of Atomic Radiation. https://www.unscear.org/. Accessed April 25, 2023.

114. Zimmerman JF. Regulating Atomic Energy in the American Federal System. *Publius.* 1988; 18(3): 51-65.

115. Burney RM. *Conference of Radiation Control Program Directors, Inc. (CRCPD) - A parternship dedicated to radiation protection.* Frankfort, Kentucky: Conference of Radiation Control Program Directors, Inc; 2020.

116. Conference of Radiation Control Program Directors. https://www.crcpd.org/page/About. Accessed April 28, 2023.

117. Nuclear Regulatory Commission. Atomic Energy Commission. 2021 https://www.nrc.gov/reading-rm/basic-ref/glossary/atomic-energy-commission.html. Accessed April 30, 2023.

118. Nuclear Regulatory Commission. History. 2021 https://www.nrc.gov/about-nrc/history.html. Accessed April 30, 2023.

119. Nuclear Regulatory Commission. Title 10 of the Code of Federal Regulations, §20.1003, Definitions. 2021 https://www.nrc.gov/reading-rm/doc-collections/cfr/part020/part020-1003.html. Accessed April 30, 2023.

120. Nuclear Regulatory Commission. NRC Maps of Agreement States. 2021 https://www.nrc.gov/reading-rm/doc-collections/maps/agreement-states.html. Accessed April 26, 2023.

121. National Archives and Office of the Federal Register. Code of Federal Regulations. 2021 https://www.archives.gov/federal-register/cfr. Accessed April 26, 2023.

122. Nuclear Regulatory Commission. Title 10 of the Code of Federal Regulations, §20, Standards for protection against radiation https://www.nrc.gov/reading-rm/doc-collections/cfr/part035/index.html. Accessed August 29, 2022.

123. Nuclear Regulatory Commission. Title 10 of the Code of Federal Regulations, §35.3045, Report and notification of a medical event. https://www.nrc.gov/reading-rm/doc-collections/cfr/part035/part035-3045.html. Accessed April 26, 2023.

CHAPTER 23

Introduction to Unsealed Radionuclides for Radiopharmaceutical Therapy

CONTENTS

Contributed by Jacqueline E. Zoberi, Ph.D., and Jose L. Garcia-Ramirez, M.S., Washington University School of Medicine, St. Louis

A radionuclide is an unstable form of an element that releases radiation in the form of energetic emissions (gamma rays, x-rays, or electrons) in order to become more stable. Radionuclides used for brachytherapy treatment as described in Chapter 22 are typically sealed, or encapsulated within some metallic material, allowing the resulting sealed source to be physically placed, or implanted, very close to or in contact with the treatment site. Radionuclides can also be unsealed, typically in liquid or powder form. When in these forms, they are called *unsealed radionuclides.* They can be administered orally or injected or infused into the bloodstream to travel through the body to the intended treatment site. While the use of sealed source brachytherapy is for more localized delivery of the radiation, the use of unsealed radionuclides to deliver radiation can be especially advantageous in cases where the treatment site is diffusely spread throughout the body or located in areas not immediately accessible to the implantation of sealed brachytherapy sources. In this chapter we focus on unsealed radionuclides.

Although the first use of an unsealed radionuclide for therapy dates back to the 1940s, the use of unsealed radionuclides has historically been more focused on nuclear medicine imaging for diagnosing (identifying) rather than treating disease. Since the 1990s, there has been an increasing trend in the use of unsealed radionuclides for therapy, as demonstrated by the development of novel radioactive drug compounds, or *radiopharmaceuticals*, for a number of different cancers. More recent

DOI: 10.1201/9781003477457-23

efforts have focused on the development of more targeted unsealed radionuclide therapy approaches to maximize the dose (energy absorbed per unit of mass) to the tumor while sparing, or limiting dose to, normal tissues. Here, we provide an overview of unsealed radionuclides, namely radiopharmaceuticals, specifically for therapeutic use and briefly outline the role of nuclear medicine imaging solely in the context of radiopharmaceutical therapy. For further reading on nuclear medicine imaging, see Chapter 12.

Before proceeding to the next section, it might be helpful to review Chapters 5 and 7 on Auger electrons, radioactive decay, isomeric transitions, and electron capture.

23.1 CHARACTERISTICS OF RADIONUCLIDES FOR RADIOPHARMACEUTICAL THERAPY

There are several considerations when selecting a radionuclide for radiopharmaceutical therapy, all based on the following characteristics and discussed below:

I. Particle Characteristics
II. Imaging Capabilities
III. Production Methods
IV. Pharmacokinetic Process and Radiolabeling
V. Half-life

Particle Characteristics
Particle characteristics include the types, intensities, and energies of particles emitted by the radionuclide. For radiopharmaceutical therapy, selected radionuclides include those that emit beta particles (electrons), alpha particles (helium nuclei), or Auger electrons, and can have a photon (gamma or x-ray) component. The therapeutic effects of the radiopharmaceuticals via dose deposition will depend on particle type and energy which is tied to the size of the area that is being targeted and the distance of the radionuclide to the targeted molecule that will cause cell death (DNA damage), as explained below.

Auger Electron Emitters Radionuclides that decay by electron capture or isomeric transition emit low-energy Auger electrons and characteristic x-rays. The characteristic x-rays have a limited use for imaging the distribution of the radionuclide within the body, as the energy is low ($\sim$20-30 keV). The Auger electrons have very short range ($< 1\,\mu$m) and low energy (< 40 keV) and therefore are only of use in therapy if the radionuclide is attached to, or very close to, the cell nucleus.

Beta Emitters Most radionuclides selected for radiopharmaceutical therapy are beta emitters. During beta minus ($\beta-$) decay, negatively charged electrons are emitted from the nucleus as beta particles with a continuous energy spectrum ranging from zero up to a maximum energy, and an average energy of about one third of the maximum energy. Beta emitters offer a wide selection in terms of particle energy (range) and chemical properties. It is useful to classify beta emitting radionuclides into three groups according to beta particle energy and, hence particle range, which should be matched to the size of the tumor. *Low* *energy* beta particle emitting radionuclides have average energies in the range of 100–200 keV, and mean ranges of 0.4–0.9 mm.[1,2] This makes them useful for tumor diameters in the range of approximately 1–2 mm.[1,2] *Medium energy* beta emitting radionuclides have average energies in the range of 200–400 keV, and mean ranges of 1.2–1.8 mm. This makes them useful for tumor diameters in the range of approximately 2–4 mm. *High energy* beta emitting radionuclides have average energies in the range of 500–1000 keV, with mean ranges of 2–5 mm. This makes them useful for tumor diameters of approximately 10 mm.[1,2] It should be noted that beta particles are referred to as low LET (linear energy transfer) radiation that yield a low specific ionization, referring to the number of atoms ionized by these particles per unit path length. The higher the beta particle energy, the larger the beta particle range and the less dense the specific ionization, which in turn causes the particles to be less biologically effective in terms of causing DNA damage and cell death. Table (23.1) lists properties of beta emitters used for radiopharmaceutical therapy, including the energies and ranges of the beta particles, and, if present, the energies of photon emissions in the form of gamma rays.

Alpha Emitters Alpha-emitting radionuclides are becoming more popular for radiopharmaceutical therapy, as will be discussed in §23.5 below. Alpha particles have a high LET and, thereby, tend to have a higher relative biological effectiveness (RBE) than low LET beta-emitting radionuclides, where the RBE is the ratio of biological effectiveness of one type of ionizing radiation relative to another, for the same amount of absorbed energy. The amount of destruction caused by a traversing alpha particle can be one thousand times as large as the destruction capacity caused by a beta particle. On the down side, the range of the alpha particles is so short that very close cellular targeting is required. Thus, for target distances or tumor diameters that are small (50-100 μm), alpha particles may be preferred.

Imaging Capabilities

Photon (gamma or x-ray) radiation emitted by therapeutic radionuclides contribute little to the therapeutic effect of the radionuclide. However, if the photon energy is in the "useful" range for diagnostic imaging (100-500 keV), then it is possible to localize, or determine the regions of, the uptake (absorption) of the radionuclide in the body via nuclear medicine imaging and to perform dosimetry estimates to target and non-target areas. Emissions of gamma rays outside the energy range appropriate for imaging only serve to increase the radiation exposure (and hence dose) to non-target areas and, therefore, to the whole body, as well as increase the dose to other individuals in proximity to patients who have received radiopharmaceutical therapy. Beta-emitting radionuclides with useful gamma-ray emissions include samarium-153 (Sm-153), lutetium-177 (Lu-177), copper-67 (Cu-67) and iodine-131 (I-131) (see Table 23.1). If gamma-ray emitters are used, the gamma-ray abundance should be low; however, a low abundance of photon emissions should provide sufficient photons for imaging.[3]

TABLE 23.1: Beta emitters for radiopharmaceutical therapy

Radionuclide	Half-Life[1] (days)	Beta Energy[1] (keV) Mean (Max*)	Beta Range[2] (mm water) Mean (Max)	Gamma Energy[1] (keV) Major* (Max*)
Iodine-131 (I-131)	8.02	182 (606)	0.4 (2.0)	364 (723)
Lutetium-177 (Lu-177)	6.64	134 (497)	0.2 (1.5)	208 (321)
Copper-67 (Cu-67)	2.6	141 (562)	0.2 (1.8)	185 (394)
Samarium-153 (Sm-153)	1.9	225 (808)	0.5 (2.9)	103 (103)
Yttrium-90 (Y-90)	2.7	932 (2278)	3.5 (11.2)	—
Strontium-89 (Sr-89)	50.6	587 (1500)	1.9 (6.5)	—
Phosphorus-32 (P-32)	14.3	695 (1710)	2.4 (7.7)	—

(1) National Nuclear Data Center, Brookhaven National Laboratory. Accessed at https://www.nndc.bnl.gov/nudat3/mird/.
(2) Radiological Health Handbook, Rockville, MD U.S. Department of Energy, H.W.E. 1970, p. 123 "Beta Particle Range Energy Curve". Shielding of the beta component can be achieved by about 1–1.5 cm of plastic.
*Max beta energy is reported as the maximum energy of beta emissions of at least 1% abundance (1). Major gamma energy is reported as the energy of the most abundant gamma emissions (1). Max gamma energy is reported as the maximum energy of gamma emissions of at least 0.1% abundance (1).

Production Methods

Radionuclides can be produced via nuclear reactors, accelerators, and generators. In reactors, the neutron flux associated with nuclear fission is utilized to irradiate a target of some stable nuclide and form a radioactive nuclide that decays by various ways to the final radioactive nuclide product (as discussed in Chapter 7). Particle accelerators like the cyclotron accelerate a charged particle (proton, alpha or deuteron) to high speeds or energies on the order of MeV, causing them to impinge on a stable target material. Accelerators are used to produce neutron deficient radionuclides, which in turn decay by electron capture or by emitting a positron ($\beta+$ particle), in contrast to the $\beta-$ particle-emitting radionuclides produced in nuclear reactors. The radionuclide generator makes use of the decay of a long half-life parent radionuclide to a short half-life daughter radionuclide which can be separated or "milked" from its parent (half-life is discussed below). Beta and alpha particle emitting radionuclides can be obtained from generator systems.

Pharmacokinetic Process and Radiolabeling

Radiopharmaceutical drugs for therapy can be administered to the patient either orally or by injection or infusion into the bloodstream. The pharmacokinetic process describes how the drug moves through the body, starting with uptake or absorption of the drug from the blood stream or stomach to the site of action, followed by distribution of the drug in the body, and finally clearance (excretion) of the drug from the body. The pharmacokinetic process is affected by the chemical properties of the drug which are dependent on a process referred to as radiolabeling. Simply put, radiolabeling involves the "labeling" of molecules with a radioactive isotope to create the radiopharmaceutical drug compound. There are different methods for radiolabeling. For example, it may involve substituting a non-radioactive atom in a molecule or compound by its radioactive counterpart. In another methodology, the molecule can be conjugated (or joined) to a radionuclide. The molecule essentially carries the radioisotope through the body and can be referred to as a "carrier molecule". Radiolabeling ultimately plays an important role in defining clinical applications of the radiopharmaceutical drug, described in §23.5.

Half-life

The *physical half-life*, which is defined in Chapter 7 as the time it takes for the level of radioactivity in a sample of the radionuclide to drop to one half of its initial value, is an important consideration in the design of radionuclide therapy. From a practical standpoint, the half-life of the radionuclide should permit widespread distribution from production facilities. Generally, radionuclide half-lives of approximately 2 days or longer should provide adequate time for production, processing, formulating agents, and shipping to research or clinical sites without excessive physical decay. From an imaging standpoint, and for radionuclides with a photon component, a desired quality in the half-life is that it should be long enough to allow for imaging for detection and for dosimetry purposes over a period of 1–3 days. From a radiation safety perspective, a radionuclide with a short half-life is preferred. This is because it will have an impact on whether to confine or shield patients that have been infused with the therapeutic radionuclide in order to protect the general public from radiation exposure.

The physical half-life may also have a major influence on the biological effectiveness of these radiopharmaceutical drugs. Higher dose rates given over shorter times (shorter half-lives) are more biologically effective at producing DNA damage (tumor cell death) than lower dose rates delivered over longer times. Thus, a radionuclide with a shorter half-life will tend to be more biologically effective than one with a similar emission energy but longer half-life.

In addition to the physical half-life, one must also account for the *biological half-life*, which is defined as the time it takes for the clearance of half of the drug from the body via natural, biological processes. The biological half-life of the "carrier" molecules that are targeting tumor tissues and being cleared from the rest of the body must be balanced against the physical half-life of the radionuclide to maximize the therapeutic benefit. Thus, the half-life may also have a major influence on the therapeutic ratio, which describes the trade-off between tumor control and toxicity of these agents. The greater the therapeutic ratio, the greater the tumor control relative to the toxicity, and, hence, the greater the therapeutic benefit of the radiopharmaceutical. The best therapeutic ratio is obtained when the physical half-life of the radionuclide is roughly 1.5 to 3 times the biological half-life of the carrier molecule.[4]

23.2 DOSIMETRY FOR RADIOPHARMACEUTICAL THERAPY

To ensure the safe use of radioactively labeled drugs in medical practice, it is necessary to perform dosimetry, that is, calculate the radiation dose received by the different organs in the patient. Because these radiation doses are received from radioactive materials deposited within different organs in the body, they are normally referred to as *internal doses*. Several methodologies can be used to estimate internal organ doses. The most widely used methodology (or schema) was developed by the Medical Internal Radiation Dose (MIRD) Committee of the Society of Nuclear Medicine.[5,6] This methodology utilizes measured (from a small population sample) or estimated (from animal data) pharmacokinetic models to determine or estimate the distribution, retention, and excretion of radiopharmaceutical activity in the body. In addition, the MIRD schema utilizes standardized human anatomical models and Monte-Carlo-derived particle energy depositions (mathematical computational techniques that model the particle interactions in a medium and the energy deposition). As a result of the assumptions used in dosimetry estimates, radiopharmaceutical therapy dosimetry is inherently inaccurate. To improve the accuracy of dosimetry estimates, patient-specific radiopharmaceutical bio-distributions in conjunction with patient-specific anatomical descriptions are necessary in order to minimize the number of assumptions and improve dosimetry estimates. This is the direction that current radiopharmaceutical dosimetry is moving toward. Even in the context of patient-specific-acquired information, the MIRD schema for dosimetry estimates is still applicable.

The MIRD schema uses a unique set of symbols and quantities to calculate the absorbed dose of radiation in any target organ per radioactive decay in any source organ (defined below). The calculations involve the energy emitted per radioactive decay (disintegration), the fraction of the emitted energy that is absorbed in various target organs, the masses of these target organs, and both the physical decay and biologic clearance of the administered radioactive material (the ingested, injected, or infused radiopharmaceutical drug) in the source organ.

As depicted in Fig. (23.1), there are two possible relationships between a "target" organ (the organ we wish to calculate the dose to) and a "source" organ (the organ that contains the radiopharmaceutical drug):

I. Source organ is the same as the target organ.
II. Source organ is different from the target organ.

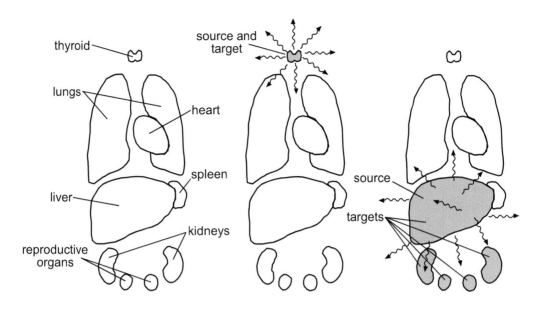

FIGURE 23.1: (Left) Various structures in the human anatomy. (Center) The source and target are the same (thyroid). (Right) The source organ is the liver with multiple target organs (liver, kidneys, reproductive organs).

For each pair of source-target organs, the mean absorbed organ dose to the target organ from the source organ can be computed by Eq. (23.1):

$$D_{t \leftarrow s} = \tilde{A}_s \left(\frac{1}{m_t} \sum_i \Delta_i \phi_i \right), \qquad (23.1)$$

where $\tilde{A}_s$ is the *cumulated activity* and can be defined as the total number of radioactive disintegrations in the source organ. The cumulated activity depends on the initial administered activity of the drug and the amount of time that the drug spends in the body, which is dependent on both the physical and biological half-lives, and can range from a few hours to a few days, sometimes weeks. The cumulated activity is also the area under a "time-activity curve", which is a graphical display of activity versus time, as shown in Fig. 23.2. The time-activity curve is reconstructed from a series of imaging measurements using nuclear medicine equipment like gamma cameras and SPECT/CT to quantify the radioactivity levels at different time-points.[7] m_t is the mass of the target organ, which can be based on standard reference phantom geometries or on more patient-specific estimates based on contouring of the organs on the images mentioned above.

The quantity Δ_i in Eq. (23.1) represents the amount of energy emitted by the ith particle per disintegration. This quantity is a characteristic of the isotope and its decay spectrum. ϕ_i is the *absorbed dose fraction*, which is the fraction of the emitted energy by the ith particle that is absorbed in the target organ. This depends on the type of particle that is being emitted and on the energy of the particle. If the particle is an electron (also referred to as non-penetrating radiation), then its

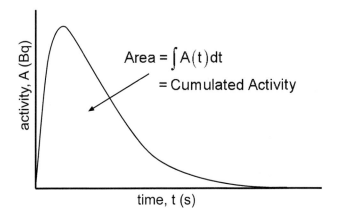

FIGURE 23.2: A "time-activity curve" displaying the activity of the administered radio-pharmaceutical drug as a function of time spent in the body as the drug undergoes physical decay as well as pharmacokinetic processing through the body. The area under the curve is the cumulated activity, $\tilde{A}_s$.

value will depend on the relationship between the target and the source organs. If the source is the same as the target, then $\phi_i = 1$. If the source and target organs are different and separated geometrically, then $\phi_i = 0$. If the target and source organs are adjacent to each other, then at the boundary we can use $\phi_i = 1/2$. If the particle being emitted is a photon (also referred to as "penetrating radiation"), then the value of ϕ_i can range from 0 to 1, depending on the energy of the photon, the geometry between the target and source, the compositions of the target and source organs and the composition of the volumes in between the target and source.

The quantity in parentheses in Eq. (23.1) has been calculated for a selected number of isotopes and assumed phantom configurations and organ compositions.[8] This quantity is referred to as the "S-Factor" and is denoted $S_{t \leftarrow s}$ in Eq. (23.2). It is also known as the *mean absorbed dose per unit of cumulated activity*. It is calculated using Monte-Carlo techniques, and the assumed anatomical geometries and tissue compositions based on standard reference phantom geometries. We thus have that the S-Factor is given by:

$$S_{t \leftarrow s} = \frac{1}{m_t} \sum_i \Delta_i \phi_i . \tag{23.2}$$

Using the definition of the S-factor as given in Eq. (23.2), the equation for the mean absorbed dose to the target organ from the source organ can be rewritten as:

$$D_{t \leftarrow s} = \tilde{A}_s S_{t \leftarrow s} . \tag{23.3}$$

If there are multiple source organs that uptake radiopharmaceuticals, then the dose to the target organ must be the sum of the doses from all the source organs that are taking up activity.

23.3 NUCLEAR MEDICINE IMAGING FOR RADIOPHARMACEUTICAL THERAPY

Nuclear medicine imaging in the context of radiopharmaceutical therapy can be done at different time points relative to the therapeutic administration to provide information that can be used in a number of different settings. The most common scenario is to acquire *pre-therapy scans* like whole-body camera images immediately after administration of some tracer (or small) amount of a radiopharmaceutical—either the drug itself or some radiopharmaceutical that mimics the uptake of the drug. Regions of the body that uptake the drug are captured on these pre-therapy scans. The activity counts in these regions of uptake can be evaluated along with anatomic imaging scans, like CT and MRI, to diagnose disease and qualitatively assess the potential of the radiopharmaceutical to target the disease and spare normal tissues. In some cases, one can take this evaluation further by performing more quantitative analyses via dosimetry calculations to the target and to the normal tissues, also referred to as organs-at-risk (*OARs*).

This pre-therapy dosimetry can be used, for example, to verify that dosing with the radiopharmaceutical is safe, and if not, whether the activity should be modified to achieve the OAR dose constraints. Quantitative analyses like this can be a fairly intensive process requiring numerous steps including calibration of imaging equipment, processing of image data, contouring of structures (target, OARs), and MIRD-based calculations of dose to the structures. Furthermore, the *pre-therapy imaging may be repeated at multiple time-points* over a period of days, for example, immediately after administration, 24 hours later, and so on, to determine the time spent by the drug in certain organs on a per-patient basis. Such information can then be used to determine the cumulated activity mentioned above in the MIRD dosimetry formalism as given by Eq. (23.1). In another scenario, *post-therapy scans* can be acquired and, similar to the pre-therapy imaging scenarios, can be evaluated qualitatively to verify distribution of the radiopharmaceutical and quantitatively for dosimetry.

23.4 ESTABLISHMENT OF A RADIOPHARMACEUTICAL THERAPY PROGRAM

Major steps for implementing a new radiopharmaceutical therapy program in the United States are described here, starting with satisfaction of regulatory requirements and the allocation of resources, i.e., staff, equipment, and space. Regulatory requirements from the appropriate governing body, i.e., either the Nuclear Regulatory Commission (NRC) or the appropriate state-governed agency, are designed to ensure safe medical use of radioactive material (*RAM*).[9] A RAM license, granted by the regulatory body, is required for the possession and medical use of RAM. Physicians listed as Authorized Users (*AUs*) on the RAM license, are allowed to administer RAM for medical use, and must have satisfied training requirements as specified in the regulations. Supporting staff, e.g., medical physicists, health physicists, technologists, and nurses, can be designated to perform tasks under the AU's supervision with the appropriate training. The administration of sufficiently high levels of activity of RAM must be prescribed by the AU using a RAM prescription, referred to as the "Written Directive", which must be documented in a manner specified by the regulations. Equipment for drug handling (receipt, storage and disposal, drug administration), and for patient handling (preparation, administration, monitoring and, if needed, isolating after treatment) must be acquired. Radiation measurement equipment (radiation exposure survey meters, activity measuring dose calibrators, contamination control well-type counters) must be acquired and meet calibration and quality assurance regulatory requirements. Space for drug and patient handling also needs to be identified, and these designated areas must satisfy regulatory requirements for safe radiation exposure levels. Support from radiation safety experts, e.g., the radiation safety officer, medical physicists, and health physicists, is key to ensuring regulatory requirements are met by the radiopharmaceutical therapy program.

Operational procedures must be written and maintained to ensure that handling of RAM is done in a manner that satisfies regulatory requirements and aligns with best practice. Regulatory requirements would include those published by the NRC, for example, Title 10 of the Code of Federal Regulations Part 35 (referred to as 10 CFR Part 35), entitled "Medical Use of Byproduct Material".[9] Best practice would come from technical standards and joint statements published by professional societies.[10] The procedures should describe the radiopharmaceutical drug itself, including a description of the properties of the isotope and of the radiolabeled drug compound. The procedures should describe the treatment schedule (the dosage or amount of activity per fraction, number of fractions, and time interval between fractions). The procedures should describe storage and handling requirements upon receipt of the drug as the nature of the compound itself may require certain storage conditions to ensure a certain shelf life. There may also be drug preparation procedures that would include dispensation, e.g., drawing of the drug from a vial into a syringe, and will also involve an independent verification of the drug activity via an assay (measurement) using specially calibrated measurement equipment, i.e., well-chamber-type dose calibrators.

The operational procedures should also describe processes to ensure that the administration of RAM to the patient is done in a manner that minimizes radioactive *exposure* and *contamination* risks to other individuals in contact with the patient, that is, to the treating staff and members of the general public.

Exposure risks are mainly dependent on the activity of and emission spectra from the radioisotope. Exposure risks can generally be managed by applying the concepts of time, distance, and shielding to keep the effective dose received by exposed individuals to levels indicated in NRC regulations, specifically Title 10 of the Code of Federal Regulations Part 20 (referred to as 10 CFR Part 20), entitled "Standards for Protection Against Radiation".[11] Furthermore, the effective dose received by exposed individuals should also be kept as low as is reasonably achievable (ALARA).[11] Time of exposure is dictated by length of time around the drug and the infused patient and should be minimized as much as possible. To further reduce exposure, shielding and distance should be utilized. Shielding measures may include the use of lead and/or plastic, depending on the emission type (for example, electrons versus photons) and the energies of these emissions. Shielding can come in different forms, for example, as containers for a vial or syringe, mobile shields that can be placed around the patient/drug, and shielding built into the walls of the treatment area. Distancing measures may include treating in an area that can be restricted from public access.

Contamination risks are mainly dependent on the chance for leaks or spills during drug handling and infusion, as well as dependent on excretion pathways and contact with bodily fluids. Prior to treatment, areas will require preparation to capture any contamination and prevent its spread, for example, by using absorbent coverings on equipment, countertops, floors, furniture, and so on. Such areas will also require some level of isolation from public access. If areas are used by the public, then these areas need to be cleared of any contamination and be at safe levels of radiation exposure prior to release for general use. There should be procedures to describe the disposal after administration of any remaining drug waste or contaminated items, usually requiring a decay-in-storage (*DIS*) program to store any radioactive waste until its decayed activity yields low enough exposure levels so it can be safely disposed of as routine trash, or transferred to a radioactive waste facility for further processing.

After treatment administration, patients typically are placed in isolation (in an area that can be restricted from public access) for the purpose of exposure and contamination control until they are considered releasable. Radioactive patients are considered releasable if the total effective dose equivalent (*TEDE*) to exposed individuals is not likely to exceed 5 mSv as stated in section 75 of 10 CFR Part 35 "Release of Individuals Containing Unsealed Byproduct Material or Implants Containing Byproduct Material" (referred to as 10 CFR Part 35.75).[9] Methodologies for making this determination for release are described in the NRC regulatory guide "Consolidated Guidance about Materials Licenses" (referred to as NUREG-1556)[12] and can be based on the amount of activity administered to the patient, or the measured exposure rate from the patient at one meter, or estimates of the TEDE from the released patients based on patient-specific factors, such as uptake and elimination of the drug. If the TEDE from a released patient is estimated to be at least 1 mSv, then radiation safety instructions are also provided to the patient to help ensure exposures are low to other individuals in contact with the patient. Such instructions may include maintaining a certain distance (typically one meter) from others, and preventing contamination by urinating in a seated position and double-flushing, good hand hygiene, and frequent showers. Each instruction is followed by the released patient for some amount of time based on the drug characteristics and biologic half-life.

23.5 EXAMPLES OF RADIOPHARMACEUTICAL THERAPIES

Below we summarize some key radiopharmaceutical therapies in time-line order by year of introduction for clinical use; these therapies are also listed in Table (23.2). Energies and ranges associated with particles emitted by the radionuclides quoted below can be found in Table (23.1).

Thyroid Disorders and Thyroid Ablation

In the 1940s after World War II, the Atomic Energy Commission (AEC) was created by Congress to direct the development of peaceful uses of nuclear energy. National

TABLE 23.2: Examples of radiopharmaceutical therapies

Radionuclide	Radiopharmaceutical	Mechanism of Action	Application(s)
Iodine-131	Sodium iodide (NaI) I-131	Oral ingestion, preferential uptake by thyroid gland	Thyroid disorders and thyroid ablation
Iodine-131	Iobenguane I-131	Intravenous infusion, norepinephrine analog (MIBG) targets norepinephrine-transporter proteins on NET cells	Paragangliomas and pheochromocytomas (neuroendocrine tumors – NETs)
Yttrium-90	Y-90 ibritumomab tiuxetan	Intravenous infusion, monoclonal antibody (ibritumomab) targets protein (CD20 antigen) expressed on the surface of B-cell NHL tumors	B-cell non-Hodgkin lymphoma
Samarium-153	Sm-153 EDTMP (Sm-153 lexidronam)	Intravenous infusion, mineral-like molecule (EDTMP) seeks bone	Bony metastases from primary cancers (for example breast cancer)
Lutetium-177	Lu-177 DOTATATE	Intravenous infusion, peptide (DOTATATE) targets somatostatin receptors over-expressed on NET cells	Gastroenteropancreatic (GEP) neuroendocrine tumors (NETs)
Yttrium-90	Y-90 microspheres*	Fluoroscopic-guided intervention, directly infused through the hepatic artery to preferentially target the tumor due to its increased vascularity	Primary liver tumors or liver metastases from primary colorectal cancers
Radium-223	Ra-223 dichloride	Intravenous infusion, radium acts as a calcium analog targeting areas of new bone growth	Bony metastases for castration-resistant prostate cancer
Lutetium-177	Lu-177 vipivotide tetraxetan	Intravenous infusion, ligand targets proteins (prostate-specific membrane antigen) over-expressed on the surface of prostate cancer cells	Bony and soft tissue metastases for castration-resistant prostate cancer

*Although considered as a radiopharmaceutical therapy, Y-90 microspheres are regulated as brachytherapy sealed sources and devices.

laboratories were created in Oak Ridge, TN and in Los Alamos, NM, and one of the earliest radioactive substances available for purchase was sodium iodide iodine-131 (NaI I-131).[13] The first reported use of NaI I-131 for the treatment of thyroid cancer was in 1945 and is one of the earliest reported examples of targeted radiopharmaceutical therapy.[14] Today, NaI I-131 is commonly prescribed for the management of thyroid cancer to ablate any functioning thyroid tissue remaining after near-total surgical removal of the thyroid gland. The NaI I-131 is administered orally, as a liquid solution or as a powder within a capsule, and quickly absorbed from the gastrointestinal tract and then trapped within the residual functioning thyroid tissues. The NaI I-131 undergoes beta decay to stable xenon-131, releasing beta particles and gamma rays during this process. The therapeutic dose is delivered by the beta particles, which have a maximum energy of 606 keV, depositing most of their energy within 2 mm.[15] The gamma rays are useful for nuclear medicine imaging to verify the distribution of the NaI I-131 within the body. The activity of NaI I-131 prescribed is based on disease type and stage, and can be administered orally, typically in an out-patient setting with appropriate radiation safety instruction.

Metastatic Bone Pain Palliation

Fast forward to the 1990s when most radiopharmaceuticals, with the exception of NaI I-131, were used solely for diagnostic applications (not discussed here). However, some radiopharmaceuticals made their way into the therapeutic arena, namely sodium phosphate phosphorus-32 (P-32), strontium-89 (Sr-89) chloride, and samarium-153 (Sm-153)-ethylene diamine tetramethylene phosphonate (-EDTMP) for palliative therapy (pain relief) of bony metastases which occur when cancer cells have relocated to the bone from primary tumors in sites such as prostate and breast.[16] All of these radiopharmaceuticals are bone-seeking agents. Strontium is a calcium analog, meaning it mimics calcium in the body. Phosphorus, like calcium, is essential for the formation of healthy bones. Sm-153 is combined with EDTMP, a mineral-like molecule, to make it a bone-seeking agent. P-32 and Sr-89 were investigated as early as the 1940s but interest was renewed in the 1980s and 1990s and they received Food and Drug Administration (FDA) approvals for medical use in the 1990s. Both Sr-89 and P-32 are beta emitters yielding highly energetic beta particles with average ranges between $2\,mm$ to $3\,mm$. As a consequence, these beta particles can penetrate beyond the bone and into the marrow cavities, and hence there is a potential for toxicity to the marrow (myelotoxicity). Of note, P-32 is currently not available. Sm-153 yields a less energetic beta particle with a relatively shorter range, about $0.5\,mm$ on average, yielding good bone-to-marrow dose ratios. Sr-89 is prescribed at a fixed activity level, and Sm-153 is prescribed based on patient weight (mCi/kg); both infused intravenously (injected into the veins) in an out-patient setting.

Radioembolization of Liver Malignancies

Moving on to the years 1999–2002, radioembolization drugs became approved for the treatment of malignant liver lesions, namely primary liver tumors or metastases from primary colorectal cancers. Embolization, done under fluoroscopic guidance, involves the insertion of a catheter into an artery supplying blood to some abnormal tissue (tumor) followed by infusion of tiny particles to create a blockage within that artery and starve the tumor of its blood supply. Radioembolization takes this therapy one step further, by radiolabeling the particles with a beta-emitting radionuclide. Millions of these particles or "microspheres" with sizes on the order of 20–60 μm are infused into the hepatic artery with the intent of preferentially targeting tumors due to their increased vascularity while maintaining sublethal doses to the surrounding normal liver. Two such types of microspheres manufactured currently are available in either glass or resin form, both labeled with yttrium-90 (Y-90). Y-90 undergoes beta decay to stable zirconium-90, releasing beta particles with an average energy of 932 keV and a maximum energy of 2278 keV, with a mean tissue penetration of 3.5 mm and a maximum of 11 mm. It should be noted that Y-90 microspheres are regulated under 10 CFR 35.1000 "Other Medical Uses of Byproduct Material or Radiation from Byproduct Material" as brachytherapy sealed sources and devices for permanent implantation as they do not metabolize within the body.[9] In practice, however, they are implemented similar to other radiopharmaceutical therapies. Different techniques of calculating the activity of microspheres required for treatment include models based on body-surface area, partition models, and on the MIRD formalism, which is specifically addressed in §23.2 above. In addition to dose to normal liver parenchyma, the dose to the lungs due to "shunting", or flow, of activity from the liver to the lungs is also accounted for in these techniques. Treatments are typically administered via catheterization under fluoroscopic guidance in an interventional unit, with patients discharged once medically stable.[17,18]

Radioimmunotherapy of B-cell Non-Hodgkin Lymphoma

During the years of 2003–2006, radioimmunotherapy agents were approved for the treatment of B-cell non-Hodgkin lymphoma (NHL), a malignancy of the immune system. Immunotherapy involves the use of a laboratory-created monoclonal antibody designed to recognize and bind to a specific protein found on tumor cells. One such protein is the CD20 antigen expressed on the surface of B-cell NHL tumors. *Radio*immunotherapy takes advantage of this targeting mechanism by conjugating (joining) a beta-emitting radionuclide with the monoclonal antibody. Two such antibodies manufactured for targeting the CD20 antigen are ibritumomab and tositumomab, each linked to their respective radioisotope, Y-90 and I-131. The ranges of the emitted particles allow for the irradiation of tumor cells that are bound to these antibodies as well as nearby tumor cells. Treatment with I-131 tositumomab requires individualized dosimetry to determine the therapeutic activity as the biologic clearance of the drug varies between patients, and involves long treatment times via slow infusions, and exposure/contamination hazards. Of note, the I-131 tositumomab is no longer manufactured. For Y-90 ibritumomab, the therapeutic activity can be calculated based on body weight, and can administered intravenously in an outpatient setting. The patient also must have a sufficient platelet count prior to infusion as treatment can lead to depletion (thrombocytopenia).[19,20,21]

Alpha Particle Therapy for Bone Metastases

Since 2010, there has been a rapid increase in the number of new radiopharmaceutical therapies. In 2013, the first alpha-emitting radiopharmaceutical, radium-223 (Ra-223) dichloride, was approved for therapeutic use specifically for the treatment of bone metastases in patients with metastatic castration-resistant prostate cancer (mCRPC). This is an advanced form of prostate cancer that has spread beyond the prostate gland and for which hormone therapy (using chemicals travelling through the bloodstream to have a specific effect on the activity of other cells or organs) is no longer effective. Ra-223 acts as a calcium analog targeting areas of new bone growth which surround bone metastases. Ra-223 decays by alpha emission to a stable isotope of lead (Pb-207). The alpha particles have a range of about 50–100 μm (versus several millimeters for alternative radiopharmaceuticals emitting beta particles) and a high linear transfer of energy of about $100 \, \text{keV}/\mu\text{m}$ (vs. $0.2 \, \text{keV}/\mu\text{m}$ for beta particles), delivering more lethal damage concentrated to bone metastatic tumor sites and yielding less myelotoxicity than its beta-emitting counterparts discussed above. Therapeutic activities of Ra-223 are weight-based and are delivered intravenously in an out-patient setting. Currently, there are a number of trials investigating Ra-223 paired with other cancer therapy agents.[22]

High-activity I-131 Therapies

Moving on to 2018, iobenguane I-131, a form of meta-iodobenzylguanidine (MIBG), became FDA-approved for the therapy of paraganglioma and certain types of pheochromocytoma, both neuroendocrine tumors (NETs) that can affect the levels of certain hormones like norepinephrine which gives the brain and body the energy it needs to respond to stress. These particular NETs highly express a transmembrane protein responsible for transporting norepinephrine across the cell membrane into these tumors. MIBG is a norepinephrine analog that can seek this protein resulting in cellular uptake.[23] I-131 MIBG was not an entirely new radiopharmaceutical as it was used as an imaging agent for neuroblastoma, pheochromocytoma, and paragangliomas in the 1990s and was evaluated in clinical trials for thyroid carcinoma in the 1990s, as well. Currently, there are several trials underway for treatment of adult and pediatric patients for neuroblastoma, paraganglioma, and pheochromocytoma. One unique aspect of this therapy is that high activities may be required for treatment as the dosing scheme is based on weight, and can range for example from 100 mCi in pediatric patients to 1200 mCi in adults.[24] The handling of such high activities of I-131 poses radiation exposure and contamination risks and, hence, requires processes and procedures to minimize these risks (as described in §23.4 above).

Peptide Receptor Radionuclide Therapy for Neuro-endocrine Tumors

Also in 2018, peptide receptor radionuclide therapy (PRRT) using Lu-177 DOTATATE for the treatment of somatostatin receptor-positive gastroenteropancreatic (GEP) neuro-endocrine tumors (NETs) was approved in the United States. These NETs are specifically those affecting the pancreas or gastrointestinal tract where the tumor cells have proteins called somatostatin receptors over-expressed on their surface. DOTATATE is a peptide designed to seek and bind to these receptors, and when paired with lutetium-177 (Lu-177) becomes a radiopeptide capable of delivering radiation directly to these cells. Lu-177 undergoes beta decay emitting beta particles with a maximum energy of 497 keV depositing most of its energy in tissue to within 1.5 mm.[25] Lutetium-177 also emits some gamma rays, which are useful for nuclear medicine imaging to verify the biologic distribution of the Lu-177 post-therapy. Therapeutic activities are currently fixed at a standard dosing level and delivered intravenously over 30-40 minutes. A unique aspect of this therapy is that it is delivered alongside an amino acid solution that is infused intravenously over a duration of several hours to help protect against renal toxicity. Because patients will remain in isolation and will need to void during this long treatment time of several hours, this therapy poses contamination risks requiring processes and procedures to minimize these risks (as described in §23.4 above). After completion of amino acid infusion, patients can be discharged once medically stable.[26,27]

Radioligand Therapies for Prostate Cancer

Since about 2017 there has been a wave of clinical trials investigating radioligand therapy of patients with metastatic prostate cancer, with approval of a Lu-177-based therapy (Lu-177 vipivotide tetraxetan) for mCRPC in the United States in March of 2022. The ligands for this application are molecules developed specifically for targeting prostate specific membrane antigen (PSMA), a protein over-expressed on the surface of prostate cancer cells.[28] Other radioisotopes besides Lu-177 include I-131, copper-67 (Cu-67), and actinium-225 (Ac-225) (an alpha emitter), all of which are being investigated, and with procedural aspects related to these therapies under development.

23.6   QUESTIONS, EXERCISES, & PROBLEMS

23-1. It is stated in §23.1 that beta particles have a low LET value, while alpha particles have a high LET value. Explain why you would expect this to be the case. (Hint: You may want to review the discussion of LET in §2.5 before attempting to answer this.)

23-2. There are two types of half-lives discussed in this chapter. Name these two types and describe the difference between them.

23-3. Write down Eq. (23.1) and explain the meaning of each symbol in the equation. (b) What is the significance of the summation over i in this summation? That is, what is being summed over? (c) Explain why this equation makes sense. Use sketches to help clarify your explanation.

23.7   REFERENCES

1. Zweit J. Radionuclides and carrier molecules for therapy. *Phys Med Biol.* 1996; 41(10): 1905-1914.
2. Howell RW, Rao DV, Sastry KS. Macroscopic dosimetry for radioimmunotherapy: nonuniform activity distributions in solid tumors. *Med Phys.* 1989; 16(1): 66-74.
3. Volkert WA, Goeckeler WF, Ehrhardt GJ, et al. Therapeutic radionuclides: production and decay property considerations. *J Nucl Med.* 1991; 32(1): 174-185.
4. Wessels BW, Rogus RD. Radionuclide selection and model absorbed dose calculations for radiolabeled tumor associated antibodies. *Med Phys.* 1984; 11(5): 638-645.
5. Loevinger R, Berman M. A Revised Schema for Calculating the Absorbed Dose from Biologically Distributed Radionuclides. *MIRD Pamphlet No. 1. Revised ed.* New York, NY: Society of Nuclear Medicine; 1976.
6. Loevinger R, Budinger T, Watson E. *MIRD Primer for Absorbed Dose Calculations. Revised ed.* New York, NY: Society of Nuclear Medicine; 1991.

7. Siegel JA, Thomas SR, Stubbs JB, et al. MIRD pamphlet no. 16: Techniques for quantitative radiopharmaceutical biodistribution data acquisition and analysis for use in human radiation dose estimates. *J Nucl Med.* 1999; 40(2): 37S-61S.

8. Snyder W, Ford M, Warner G, et al. "S," Absorbed Dose per Unit Cumulated Activity for Selected Radionuclides and Organs. *MIRD Pamphlet No. 11.* New York, NY: Society of Nuclear Medicine; 1975.

9. U.S. NRC Regulations Title 10, CFR Part 35 Medical Use of Byproduct Material. https://www.nrc.gov/reading-rm/doc-collections/cfr/part035/index.html. Accessed June 12, 2022.

10. American College of Radiology. ACR practice parameter for the performance of therapy with unsealed radiopharmaceutical sources. Revised 2019. https://www.acr.org/-/media/ACR/Files/Practice-Parameters/UnsealedSources.pdf. Accessed August 10, 2022.

11. U.S. NRC Regulations Title 10, CFR Part 20 Standards for Protection Against Radiation. https://www.nrc.gov/reading-rm/doc-collections/cfr/part020/index.html. Accessed August 10, 2022.

12. U.S. NRC NUREG-1556, Vol. 9, Rev.3 Consolidated Guidance About Materials Licenses, Program-Specific Guidance About Medical Use Licenses: Appendix U. https://www.nrc.gov/reading-rm/doc-collections/nuregs/staff/sr1556/v9/index.html. Accessed August 10, 2022.

13. Staum MM. Landmarks and Landmines in the Early History of Radiopharmaceuticals. *Journal of Nuclear Medicine Technology.* 1992; 20: 209-213.

14. Parthasarathy KL, Crawford ES. Treatment of thyroid carcinoma: emphasis on high-dose ^{131}I outpatient therapy. *J Nucl Med Technol.* 2002; 30(4): 165-171; quiz 172-163.

15. Bender J, Dworkin H. Iodine-131 as an Oncology Agent. *Journal of Nuclear Medicine Technology.* 1993; 21(3): 140-150.

16. Atkins H, Srivastava, SC. Radiopharmaceuticals for Bone Malignancy Therapy. *J Nucl Med Technol.* 1998; 26(2): 80-83.

17. Dezarn WA, Cessna JT, DeWerd LA, et al. Recommendations of the American Association of Physicists in Medicine on dosimetry, imaging, and quality assurance procedures for ^{90}Y microsphere brachytherapy in the treatment of hepatic malignancies. Med Phys 2011; 38(8): 4824-4845.

18. Westcott MA, Coldwell DM, Liu DM, et al. The development, commercialization, and clinical context of yttrium-90 radiolabeled resin and glass microspheres. Adv Radiat Oncol 2016; 1(4): 351-364.

19. Fink-Bennett DM, Thomas K. ^{90}Y-ibritumomab tiuxetan in the treatment of relapsed or refractory B-cell non-Hodgkin's lymphoma. J Nucl Med Technol 2003; 31(2): 61-68; quiz 69-70.

20. Macklis RM, Pohlman B. Radioimmunotherapy for non-Hodgkin's lymphoma: a review for radiation oncologists. Int J Radiat Oncol Biol Phys 2006; 66(3): 833-841.

21. Seldin DW. Techniques for using Bexxar for the treatment of non-Hodgkin's lymphoma. J Nucl Med Technol 2002; 30(3): 109-114.

22. Shore ND. Radium-223 dichloride for metastatic castration-resistant prostate cancer: the urologist's perspective. Urology 2015; 85(4): 717-724.

23. Pandit-Taskar N, Modak S. Norepinephrine Transporter as a Target for Imaging and Therapy. J Nucl Med 2017; 58(Suppl 2): 39S-53S.

24. de la Guardia M, McCammon S, Nielson K, et al. Administration of (1)(3)(1)I-Metaiodobenzylguanidine Using the Peristaltic Infusion Pump Method. J Nucl Med Technol 2014; 42(2): 109-113.

25. Mantel E, Williams J. An Introduction to Newer PET Diagnostic Agents and Related Therapeutic Radiopharmaceuticals. J Nucl Med Technol 2019; 47(3): 203-209.

26. Hope TA, Abbott A, Colucci K, et al. NANETS/SNMMI Procedure Standard for Somatostatin Receptor-Based Peptide Receptor Radionuclide Therapy with (177)Lu-DOTATATE. J Nucl Med 2019; 60(7): 937-943.

27. Maughan NM, Kim H, Hao Y, et al. Initial experience and lessons learned with implementing Lutetium-177-dotatate radiopharmaceutical therapy in a radiation oncology-based program. Brachytherapy 2021; 20(1): 237-247.

28. Kratochwil C, Giesel FL, Stefanova M, et al. PSMA-Targeted Radionuclide Therapy of Metastatic Castration-Resistant Prostate Cancer with ^{177}Lu-Labeled PSMA-617. J Nucl Med 2016; 57(8): 1170-1176.

CHAPTER 24

Radiation Protection and Quality Assurance

CONTENTS

As we have stated several times throughout this text, ionizing radiation has been shown to be useful for medical diagnosis as well as for treatment. However, radiation has its harmful side as well. Full body doses of around $4.5\,Gy$ to $5\,Gy$ have been observed to be fatal. Higher doses to specific organs can cause adverse reactions specific to that organ. For example, a dose of $20\,Gy$ to the lungs can result in pneumonitis, whereas a dose of $45\,Gy$ to the spinal cord can cause myelitis and eventual paralysis. Lower doses of radiation are also harmful, increasing the risk of cancer induction after a latency period. Even lower doses to a developing fetus have been observed to cause fetal malformations.

In light of these risks, should we abandon the use of radiation? If we did, this book would be much shorter. More importantly, we would not be able to image internal anatomy and tumors. Our diagnostic abilities would be severely diminished. Internal organs might have to be viewed directly in a surgical procedure, as they often were in pre-CT days, increasing the risk to the patient. Nor would we have the powerful weapon of ionizing radiation to treat tumors, resulting in poorer outcomes for the patient. Instead of abandoning the use of radiation, we adopt a philosophy of *benefit vs. risk*. We accept some risk in the use of ionizing radiation because of the potential benefit that is derived from its use. We accept a low probability of cancer induction or minor damage to uninvolved tissue with the knowledge that with the radiation we are able to diagnose and/or treat many kinds of diseases. This is not a unique application of benefit vs. risk. We accept a small amount of risk every time we step into an automobile to drive anywhere. Even though there is the risk of becoming involved in a fatal automobile accident when we drive, we recognize that, without our automobiles, we might not be able to get to school or to our job. The basis of radiation protection is that we need to implement methods that protect the patient,

DOI: 10.1201/9781003477457-24

the radiation worker, and the general public against any radiation other than that which is used for diagnosis and treatment.

In addition to protecting the public from unwanted radiation, we must also protect the patient. This is done by verifying that the radiation that is planned to be delivered is accurately being delivered throughout the course of radiation treatment, both in quantity and in location. The final section in this chapter addresses the issue of quality assurance and quality improvement in the management of the radiation delivered to patients.

24.1   LINEAR NON-THRESHOLD HYPOTHESIS

A great deal of information exists relating biological and clinical effects of exposure to large amounts of ionizing radiation; however, very little data exists on the effects of low doses of radiation. These low doses of radiation are the doses that one would expect an individual to receive while using, rather than receiving, radiation for practical applications. Consequently, in radiation protection, we focus on radiation workers and the general public, rather than on patients.

Several factors complicate the problem of determining the effects of low doses of radiation. The first factor is that, because of the stochastic response of tissue to low doses of radiation, it is not possible to determine low-level radiation effects on single individuals; one needs to look at a population. Moreover, the late effects of radiation, such as cancer induction, cannot be differentiated from the same effects, but may be caused by other factors, such as genetics, exposure to asbestos, or smoking. Consequently, in order to determine the dose-response relationship of radiation, it is necessary to examine increases in frequency of late effects as a result of exposure. Next, the data on late effects is very limited and the dosimetry is not necessarily accurate. It is, of course, unethical to intentionally expose individuals to known amounts of radiation; the data used to determine late effects comes from incidental exposure to radiation—for example, dose received by the survivors of the atomic-bomb from Hiroshima and Nagasaki and the survivors of the nuclear plant incidents in Chernobyl and Fukushima. The amount of radiation to which individuals were exposed could not be measured; radiation dose had to be estimated. Finally, political issues may have made acquisition of data difficult.

With limited dose-response data at moderate doses it is necessary to extrapolate the extent of radiation effect to zero dose. Extrapolation of data is fraught with danger and is based on the model used to determine dose responses. The most widely accepted extrapolation model is based on the *linear non-threshold* (LNT) hypothesis. The LNT hypothesis says that extrapolation of dose response should be linear, and intersect zero response at zero dose. The hypothesis is based on the idea that a break in a single DNA strand may cause biological effects. (See Chapter 2.) Other hypotheses exist, however. Some advocate the existence of a threshold dose below which there are no biological effects. Some even advocate the concept of *radiation hormesis*—the idea that very low doses of radiation are beneficial. Consequently, there is still a great deal of controversy regarding the biological effects of very low doses of radiation, but the LNT hypothesis is the most widely accepted.

24.2   EFFECTS OF RADIATION

Depending on the dose of radiation, two classes of effects are critical to the study of radiation protection: stochastic effects and deterministic effects. *Stochastic effects* are those observed at very low doses of radiation. Characteristics of stochastic effects include the absence of a dose threshold below which no effects are observed and an increase in the probability of dose response with increase of dose. For stochastic effects the severity of dose response is independent of the dose—there either is or is not a response. The most common stochastic effect of radiation is cancer induction, but other stochastic effects include induction of birth defects or genetic defects. As mentioned in the previous section, cancer, birth defects, and genetic defects can all occur independently of irradiation; consequently, in order to estimate the dose-response effect in the stochastic range of doses, one must determine the excess incidence of these occurrences. The determination of the excess incidence of occurrences at very low doses causes a great deal of uncertainty in the quantitation of the dose-response effect.

Deterministic effects, on the other hand, occur at much greater doses of radiation. Deterministic effects, such as inflammation and tumor killing, include the presence of a threshold dose, with the extent of damage dependent on the dose. Most of the issues involved in treatment planning are based on the goal of reducing the extent of deterministic effects of the radiation, whereas a great deal of the efforts in radiation protection are based on reducing the extent of the stochastic effects.

24.3   DOSE LIMITS

In recognition of the potential harm of low doses of radiation, various organizations have established recommended limits on the amount of radiation an individual might receive. Dose limits are set based on the concept of benefit vs risk; we are willing to tolerate the risk of a small dose of radiation in order to derive the benefit to be gained by exposure. Moreover, we must recognize that people are continually exposed to a small amount of background radiation ($\sim 3\,mSv/y$) simply by living on the Earth.

In addition to the actual dose received by an individual, we must also take into account the nature of the radiation and the specific organs that are irradiated. Consequently, before assessing whether there is adequate protection from radiation, we first must weight the mean dose, $\overline{D_r}$, from radiation type r, by an appropriate radiation-specific quality factor Q_r, giving a mean dose equivalent $\overline{H}$, or

$$\overline{H} = \sum Q_r \, \overline{D_r}. \tag{24.1}$$

The quality factor is a measure of the approximate linear energy transfer of the incident radiation. (See §2.5 for a discussion of linear energy transfer.) It is set to 1 for x-rays, gamma rays, and electrons. It is set to 2 for high-energy protons, 5 for high-energy neutrons, and 20 for alpha particles.

Dose limits, or more precisely, equivalent dose limits, are recommended by scientific organizations and mandated into law by regulatory bodies. Two major scientific organizations recommend dose limits. These are the *International Commission on*

Radiological Protection (ICRP) and the *National Council on Radiation Protection and Measurements* (NCRP). As their names imply, the ICRP is an international body whereas the NCRP is an organization based in the United States. Both organizations publish reports addressing various aspects of radiation protection, including medical radiation. These reports do not have the force of legislation; however, the recommended dose limits are often adopted by regulatory bodies. In the United States, regulation of the use of radioactive isotopes and naturally occurring radioactive materials is the purview of the U.S. *Nuclear Regulatory Commission* (NRC); regulation of naturally-occurring radioactive materials and accelerator-produced radiation is handled by the radiation regulatory agencies of the individual states. In many cases, a state will enter into a compact with the NRC to regulate the use of certain radioactive materials under specified conditions, in particular, for medical applications. These states are often referred to as "Agreement States".

In setting radiation dose limits, two different classes of individuals are identified. Individuals who work with radiation have been specifically trained in the safe use of radiation and are monitored for the amount of radiation to which they are exposed, whereas the general public is assumed not to have training in radiation protection, nor are they monitored. The NCRP gives recommended limits for whole body dose to be $50\,mSv/y$ for radiation workers and $1\,mSv/y$ for the general public.[1] In addition, an effective dose limit for pregnant occupational exposure has been set to be $0.5\,mSv$ in each month of pregnancy. These are dose limits for whole body dose; other limits have been set for individual organs such as skin or lens of the eye.

24.4 SHIELDING

The amount of radiation received by an individual is based on three factors—time, distance, and shielding—each one of which can be adjusted to reduce radiation dose. Time is simply the amount of time that an individual is exposed to the radiation. Dose is linearly dependent on time, so that a reduction in time spent near a radiation source will reduce the radiation dose received by an individuals. Dose is inversely proportional to the square of the distance for point radiation sources, as well as decreasing with distance for extended sources; thus increasing the distance from a radiation source will also decrease the received dose. Shielding takes advantage of the approximate exponential attenuation of an x-ray beam as it passes through absorption material. The remainder of this section will address how the amount of shielding required to reduce radiation dose to acceptable levels is determined.

Shielding of the area surrounding the source of radiation is incorporated to limit radiation exposure to radiation workers and the general public. It should be noted that one must refer to limiting radiation exposure to an acceptable level, and not to zero exposure. To limit radiation to zero exposure is an impossible task that would make the medical use of radiation impossible. However, as we saw earlier in this chapter, exposure to a small amount of radiation when there is benefit to be gained is deemed acceptable.

Regions in a typical radiation facility are identified as belonging to two areas. A *controlled area* is a region in which the occupational exposure to radiation is under the supervision of an individual in charge of radiation protection. Typically these are the areas in and around the radiation-producing equipment. Individuals who have to occupy controlled areas are specifically trained in the safe use of radiation and are monitored for exposure to radiation. Access to these areas is generally restricted to radiation workers. If a member of the general public (patients and their companions) or a non-radiological hospital worker enters a controlled area, they do so only for a short period of time. Regions in the radiation facility that are not controlled areas are designated as *uncontrolled areas*. Uncontrolled areas are accessible to the general public, untrained in the safe use of radiation and unmonitored.

Because of the difference between controlled areas and uncontrolled areas, shielding for the different regions is designed for different radiation dose limits. Shielding for a controlled area must be designed to reduce doses to $0.1\,mGy/wk$ ($5\,mGy/y$), whereas shielding for an uncontrolled are must reduce doses to $0.02\,mGy/wk$ ($1\,mGy/y$).

The following assumptions are made in designing shielding for radiation facilities:

I. Attenuation of the primary beam by the patient is neglected. However, the patient is considered to be the source of scattered radiation.

II. Perpendicular incidence of radiation on the shielding is assumed. Thus the radiation takes the shortest path through the attenuating material.

III. The presence of additional attenuating materials, such as lead aprons, equipment cabinets, *etc.*, is ignored.

IV. Radiation leaking through the head of the radiation-producing machine is assumed to be the maximum value allowed by federal standard, which is $0.876\,mGy/h$.

V. The field size and phantom used for scatter calculations is assumed to be very large.

VI. The uncontrolled areas are occupied continuously. (*We will discuss occupancy shortly.*)

VII. The minimum distance from a shielded wall to an area that is occupied is assumed to be $0.3\,m$.

In designing shielding for external-beam radiation, one must consider three types of radiation: primary, scatter, and leakage. *Primary radiation* is that radiation coming directly out of the radiation-producing machine. It should be noticed, however, that, in many cases, the presence of a beam stopper in a linear accelerator results in sufficient attenuation of the primary beam that primary radiation can be ignored. *Scattered radiation* is the result of Compton scatter within the patient, while *leakage* results from radiation penetrating the housing of the machine producing the radiation.

In performing shielding calculations, it is customary to look at radiation scattered 90° from the central axis of the incident beam. Generally, the energy of the scattered radiation is considerably different from the energy of the primary and leakage radiation, so the amount of shielding for scattered radiation must be calculated separately from the calculation for primary and scatter.

The calculation of the amount of shielding required is relatively straightforward. One first calculates the radiation dose that would be received in the absence of shielding, then calculates the amount of shielding required to bring the dose to acceptable levels. In the absence of shielding, the unshielded dose rate is given by the relation

$$D^{unshielded} = \frac{W \cdot U \cdot T}{d^2}.$$
(24.2)

In this relation, W is the *workload*, U is the *use factor*, T is the *occupancy factor*, and d is the distance from the radiation source. These quantities are explained below.

The *workload*, W, is a measure of how much radiation is produced. If known, W is the absorbed dose delivered to the isocenter in one week, based on number of patients treated and an estimate of the weekly dose during physics procedures. If, on the other hand, W is not known, then NCRP Report 49[2] recommends a value of $1000\,Gy/wk$ for machines with energies up to 10 MeV, and NCRP Report 51[3] recommends a value of $500\,Gy/wk$ for machines with energies above 10 MeV. Leakage and scatter are generally estimated to be 0.1% of the primary radiation.

The second factor, U, is the *use factor*, indicating what fraction of time the radiation beam is directed at a barrier. For the primary beam, one generally uses 0.5 for the floor and ceiling of the radiation room and 0.25 for walls. It should be noted that the primary beam may be partially attenuated by a beam stop or other device. For leakage and scatter, one uses a U value of 1.0.

The third factor, T, is the *occupancy factor*, a measure of the fraction of time a particular area is occupied. For offices, treatment control rooms, and treatment planning rooms, a recommended T-value is 1.0, indicating that these rooms are generally occupied full time during the working day. For rooms adjacent to a treatment room, not included in the previous assessment, a value of 0.5 is recommended. For corridors, lounges, rest rooms, etc., near the treatment room, a value of 0.2 is recommended. A more complete set of recommended values of T can be found in the NCRP Reports.

Combining the three factors of workload, use, and occupancy, and dividing by the square of the distance from the barrier to the radiation source gives us the unshielded dose rate at the barrier. It is now necessary to design the barrier. The first issue is that of the shielding material. For x-rays of energies used in diagnostic imaging, the main interaction is the photoelectric effect. The attenuation coefficient for the photoelectric effect is highly dependent on the atomic number, Z, of the barrier material, so we would want to use high-Z materials such as lead in our barriers. For energies used in radiation therapy, the Compton interaction is the predominant interaction. (See Chapter 8 for a discussion of the photoelectric and Compton effects.) Because the attenuation is independent of Z, the thickness of lead required to provide adequate shielding at these energies is so large to make it impractical for use as a building material, so one uses a typical building material, such as concrete to shield the regions adjacent to the therapy room.

24.5 QUALITY ASSURANCE AND QUALITY IMPROVEMENT

One of the major roles of the medical physicist in radiation oncology is to verify that the correct amount of radiation is delivered to correct region in the patient, that is, the target volume receives the prescribed dose and doses to uninvolved tissue are kept to within acceptable limits. However, no dose delivery is exactly as prescribed. Uncertainties in the calculation of dose in the treatment plan and in the measurement of dose from the treatment machine combine to result in an overall uncertainty in the dose delivered to the patient.

But just what is an acceptable uncertainty? In the radiation oncology world the magic number for dose uncertainty is taken to be 5%. Clinical experience has shown that appropriate tumor control may be a very steep function of dose as is normal tissue complications, and that a dose difference that may be as small as 5% can be the difference between tumor control and normal tissue complications. Moreover, various events in the history of radiation oncology have shown that a skilled clinician can observe difference in tumor response to a dose difference of 5%.

Originally, a *quality assurance* (QA) program was directed toward the radiation treatment equipment that would deliver dose to the patient, with the goal of assuring that machine characteristics and practice do not deviate significantly from baseline values obtained at time of commissioning. Many causes of change in these machine parameters are possible, including machine malfunction, mechanical breakdown, physical accidents, and component failure. Changes in machine parameters may also be the result of replacement of major components of the equipment or of aging of machine components.

In this section, we shall focus on QA as applied to radiation oncology equipment because accuracy in delivery of radiation is much more critical in radiation oncology. However, QA of diagnostic radiation equipment is also a significant component of the role of the medical physicist in imaging.

The practice of QA currently in the United States is described in reports by various Task Groups of the *American Association of Physicists in Medicine* (AAPM). These Task Group reports are continually being revised and updated to reflect current knowledge and practice in QA. In this section, we shall describe three of these reports.

The first two of these Task Group reports, AAPM Report 46[4] and AAPM Report 142[5], focus on QA of radiation oncology equipment whereas the third report, AAPM Report 283[6], addresses the more general issue of quality management (QM), and focuses more on the entire radiation oncology process.

Radiation equipment needs to be tested on a regular basis. The frequency of testing represents a balance between resources and risk. For example, parameters affecting the patient dose by either dosimetric or geometric means are typically evaluated on a daily basis by the radiation therapist as part of the machine warm-up procedure. Dosimetric tests are typically consistency checks with tolerance levels and action levels explicitly identified. In addition, safety tests such as verifying the operation of door interlocks and the equipment for audiovisual monitoring of patient are also performed daily by the radiation therapist.

Tests performed on a less frequent basis monitor issues that have a lower likelihood of change, for example, tray position, beam profiles, and respiratory gating equipment. These less frequent tests are generally performed by a qualified medical physicist or a physicist assistant working under the supervision of the qualified medical physicist. Finally, on an annual basis, the medical physicist performs a subset of the acceptance testing and commissioning procedures.

Identification of these tests and the frequency of performance can be found in various task group reports. These reports are continually being reviewed and, if necessary, revised. Revisions to these reports are necessary because radiation oncology is a rapidly-advancing field. Many technologies presently used in the clinic were unheard of a decade ago, and tests needed to be developed to ensure the reproducibility of radiation delivery. In addition, developments in the principles of QA and continuous quality improvement (CQI) cause changes in the way quality testing is done.

As equipment is becoming more and more complex, the amount of resources expended on QA increases. In order to develop a more proactive rather than reactive approach to QA, and to integrate QA of machine performance as part of a larger system of quality management of the entire radiation treatment process, the AAPM Report 283 takes a risk analysis approach.[6] Rather than explicitly identifying tests and tolerances, the Task Group report describes a methodology for analyzing a procedure in radiation oncology, identifying possible points in the procedure where a deviation from intent might occur, and assessing the risk and consequences of such a deviation. A specific example of the application of this methodology to intensity-modulated radiation therapy (IMRT) is given, with the recommendation that each facility develop its own risk-aware quality management program for all clinical procedures. Furthermore, quality assurance procedures should be prioritized based on risk of failure, severity of effects of failure, and intensity of resources.

24.6   QUESTIONS, EXERCISES, & PROBLEMS

24-1. (a) Explain the LNT hypothesis. (b) Explain why the LNT hypothesis follows from the idea that a *singe* DNA strand break may result in biological effects.

24-2. Compare and contrast stochastic and deterministic effects of radiation.

24-3. This chapter contains the statement, "Most of the issues involved in treatment planning are based on the goal of reducing the extent of deterministic effects of the radiation, whereas a great deal of the efforts in radiation protection are based on reducing the extent of the stochastic effects". Explain this statement.

24-4. List and explain the three factors that affect the amount of radiation received by a person.

24-5. Work out the details of the following shielding examples in Chapter 5 of the NCRP Report 147.[7] You will need to do some studying of the equations and terms that are referred to in the example solutions. Be sure to explain the equations and terms associated with these solutions as presented in the Report. (a) Work through the example on p. 92 dealing with a mammography suite. (b) Work through the example on p. 96 dealing with the multi-slice scanner. (c) Work through the example on p. 99 applying the Dose-Length Product Method. (d) Work through the example on p. 101 dealing with the fan beam unit.

24-6. Work out the details of the following examples in Chapter 7 of the NCRP Report 151.[8] You will need to do some studying of the equations and terms that are referred to in the example solutions. Be sure to explain the equations and terms associated with these solutions as presented in the Report. (a) Example 7.1.1 on p. 105. (b) Example 7.1.3 on p. 109. (c) Example 7.1.4 on p. 111.

24.7   REFERENCES

1. NCRP. *Limitation of Exposure to Ionizing Radiation, NCRP Report No. 116.* Bethesda, MD: NCRP; 1993.
2. NCRP. *Structural Shielding Design and Evaluation for Medical Use of X Rays and Gamma Rays of Energies up to 10 MeV, NCRP Report No. 49.* Bethesda, MD: NCRP; 1976.
3. NCRP. *Radiation Protection Design Guidelines for 0.1-100 MeV Particle Accelerator Facilities, NCRP Report No. 51.* Bethesda, MD: NCRP; 1977.
4. Kutcher GJ, Coia L, Gillin M, et al. Comprehensive QA for radiation oncology: Report of AAPM Radiation Therapy Committee Task Group 40. *Med Phys.* 1994; 21(4): 581-618.
5. Klein EE, Hanley J, Bayouth J, et al. Task Group 142 report: Quality assurance of medical accelerators. *Med Phys.* 2009; 36(9): 4197-4212.
6. Huq MS, Fraass BA, Dunscombe PB, et al. The report of Task Group 100 of the AAPM: Application of risk analysis methods to radiation therapy quality management. *Med Phys.* 2016; 43(7): 4209-4262.
7. NCRP. *Structural Shielding Design for Medical X-Ray Imaging Facilities, NCRP Report No. 147.* Bethesda, MD: NCRP; 2004.
8. NCRP. *Structural Shielding Design and Evaluation for Megavoltage X- and Gamma-Ray Radiotherapy Facilities, NCRP Report No. 151.* Bethesda, MD: NCRP; 2005.

Evolving Topics in Medical Physics

CONTENTS

Medical physics is an evolving field. The practice of medical physics is very different now from what it was a generation ago, or even a few years ago. New modalities are being introduced both for diagnosis and treatment, new techniques are being introduced to analyze images and improve the quality of radiation treatment, and the definition of "medical physics" has been expanded beyond conventional radiological physics. In this chapter, we present information about several new fields that are developing in which medical physicists play a significant role.

The new fields being discussed in this chapter are informatics, radiomics, machine learning, and Flash radiotherapy. All are being introduced into the clinical practice of medical physics and have been made feasible by the development of high-speed computers, large storage capabilities, and fast data transfer.

25.1 INFORMATICS

The past several years have seen a significant increase in information confronting the clinician in patient diagnosis and treatment. Consequently, there has been a need to systematize the acquisition, processing, and interpretation of information. The science of understanding these tasks is the role of informatics. *Informatics*, as applied to medicine, is defined to be the study of information in medical decision making. The various types of information confronting the clinician includes textual information such as patient demographics and physician reports, image information such as radiographic images and histopathological images, statistical information such as treatment records, and lexicographic information such as clinical and radiographic nomenclature.

One of the tasks of informatics is to formalize the description of information flow in radiation oncology. In order to do this we need to establish an *ontology*, defined as "a technology that is used to represent knowledge and information within a specified

DOI: 10.1201/9781003477457-25

domain or area of interest".[1] An ontology provides an organized way to collect and represent medical knowledge.

Let us identify some of the components of an ontology for a radiation oncology knowledge database. The names we give to these components should be self-evident. One such entity is *Concepts*. Concepts includes such components as "Case", "PTV", and "TreatmentBeam". Another entity is *Properties*, which are associated with Concepts. Some examples of Properties are "CreationDate" and "DoseUnits". One can then establish *Relationships* among Concepts. For example, "TreatmentPlan" and "TreatmentBeam" are related by "hasTreatmentBeam". Finally there are specific *Instances*, in which each of the Concepts and Properties are given values. With establishment of an ontology, an unambiguous understanding of concepts and their relationships can be provided.

It is important to be able to transfer information accurately across various platforms. For example, patient demographic information needs to be transferred from the hospital information system to the radiation oncology patient management system, and then to the imaging system(s), the treatment planning system, and the radiation therapy machine. It is very likely that multiple vendors are used to provide the clinic with these systems. How, then, does one transfer information from one system to another? It is analogous to a conversation in which one participant can speak and understand only English, while the second participant speaks and understands only Mandarin. Information standards provide a common language to transfer information accurately from one platform to another.

An example of such a standard is the *Digital Imaging and Communications in Medicine* (DICOM) standard, which was developed to handle radiological images. In the early 1980s, a combined effort by the *American College of Radiology* (ACR) and the *National Electrical Manufacturers Association* (NEMA) formed a committee to develop and maintain an imaging standard. Since that time many modifications have been made in the DICOM standard to accommodate new imaging modalities and expanded applications.

The image information is stored in a file as a two-dimensional array, but the file also has a header that provides additional information such as patient identification, image source, image resolution, *etc*. DICOM also identifies services that involve data transmission, such as storage into a *Picture Archival and Communications System* (PACS), query a database and retrieve images from the database, and modality worklist, a list of imaging procedures that have been scheduled to be performed.

In 1997, the DICOM Standard was extended to include objects used in radiation oncology, forming the DICOM-RT Standard. This extension include objects used specifically in radiation oncology, such as "RT Structure Set", "RT Dose", "RT Plan", and "RT Treatment Record". The meanings of each of these objects should be relatively self-evident. Manufacturers of systems that use the DICOM-RT Standard meet regularly in a *connectathon* to verify that information is transferrable. An organization known as *Integrating the Healthcare Enterprise in Radiation Oncology* (IHE-RO) oversees these connectathons, which test interoperability through the use of test cases.

Let us examine more closely the issue of information flow in a radiation oncology clinic. The paradigm for assessing the quality of information flow is the paper chart. On the paper chart, an individual records patient demographic information, dose prescription, and treatment record. In a separate record, one might have the treatment plan, and in yet another record, one might have the results of clinical examination. The paper chart has the advantage of being fast, easy to use and modify, adaptable for needs and workflow, and inexpensive. There is a high comfort level among users. On the other hand, the paper chart is not secure, nor is it conducive to real-time, collaborative decision making and outcome analysis.

Important for systematizing information transfer is a well-defined workflow. Radiation oncology handles many sources of data, many types of interactions using the data, and many users of the data. In addition, the radiation oncology practice handles many activities, including determining dose prescriptions, scheduling appointments, developing treatment plans, *etc.* These activities must be associated with appropriate users, and the point in the workflow in which the information is needed must be identified.

What, then, are the basic processes that make up workflow in the radiation oncology clinic?[2,3] Although most of the processes may seem obvious, it is necessary to identify the processes, identify what information is acquired in each process, and identify where the information goes after the process. We start with patient registration, the acquisition of relevant demographic information. This information is generally acquired prior to the first encounter the patient has with the clinic. Although this information was originally acquired directly from the patient and entered manually into the radiation oncology information system, a more desirable process integrates the patient information system with the hospital information system and transfers the data to the patient information system.

The next step in the workflow is the consultation with the radiation oncologist. In the consultation, the clinical information, including images used in treatment planning, is acquired and entered into the information system. The treatment plan is then developed based on the clinical information combined with the judgment of the radiation oncologist. Plan parameters are entered into the information system, where they can be transferred to the treatment machine and evaluated by the radiation oncologist. Finally, the radiation oncologist generally meets on a regular basis with the patient to monitor the clinical outcome.

A process that is run concurrently with the acquisition of patient information is the task of departmental scheduling. Scheduling of patient-related activities such as treatment delivery and chart review is important both in the radiation oncology clinic as well as in other departments and clinics. No longer is it necessary for the radiation oncology clinic personnel to go on a scavenger hunt for charts that may be sitting in another department, awaiting some sort of action from that department, while the patient is preparing for treatment in the busy radiation oncology clinic. Scheduling aids in the task of coordinating staff and resources, both in radiation oncology as well as in other departments and clinics. It would be highly desirable for the department scheduling system to be integrated with the hospital information system on a single server, ensuring that personnel in other departments are fully aware of what is happening to the patient in the radiation oncology clinic.

All of this information must be recorded; the way recording has traditionally been done is to use a chart. The process of charting records all data pertaining to the radiation treatment—for example, the patient history and physical, pathology, nursing notes, treatment record, and recorded images.

The next process is treatment simulation. This process involves the acquisition of images to delineate the target, identify the critical structures, and define the isocenter for patient setup. This process is described in much greater detail in Chapter 20 of this text. After simulation, the information acquired during simulation must then be transferred to the treatment planning computer.

Once these simulation images are acquired and transferred to the treatment planning computer, the process of treatment planning begins. In this process machine parameters for treatment such as table location, gantry angle, collimator angle, collimator setting, and monitor units, are determined. The process of treatment planning is also described in much greater detail in Chapter 20. Information acquired during treatment planning must then be transferred to the treatment machine.

The patient comes to the treatment machine for anywhere from one session to over thirty sessions. In these sessions the planned treatment is delivered, and the information regarding the machine settings, including the dose delivered, is transferred to the record and verify system.

Administrative services, such as billing, patient education, report generation, and data collection, are also part of the radiation oncology workflow. In addition, it is highly desirable to link patient billing to patient scheduling and code capture.

Quality assurance for the radiation oncology processes is performed on a regular basis, as identified in the previous chapter. Originally, quality assurance meant determining machine performance, but now it is necessary to include quality assurance of information flow and workflow.

With the workflow for the radiation oncology process established, it is also necessary to examine the information flow associated with this workflow and how this information is represented.[4] The first step in this information flow is the representation of volumetric image information, typically acquired via CT scanning. The image information is a data set that consists of a set of voxels (volume elements), each containing a number—the CT number—which can be correlated to the mean electron density in the patient volume element corresponding to the voxel. The image data then must be transferred to the treatment planning system. The amount of data to be transferred is worth noting; a typical CT study can consist of up to $100 \, MB$ of data; a four-dimensional CT study can take up to $1 \, GB$.

Next the radiation oncologist and treatment planner define target volumes and critical structure volumes on the image data set. Several representations of volumes are used in treatment planning. The volumes can be represented as contours on axial images, in the manner they are usually delineated. However, the volumes can also be represented as a polygonal mesh, which defines the surface of the volume. Another way to represent a volume of a structure is via bit coding, in which a voxel receives a value of 1 in the ith bit of a binary code number if the voxel is in the ith structure.

Thus, if a voxel lies inside structure 1, say the patient volume, and inside structure 4, say the left lung, then the bit code for that voxel is 00001001 in binary, or 9 in decimal form. Often multiple imaging modalities are used to assist in determining a structure set, for example, using CT to determine most patient anatomy, and ^{18}FDG-PET to determine volumes of high metabolic activity, characteristic of tumors. Accurate image registration is necessary in planning based on multi-modality imaging, and this registration may be either rigid or deformable, depending on the anatomy being imaged.

Based on the geometry of the target volume and the critical structures, the planner then determines the appropriate machine parameters. These parameters include the machine type, beam energy, the gantry and collimator angles, and the beam aperture. Often a *digitally reconstructed radiograph* (DRR) is obtained for each beam by tracing rays from a virtual point source, located at the position of the machine source, through the CT image, attenuating the beam intensity based on the value in the CT voxels along the ray path, and displaying the distribution of ray intensities in the plane of the image receptor. In addition, one often superimposes a projection of the target volume onto the DRR to ensure that the radiation field adequately covers the target volume.

Once the beam parameters have been determined, the radiation dose is calculated. A rectangular grid is set up to encompass the patient anatomy and some sort of dose model, as described in Chapter 18, is used to calculate the dose at each point on the grid. If it is necessary to account for motion, the dose is calculated on each phase of motion (see Chapter 21); the grid is then deformed on each phase, and the doses at each point on a reference grid are interpolated, and then accumulated.[5]

The resulting dose distributions can then be depicted either as isodose lines, dose clouds, or dose-volume histograms (DVH), enabling the radiation oncologist to review the plan and, if appropriate, approve it. The plan information is then transferred to the information system from which it is further transferred to the treatment machine.

We conclude this section by identifying two trends in informatics.[6] One of these trends is the opportunity for data aggregation. As long as data is stored in an information system and a common protocol exists for representation of the data enabling accurate inter-institutional transfer of data, then it is feasible to collect and analyze "big data" from many patients and multiple institutions. The second trend is to use cloud-based information systems with a common server for storage of plan information. Storing patient and plan information in the cloud would significantly facilitate multi-institutional studies that may not be feasible at present because of data limitations.

25.2   RADIOMICS

Radiomics is a process based on the principle that the image appearance of a tumor is somewhat related to the tumor phenotype and hence, to the outcome of treatment when the radiation is delivered. When applying principles of radiomics to an image, one extracts a large number of imaging features from a radiographic image and associates these imaging features with disease traits. Radiomics has several distinct advantages over biopsy for determining disease traits. Application of radiomics, unlike acquiring a biopsy, is a non-invasive procedure, but gives a total 3D picture of the tumor. The application of radiomics is based on images already acquired in the clinic, and if the images are acquired multiple times during the course of treatment, and we can demonstrate a correlation between image features and tumor features, we are able to capture the tumor's appearance over time and space.

There are some challenges to the use of radiomics in assessing tumors. Radiomics is image-based, and digitized images have a finite resolution, certainly no better than $1\,mm$ for most imaging modalities. Histopathology, on the other hand, is analyzed on a microscopic level, so the question remains whether or not a macroscopic assessment of the tumor is valid on a microscopic level. A second concern is that patients are heterogeneous, requiring a large amount of data to make any sort of viable correlations. This concern may be alleviated, however, by the use of "big data", as discussed in the next section of this chapter. Finally, image acquisition protocols are heterogeneous, not only among institutions but also among modalities within the same institution. Consequently, comparisons between protocols may be difficult; even comparisons between the same patient at different points in their treatment may also be difficult.

Radiomics is thus based on the hypothesis that quantitative image features are related to underlying gene expression and phenotype. If the hypothesis is verified, these image features can be used to provide a comprehensive quantification of the tumor and provide patient-specific predictions of the outcome of a specific treatment, the outcome being genetic expression, treatment response, overall survival, or freedom from metastases.

The radiomics workflow is as follows: First, the patient is imaged, generally using a three-dimensional imaging modality such as CT, MRI, or PET.

Next, *regions of interest* (ROI), from which features are measured, are segmented. Several techniques exist for image segmentation. One such technique allows an expert to delineate the ROI manually. One issue that persists in manual segmentation is both inter-observer as well as intra-observer variability. Alternatively, a semi-automatic segmentation method can be used, in which the observer selects a seed point, known to be in the ROI, and the segmentation algorithm continues to delineate the boundary between voxels inside the ROI and those outside the ROI. Finally, in fully automated segmentation, there is no observer intervention. The segmentation method can affect the determination of features; it might be necessary to eliminate some features because of non-reproducibility. The use of semi-automatic or automatic segmentation may increase reproducibility, but the choice of segmentation algorithm may affect the radiomics features. Moreover, some features are volume-dependent, and one may have to incorporate a volume-dependent normalization factor into the evaluation of the selected features. Finally, segmentation can affect features. Inconsistent contouring of the ROI can result in large changes for certain features.[7] Even different autosegmentation algorithms can yield different results. Consequently, when performing a radiomics study, it is recommended that the same algorithm be used for all images in a study.[8]

The next step in the radiomics workflow is image processing, used to reduce noise, improve feature usefulness, and increase reproducibility. Image processing includes such tasks as smoothing, enhancement, deblurring, thresholding, and adjusting the bin width in the histogram used to reduce the bit length of the image voxel values. Adaptive histogram equalization, a process by which the bin widths are adjusted so that the same number of voxels are in each bin, can also be used to process the image. Image processing affects texture matrices and thus feature values. The differences in feature values due to differences in the imaging device can be removed with appropriate processing.

The core of the radiomics workflow is feature extraction. Many features can be extracted from a digitized image. Figure (25.1) illustrates an example of a digitized image consisting of a set of pixels with their intensities identified, along with a histogram of pixel values. Common features include first-order statistics based on the histogram of voxel values. Such features include maximum, minimum, mean, standard deviation, entropy, skewness, and kurtosis. Here one might use all or part of the intensity distribution in the ROI; the spatial distribution is not evaluated. One hopes that there will be a difference in the shape of histograms for tumors with and without the specific features one is seeking.

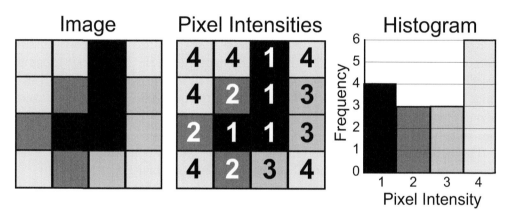

FIGURE 25.1: An "image" along with its pixel intensities labeled and then depicted in a histogram.

One can then extract second-order statistics that assess the *texture* of the ROI voxels, characterizing the spatial relationships between pixel intensities. One example of a second-order textural feature is the *Gray Level Co-occurrence Matrix* (GLCM or COM). The COM is a plot of frequencies of spatial relationships. It is analogous to the histogram in that the histogram is a plot of frequencies of voxel intensities. The COM is directional and step-size dependent and is typically symmetric. There are various ways to define a COM; we shall consider a very simple one.

Consider the simple 4×4 image shown at the top of Fig. (25.2). The numbers in the boxes represent the pixel intensities in the image. We imagine drawing a horizontal line through the first row of intensities, representing an angle of 0°. We can move from one pixel to the next along this line, either toward the right or toward the left. Since the pixel values range from 1 through 4, there are four possible pixel values, which means that the COM will be a 4×4 matrix. We will consider a step size of 1 pixel in this simple definition of the COM (this is the "1" after the angle in the COM heading). The (row,column) = (1,1) element in the $(0^o,1)$ COM will be the

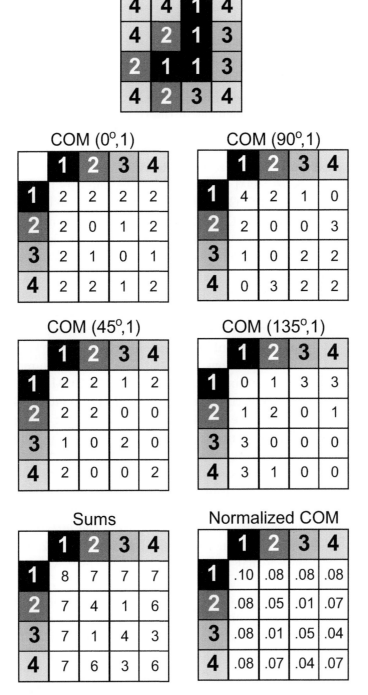

FIGURE 25.2: Co-occurrence matrices (COMs) evaluated at 0°, 45°, 90°, and 135°. (All angles are measured counter-clockwise from the horizontal.) Also shown are the matrix of sums and the normalized matrix.

number of times we move from a pixel value of 1 to another pixel value of 1 when we take one step toward the right or left within the image matrix. In the first row of the image matrix, there are two instances of moving from 1 to 1: one when we move toward the right and one when we move toward the left. In this case, both of these instances involve the same two pixels in the image. Moving our horizontal line down to each of the other rows shows that there are no other occurrences of moving from 1 to 1 in either direction. Thus, the total number of $1 \rightarrow 1$ occurrences for a 0° line in the image is 2. This is then the value of the (1,1) element in the (0°,1) COM.

Let's now look at the (2,3) element in the (0°,1) COM, so we are looking for a pixel-value change from 2 to 3. In the first row of the image matrix there is no such occurrence; no is there such an occurrence in the second or third rows. However, there is 1 such occurrence moving from left to right in the fourth row. The value of the (2,3) element in the 0° COM is therefore 1. The numbers in the white boxes in the upper-left matrix labeled "COM (0°,1)" (the COM for the 0° line with a 1-pixel step size) represent the values of the 0° 1-pixel-step-size component of the full COM. Note that the (1,1) element equals 2 and the (2,3) element equals 1, as we determined above. In like manner, you should be able to verify the remaining values shown in the 0° COM. Figure (25.2) also shows the COM components corresponding to lines drawn at 45°, 90°, and 135°, where all angles are measured counter-clockwise from the horizontal; you should verify the values in all of these matrices.

The four component matrices shown in Fig. (25.2) contain a good bit of data, even for this simple 4×4 image with only four possible pixel values. Keep in mind that these values tell us about the relations between pixels and their immediate neighbors as a result of our simple single-pixel step size rule for the COM. The values in these four component matrices can be combined into a single 4×4 matrix—the full COM—by adding together all four of the COMs and then normalizing the resulting matrix so that the sum of all of its values is 1. Fig. (25.2) shows the matrix of sums as well as the normalized COM (rounded to two decimal places).[a] Note that this final COM is symmetric, as mentioned above. Since the normalized sum of the COMs involves moving horizontally, vertically and diagonally from a given pixel intensity in the image, the elements in the normalized COM represent the probabilities of the corresponding change in intensity, which contributes to the *texture* of the image. For example, the (3,1) element of the normalized COM in Fig. (25.2) is 0.08, telling us that there is an 8% chance that an image pixel of intensity value 3 has a nearest neighbor pixel in any direction that has an intensity value of 1.

Even though we have combined four COMs into one normalized matrix, there can still be a lot of data within that matrix for a real image. The data in the normalized matrix can be combined into single values that can reflect various types of texture in the image. These numerical values are called *Haralick texture features* and can quantify features such as homogeneity and contrast in the image.[9,10]

Another textural feature is the *gray-level run-length matrix* (GLRLM or RLM). Many features of the RLM correlate with those of the COM. To evaluate the RLM,

---

[a]Each element in the Sums matrix is the sum of all of the corresponding elements in the four component COMs. The sum of all of the elements in the Sums matrix is 84. Dividing each element in the Sums matrix by 84 then yields the full normalized COM.

RLM (0°)

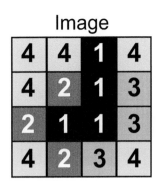

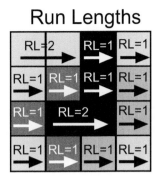

FIGURE 25.3: The matrix on the left is the 4×4 image matrix of pixel intensity values. In the center is the image showing the horizontal run-length regions for different pixel intensity values. The 4×3 matrix of white boxes on the right is the corresponding $0°$ gray-level run-length matrix.

one starts by determining the $0°$ (horizontal) RLM. For example, in the image matrix illustrated in Fig. (25.3), there are 4 pixels with an intensity value of 1; the horizontal run length of 2 of these pixels is 1, and 1 set of 2 pixels has a run length of 2 (two in a row). Consequently, the entry in the first row (corresponding to a pixel intensity value of 1) and first column (corresponding to the run length of 1) has a value of 2, and the first row-second column entry is 1. (Note that a pixel value of 1 with a run length of 2 cannot also count as two pixel values of 1 with run lengths of 1—we only use the longest run length corresponding to a given set of pixels.) Next, there are 3 pixels with a value of 2 and $0°$ run length 1, and no pixels with a value of 2 and run length 2, so the second row has a value of 3 in column 1 and 0 in column 2. In a similar manner, the remainder of the RLM is filled. The number of rows in the RLM is determined by the number of pixel values, whereas the number of columns is determined by the maximum run length of pixel values in the image. Analogous to the calculation of the COM, we calculate run lengths at angles of $0°$, $45°$, $90°$, and $135°$, and then combine and normalize the results. (We kept 3 columns in the RLM of Fig. 25.3, corresponding to a maximum value of RL = 3, since the $90°$ RLM has a single RL = 3 value for a pixel value of 1.) Many features can be extracted from the RLM depending on whether one wishes to emphasize noise (emphasis on short runs) or signal (emphasis on long runs).

Another feature incorporated in a radiomics study is the *gray-level size zone matrix* (GLSZM), designed to quantify regions of contiguous pixels in image. The GLSZM is similar to the GLRLM, but with *zone* sizes instead of run lengths as columns. For a pixel to be in the same zone as another pixel, it must be adjacent to that pixel horizontally, vertically, or diagonally. Thus, for example, in Fig. (25.4), we see that, for a pixel value of 1, there is a single zone containing 4 pixels. Consequently, the values placed in row 1 of the GLSZM are all zero with the exception of column 4, whose value is 1 (since there is 1 zone of size 4). Make sure you understand the remaining entries in the GLSZM shown in Fig. (25.4).

The GLSZM does not have to be calculated for multiple directions since it already incorporates all directions in the image matrix. Features extracted from the GLSZM are the same as the features extracted from the RLM.

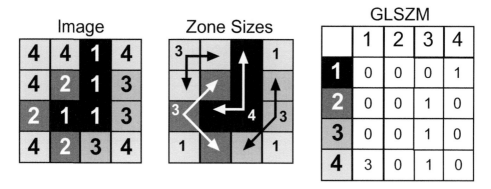

FIGURE 25.4: The matrix on the left is the 4×4 image matrix of pixel intensity values. In the center is the image showing the different zone sizes for the various pixel intensity values. The 4×4 matrix of white boxes on the right is the corresponding gray-level size zone matrix (GLSZM).

The final second-order statistical quantity that we shall address is the *neighborhood gray-tone difference matrix* (NGTDM or NDM). The NDM is a matrix consisting of a single column, each row of which corresponds to a different pixel intensity value. The value placed in a cell of this column matrix is the difference between the pixel intensity value and the average value of pixel intensities in the neighborhood around the selected intensity value. The NDM is specific to a chosen neighborhood size—for example, one could select a neighborhood three pixels deep surrounding a given pixel to generate the NDM. The method for calculating the NDM is as follows:

I. Ignore pixels on the boundary of the image and only include pixels that have a full neighborhood surrounding them.

II. Select a pixel intensity value to evaluate and identify a pixel with that intensity value.

III. Calculate the average value of the intensity of the pixels in the neighborhood surrounding the selected pixel.

IV. For each pixel with an intensity of the specified value, calculate the difference between pixel intensity value and average neighborhood values.

V. Sum the differences to obtain the value for the row in the NDM corresponding to the selected pixel intensity.

Parameters that one can adjust in the calculation of the NDM include pixel intensity binning, neighborhood size, the choice of averaging over a two-dimensional neighborhood versus a three-dimensional neighborhood, and whether or not to include border pixels.

So far, we have calculated global features, calculated once for the segmented tumor. However, one could also calculate these features locally in neighborhoods of predetermined size covering the tumor. One could then perform a statistical analysis on quantities calculated in the local neighborhoods to determine the heterogeneity of the tumor.

Higher-order statistics can also be used, in which filters such as wavelets or Laplacian of Gaussian filters, are applied to extract repetitive or non-repetitive data. First or second order features are then calculated after filtering. The *Laplacian of Gaussian* (LoG) filter, for example, is used to highlight edges in an image. The filter has the form

$$LoG\,(x,y) = -\frac{1}{\pi\sigma^4}\left[1 - \frac{x^2+y^2}{2\sigma^2}\right]exp\left(\frac{x^2+y^2}{2\sigma^2}\right),\qquad(25.1)$$

but is normally discretized into a matrix, which is then convolved with the image matrix. The LoG takes the second derivative of the image so that where the image is uniform, the LoG will give zero, but at edges, the LoG will give a value of 0 away from the edge, positive just on one side of the edge, negative just on the other side, and 0 on the edge itself. The parameter σ, a measure of the width of the Gaussian, changes the filter scale. Using a small value of the Gaussian width gives a sharper image, but one that is rather noisy, whereas, using a larger value reduces the noise but also reduces the sharpening. Once the image has been filtered using the LoG, one can then calculate features from the filtered image histogram or texture.

A wavelet transform can also be used to process the image. Wavelet transforms are analogous to Fourier transforms, but, unlike the sines and cosines of Fourier transforms, wavelets have finite support, that is, they only go to 0 at some finite distance from the center. Figure $(25.5)^{11}$ illustrates an example of a wavelet basis. Analogous to the use of the LoG, the wavelet transform filters the image matrix, from which can once again calculate features from the filtered image histogram or texture.

Shape features can also be used to characterize a segmented image. For example, less spherical tumors are commonly believed to correlate with a higher probability

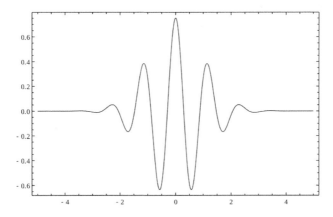

FIGURE 25.5: An example of a wavelet that can be convolved with an image to highlight edges of regions of interest. (Open Source.)

of metastasis and poorer outcome so attempts can be made to quantify a structure's deviation from a sphere and correlate it with the likelihood of metastatic disease. Examples of shape parameters include volume, surface area, mass, maximum diameter, and so forth.

Although most radiomics studies have been based on CT images, studies have also used various other imaging modalities. One significant problem when using multiple modalities is reproducibility of features extracted from these images acquired under different conditions. One study has shown, however, that variations in imaging features acquired on multiple scanners were comparable to variations from images on the same scanner, and that variations due to differences in pixel size are correctable with appropriate image processing.[12] A more significant problem has been observed in variability of image features extracted from PET images.[13] Another study examined features of MR images of various phantoms acquired under different protocols and found that wavelet and COM features correctly differentiated images regardless of imaging parameters.[14]

Clinical applications of radiomics include patient stratification to determine alternative treatments, early prediction of treatment response, and monitoring of treatment efficacy. In one example of the use of radiomics, the investigators analyzed retrospective data from a protocol that examined the effects of dose escalation on lung cancer patients.[15] The study found no benefit and possible harm in dose escalation for these patients. However, a radiomics study found features that identified sub-groups of patients whose survival time increased from dose escalation and another sub-group of patients whose survival time decreased by dose escalation. Another study examined the use of radiomics to achieve a more accurate prediction of malignant nodules from screening CT images for lung cancer.[16] A problem with screening CT images is the high number of false positives. Fewer than 4% of the pulmonary nodules detected on these images are actually cancers. The application of radiomics increased the accuracy of some patient groups (around 55% of patients) to over 90%.

Radiomics is a potentially useful tool for improving risk stratification, understanding genetic expression, and predicting patient-specific response to treatment. The advantages of radiomics are that it is non-invasive and uses routinely obtained images. However, some unknowns remain. It is not known, for example, why some features provide prognostic capability while other features may not have relevance. Nor is it known how to optimize features algorithmically. The role of multimodality imaging is not yet clearly defined, nor is the role of machine learning. Consequently, radiomics remains an open book whose role in the clinic is not yet specified.

25.3 MACHINE LEARNING

Machine learning (ML) is the third topic we will address in this chapter on evolving topics in medical physics. Machine learning is one approach toward the use of artificial intelligence (AI). Early forms of AI were rule-based, that is, the logic path followed the algorithm "If A, then B". In contrast to rule-based AI, ML is an application of AI that provides systems with the ability to automatically learn and improve from experience without being explicitly programmed. In that respect, ML is very different from traditional programming. In traditional programming, data and programs are provided as input, while the computer generates the output, whereas in ML, data and output from a training set of input are provided as input; the computer then generates the program to handle new data.

There are two types of ML, *supervised learning* and *unsupervised learning*. Supervised learning uses data sets that have specific inputs and specific outputs. The ML algorithm used in supervised learning is iterative. An initial guess is made as to the parameters in the algorithm and an output is calculated. The parameters are then adjusted according to the algorithm to improve the fit, and the calculation is repeated. Adjustment of parameters, calculation of output, and comparison of calculated output with true output is the repeated until a desired degree of accuracy is achieved.

Supervised ML consists of the steps of training, feature extraction, algorithm implementation, and machine prediction. In the training step, input data is entered into the ML algorithm as well as output data. The features of note are then extracted from the input data. By adjusting the parameters in the ML algorithm, the algorithm tries to fit the calculated output data to the actual output data. Finally, the algorithm along with its new parameters is tested against another set of output data to assess the predictive ability of the model.

A form of ML that has drawn some attention in medical physics is *deep learning* (DL). DL differs from ML in that in DL, several layers of hidden nodes are used rather than a single hidden layer.

In the validation of the ML algorithm, one takes a series of known inputs and compares the predicted output values to the actual output values. However, before we discuss what the ML algorithm does with that comparison, we need to define several terms that describe the differences between predicted output and actual output. Consider a situation in which output is binary, with values of either "true" or "false". Four possible outcomes exist: If the prediction is "true", and the reality is "true", we have a *true positive* (TP). A prediction of "false" combined with a reality of "true" gives us a *false negative* (FN). A predicted value of "true" combined with a "false" reality is a *false positive* (FP), whereas a prediction of "false" and an actual value of "false" gives us a *true negative* (TN). With these four outcome values, we can define four measures of accuracy. *Model accuracy* is defined as the number of correct predictions (TP+TN) divided by the total number of predictions (TP+FP+TN+FN). The opposite of model accuracy is *misclassification rate*, defined as the number of incorrect predictions (FP+FN) divided by the total number of predictions. The *sensitivity* is defined as the number of true positives divided by the total number of true positives plus false negatives, whereas the *specificity* is defined to be the number of true negatives divided by the total number of true negatives plus false positives. To summarize,

$$\text{Model Accuracy} = \frac{TP + TN}{TP + FP + TN + FN}; \tag{25.2}$$

$$\text{Misclassification Rate} = \frac{FP + FN}{TP + FP + TN + FN}; \tag{25.3}$$

$$\text{Sensitivity} = \frac{TP}{TP + FN} \; ; \tag{25.4}$$

$$\text{Specificity} = \frac{TN}{TN + FP} \; . \tag{25.5}$$

The next step in assessing accuracy of the algorithm is to vary the discrimination threshold and generate a *Receiver Operating Characteristic* (ROC) curve, which is a plot of *Sensitivity vs.* $(1 - Specificity)$, as the discrimination threshold is varied. Since the *Sensitivity* is also called the *True Positive Rate* (TPR), and $(1-Specificity)$ is also called the *False Positive Rate* (FPR), we can also say that the ROC curve is a plot of *TPR vs. FPR*. An ideal ROC curve would be close to the upper left corner of the plot, with the Sensitivity and Specificity both equal to 1. The *area under the ROC* curve (AUROC or AUC, for *Area Under the Curve*) is a measure of the quality of the algorithm. Figure (25.6) shows examples of ROC curves.[17]

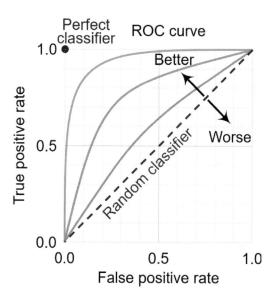

FIGURE 25.6: Examples of ROC curves. Note that the closer a curve is to the 45° line, the less reliable the algorithm. (Open Source.)

In validating a model, one withholds a sample of data from the training data set to perform the model testing. Generally one has insufficient data to do a complete validation, so some compromises are necessary, generally using some of the training data to add to the testing data set. Finally, once a model has been determined, it is necessary to check if the model is still behaving as intended; if not, it may be necessary to rebuild the model.

Unsupervised learning differs from supervised learning in that there is no classification of data; the algorithm creates its own classification.

A typical neural network used in ML consists of layers of *nodes* connected to other layers of nodes; nodes are connected to nodes by *neurons*, which are units for transferring information from one layer of nodes to another. Figure (25.7) is a schematic representation of such a neural network. The first layer receives the input data. It then transfers information to one or more hidden layers. The hidden layers perform computations on the information gathered from the input layers. Every node in the hidden layer(s) is connected with each node in the input layer. Part of the consideration in the design of a neural network is determining the optimal number of hidden layers as well as the number of neurons for each layer. Every node in the hidden layer(s) is then connected with each node in the output layer. The process of training the neural network consists of varying the weights connecting the nodes in such a manner that the values of the output nodes calculated using the neural network accurately reproduces the actual values of the output in the training set.

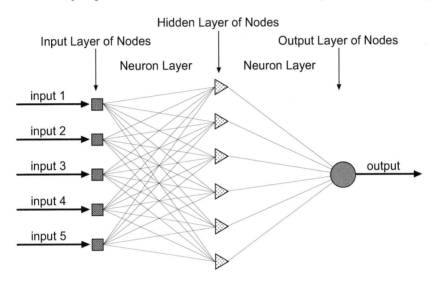

FIGURE 25.7: A typical neural network with 5 input nodes, a single output node, and a hidden layer of 6 nodes. Nodes are connected to other nodes by neurons.

The key to the operation of a neural network is the manner in which information is transferred through the hidden nodes. If we let x_i be the value in the ith input node and w_{ij} be the weight to be determined that connects the ith input node with the jth hidden node, then the value y_j that is given to the jth hidden node is a linear combination of the values in the input nodes, or

$$y_j = \sum_{i=1}^{m} x_i w_{ij} \,, \tag{25.6}$$

where m is the total number of input nodes. The value then transferred to the next layer of nodes, either another layer of hidden nodes or the output node, is 1 if y_j is greater than a threshold value and 0 if y_j is less than the threshold—that is, a step function. The "learning" component of ML is then the process of varying the weights and the threshold values so that the learned output value is equal to the actual output value from the training set. Although, in this discussion, a step function has been used as the transfer function, a more practical transfer function would be one for which the derivative can be readily calculated analytically, such as a sigmoidal function or hyperbolic tangent function.

Care must be taken in constructing an ML model, in particular, in the number of nodes and layers—and hence, the number of connection weights—in the model. If too few connection weights are present in the model, the model may exhibit insufficient flexibility, giving rise to bias. On the other hand, if too many connection weights are present, then the model will be too sensitive to the sample and may result in too much noise.

An example of the use of ML in medical physics can be found in the evaluation of portal images used in radiation oncology to verify that the patient positioning is correct and the radiation beam is irradiating the desired region. In the training phase of the ML process, a set of portal images is reviewed and labeled either "acceptable" or "unacceptable". In addition to extracting labels from the portal images, one can also extract features such as distance of field edge to specified bony landmarks. This information is then run through the ML algorithm and a predictive model is developed. In the test phase, a portal image is entered into the system and features are extracted. The input data is then run through the model and output; either "acceptable" or "unacceptable" is obtained and compared to the judgment of an expert reviewer.

Another example of ML is the detection of lesions in radiographic images. In the training set, the images are segmented and features of the image are extracted. The output is either positive (a lesion is identified) or negative (no lesion is identified). The data is then processed through the ML algorithm. The model is then tested using test images.

The study of the applicability of deep learning to medical physics is an area undergoing significant progress.

25.4 FLASH RADIOTHERAPY

Contributed by Wendy Smith, Ph.D., Director, FLASH Research Portfolio for Varian, a Siemens Healthineers company

What is FLASH Radiotherapy?

This text describes many of the advancements in radiotherapy that have improved outcomes for patients in recent decades. Unfortunately, the dose delivered by radiotherapy is still limited by the toxicity to nearby healthy tissues. Recent work suggests that delivering radiotherapy at ultra-high-dose rates may better spare normal tissues while having the same tumoricidal effect. The *FLASH Effect* is a biological effect, defined by the improved sparing of normal tissues with antitumor efficacy equivalent to that of conventional dose rate radiotherapy at the same dose level. In addition, the shorter treatment delivery time for FLASH radiotherapy may improve throughput and limit the effect of motion during irradiation. Although FLASH is a promising direction, there is much work to be done to investigate the biological mechanisms of action, understand the circumstances in which the FLASH Effect occurs and effectively bring FLASH radiotherapy into the clinic.

Ultra-high-dose rate (UHDR) irradiation is a physical definition for FLASH and is most commonly cited as a dose rate higher than $40\,Gy/s$, although we will see that defining a FLASH dose rate is a non-trivial problem. Modern linear accelerators deliver *conventional dose rates* between 600 and $2400\,MU/min$, which is 600 to $2400\,cGy/min$ (0.1 to $0.4\,Gy/s$) at isocenter at d_{max}. The FLASH dose rate is, therefore, at least two orders of magnitude greater than conventional dose rates.

History

The FLASH Effect was first reported in 1959, by Dewey and Boag.[18] Reports at that time indicated that ultra-high dose rate radiotherapy had a protective effect in bacteria and mammalian cells compared to conventional irradiation.[18,19,20] Early experiments suggested this protective effect was related to the oxygen effect (see Chapter 3). At that time, most studies were performed on cells in vitro and differential effects between tumors and normal tissues were not reported. Technological constraints on FLASH beam production also limited work at this time.

Modern FLASH

Modern interest in the FLASH Effect was re-ignited in 2014 by a paper by Favaudon[21] by examining the FLASH Effect on both normal tissues and tumors in mice. They compared acute pneumonitis and late lung fibrosis after bilateral thorax irradiation in 240 mice that received sham irradiation or a single dose of 15 or $17\,Gy$ conventional irradiation with Cs-137 gamma rays or FLASH $4.5\,MeV$ electrons. The researchers observed a "complete lack of acute pneumonitis and late lung fibrosis" in mice treated with FLASH at the same doses that cause pulmonary fibrosis at conventional dose rates. Their dose escalation study of 16 to $30\,Gy$ FLASH demonstrated that a $30\,Gy$ FLASH dose produced lung fibrosis similar to a $17\,Gy$ conventional dose. Finally, the scientists irradiated three different tumor models in mice and found that tumor growth after FLASH irradiation was comparable to that after conventional irradiation.

Since this publication, various studies have demonstrated the FLASH Effect in a variety of assays, animals (including wild-type mice, zebrafish embryos, mini-pigs and cats) and tumor models, for ultra-high dose rate x-ray, proton and electron irradiation. The magnitude of the FLASH Effect probably depends on the organs affected, but it has been seen in both acute-responding organs (gut, hematopoietic system) and late-responding organs (brain, lung, skin). Reviews such as those by Wilson, Friedl, Bouhis, and Schüler helpfully summarize this work.[22,23,24,25]

The magnitude of the FLASH Effect is a matter for on-going investigation. Perhaps the most comprehensive trial to date was conducted by Sørensen.[26,27] This group investigated tumor control and normal tissue toxicity of proton FLASH in a mouse model. In the first paper (2021), hind legs of 301 mice were treated with transmission proton pencil beam scanning (the target was in the entrance plateau not the Bragg Peak region) using $244\,MeV$ conventional dose rate field or a $250\,MeV$ FLASH. Single fraction doses were delivered: conventional 23.2 to $39.2\,Gy$; FLASH 31.2 to

$53.5\,Gy$. The severity of acute moist desquamation to the skin of the foot within 25 days post irradiation was evaluated and full dose response curves were generated with 7 to 21 mice per dose point. 44–58% higher dose with FLASH produced the same biological response as compared to the conventional dose rate. In their second paper (2022), the feet of 162 mice were subcutaneously implanted with mammary carcinoma, and the feet were irradiated with physical doses of 40–$60\,Gy$ (8 to 14 mice per dose point). Tumor control was similar for conventional and FLASH. Radiation induced fibrosis (a late radiation effect) was also investigated in mice whose tumors were controlled and a normal tissue sparing effect of FLASH was found, with a dose modifying factor of 1.14. (*Dose modifying factor* is the ratio of doses with and without modifying agents, causing the same level of biological effect.) In contrast, Diffenderfer[28] examined proton FLASH in the small intestine of mice. They found a stronger FLASH Effect in fibrosis (a late effect) compared to crypt proliferation (an early effect).

There are certainly limits to the FLASH Effect, as demonstrated in a recent series of papers by Vozenin.[29,30] This group estimate the FLASH Effect in their first paper. They reported treating six companion animal cats with histologically confirmed nasal squamous cell carcinoma with a single-fraction radiotherapy under a dose-escalation scheme (25 to $41\,Gy$). Complete responses were observed for all cats (100%) at 6 months, although two cats later recurred. All of the cats experienced permanent depilation in the radiation field, but the authors reported "No other permanent, late toxicity, or outside-radiation field side effect has been observed", in up to 1 year follow up. Based on this study, the same group began a trial comparing a standard-of-care veterinary treatment having 10 fractions of $4.8\,Gy$ each (90% isodose) to a single-fraction FLASH treatment of $30\,Gy$ (90% isodose). In the FLASH treatment arm, retrospective dose calculations indicated hot spots of up to $42\,Gy$ for the single-fraction dose. The trial was prematurely interrupted due to maxillary bone necrosis, which occurred 9 to 15 months after radiotherapy in 3 of 7 cats treated with FLASH-radiotherapy (43%), as compared with 0 of 9 cats treated with standard-of-care. All cats were tumor-free at 1 year in both arms, with one cat progressing later in each arm. This result reminds us of the realistic limitations of FLASH-radiotherapy.

Humans

The first patient was treated with FLASH in 2019 with positive results.[31] Other clinical trials are in progress; current U.S. trials can be identified by searching for "FLASH Radiation" on the U.S. National Library of Medicine Clinical Trials website.[32]

FLASH Dose Rate Definitions

The induction of the FLASH Effect may depend on dose rate, total dose, pulse rate, fractionation, and modality of radiation. The complex physics of FLASH beams and the multiple definitions of dose rate may contribute to some studies not showing the FLASH Effect in their biological systems.[22,25,33] With a variety of irradiation types being investigated for FLASH, it becomes difficult to ensure consistent definition of an ultra-high dose rate.

The simplest and most stringent definition of dose rate is the average or *field dose rate*, which is simply the total dose divided by the time it takes to deliver that dose. The most common quoted value for a FLASH dose rate is $40\,Gy/s$. FLASH beams may be pulsed, quasi-continuous or continuous. For pulsed beams, parameters such as the dose per pulse, duty cycle and pulse length may influence the FLASH Effect.[34,25] Bourhis[33] reviewed a number of flash papers and found that whether the FLASH Effect was observed or not appeared to depend not only on the average dose rate but also dose, dose-rate within the pulse, and overall time of irradiation. A variety of FLASH dose rate definitions are currently being used, including instantaneous and local or voxel-based dose rates. Overall treatment times for FLASH are generally of the order of a few hundred milliseconds for FLASH and seconds or minutes for conventional dose rates.

Delivery Mechanisms

The majority of FLASH animal studies to date have used pulsed electron beams. (See Chapter 15 for a discussion of treatment beam generation.) Electron FLASH beams may be generated using modified high energy linear accelerators or intraoperative irradiators. In FLASH, each pulse may deliver $1\,Gy$ or more in a few milliseconds, with extremely high dose rates within these pulses ($> 10^5\,Gy/s$). The delivered dose rate will depend on the pulse length, dose per pulse, frequency (or repetition rate) of the pulses, and so on. A complete description of electron FLASH beams should include beam energy, beam structure, total dose, mean dose rate, instantaneous (intra-pulse) dose rate, pulse repetition frequency, dose per pulse, pulse width, duration of exposure, field size, percentage depth dose, dose profiles, and irradiated volume. Unfortunately, complete parameters are not available for all studies.[25]

The majority of patient radiotherapy treatments today use photons. Photons are produced by an electron beam hitting a high atomic number target. The conversion process is inefficient and heats the target, limiting the dose rate of the photons. Synchrotrons provide alternative beam sources, although access to these is limited. X-ray FLASH sources are of great interest, particularly for small animal irradiators and multiple system types have been proposed. The beam properties depend on the mechanism of generating x-rays—see, for example, the work by Montay-Gruel.[35]

Proton beams are produced in cyclotrons, which generate a beam with a single fixed energy. The lower energies to position the Bragg Peak within the patient are generated using a beam degrader and an energy selection system. This process results in a significant loss in beam current for lower energies. Some proton FLASH studies[26,27] use the transmission mode at the maximum energy (treat using the plateau region of the beam) rather than the Bragg peak. Isochronous cyclotron proton beams are pulsed beams having high frequency, short pulses with lower dose rates within each micropulse, and so are considered *quasi-continuous*, while synchrocyclotron beams are considered *pulsed* with shorter, higher-dose pulses.

Many proton systems use pencil beam scanning (PBS) to deliver dose, meaning that the dose to a point in the tissue is accumulated from dose delivery to nearby spots, while distant spots may not contribute any significant dose to that point. In such cases, a voxel-based dose rate may be appropriate. For example, PBS dose rate is defined as a voxel's dose divided by an effective irradiation time.[36] Each voxel's effective irradiation time starts when the cumulative dose rises above a chosen threshold value, and stops when its cumulative dose reaches its total dose minus the same threshold value. The overall dose rate for a volume is further quantified by the percentage of voxels with this value exceeding a flash dose rate, e.g., $40\,Gy/s$.

Clinical Implementation of FLASH

FLASH is a promising technique, but more work remains to be done to allow its transition to the clinic. While the FLASH Effect has been shown in a wide variety of animal models and tissues, many unanswered questions remain, including investigating the impact of delivering dose with multiple beams. Few studies have investigated fractionated delivery. Some have suggested that a minimum dose per fraction may be required to elicit the FLASH Effect, or that the FLASH Effect may increase with dose.[37] The generation of FLASH treatment plans with plan quality equivalent to current clinical plans continues to be an active area of research.

Dose measurement is also a challenge because many conventional dosimeters saturate and behave non-linearly at ultrahigh dose rates. In slower, fractionated conventional treatments, positioning and motion errors may average out over the course of treatment, but that is not the case for FLASH, which might someday be delivered in a handful or even a single delivery lasting a few hundred milliseconds. Emergency procedures also must evolve for the extremely short beams.

Oxygen Depletion Hypothesis

The fast delivery of FLASH fields also applies a new approach in radiochemistry and radiobiology. The deposition of energy from radiation interactions in tissue takes under $10^{-15}\,s$, physical-chemical interactions between 10^{-15} and $10^{-12}\,s$, various chemical interactions between 10^{-12} and $10^{-5}\,s$ (see Fig. 25.8, from Vozenin).[38] The free radicals have a lifetime around $10^{-5}\,s$. In FLASH, the total delivery time is much shorter than the time for oxygen to rediffuse.[29] Recall from Chapter 3 that oxygen is a potent radiosensitizer, and that well oxygenated cells are more sensitive to radiotherapy than fully hypoxic cells by up to a factor of three (the oxygen enhancement ratio).

In the early days of FLASH research, it was proposed that FLASH affected cells differently from conventional irradiation by causing transient local oxygen depletion (see the references in Schüler[25]). If tumors are already hypoxic, this might explain how FLASH beams have the same effect on tumors but less effect on oxygenated normal tissue. This theory continues to be hotly debated in the literature. Montay-Gruel[39] indicated that FLASH produced lower levels of reactive oxygen species when examining the neurocognitive effects of FLASH in mice. They showed that doubling the oxygen concentration in the mouse brain through carbogen breathing reversed the neurocognitive benefits of FLASH-RT. In zebrafish embryos, using antioxidants protected somewhat from radiation damage for conventionally irradiated samples, but not for FLASH irradiated.

In water, oxygen consumption depends on dose, dose rate and linear energy transfer. It is challenging to accurately measure oxygen depletion *in vitro* on short time

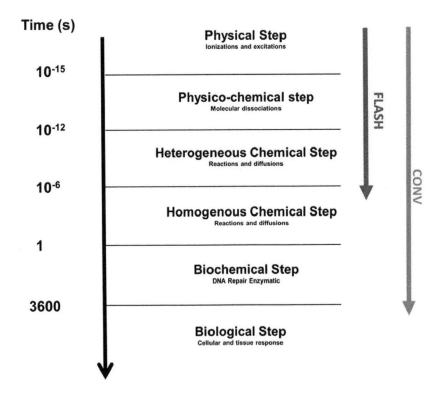

FIGURE 25.8: Comparison of time frames for various mechanisms of action for FLASH and conventional radiotherapy. (Elsevier, with permission.)

scales due to reoxygenation from the blood. Hypoxic tissues, such as some tumors, have an O_2 concentration lower than 0.5% atm while normal tissues have an O_2 concentration of 1–11%.[26] Jansen[40] tested $10\,Gy$ irradiations by photons, protons and carbon ions and found the maximum oxygen depletion was only 0.25% atm, and was saturated by self-interactions of free radicals, which suggests that oxygen depletion is not the whole story. Some studies have reported oxygen depletion in cell cultures, but Cao[41] performed bulk tissue measurements that suggest radiologically relevant levels of hypoxia are unlikely to occur during FLASH irradiation.

In all likelihood, oxygen and the production of reactive oxygen species play an important role in mediating, but may not fully explain, the FLASH Effect. Other, possibly complementary, theories suggest that FLASH may alter the yields of other free radicals and downstream processes to impact later biological responses.[39] Other mechanisms suggested include an altered inflammatory cellular signaling, the sparing of circulating immune cells and the altered probability of interactions between free radicals at ultrahigh dose rates.[42,43,44,45,46]

Future Challenges

If FLASH is transitioned to the clinic, it may offer radiotherapy treatments with fewer side effects. Alternatively, it could be used to deliver more dose to tumors with the same toxicity, which could, in some cases, improve the probability of tumor control or even of curing the patient. Some have suggested combining FLASH capabilities with high-dose spatial fractionation like GRID or microbeams.[47] Others hope it will enable a renewed interest in combining radiotherapy with immunotherapy.

25.5   A CLOSING NOTE

Radiation Oncology continues to be a field where improving hardware and software technology and cutting edge scientific developments are improving the care for cancer patients. The innovations needed for future improvements will be in the hands of the next generation of medical physicists and oncologists. Perhaps the discussions in this book have inspired you to dig more deeply into these topics, or even to pursue a career in medical physics. If so, we wish you the best of luck, and welcome you to the challenging and rewarding field of radiation oncology physics.

25.6   QUESTIONS, EXERCISES, & PROBLEMS

25-1. Verify the numbers given in the four COM matrices and in the Normalized matrix of Fig. (25.2).

25-2. Verify the numbers in the RLM matrix of Fig. (25.3).

25-3. Explain the definitions of *Model Accuracy*, *Misclassification Rate*, *Sensitivity*, and *Specificity* as given in Eqs. (25.2) through (25.5)—that is, why are they defined as they are in these equations?

25-4. Figure (25.9) shows an image matrix containing pixel intensity values. Determine the 0°, 45°, 90°, and 135° COMs. Then determine the full normalized COM, as was done in Fig. (25.2).

FIGURE 25.9: An image matrix of pixel intensity values for COM and GLSZM problems.

25-5. Figure (25.3) shows the 0° RLM for the given image. Determine the 45°, 90°, and 135° RLMs. Then determine the full normalized RLM.

25-6. Figure (25.10) shows an image matrix containing pixel intensity values. Determine the 0°, 45°, 90°, and 135° RLMs. Then determine the full normalized RLM.

25-7. The discussion on radiomics in §25.2 refers to first- and second-order statistics associated with pixel-intensity values for images. Explain the difference between first-order and second-order statistics in this discussion.

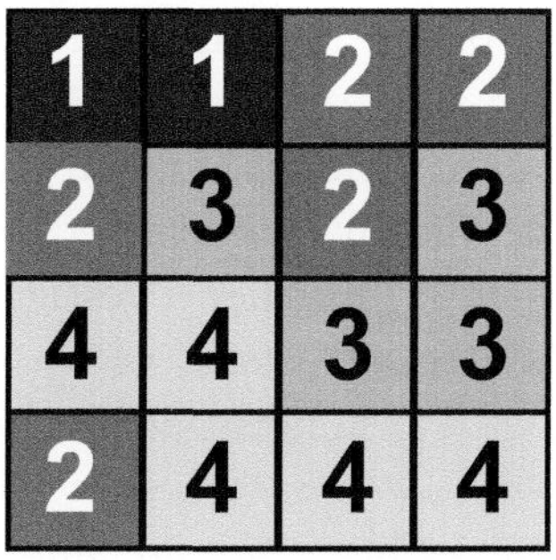

FIGURE 25.10: An image matrix of pixel intensity values for RLM problem.

25-8. The ROC graph plots the *Sensitivity vs.* (1 − *Specificity*). (a) The *Sensitivity* is also called the *True Positive Rate* (TPR). Explain why. (b) (1 − *Specificity*) is also called the *False Positive Rate* (FPR). Explain why.

25-9. A 45° line in an ROC curve, extending from (0,0) to (1,1), is interpreted as corresponding to random results, meaning a useless algorithm. Explain why this line has that interpretation.

25-10. (a) The upper-left point in the ROC plot in Fig. (25.6) is labeled "Perfect Classifier". Explain why. (b) Explain the "Better" and "Worse" arrows in the plot. (c) What is the AUC (Area Under the Curve) of an ROC curve corresponding to the best possible algorithm? (d) What is the AUC of a useless algorithm that simply outputs random predictions?

25-11. Discuss how FLASH radiotherapy differs from conventional radiotherapy.

25-12. Discuss the *FLASH Effect*. What is it? What types of studies have demonstrated this effect? (You may want to do some online research to answer these questions.)

25-13. Section 25.4 on FLASH radiotherapy discusses work done by Vozenin *et al.*[29,30] involving the treatment of cats having nasal squamous cell carcinomas. Their work compared the results of a standard radiotherapy treatment with those of a FLASH radiotherapy treatment. In this problem and the next, we will dig more deeply into the results they obtained.

The *Biologically Effective Dose* (BED) is a measure of the dose required to achieve a given biological effect. It provides a useful means of comparing different fractionation schedules for dose delivery. The BED is given by

$$BED = D \left(1 + \frac{d}{D_{\alpha\beta}} \right), \tag{25.7}$$

where D is the total prescribed dose to be delivered, d is the dose per fraction, and $D_{\alpha\beta}$ is the crossover dose, given by $D_{\alpha\beta} = \alpha/\beta$. (See §2.9 for a discussion of the crossover dose.) Vozenin's group compared results for normal early-responding ($D_{\alpha\beta} = 10\,Gy$) and late-responding ($D_{\alpha\beta} = 3\,Gy$) tissues. (See §3.5 for a discussion of early- and late-responding tissue.)

The standard veterinary treatment consisted of 10 fractions of radiation treatment with $4.8\,Gy$ delivered per fraction. The FLASH treatment consisted of a single fraction delivering a dose of $30\,Gy$. All of the treatments resulted in complete responses in the cats after 6 months.

(a) Compute the BED associated with the standard treatment for early- and late-responding tissue. (b) Compute the BED associated with the FLASH treatment for early- and late-responding tissue. (c) Further investigation of the FLASH treatment showed that the cats received hot-spot doses of up to $42\,Gy$ in a single fraction. Compute the BED associated with such hot spots for both early- and late-responding tissue.

25-14. *This problem is a continuation of the previous problem.* The *Dose Modifying Factor* (DMF) is the ratio of two doses resulting in the same biological effect, where one of the doses is delivered with a modifying agent and the other dose is delivered without the agent. For our purposes, the modifying agent will be taken to be the FLASH treatment regime; the standard veterinary treatment will be the treatment without the modifying agent. The doses we will compare are the BEDs, so we will take $DMF = BED_{FLASH}/BED_{standard}$.

(a) Compute the *DMF* for early- and late-responding tissue for the $30\,Gy$ FLASH treatment. (b) Compute the *DMF* for early- and late-responding tissue for the $42\,Gy$ hot spots resulting from the FLASH treatment. (c) What is the range of DMF values from the mouse experiments described in this chapter and from information that you can find in the literature? Does the DMF that you calculated in (b) for treatment in cats fall within the same range, or is it larger or smaller than that? Given this, do you expect more or less toxicity in the FLASH treatment described in the Vozenin experiment compared to the veterinary standard of care?

Note: The remaining three problems require some skill in computer programming and access to appropriate computer software.

25-15. *(This problem is needed for the following two problems.)* Generate a set of four artificial CT "images", say, of size 16×16 or 32×32. Let the images be pictures of various solid 2-D geometric shapes: one a triangle, one a square, one a rectangle, and one a circle. Make several copies of each set, varying the size and position of the geometric shape in the image. Add some noise to each image in one of the sets, varying the degree of noise. Feel free to generate additional sets with varying characteristics (size, orientation, noise), as you wish. You will use these image sets in the following problems.

25-16. Write a program that calculates the radiomics quantities COM (at two different angles), RLM, and GLSZM discussed in §25.2, and determine if those quantities are sufficient to differentiate the various geometric shapes.

25-17. Using a deep learning software package (e.g., MATLAB), train the software to extract shape information from your image data set, and determine how effectively the software is at identifying shapes.

25.7 REFERENCES

1. McShan DL. Ontology for Radiation Oncology. In: Siochi RAC, Starkschall G, eds. *Informatics in Radiation Oncology*. London: Taylor & Francis; 2013.
2. Brooks K. Radiation Oncology Information Management System. In: Van Dyk J, ed. *The Modern Technology of Radiation Oncology*. Madison, WI: Medical Physics Publishing; 1999.

3. Brooks KW, Fox TH, Davis DL. Advanced Therapy Information Management Systems: An Oncology Information Systems RFP Toolkit. In: Hazle JD, Boyer AL, eds. *Imaging in Radiation Therapy.* Madison, WI: Medical Physics Publishing; 1998.

4. Mageras GS, Hu Y-C, McNamara S, Pham H, Xiong J-P. Imaging for Radiation Treatment Planning. In: Siochi RAC, Starkschall G, eds. *Informatics in Radiation Oncology.* London: Taylor & Francis; 2013.

5. Starkschall G, Britton K, McAleer MF, et al. Potential dosimetric benefits of four-dimensional radiation treatment planning. *Int J Radiat Oncol Biol Phys.* 2009; 73(5): 1560-1565. PMID: 19231098.

6. Moore KL, Kagadis GC, McNutt TR, Moisenko V, Mutic S. Automation and advanced computing in clinical radiation oncology. *Medical Physics.* 2014; 41(1): 010901. doi:10.1118/1.4842515.

7. Zhao B, Tan Y, Tsai W-Y, et al. Reproducibility of radiomics for deciphering tumor phenotype with imaging. Scientific Reports 2016; 6: 23428. doi: 10.1038/srep23428.

8. Kalpathy-Cramer J, Zhao B, Goldgof D, et al. A comparison of lung nodule segmentation algorithms: methods and results from a multi-institutional study. *J Digit Imaging.* 2016; 29(4):476-487. doi: 10.1007/s10278-016-9859-z.

9. Haralick RM, Shanmugam K, Dinstein I. Textural Features for Image Classification. *IEEE Transactions on Systems, Man, and Cybernetics.* 1973; 3: 610-621. doi:10.1109/TSMC.1973.4309314.

10. Brynolfsson P, Nilsson D, Torheim T, et al. Haralick texture features from apparent diffusion coefficient (ADC) MRI images depend on imaging and pre-processing parameters. *Sci Rep.* 2017; 7: 4041. https://doi.org/10.1038/s41598-017-04151-4

11. JonMcLoone (https://commons.wikimedia.org/wiki/File:MorletWaveletMathematica.svg), "MorletWaveletMathematica", https://creativecommons.org/licenses/by-sa/3.0/legalcode

12. Mackin D, Fave X, Zhang L, et al. Measuring CT scanner variability of radiomics features. *Investigative Radiology.* 2015; 50(11): 757-765. Doi: 10.1097/RLI.0000000000000180.

13. Galavis PE, Hollensen C, Jallow N, Paliwal B, Jeraj R. Variability of textural features in FDG-PET images due to different acquisition modes and reconstruction parameters. *Acta Oncologica.* 2010; 49(7): 1012-1016. https://www.tandfonline.com/doi/epdf/10.3109/0284186X.2010.498437?needAccess=true.

14. Waugh SA, Lerski RA, Bidaut L, Thompson AM. The influence of field strength and different clinical breast MRI protocols on the outcome of texture analysis using foam phantoms. *Med Phys.* 2011; 38(9): 5058-5066. Doi: 10.1118/1.3622605.

15. Fried DV, Mawlawi O, Zhang L, et al. Potential use of ^{18}F-fluorodeoxyglucose positron emission tomography-based quantitative imaging features for guiding dose escalation in Stage III non-small-cell lung cancer. International *J Rad Onc Phys Biol.* 2016; 94(2): 368-376.

16. Hawkins S, Wang H, Liu Y, et al. Predicting Malignant Nodules from Screening CT Scans. *J Thoracic Oncology.* 2016; 11(12): 2120-2128.

17. cmglee, MartinThoma (https://commons.wikimedia.org/wiki/File:Roc_curve.svg), https://creativecommons.org/licenses/by-sa/4.0/legalcode

18. Dewey DL, Boag JW. Modification of the Oxygen Effect When Bacteria Are Given Large Pulses of Radiation. *Nature.* 1959; 183(4673): 1450. doi:10.1038/1831450a0.

19. Town CD. Effect of High Dose-Rates on Survival of Mammalian Cells. *Nature.* 1967; 215(5103): 847-848. doi: 10.1038/215847a0.

20. Berry RJ, Hall EJ, Forster DW, Storr TH, Goodman MJ. Survival of Mammalian Cells Exposed to X Rays At Ultra-High Dose-Rates. *Br J Radiol.* 1969; 42(494): 102-107. doi: 10.1259/0007-1285-42-494-102.

21. Favaudon V, Caplier L, Monceau V, et al. Ultrahigh dose-rate FLASH irradiation increases the differential response between normal and tumor tissue in mice. *Sci Transl Med.* 2014; 6(245): 245ra93. doi: 10.1126/scitranslmed.3008973. Erratum in: *Sci Transl Med.* 2019; 11(523):eaba4525. doi: 10.1126/scitranslmed.aba4525. PMID: 25031268.

22. Wilson JD, Hammond EM, Higgins GS, Petersson K. Ultra-High Dose Rate (FLASH) Radiotherapy: Silver Bullet or Fool's Gold? *Front Oncol.* 2020; 9:1563. doi: 10.3389/fonc.2019.01563. Erratum in: Front Oncol. 2020; 10: 210. PMID: 32010633; PMCID: PMC6979639.

23. Friedl, AA, Prise, KM, Butterworth, KT, Montay-Gruel, P, Favaudon, V. Radiobiology of the FLASH Effect. *Med Phys.* 2022; 49(3): 1993-2013. https://doi.org/10.1002/mp.15184.

24. Bourhis J, Montay-Gruel P, Gonçalves Jorge P, et al. Clinical translation of FLASH radiotherapy: Why and how? *Radiother Oncol.* 2019; 139: 11-17. doi: 10.1016/j.radonc.2019.04.008. Epub 2019 Jun 25. PMID: 31253466.

25. Schüler E, Acharya M, Montay-Gruel P, Loo BW Jr, Vozenin MC, Maxim PG. Ultra-high dose rate electron beams and the FLASH Effect: From preclinical evidence to a new radiotherapy paradigm. *Med Phys.* 2022; 49(3): 2082-2095. doi: 10.1002/mp.15442. Epub 2022 Jan 19. PMID: 34997969; PMCID: PMC9032195.

26. Sørensen BS, Sitarz MK, Ankjærgaard C, et al. Pencil beam scanning proton FLASH maintains tumor control while normal tissue damage is reduced in a mouse model. *Radiother Oncol.* 2022; S0167-8140(22): 00254-7. doi: 10.1016/j.radonc.2022.05.014. Epub ahead of print. PMID: 35595175.

27. Singers Sørensen B, Krzysztof Sitarz M, Ankjærgaard C, et al. In vivo validation and tissue sparing factor for acute damage of pencil beam scanning proton FLASH. *Radiother Oncol.* 2022; 167: 109-115. doi: 10.1016/j.radonc.2021.12.022. Epub 2021 Dec 22. PMID: 34953933.
28. Diffenderfer ES, Verginadis II, Kim MM, et al. Design, Implementation and in Vivo Validation of a Novel Proton FLASH Radiation Therapy System. *Int J Radiat Oncol Biol Phys.* 2020; 106(2): 440-448. doi: 10.1016/j.ijrobp.2019.10.049. PMID: 31928642; PMCID: PMC7325740.
29. Vozenin MC, De Fornel P, Petersson K, et al. The Advantage of FLASH Radiotherapy Confirmed in Mini-pig and Cat-cancer Patients. *Clin Cancer Res.* 2019; 25(1): 35-42. doi: 10.1158/1078-0432.CCR-17-3375. Epub 2018 Jun 6. PMID: 29875213.
30. Rohrer Bley C, Wolf F, Gonçalves Jorge P, et al. Dose and volume limiting late toxicity of FLASH radiotherapy in cats with squamous cell carcinoma of the nasal planum and in mini-pigs. *Clin Cancer Res.* 2022; 28(17): 3814-3823. doi: 10.1158/1078-0432.CCR-22-0262. PMID: 35421221.
31. Bourhis J, Sozzi WJ, Jorge PG, et al. Treatment of a first patient with FLASH-radiotherapy. *Radiother Oncol.* 2019; 139: 18-22. doi: 10.1016/j.radonc.2019.06.019. Epub 2019 Jul 11. PMID: 31303340.
32. U.S. National Library of Medicine Clinical Trials. https://clinicaltrials.gov/. Accessed July 17, 2022.
33. Bourhis J, Montay-Gruel P, Gonçalves Jorge P, et al. Clinical translation of FLASH radiotherapy: Why and how? *Radiother Oncol.* 2019; 139: 11-17. doi: 10.1016/j.radonc.2019.04.008. Epub 2019 Jun 25. PMID: 31253466.
34. Darafsheh A, Hao Y, Zwart T, et al. Feasibility of proton FLASH irradiation using a synchrocyclotron for preclinical studies. *Med Phys.* 2020; 47(9): 4348-4355. doi: 10.1002/mp.14253. Epub 2020 Jun 15. PMID: 32452558.
35. Montay-Gruel P, Corde S, Laissue JA, Bazalova-Carter M. FLASH radiotherapy with photon beams. *Med Phys.* 2022; 49(3): 2055-2067. doi: 10.1002/mp.15222. Epub 2021 Nov 7. PMID: 34519042.
36. Folkerts MM, Abel E, Busold S, Perez JR, Krishnamurthi V, Ling CC. A framework for defining FLASH dose rate for pencil beam scanning. *Med Phys.* 2020; 47(12): 6396-6404. doi: 10.1002/mp.14456. Epub 2020 Nov 15. PMID: 32910460; PMCID: PMC7894358.
37. Böhlen TT, Germond JF, Bourhis J, et al. Normal tissue sparing by FLASH as a function of single fraction dose: A quantitative analysis. *Int J Radiat Oncol Biol Phys.* 2022: 114(5); 1032-1044. doi: 10.1016/j.ijrobp.2022.05.038. PMID: 35810988.
38. Vozenin MC, Hendry JH, Limoli CL. Biological Benefits of Ultra-high Dose Rate FLASH Radiotherapy: Sleeping Beauty Awoken. *Clin Oncol (R Coll Radiol).* 2019; 31(7): 407-415. doi: 10.1016/j.clon.2019.04.001. Epub 2019 Apr 19.
39. Montay-Gruel P, Acharya MM, Petersson K, et al. Long-term neurocognitive benefits of FLASH radiotherapy driven by reduced reactive oxygen species. *Proc Natl Acad Sci U S A.* 2019; 116(22): 10943-10951. doi: 10.1073/pnas.1901777116. Epub 2019 May 16. Erratum in: Proc Natl Acad Sci U S A. 2020 Oct 13;117(41):25946-25947. PMID: 31097580; PMCID: PMC6561167.
40. Jansen J, Knoll J, Beyreuther E, et al. Does FLASH deplete oxygen? Experimental evaluation for photons, protons, and carbon ions. *Med. Phys.* 2021; 48: 3982-3990. https://doi.org/10.1002/mp.14917.
41. Cao X, Zhang R, Esipova TV, et al. Quantification of Oxygen Depletion During FLASH Irradiation In Vitro and In Vivo. *Int J Radiat Oncol Biol Phys.* 2021; 111(1): 240-248. doi: 10.1016/j.ijrobp.2021.03.056. Epub 2021 May 18. PMID: 33845146; PMCID: PMC8338745.
42. Durante M, Bräuer-Krisch E, Hill M. Faster and safer? FLASH ultra-high dose rate in radiotherapy. *Br J Radiol.* 2018; 91(1082): 20170628. doi: 10.1259/bjr.20170628. Epub 2017 Dec 15. PMID: 29172684; PMCID: PMC5965780.
43. Buonanno M, Grilj V, Brenner DJ. Biological effects in normal cells exposed to FLASH dose rate protons. *Radiother Oncol.* 2019; 139: 51-55. doi: 10.1016/j.radonc.2019.02.009. Epub 2019 Mar 5. PMID: 30850209; PMCID: PMC6728238.
44. Borghini A, Vecoli C, Labate L, Panetta D, Andreassi MG, Gizzi LA. FLASH ultra-high dose rates in radiotherapy: preclinical and radiobiological evidence. *Int J Radiat Biol.* 2022; 98(2): 127-135. doi: 10.1080/09553002.2022.2009143. Epub 2021 Dec 16. PMID: 34913413.
45. Pratx G, Kapp DS. Ultra-High-Dose-Rate FLASH Irradiation May Spare Hypoxic Stem Cell Niches in Normal Tissues. *Int J Radiat Oncol Biol Phys.* 2019; 105(1): 190-192. doi: 10.1016/j.ijrobp.2019.05.030. Epub 2019 May 27. PMID: 31145965.
46. Fouillade C, Curras-Alonso S, Giuranno L, et al. FLASH Irradiation Spares Lung Progenitor Cells and Limits the Incidence of Radio-induced Senescence. *Clin Cancer Res.* 2020; 26(6): 1497-1506. doi: 10.1158/1078-0432.CCR-19-1440. Epub 2019 Dec 3. PMID: 31796518.
47. Griffin RJ, Prise KM, McMahon SJ, Zhang X, Penagaricano J, Butterworth KT. History and current perspectives on the biological effects of high-dose spatial fractionation and high dose-rate approaches: GRID, Microbeam & FLASH radiotherapy. *Br J Radiol.* 2020; 93(1113): 20200217. doi: 10.1259/bjr.20200217. Epub 2020 Jul 30. PMID: 32706989; PMCID: PMC7465857.

Index

For Product Safety Concerns and Information please contact our
EU representative GPSR@taylorandfrancis.com Taylor & Francis
Verlag GmbH, Kaufingerstraße 24, 80331 München, Germany